MW01226557

Advanced
CARDIOVASCULAR MEDICINE

Advanced
CARDIOVASCULAR MEDICINE

Editors

Ashok Seth
FRCP (London, Edin, Irel) FACC FESC FSCAI (USA)
FCSI DSc (Honoris Causa) DLitt (Honoris Causa)
Chairman
Fortis Escorts Heart Institute
Chairman
Cardiology Council
Fortis Group of Hospitals
New Delhi, India

Sameer Shrivastava
MD DM FISCU FESC FIAE FISC
Director
Noninvasive Cardiology
Fortis Escorts Heart Institute and
Research Center
New Delhi, India

Upendra Kaul
MD DM FCSI FICC FACC FSCAI FAMS
Executive Director
Interventional Cardiology
Fortis Escorts Heart Institute and
Research Center
New Delhi, India

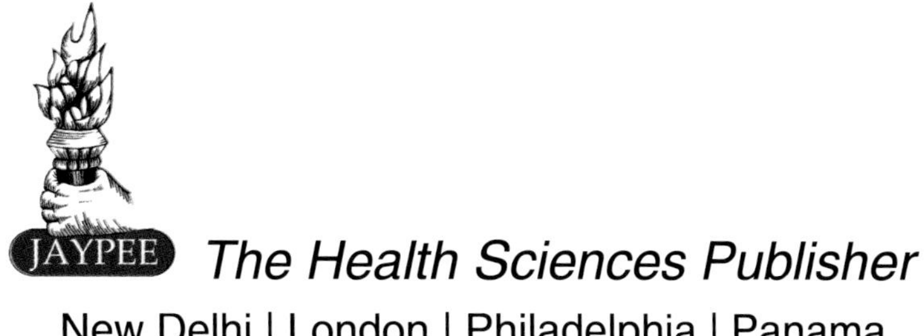

The Health Sciences Publisher
New Delhi | London | Philadelphia | Panama

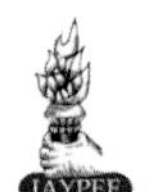

Jaypee Brothers Medical Publishers (P) Ltd.

Headquarters
Jaypee Brothers Medical Publishers (P) Ltd.
4838/24, Ansari Road, Daryaganj
New Delhi 110 002, India
Phone: +91-11-43574357
Fax: +91-11-43574314
E-mail: jaypee@jaypeebrothers.com

Overseas Offices
J.P. Medical Ltd.
83, Victoria Street, London
SW1H 0HW (UK)
Phone: +44-20 3170 8910
Fax: +44 (0)20 3008 6180
E-mail: info@jpmedpub.com

Jaypee-Highlights Medical Publishers Inc.
City of Knowledge, Bld 235, 2nd Floor
Clayton, Panama City, Panama
Phone: +1 507-301-0496
Fax: +1 507-301-0499
E-mail: cservice@jphmedical.com

Jaypee Medical Inc.
325, Chestnut Street
Suite 412
Philadelphia, PA 19106, USA
Phone: +1 267-519-9789
E-mail: support@jpmedus.com

Jaypee Brothers Medical Publishers (P) Ltd.
17/1-B, Babar Road, Block-B
Shaymali, Mohammadpur
Dhaka-1207, Bangladesh
Mobile: +08801912003485
E-mail: jaypeedhaka@gmail.com

Jaypee Brothers Medical Publishers (P) Ltd.
Bhotahity, Kathmandu, Nepal
Phone: +977-9741283608
E-mail: kathmandu@jaypeebrothers.com

Website: www.jaypeebrothers.com
Website: www.jaypeedigital.com

Inquiries for bulk sales may be solicited at: jaypee@jaypeebrothers.com

Advanced Cardiovascular Medicine

First Edition: **2016**

ISBN: 978-93-5152-437-3

Printed at Replika Press Pvt. Ltd.

Dedicated to

All our friends
and well-wishers

CONTRIBUTORS

Ajay Kaul MCH
Chairman and Head
Department of Cardiothoracic and Vascular Surgery
BLK Center for Cardiac Sciences
BLK Super Specialty Hospital
New Delhi, India

AK Khera MD DNB MNAMS
Principal Consultant in Non-invasive Cardiology
Fortis Escorts Heart Institute
New Delhi, India

AK Singh MD (Respiratory Medicine)
Consultant
Department of Pulmonology
Sleep Medicine and Critical Care
Fortis Escorts Heart Institute
New Delhi, India

Amit Varma MBBS MD
Director
Department of Critical Care Medicine
Fortis Escorts Heart Institute
New Delhi, India

Amitesh Chakravarty MD
Fortis Escorts Heart Institute and Research Center
New Delhi, India

Anil Karlekar MD
Executive Director and Head
Department of Cardiac Anesthesiology and Critical Care
Fortis Escorts Heart Institute
New Delhi, India

Ankush Sachdeva MD
Associate Consultant
Department of Cardiology
Fortis Escorts Heart Institute
New Delhi, India

Anumeha Omar MBBS
Resident
Non-invasive Cardiology
Fortis Escorts Heart Institute
New Delhi, India

Aparna Jaswal MD DNB CCDS FHRS FACC
Heart Rhythm Society-IBHRE World Ambassador
Senior Consultant Electrophysiologist
Fortis Escorts Heart Institute
New Delhi, India

Arvind Sethi MD DNB
Chairman
Interventional Cardiology
Fortis Escorts Heart Institute
New Delhi, India

Aseem Dhall MD DM (Cardiology)
Senior Intervention Cardiologist
Department of Cardiology
Fortis Escorts Heart Institute and
Research Center
New Delhi, India

Ashok K Omar MD FESC FIAE FASE FCSI
Director
Non-invasive Cardiology
Head
Heart Command and Emergency
Fortis Escorts Heart Institute
New Delhi, India

Ashok Seth FRCP (London, Edin, Irel) FACC FESC FSCAI (USA) FCSI DSc (Honoris Causa) DLitt (Honoris Causa)
Chairman
Fortis Escorts Heart Institute
Chairman, Cardiology Council
Fortis Group of Hospitals
New Delhi, India

Ashutosh Marwah MD FNB
Principal Consultant
Department of Pediatric and
Congenital Heart Diseases
Fortis Escorts Heart Institute
New Delhi, India

Atul Verma MBBS DRM
Principal Consultant and Head
Nuclear Medicine
Fortis Escorts Heart Institute
New Delhi, India

Avinash Verma MD DNB
Junior Consultant
Department of Electrophysiology
Fortis Escorts Heart Institute
New Delhi, India

Bhumika S Anand
Physician Assistant
Fortis Escorts Heart Institute
New Delhi, India

Biswajit Paul MD DNB
Consultant Cardiologist
Department of Non-invasive Cardiology
Fortis Escorts Heart Institute
New Delhi, India

Devesh Dutta MD FNB
Junior consultant
Department of Anesthesia and
Critical Care Medicine
Fortis Escorts Heart Institute
New Delhi, India

Dheeraj Gandotra MD DNB (Cardiology)
Junior Consultant
Interventional Cardiology
Fortis Escorts Heart Institute
New Delhi, India

Kenneth Lee Harris MS
Fortis Totipotent RX Center for Cellular Medicine
Fortis Memorial Research Institute
Gurgaon, Haryana, India

Khushboo Choudhury MSc
Fortis Totipotent RX Center for Cellular Medicine
Fortis Memorial Research Institute
Gurgaon, Haryana, India

KK Sharma MD
Anesthesiologist
Department of Anesthesiology and Intensive Care
Fortis Escorts Heart Institute
New Delhi, India

Krishna S Iyer MBBS MS MCH
Executive Director
Pediatric and Congenital Heart Surgery
Fortis Escorts Heart Institute
New Delhi, India

Lal C Daga DNB (Fellow) DNB (Cardiology)
Junior Consultant
Fortis Escorts Heart Institute
New Delhi, India

Malay Shukla MD DM
Junior Consultant
Fortis Escorts Heart Institute
New Delhi, India

Mitu A Minocha MD
Associate Consultant
Department of Cardiology
Fortis Escorts Heart Institute and Research Center
New Delhi, India

Mona Bhatia MD
Head
Department of Radiodiagnosis and Imaging
Fortis Escorts Heart Institute
New Delhi, India

N Dalal MBBS MD
Associate Consultant
Department of Pulmonology, Sleep Medicine and Medical Critical Care
Fortis Hospital, Vasant Kunj, New Delhi, India
Fortis Escorts Heart Institute
New Delhi, India

Neel Bhatia MD
Junior Consultant
Fortis Escorts Heart Institute
New Delhi, India

Neeraj Awasthy MD DM
Associate Consultant
Department of Pediatric Cardiology and
Congenital Heart diseases
Fortis Escorts Heart Institute
New Delhi, India

Nishant Kumar MBBS PGDCC
Clinical Assistant
Non-invasive Cardiology
Fortis Escort Heart Institute
New Delhi, India

Nishith Chandra MD DM
Director
Interventional Cardiology
Fortis Escort Heart Institute
New Delhi, India

Niti Chadha MD DM (Cardiology)
IBHRE Certified EP Specialist
Department of Pacing and Electrophysiology
Fortis Escorts Heart Institute
New Delhi, India

Parvathi U Iyer MBBS MD FICU
Director
Pediatric Intensive Care
Fortis Escorts Heart Institute
New Delhi, India

Peeyush Jain MD (Med) DM (Cardiology)
Head
Department of Preventive and Rehabilitative Cardiology
Fortis Escorts Heart Institute
New Delhi, India

Poonam Khurana MD
Principal Consultant
Department of Radiodiagnosis and Imaging
Fortis Escorts Heart Institute
New Delhi, India

Pradyut Bag MD IDCCM FNB EDIC
Consultant
Critical Care Medicine
Fortis Escorts Heart Institute
New Delhi, India

Pramod Joshi MD DNB
Junior Consultant
Fortis Escorts Heart Institute
New Delhi, India

Rajat Agrawal MBBS MD
Senior Consultant
Critical Care Medicine
Fortis Escorts Heart Institute
New Delhi, India

Rajat Gupta DNB FNB
Associate Consultant
Fortis Escorts Heart Institute
New Delhi, India

Rajeev Dhalwani MD
Junior Consultant
Non-invasive Cardiology
Fortis Escorts Heart Institute
New Delhi, India

Rajesh Chauhan MD (Anesthesia)
Principal Consultant Anesthesia
Department of Cardiac Anesthesiology
Fortis Hospital, Vasant Kunj
New Delhi, India

RC Khurana MD
Head
Transfusion Medicine
Fortis Escorts Heart Institute
New Delhi, India

Rishabh Khurana MD
Postgraduate student
Department of Radiodiagnosis
Maulana Azad Medical College
New Delhi, India

RS Chatterji MD DNB
Senior Consultant
Department of Pulmonology
Critical Care and Sleep Medicine
Fortis Escorts Heart Institute
New Delhi, India

S Radhakrishnan MD DM
Director and Head
Department of Pediatric and
Congenital Heart Disease
Fortis Escorts Heart Institute
New Delhi, India

S Yadav MBBS PGDCC
Senior Resident
Fortis Escorts Heart Institute
New Delhi, India

Sachin V Chaudhary DNB Fellow (Cardiology)
Department of Cardiology
Fortis Escorts Heart Institute and Research Center
New Delhi, India

Sameer Shrivastava MD DM FISCU FESC FIAE FISC
Director
Non-invasive Cardiology
Fortis Escorts Heart Institute and
Research Center
New Delhi, India

Sanjay Gupta MD DNB
Associate Director
Department of Cardiac Anesthesiology
Principal Consultant
Department of Cardiac Surgery
Fortis Flt Lt Rajan Dhal Hospital, Vasant Kunj
New Delhi, India

Sanjeev Pandey MBBS DRM
Consultant
Nuclear Medicine
Fortis Escorts Heart Institute
New Delhi, India

Sanjiv Bharadwaj MD DM
Senior Consultant
Invasive Cardiology
Fortis Escorts Heart Institute
New Delhi, India

Saramma Thomas MRS
Head
Regional Nursing
Fortis Escorts Heart Institute
New Delhi, India

Satyendra Kumar Tiwari DNB Fellow (Cardiology)
Department of Cardiology
Fortis Escorts Heart Institute and Research Center
New Delhi, India

Savitri Srivastava MD (Med) DM (Card) FAMS FACC
Director
Pediatric and Congenital Heart Disease
Fortis Escorts Heart Institute
New Delhi, India

Seema Thakur DM (Medical Genetics)
Senior Consultant
Genetics and Fetal Medicine
Fortis Hospitals
New Delhi, India

Smita Mishra MD (Pediatrics) FDNB (Ped Cardiology)
Senior Consultant
Pediatric Cardiologist
Fortis Escorts Heart Institute
New Delhi, India

Subhash Chandra MD DM (AIIMS) DNB
Associate Director
Interventional Cardiology
Fortis Escorts Heart Institute
New Delhi, India

Sujeet Narain MD DNB (Cardiology)
Junior Consultant
Fortis Escorts Heart Institute
New Delhi, India

Suman Bhandari MD DM FSCAI
Chairman
Interventional Cardiology
Saket City Hospital
New Delhi, India

Syed Asrar Ahmed Qadri MCH
Department of Cardiovascular Surgery
Escorts Heart Institute and Research Center
New Delhi, India

TS Kler MD DM (Cardiology)
Executive Director and Head
Department of Cardiology
Fortis Escorts Heart Institute
New Delhi, India

Upendra Kaul MD DM FCSI FICC FACC FSCAI FAMS
Executive Director
Interventional Cardiology
Fortis Escorts Heart Institute and
Research Center
New Delhi, India

V Nangia MD FCCP
Fellowship in Sleep Medicine (Standford) (USA)
Diploma in Interventional Bronchoscopy (Spain)
MSc in Infectious Diseases (UK)
Director and Head
Pulmonology
Sleep Medicine and Medical Critical Care
Fortis Hospital, Vasant Kunj
Fortis Escorts Heart Institute
New Delhi, India

Venkatesh Ponemone PhD
Director
Laboratory and Clinical Research Affairs
Fortis Totipotent RX Center for
Cellular Medicine
Fortis Memorial Research Institute
Gurgaon, Haryana, India

Vibhu Ranjan Gupta MBBS MPhil
Medical Director
Fortis Escorts Heart Institute and Research Center
New Delhi, India

Vijay Kumar MD DNB (Cardiology)
Senior Consultant Cardiologist
Fortis Escorts Heart Institute and Research Center
New Delhi, India

Vinay Kumar Sharma MD DM
Senior Consultant
Department of Non-invasive Cardiology
Fortis Escorts Heart Institute
New Delhi, India

Vinay Sanghi MD DM
Associate Director
Department of Interventional Cardiology
Fortis Hospital, Shalimar Bagh
New Delhi, India

Vishal Rastogi MD DM FSCAI
Senior Interventional Cardiologist
Fortis Escorts Heart Institute
New Delhi, India

Vivek Kumar MD
Principal Consultant Cardiologist
Fortis Escorts Heart Institute
New Delhi, India

Yugal K Mishra MBBS MS PhD
Director
Department of Cardiovascular Surgery
Fortis Escorts Heart Institute and Research Center
New Delhi, India

PREFACE

The last 25 years have witnessed unprecedented scientific advancements in the field of cardiology. Every year, new drugs, new devices and new technologies continue to improve outcomes and prolong lives of our patients with heart disease. Every year, robust clinical trials influence our management of life-threatening cardiac conditions to save lives. To the extent that the way, we practice cardiology today, is distinctly superior and different from what we practiced even 3-5 years ago.

'Staying updated' with the present knowledge has become never as more important than before to benefit our patients and do justice to our profession and receive satisfaction in doing so.

Advanced Cardiovascular Medicine brings you the 'up-to-date' knowledge of the art and science of management of the most important cardiac conditions, we face in our clinical practice. We have ensured that the book covers a vast variety of relevant topics, which would be very useful to all physicians and cardiologists in their daily care of patients. Each chapter has been written by acknowledged international and national authorities in the field, who have ensured that their presentation of advanced science and technology is combined with their own vast experience of its applications to the Indian Clinical Scenario.

As we continue to look beyond the horizon and strive for the ultimate advancements of *gene therapies and genomics, artificial blood, organ regeneration in laboratory,* etc. We believe that this book will become an inseparable companion to us for delivering our best to our patients in 2016 and beyond.

Wish you a very successful and fruitful professional journey with *Advanced Cardiovascular Medicine*.

Ashok Seth
Sameer Shrivastava
Upendra Kaul

ACKNOWLEDGMENTS

We acknowledge all those people who are part of this project and have helped us in making *Advanced Cardiovascular Medicine* see the light of the day.

Working with such multitalented personalities and an excellent team has indeed been an honor and it is hard to pen down words for the enormous care, empathy and affection they bestowed upon us!!

We are grateful to all our residents and juniors for their valuable suggestions, unmatched enthusiasm, constructive criticism and constant efforts. We would like to thank all the staff from our department for their persistent support.

We also express our highest regards to our parents and our families for their prayers and blessings.

We are thankful to M/s Jaypee Brothers Medical Publishers (P) Ltd, New Delhi, India, and their dedicated staff for the skillful and admirable production qualities of the book.

Last but not least, our sincere thanks to all our patients without whose participation this book would not have been possible.

CONTENTS

1

Rheumatic Fever: Time for Newer Recommendations

Ashutosh Marwah

INTRODUCTION

Acute rheumatic fever (ARF) is a unique nonsuppurative complication of pharyngeal infection with group A *Streptococcus*. It affects major joints, central nervous system, subcutaneous tissue, and the heart. All except cardiac effects are reversible without leaving any long-term sequelae. Cardiac manifestations are the cause of long-term morbidity and mortality in young adults and children.

BURDEN OF RHEUMATIC FEVER AND RHEUMATIC HEART DISEASE IN INDIA

The true incidence of rheumatic heart disease (RHD) and rheumatic fever (RF) remains unknown in India. Our estimates are based on hospital admissions and small sample surveys. According to various authors, RF is endemic and remains one of the major causes of cardiovascular disease, accounting for nearly 25-45% of the acquired heart disease. We are also observing a decline in the overall incidence of RF similar to that in Western countries. Perhaps the decline is more in the urban population as compared to rural areas. Population-based surveys for prevalence are very few and scattered. In a study in rural Haryana, prevalence of RHD was found to be 2.2/1000 in 5-30 years old subjects.[1] In a study of the urban population of Agra, Mathur et al. found RHD in 1.8/1000 in the same age group.[2] Berry[3] studied the urban population of Chandigarh and found RHD in 1.23/1000 male and 2.07/1000 in the female population of all age groups. The incidence has been quoted to be 0.5/1000 in a study conducted by Misra et al. in Uttar Pradesh on 1,18,212 school children 4-18 years in age.[4]

The ICMR has conducted three major surveys in school going children between the years 1970 and 2010. In the first study (1972-1975), 1,33,000 children were evaluated and the prevalence of RHD varied from 0.8 to 11/1000 (overall 5.3/1000). The second study (1984-1987) included 53,786 children and the prevalence ranged from 1.0 to 5.6/1000 (overall 2.9/1000). The third and the largest study included 1,76,904 school children with a prevalence varying from 0.13 to 1.5/1000 (overall 0.9/1000) in the 5-14 years age range.[5] Though the data suggests the declining trends, various authors, however, have refuted this claim.

REVISED JONES CRITERIA FOR ACUTE RHEUMATIC FEVER[6-9]

Diagnosis of RF is based on Jones criteria, which were first published in 1944, and have been modified three times since then. The latest modification was published in 1992 and has remained unchanged. A definitive diagnosis requires that two major or one major and two minor criteria are satisfied, in addition to evidence of recent streptococcal infection.

Major Criteria

- *Carditis*: All layers of cardiac tissue are affected (pericardium, epicardium, myocardium, endocardium). The patient may have a new or changing murmur, with mitral regurgitation being the most common followed by aortic insufficiency.
- *Polyarthritis*: Migrating arthritis that typically affects the knees, ankles, elbows, and wrists. The joints are very painful and symptoms are very responsive to anti-inflammatory medicines.
- *Chorea*: It is also known as Sydenham's chorea, or "St Vitus' dance". There are abrupt, purposeless movements. This may be the only manifestation of ARF and its presence is diagnostic. It may also include emotional disturbances and inappropriate behavior.
- *Erythema marginatum*: A nonpruritic rash that commonly affects the trunk and proximal extremities, but spares the face. The rash typically migrates from central areas to periphery, and has well-defined borders.
- *Subcutaneous nodules*: Usually located over bones or tendons, these nodules are painless and firm.

Minor Criteria

- Fever
- Arthralgia
- Previous RF/RHD
- *Acute phase reactants*: Leukocytosis, elevated erythrosedimentation rate (ESR) and C-reactive protein (CRP)
- Prolonged P-R interval on electrocardiogram (ECG).

EVIDENCE OF PRECEDING STREPTOCOCCAL INFECTION

Any one of the following is considered adequate evidence of infection:

- Increased antistreptolysin O (ASO) or other streptococcal antibodies
- Positive throat culture for group A β-hemolytic streptococci
- Positive rapid direct group A streptococci carbohydrate antigen test
- Recent scarlet fever.

PROBLEMS IN DIAGNOSIS OF RHEUMATIC FEVER IN INDIAN SCENARIO USING JONES CRITERIA

Various authors have suggested that patients in India often do not present with all the manifestations of RF. In a study by Pereira et al., only 30% patients fulfilled the criteria for diagnosing ARF, requiring an evidence of group A streptococcal infection. When the essential criteria of previous streptococcal infection were disregarded, the number rose to 87.7%.[10]

There are several fallacies, which include:[11,12]

- RF cannot be diagnosed, if carditis is the only manifestation of the disease, particularly of the recurrence.
- Patients with subclinical carditis can often be missed on clinical evaluation.
- Migratory polyarthritis that is major criteria for making diagnosis is often absent in our population. More than 50% patients do not give typical history. However, monoarthritis and arthralgias are more commonly seen in our population.
- Erythema marginatum is often missed in our population owing to darker skin and transient nature of the manifestation.
- Subcutaneous nodules also included in major criteria are seen on one-third cases of RF. However, when present they are almost always associated with carditis. Similar nodules may be found in adults with rheumatoid arthritis.
- Further, in our population, there is higher incidence of carrier state for streptococci, elevation of ASO may not be specific for RF, and an elevated ASO titer is found in only in 75–80% of cases. An elevated ASO may be found in 20% normal population. A single low ASO titer does not exclude RF.

WHO GUIDELINES[13]

Based on Jones criteria WHO has come out with guidelines 2002–2003 to help in facilitating the diagnosis of the following groups:

Primary Episode of Rheumatic Fever and Recurrent Episode of Rheumatic Fever without RHD

- Two major manifestations
- One major and two minor manifestations
- Plus evidence of preceding streptococcal infection.

Recurrent Episode of Rheumatic Fever with Established RHD

- Two minor manifestations
- Plus evidence of preceding streptococcal infection.

Rheumatic Chorea and Insidious Onset Carditis

Other manifestations or evidences of streptococcal infection are not required.

Chronic Valve Lesions of RHD in Patients Presenting for the First Time

Do not require other criteria to be diagnosed as having RHD.

Further WHO Guidelines

1. Patients may present with polyarthritis (or with only polyarthralgia or monoarthritis) and with several (3 or more) other minor manifestations, together with evidence of recent group A streptococcal infection. Some of these cases may later turnout to be RF. It is prudent to consider them as cases of 'probable rheumatic fever' (once other diagnoses are excluded) and advise regular secondary prophylaxis. Such patients require close follow-up and regular examination of the heart. This cautious approach is particularly suitable for patients in vulnerable age groups in high incidence settings.

2. Patients with previous RHD may not completely satisfy all criteria.
3. Infective endocarditis and congenital heart disease should be excluded.

OTHER INVESTIGATIONS TO AID DIAGNOSIS OF RHEUMATIC FEVER

Since Jones criteria are insufficient in diagnosing RF, other modalities have been evaluated for making a definitive diagnosis. The three main contenders are myocardial biopsy, radionuclide scanning, and echocardiography. All three have been discussed here:

Role of Myocardial Biopsy for Diagnosis of RF[14,15]

Since carditis is essential component of cardiac involvement in RF, role of myocardial biopsy has been studied for diagnosing carditis. Myocardial biopsies from patients were compared with biopsies from patients with quiescent disease. The results demonstrated virtual absence of myocarditis (based on Dallas criteria). There was evidence of interstitial inflammation that ranged from perivascular mononuclear cellular infiltration to histiocytic aggregates and Aschoff nodule formation. Histiocytic aggregates and Aschoff nodules were identified in only 30% of patients. Aschoff nodules were seen in 40% of the endomyocardial biopsies taken from patients with pre-existing RHD and who developed a possible recurrence of rheumatic carditis with congestive heart failure (CHF).

These results suggested that myocardial biopsy did provide any additional diagnostic information in patients with first episode of RF and unexplained CHF in patients with established RHD, and who presented with only minor manifestations of RF and elevated ASO titers, would indicate a high probability of rheumatic carditis, and that an invasive test may not be needed for the diagnosis.

Role of Radionuclide Scanning[16-19]

Gallium-67, radiolabeled leukocytes, and radiolabeled antimyosin antibody have all been used to image myocardial inflammation. However, the results of these studies have revealed that gallium-67 imaging has better diagnostic characteristics than antimyosin scintigraphy; and the results also confirmed that rheumatic carditis is predominantly infiltrative, rather than degenerative, in nature. Although radionuclide imaging has been used successfully to identify rheumatic carditis by noninvasive means, WHO guidelines clearly state that there is not enough experience with such methods to allow them to be used for the routine diagnosis of RF.

Echocardiography for Diagnosis of RF[19-22]

Echocardiography gives excellent details of the structural abnormalities, and the Doppler allows the evaluation of functional abnormalities. Yet, echocardiography has not been included as a criterion in the diagnosis of RF. Many authors have reported a higher rate of detection of valve leak in patients with suspected carditis, when subjected to echocardiography rather than relying on auscultation alone.

Major advantage seems to be detection of subclinical carditis or so-called "echocarditis". In such cases of subclinical rheumatic carditis, annular dilatation, leaflet prolapse, and elongation of the anterior mitral chordae were observed, indicating that the valve might have been sensitized or damaged. These patients may remain asymptomatic or develop audible murmur or progress to irreversible sequelae such a mitral stenosis.

Echocardiography also can help in the evaluation of valve structure and differentiate between rheumatic and nonrheumatic structural abnormalities of cardiac valves. According to WHO, echocardiography is definitely useful to detect left-sided valvular lesions. However, making the diagnosis of subclinical rheumatic carditis solely based on this modality remains controversial. Until the results of long-term encompassing prospective studies are available to substantiate the therapeutic and prognostic importance of subclinical rheumatic carditis, the addition of echocardiography to the Jones criteria cannot be justified.

DO WE REALLY NEED NEW GUIDELINES?[23,24]

Some of the highest documented rates of ARF and RHD in the world are found in Aboriginal Australians, Maoris, Pacific Islanders in New Zealand, and Pacific Island nations. The prevalence of RHD is also high in sub-Saharan Africa, Latin America, the Indian subcontinent, the Middle East, and Northern Africa.

Indian working group came out with guidelines on diagnosis and treatment of RF in 2008. These guidelines are based on Jones criteria; however, these guidelines have failed to address the needs of Indian population. Countries like Australia and New Zealand have come out with their own guidelines for high-risk population, enabling clinicians to identify cases with incomplete manifestations of the disease and provide appropriate treatment.

MAJOR CHANGES

- The ability to diagnose a recurrence of ARF in a patient from a high-risk group who has only one major plus one minor manifestation, provided that other more likely diagnoses are excluded.

- Fever can be considered a minor manifestation based on a reliable history (in the absence of documented temperature), if anti-inflammatory medication has already been administered.
- Polyarthralgia and aseptic monoarthritis have been included as major criteria for high-risk population.
- Subclinical carditis has also been included as major criteria for the high-risk population.
- Monoarthralgia has been included as minor manifestation for the high-risk population.

A new category of probable RF has been created to include patients in whom the clinician strongly suspected RF, but all the Jones criteria could not be fulfilled or there was absence of evidence for group A streptococcal infection or serology.

In these patients, presence of subclinical carditis (i.e. evidence of valvulitis on echocardiogram, monoarthritis, and polyarthralgia) was also considered to be major manifestation of RF. Monoarthralgia and a documented history of fever have been included in minor criteria.

These cases have been categorized into two major subgroups according to the level of confidence with which the diagnosis is made.

1. Highly suspected ARF
2. Uncertain ARF

Patients falling under "Highly suspected group" are managed as ARF and are provided secondary prophylaxis for minimum of 10 years or till the age 21 years (whichever is longer).

Patients falling under "uncertain rheumatic fever group" are provided secondary prophylaxis for 12 months or until an alternative diagnosis is confirmed. These patients are reassessed, and if there is still no evidence of RHD, secondary prophylaxis is stopped. Patients are then advised to report back in case of any recurrence of symptoms. However, if after 1 year there is evidence of RF, then patient is shifted to "highly suspected group" and treated accordingly.

The guidelines clearly state that:

- Patients presenting with monoarthritis should be considered to have septic arthritis until proven otherwise.
- Patients presenting with polyarthritis or polyarthralgia should be thoroughly investigated for alternative diagnoses, including arboviral infections in regions where these diseases are prevalent.

CONCLUSION

The Jones criteria have been periodically modified and updated; the 1992 update is currently the most widely used and quoted version. Each change was made to improve the specificity of the criteria at the expense of sensitivity, largely in response to the falling incidence of ARF in the USA. As a result, the criteria may not be sensitive enough to pick up disease in high-incidence populations, where the consequences of underdiagnosis may be greater than those of over diagnosis. It is imperative that high-risk countries like India should modify the guidelines to suit the need of Indian people.

REFERENCES

1. Roy SB. Prevalence of rheumatic fever and rheumatic heart disease in Ballabhgarh. Annual Report. Indian Council of Medical Research 1968-1969. p. 52.
2. Mathur KS, Banerji SC, Nigam DK, et al. Rheumatic heart disease and rheumatic fever-prevalence in a village community of Bichpuri block Agra. J Assoc Physicians India. 1971;19:151-6.
3. Berry JN. Prevalence survey of chronic rheumatic heart disease and rheumatic fever in Northern India. Br Heart J. 1972;34: 134-49.
4. Misra M, Mittal M, Singh R, et al. Prevalence of rheumatic heart disease in school-going children of Eastern Uttar Pradesh. Indian Heart J. 2007;59(1):42-3.
5. Shah B, Sharma M, Kumar R, et al. Rheumatic heart disease: progress and challenges in India. Indian J Pediatr. 2013;80 (Suppl 1):77-86.
6. Jones TD. Diagnosis of rheumatic fever. JAMA. 1944;126:481-4.
7. Ad Hoc Committee on Rheumatic Fever and Bacterial Endocarditis of the American Heart Association. Jones criteria (revised) for guidance in the diagnosis of rheumatic fever. Circulation. 1965;32:664-8.
8. Committee on Rheumatic Fever and Bacterial Endocarditis of the American Heart Association. Jones criteria (revised) for guidance in the diagnosis of rheumatic fever. Circulation. 1984;69:203A-8A.
9. Special Writing Group of the Committee on Rheumatic Fever, Endocarditis and Kawasaki Disease of the Council of Cardiovascular Disease in the Young of the American Heart Association. Guidelines for the diagnosis of rheumatic fever: Jones criteria: 1992 update. JAMA. 1992;268:2069-73.
10. Pereira BA, da Silva NA, Andrade LE, et al. Jones criteria and under diagnosis of rheumatic fever. Indian J Pediatr. 2007;(2): 117-21.
11. Vijayalakshmi IB, Mithravinda J, Deva AN. The role of echocardiography in diagnosing carditis in the setting of acute rheumatic fever. Cardiol Young. 2005;15:583-8.
12. Vijayalakshmi IB. Association of Physicians of India. Medicine Update, Kamath S (Eds). 2012;Vol 22:199-210.
13. World Health Organization. Rheumatic fever and rheumatic heart disease: report of a WHO expert consultation, Geneva, 29 October–1November 2001. WHO technical report series 923 2004; Available from *www.who.int/entity/cardiovascular_diseases/resources/trs923/en/*.
14. Narula J, et al. Endomyocardial biopsies in acute rheumatic fever. Circulation. 1993:88:2198-205.

15. Massell BF, Narula J. Rheumatic fever and rheumatic carditis. In: Braunwal dE, Abelman WH (Eds). The Atlas of Heart Diseases. Philadelphia: Current Medicine; 1994. pp. 10.1-20.
16. Calegaro JU, et al. Galio-67 nafebrerheumatica: experiencia preliminary. [Gallium-67 in rheumatic fever: preliminary experience.] Arquivos Brasileirosde Cardiologia [Braz Arch Cardiol]. 1991;56:487-92.
17. Kao CH, Wang SJ, Yeh SH. Detection of myocarditis in dilated cardiomyopathy by Tc-99m HMPAO WBC myocardial imaging in a child. Clin Nucl Med. 1992;17:678-9.
18. Kao CH, et al. Comparison of Tc-99m HMPAO labeled white blood scanning for the detection of carditis in the differentiation of rheumatic fever and inactive rheumatic heart disease in children. Nucl Med Commun. 1992;1:478-81.
19. Narula J, Chandrashekhar Y, Rahimtoola SH. Echoes of change: diagnosis of active rheumatic carditis. Circulation. 1999;100: 1576-81.
20. Dajani AS, et al. American Heart Association Guidelines for the Diagnosis of Rheumatic Fever: Jones criteria, updated 1992. Circulation. 1993;87:302-07.
21. Ferrieri P. AHA Scientific Statement: proceedings of the Jones Criteria Working Group. Circulation. 2002;106:2521-3.
22. Shaver JA. Cardiac auscultation: a cost-effective diagnostic skill. Curr Probl Cardiol. 1995;20:441-532.
23. Carapetis J, Brown A, Maguire G, Walsh W, et al. RHD Australia (ARF/RHD writing group) National Heart Foundation of Australia and Cardiac Society of Australia and New Zealand. The Australian guidelines for prevention, diagnosis and treatment of acute rheumatic fever, 2nd edn.
24. Saxena A, Kumar RK, Gera RP, et al. Consensus Guidelines on Pediatric Acute Rheumatic Fever and Rheumatic Heart Disease. Working Group on Pediatric Rheumatic Fever and Cardiology Chapter of Indian Academy of Pediatrics. Indian Pediatr. 2008;(45):565-73.

2

Pulmonary Hypertension: Evaluation and Optimizing Therapy in the Present Era

Neeraj Awasthy

INTRODUCTION

Pulmonary arterial hypertension (PAH) is defined as a mean pulmonary artery (PA) pressure of ≥25 mm Hg at rest. Pulmonary arterial hypertension has varied etiology and clinical features. Underlying etiology of PAH determines the natural history of the disease and response to therapy. Early identification of PAH is suggested because advanced disease may be less responsive to therapy.[1-3] Although pulmonary hypertension (PH) being a vast topic in itself, it is important to understand that this chapter does not discuss the various definitions, classifications, epidemiology, pathogenesis, clinical manifestations, natural history, and prognosis. This chapter mainly discusses about how to proceed with a patient of PAH and its management. Management is essentially diagnosing the patient with PAH followed by treatment. Treatment involves the primary therapy and advanced therapy. Primary therapy is directed at the underlying cause of the PAH and advanced therapy is the therapy directed at the PAH itself. Advanced therapy includes treatment with prostanoids, endothelin receptor antagonists, phosphodiesterase type 5 inhibitors, or, rarely, certain calcium channel blockers (CCBs).

CLASSIFICATION

The World Health Organization (WHO) classifies patients with PH into five groups based upon etiology: Dana Point, 2008 (Table 2.1). While patients in group 1 are considered to have PAH, patients in the remaining four groups are considered to have PH. When all five groups are discussed collectively, PH is generally used. We adhere to this nomenclature in the discussion that follows.

CLINICAL PRESENTATION

The early symptoms of PH are often mild and may be overlapped with many other conditions. These symptoms include dyspnea, dizziness, and fatigue. At rest there may be no symptoms and no apparent signs of illness. As a result there is a lag period of about 2 years from the onset of symptoms to the diagnosis of disease.[1,2] PAH is thus frequently not recognized until the disease is relatively advanced. Insidious presentation with exercise induced dyspnea that may be progressive. Angina generally late presentation may be because of right ventricular (RV) ischemia in a hypertrophied ventricle. Syncope or near syncope occurs once the RV output becomes fixed. Once the right ventricle fails, it may present with systemic congestion. Presence of orthopnea and paroxysmal nocturnal dyspnea signifies left-sided dysfunction. Presence of chronic cough signifies pulmonary pathology. Causes of hemoptysis include underlying thromboemolism, lung infarction, superadded infection, deranged coagulation, and bleeding parameters secondary to chronic hypoxia and secondary to pulmonary edema in left-sided diseases. Hoarseness of voice may be secondary to paralysis of left laryngeal nerve by dilated pulmonary arteries.

Patients with high-risk factors and associated condition such as family history, connective tissue diseases, congenital heart disease, or a history of intake of drugs or toxins should be proactively investigated for the presence of PAH.

Clinical Signs

Physical signs of PAH include large "a" wave in jugular venous pulse, a low volume carotid arterial pulse with normal upstroke, left parasternal (or RV) lift, a systolic pulsation of the dilated pulmonary arteries may be seen in second intercostal space, an accentuated pulmonary component of second heart sound, a diastolic murmur of pulmonary insufficiency (starting with a gap from the second heart sound), and RV S3 and fourth heart sound of RV origin. In advanced disease with RV failure, there may be jugular venous distension, hepatomegaly, lower limb edema, ascites, and cool extremities.

Table 2.1 The classification of PAH as per WHO (Dana Point 2008)

Group 1	**Pulmonary arterial hypertension (PAH)**
	Idiopathic pulmonary hypertension (IPH)
	Heritable pulmonary hypertension (HPH)
	Bone morphogenetic protein receptor type 2 (BMPR2)
	Activin receptor-like kinase 1 gene (ALK1), endoglin (with or without hemorrhagic telangiectasia)
	Unknown
	Drug- and toxin-induced
	Associated with pulmonary hypertension (APH):
	– Connective tissue diseases
	– Human immunodeficiency virus (HIV) infection
	– Portal hypertension
	– Congenital heart disease (CHD)
	– Schistosomiasis
	– Chronic hemolytic anemia
	– Persistent pulmonary hypertension of the newborn (PPHN)
	– Pulmonary veno-occlusive disease (PVOD) and/or pulmonary capillary hemangiomatosis (PCH)
Group 2	**Pulmonary hypertension due to left heart diseases**
	Systolic dysfunction
	Diastolic dysfunction
	Valvular disease
Group 3	**Pulmonary hypertension due to lung diseases and/or hypoxemia**
	Chronic obstructive pulmonary disease (COPD)
	Interstitial lung disease (ILD)
	Other pulmonary diseases with mixed restrictive and obstructive pattern
	Sleep-disordered breathing
	Alveolar hypoventilation disorders
	Chronic exposure to high altitude
	Developmental abnormalities
Group 4	**Chronic thromboembolic pulmonary hypertension (CTEPH)**
Group 5	**Pulmonary hypertension with unclear multifactorial mechanisms**
	Hematological disorders: Myeloproliferative disorders, splenectomy
	Systemic disorders: Sarcoidosis, pulmonary Langerhans cell histiocytosis, lymphangioleiomyomatosis, neurofibromatosis, vasculitis
	Metabolic disorders: Glycogen storage disease, Gaucher's disease, thyroid disorders
	Others: Tumoral obstruction, fibrosing mediastinitis, chronic renal failure on dialysis

BASIC INVESTIGATIONS

Polycythemia may be seen in chronic hypoxia secondary to lung pathology or chronic right-to-left shunt lesions. Test to detect hypercoagulable state, platelet number and function should be done in appropriate patients. Abnormal liver function test (LFT) may be present in RV dysfunction. Uric acid levels are elevated in PAH. There is increased incidence of thyroid diseases in PAH.

Electrocardiogram

Electrocardiogram (ECG) changes including RV hypertrophy and right atrial overload correlate well with a diagnosis of RV hypertrophy but are not sensitive or specific for PAH. Presence of prominent left ventricular (LV) forces or left atrial overload suggests LV disease and mitral valve disease, respectively. The ECG abnormalities are relatively less pronounced in obstructive pulmonary disease because in these patients PH shows increased modest increase and also because of associated hyperinflation.

Chest Radiograph

Dilated central pulmonary arteries, with peripheral pruning of blood vessels are a classical chest X-ray finding. Right atrial and RV dilatation may be seen in advances disease. The other important features which may be seen in individual types include the following:[4-6]

- *Group 2*: Pulmonary venous hypertension may point to the left heart disease.
- *Group 3*: This may show evidence of lung disease, these may be associated with kyphoscoliosis.
- In pulmonary veno-occlusive disease, there are enlarged central pulmonary arteries with septal lines and normal left-sided chambers.
- In pulmonary capillary hemangiomatosis, there are bilateral bibasilar reticular or reticulonodular opacities with enlarged central pulmonary arteries and septal lines, and pleural effusions are unusual as compared to pulmonary veno-occlusive disease.
- In chronic thromboembolic pulmonary hypertension (CTEPH), there may be irregular shaped and asymmetrically enlarged proximal vessels and regional differences in pulmonary vascularity.

Echocardiography

Echocardiography is particularly helpful in evaluating the following aspects of PH:

1. Estimation of PA pressure to determine, if PH is present
2. Assessment of cardiac cause of pulmonary hypertension
3. Assessment of severity of RV dysfunction
4. Assessment of prognostic variables.

Estimation of PA Systolic Pressure to Determine if PH is Present

Doppler Echocardiography

It is the most commonly used modality for the estimation of PA pressures. It enables the reliable estimation of PA pressures, because in the absence of pulmonary outflow obstruction, tricuspid regurgitation peak velocity (TRV) and RV outflow tract acceleration time have linear positive and negative correlations, respectively, with systolic pulmonary artery pressures (SPAP) and mean pulmonary artery pressures (MPAP) measured by right heart catheterization (RHC).[6]

Tricuspid Regurgitation Peak Velocity (Fig. 2.1)

Tricuspid regurgitation peak velocity is estimated by calculating systolic transtricuspid gradient using modified Bernoulli equation[7] and then adding an assumed or calculated right atrial pressure (RAP).[8-14] The RAP can be calculated as in Table 2.2 (Fig. 2.2). Echocardiographic Doppler estimated RV systolic pressure has good correlations with invasively measured pressures. False positive of TRV may be seen in the following circumstances:

- Physiologic range of SPAP is dependent on age and body mass index (BMI). It may be as high as 40 mm Hg in older (age >50 years) or obese (BMI >30 kg/m^2) subjects. It is more common in patients with diabetes and is likely due to PA noncompliance or abnormal LV diastolic filling pressures occurring with aging and systemic hypertension.
- *Flow-dependent variable*: In hyperdynamic states such as in hypothyroidism, anemia, dobutamine infusion, a TRV of 3 m/s is achieved easily; on the other hand, in low output states the velocity can be underestimated.
- Agitation can give falsely high value of TRV. This is very important in children, they should be quite comfortable and hence preferably sedated.
- Multiple views searching for the best envelope and maximal velocity should be taken for TRV estimation, as TRV velocity measurements are angle dependent.
- From the apical four chamber view the position of the transducer must be angled more medially and inferiorly particularly to avoid mitral valve signal.
- Color flow Doppler is recommended to obtain the best alignment between regurgitant flow and the Doppler signal.
- The injection of contrast agents (agitated saline, sonicated albumin, air-blood-saline mixture) may be required to achieve clear delineation of the tricuspid regurgitation (TR) jet envelope. Potential overestimation of Doppler

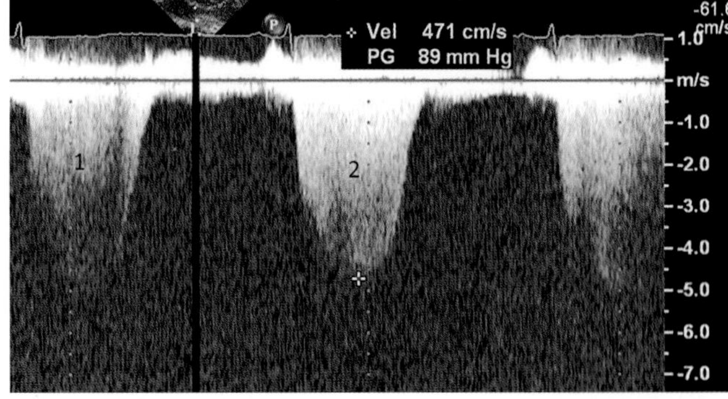

Fig. 2.1 2D Echocardiography with continuous flow Doppler across the tricuspid valve showing TR Max PG= 89 mm Hg, suggestive of significant PAH

Table 2.2 Evaluation of RAP by echocardiography

Inferior vena cava diameter	*Change with respiration*	*Estimated right atrial pressure (mm Hg)*
Small, 1.5 cm	Collapse	0
Normal, 1.5–2.5 cm	Decrease by > 50%	5
Normal	Decrease by < 50%	10
Dilated >2.5 cm (Fig. 2.2)	Decrease by < 50%	15
Dilated with dilated hepatic veins	No change	20 or more

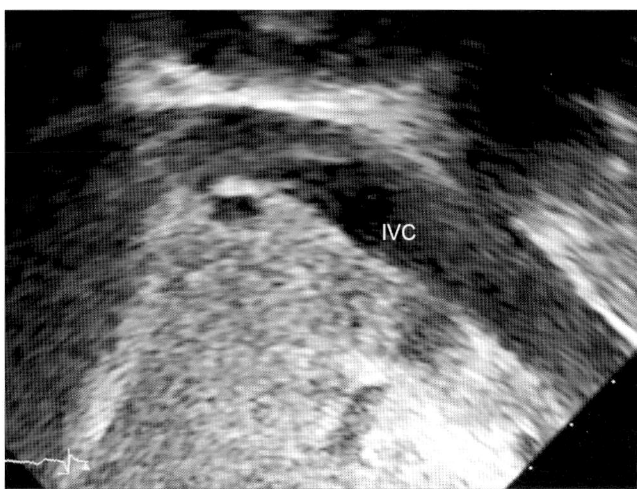

Fig. 2.2 2D echocardiography with subcoastal bicaval view showing dilated inferior vena cava (IVC). IVC may be measured in this view

velocities should be taken into account because of contrast artifacts.

- In severe TR because of early equalization of RV pressure and RAP, the peak velocity may not reflect the true RV–RAP gradient. So, the observed values have to be interpreted in the context of the clinical scenario.
- At the time of definitive diagnosis, many patients with PH show at least moderate TRV, because of annular dilation, altered RV geometry, and apical displacement of the tricuspid leaflets. The degree of TR cannot be used as a surrogate for the degree of PAP elevation.
- Another important variable of TR is d*p*/d*t*. RV d*p*/d*t* was assessed using spectral Doppler recordings from the TR signal at a sweep speed of 200 mm/s by measuring the time interval in which the regurgitant velocity increased from 0.5 m/s to 2 m/s (1–16 mm Hg). A value of <410 ms was considered a poor prognostic marker in PH. Various objective parametrs are summarized in Table 2.3.

European Society of Cardiology guidelines for the echocardiographic diagnosis and treatment of PH suggest the following:

1. PH unlikely for TRV <2.8 m/s, SPAP <36 mm Hg (assuming RAP of 5 mm Hg), and no additional echocardiographic signs of PH
2. *PH possible for:*
   a. TRV ≤2.8 m/s and SPAP ≤36 mm Hg but the presence of additional echocardiographic signs of PH
   b. TRV of 2.9–3.4 m/s and SPAP of 37–50 mm Hg with or without additional signs of PH
3. PH likely for TRV >3.4 m/s and SPAP >50 mm Hg with or without additional signs of PH[15]

Abbreviations: TRV, tricuspid regurgitation peak velocity; PH, pulmonary hypertension; SPAP, systolic pulmonary artery pressures

Pulmonary Regurgitation Velocity (Fig. 2.3)

Pulmonary valvular regurgitation is common in PH. Peak velocity of the pulmonary regurgitation signal gives an estimate of mean PAP and end-diastolic velocity can give an estimate of pressure difference between the PA diastolic and right ventricle end-diastolic pressures. Mean PAP and pulmonary end-diastolic pressure are not routinely used in the diagnosis or follow-up of PH, but may be useful when TR is absent or unreliable.

Acceleration Time (Fig. 2.4)

Pulsed-wave Doppler interrogation of the RV outflow tract in a patient of PH usually reveals an acceleration time of <100 ms, which reflects abnormal MPAP. It may be used when the tricuspid velocity cannot be measured.

- *Notching of the flow velocity envelope* may also be seen in PH. A notch seen in mid-systole is associated with severe PH and RV dysfunction.
- PVR may be calculated on echocardiography, but a PVR calculated by these methods has its limitations as compared to those calculated by cardiac catheterization.

Table 2.3 The various objective parameters for pulmonary hypertension assessment

Parameter	Normal		Abnormal
TRV (m/s)	<2.6		2.6 2.8 in obese subjects 2.9 in patients >60 years
RVOT acceleration time ms	>110	105–110	<105
RA volume index mL/m^{-2}	≤34 in males ≤27 in females		>34 in males >27 in females
RV fractional area change (%)	32–60		≤32
LV eccentricity index	1		>1 at end-diastole indicates volume loading of the RV >1 at end-systole indicates pressure loading of the RV
RV MPI (Tei index)	<0.28	0.28–0.32	>0.32
S′ wave of tricuspid annulus (cm/s)	>12	11.5–12	<11.5
IVRT (s)	<75		≥75
TAPSE (ms) (for children use charts) (Fig. 2.8)	≥20	16–20	<16
Estimated PVR wood units	<1	1–3	>3

Abbreviations: TRV, tricuspid regurgitation peak velocity; TAPSE, tricuspid annular plane systolic exertion; RA, right atrial; RV, right ventricular; LV, left ventricular; RVOT, right ventricular outflow tact; PVR, pulmonary vascular resistance; IVS, interventricular septum; IVRT, isovolumic relaxation time.

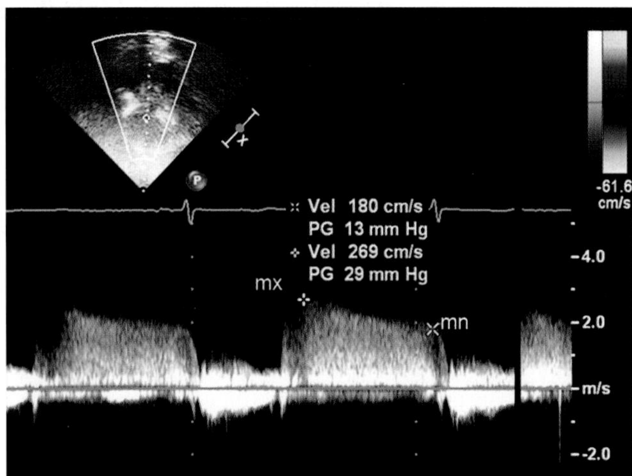

Fig. 2.3 2D echocardiography with continuous flow Doppler across the pulmonary valve measuring pulmonary regurgitation jet velocity. PR max PG of 29 mm Hg and end diastolic gradient of 13 mm Hg

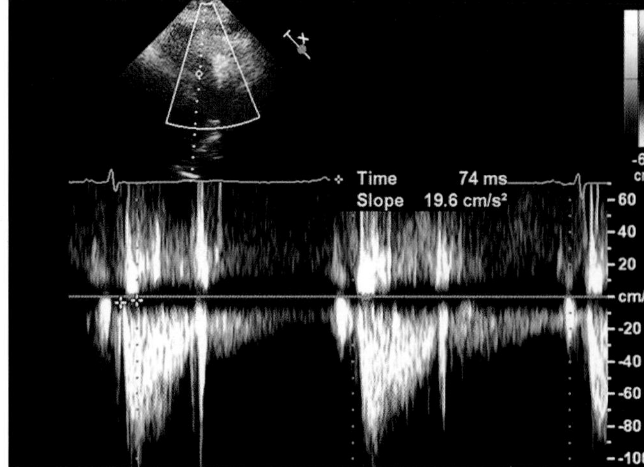

Fig. 2.4 Acceleration time

Other features of PH include (non-Doppler features of PH) the following (Figs 2.5 to 2.8):

- Enlarged right-sided chambers
- RV hypertrophy
- Increased interventricular septal thickness
- An abnormal interventricular septum/posterior LV wall ratio (>1)
- Reduced global RV systolic function

Table 2.3 summarizes various objective parameters for PH assessment:

- In a case of PH high RV pressure results in shape distortion and motion of the interventricular septum ("flattening"), which persists throughout the cardiac cycle (Fig. 2.5). As a consequence, the left ventricle appears D-shaped, with reduced diastolic and systolic volumes but preserved global systolic function.[5–8]
- Pericardial effusion (Fig. 2.8) and mitral valve prolapse have also been described in patients with PH. Pericardial effusion may be a because of impaired venous and

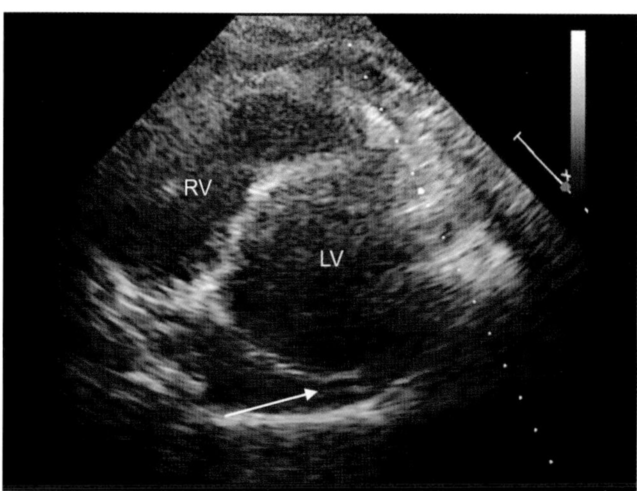

Fig. 2.5 2D echocardiography with parasternal short axis view at the level of the papillary muscles showing the flattened septal motion and presence of mild pericardial effusion (marked by arrow) in a patient with severe PAH

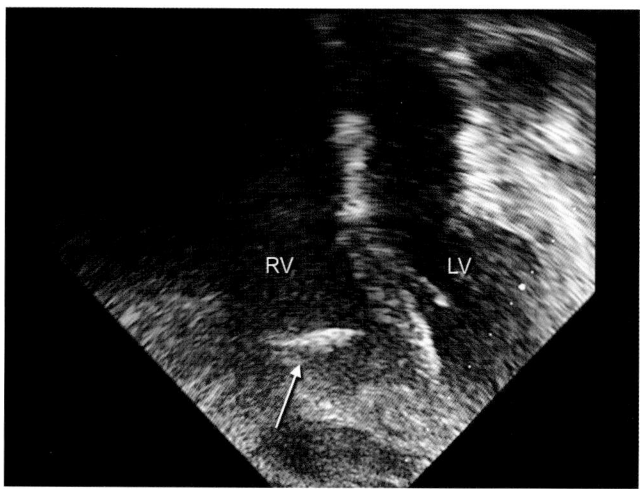

Fig. 2.6 Apical 4c view in a patient with severe PAH showing the hypertrophied RV with prominent moderator band (marked by arrow)

lymphatic drainage secondary to increased RAP. Mitral valve prolapse is related to a small left ventricle and the possible involvement of valve leaflets affected by associated connective tissue disorders, valvular heart disease.

- Because of altered RV–LV interaction, LV diastolic dysfunction may be characterized by a marked dependence of LV filling on atrial contraction, thus atrial fibrillation may not be well tolerated and vasodilating therapy may have detrimental effects on diastolic LV loading.

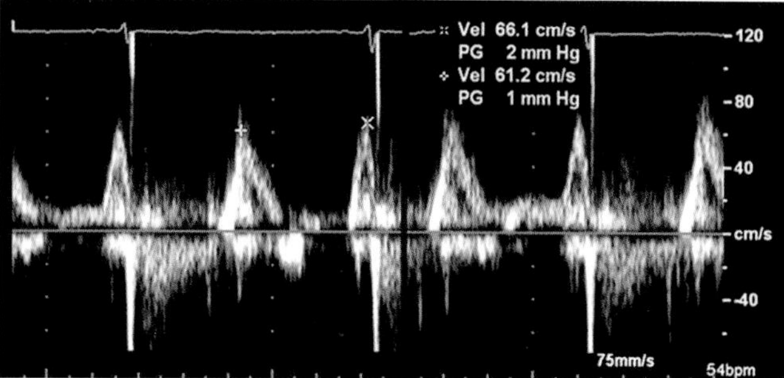

Fig. 2.7 Doppler flow echocardiography with cursor across the mitral inflow in a patient of pulmonary artery hypertension showing diastolic dysfunction of the left ventricle

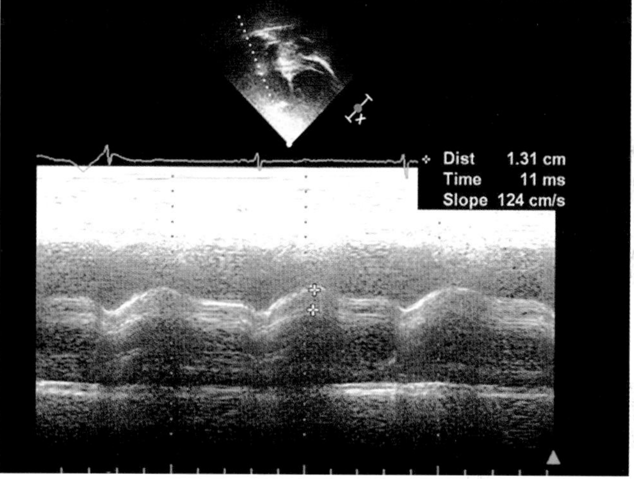

Fig. 2.8 TAPSE signal taken across the lateral annulus of the TV (as detailed in the text) showing borderline RV diastolic dysfunction with TAPSE of 13 mm in a 60-year-old lady

- Left ventricular eccentricity index is the ratio of the major axis of the LV parallel to the septum (D2) divided by the minor axis perpendicular to the septum (D1). It is measured in the parasternal short-axis view at the level of the LV papillary muscles in both end diastole and end systole.
- In a purely pressure-loaded RV, flattening of the IVS occurs in end systole, resulting in an increased end-systolic LV eccentricity index. Conversely, the eccentricity index will be increased in end diastole in pure volume loading of the RV. Left ventricular diastolic eccentricity index has been shown to be of prognostic significance particularly in patients with idiopathic PH who also have reduced RV function [tricuspid annular plane systolic exertion (TAPSE) <15 mm] (Fig. 2.8).
- Right atrial volume index is calculated from the apical four-chamber view or from the subcostal view and is measured at maximum atrial volume at the end systole.

The single plane area—length method—is used and right atrium volume is measured using the area and the long-axis length of the atrium.[24-26]

Right atrium volume index = $(0.85\ A2/L)/\text{BSA}$,

where A is the atrium area in any view (cm^2), L is the long-axis atrium length (cm), and BSA is body surface area.

- Stroke volume, cardiac output, and pulmonary vascular resistance calculated on echocardiography are not considered to be mandatory measures in PH.

Qualitative Assessment of the RV

Right ventricular dilation is assessed in multiple views including the parasternal long-axis, short-axis, and the apical four-chamber views. With chronically elevated PA pressures the RV walls become hypertrophied. Right ventricular hypertrophy is defined by RV free wall thickness of ≥0.5 mm on the apical four-chamber view. One of the first anatomical elements to become hypertrophied is the moderator band (Fig. 2.6). In contrast to other conditions affecting the RV (e.g. RV infarction or arrhythmogenic RV cardiomyopathy) where there will be regional wall motion abnormalities, contractility assessment in PH shows global RV impairment. Dilation of the RV has been shown to be linked to adverse clinical outcome and mortality.[27]

M-Mode in PH

M-mode echocardiography at the level of pulmonary valve may show diminution of a wave, fast deceleration slope, and mid-diastolic closure.

Computerized Tomography

Spiral chest computerized tomography (CT) scan is important to diagnose chronic thromboembolic PH. Besides thrombi in the pulmonary vasculatures, a mosaic pattern of variable attenuation compatible with variable pulmonary perfusion can be seen on nonenhanced CT scan. Marked variation in the size of pulmonary arteries is also a feature of chronic thromboembolism. CT scan is also important to exclude pulmonary cause of PAH.

Cardiac Catheterization

Cardiac catheterization not only establishes the severity of the disease, it is also important to adjust the response to therapy. Pulmonary artery wedge pressures are classically normal in PAH except in advanced stages when left-sided dysfunction sets in. Response to vasodilator therapy (as discussed later) is an important parameter.

Pulmonary Artery Wedge Angiogram

Pulmonary artery angiography should be done with caution with adequate precautions such as maintenance of adequate oxygenation and prevention of vasovagal reactions and rapid treatment of those that occur with intravenous atropine. Features on the wedge angiogram include the following:

- Sparsity of arborization of the pulmonary tree
- There is abrupt termination of arteries measured by measuring the length of segment over which lumen diameter narrows from 2.5 to 1.5 mm
- Tortuosity and narrowing of the small arteries
- Reduced background capillary filling.

There are certain pitfalls in the interpretation of wedge angiogram:

- In advanced vascular disease because of intimal hyperplasia there is diffuse narrowing and hence abrupt tapering may not be observed; however, background haze is absent and pulmonary circulation time is prolonged.
- The background may appear dark if the whole vessel is not filled with contrast.
- Incomplete occlusion by the balloon may also give the false impression of a dense background.
- Pulmonary stenosis or presence of previous band may give the false impression of rapid tapering.

With the advent of CT scan and the risk involved in PA wedge angiogram, it is less commonly used modality.

Other investigations summarizing the treatment of patients are given in Table 2.4.

PH Evaluation and Classification (Type, Functional Capacity, Hemodynamics)

Once the diagnosis of PH is established next step in the management involves the initiation of the therapy. Prior to initiation of the treatment a baseline investigations aimed at assessing the severity of the lesion are helpful and these would in turn aid in monitoring the response to therapy.

BASELINE ASSESSMENT

Key determinants of disease severity are functional impairment and hemodynamic derangement. The functional significance of the PH is determined by measuring exercise capacity. From the exercise capacity, the patient's WHO functional class can be determined (Table 2.5).[4]

Table 2.4 Investigations which rule out the selective subsets of pulmonary hypertension

Exclusion of group 2 (left heart disease) and group 3 (lung diseases):

- Clinical evaluation, electrocardiogram, chest radiograph, echocardiogram, pulmonary function tests, and high-resolution computed tomography (HRCT):
  - ECG may provide suggestive or supportive evidence of pulmonary hypertension by demonstrating right ventricular (RV) hypertrophy and strain, and right atrial dilatation.
  - Doppler echocardiography provides several variables that correlate with right heart hemodynamics—Doppler echocardiography should always be performed in the case of suspected pulmonary hypertension.
  - Chest radiography may show cardiomegaly and enlarged pulmonary arteries, allows the reasonable exclusion of associated moderate to severe lung diseases (Group 3) or pulmonary venous hypertension due to left heart disease (Group 2).
  - Pulmonary function tests and arterial blood gas samples to identify contribution of underlying airway or parenchymal lung disease.
  - HRCT provides evaluation of lung parenchyma. It facilitates the diagnosis of interstitial lung disease and emphysema.

Exclusion of group 4:

- If pulmonary hypertension groups 2 or 3 are not found less common causes of pulmonary hypertension should be looked for:
  - *A ventilation/perfusion lung scan:* Where there is evidence of multiple segmental perfusion defects, a diagnosis of chronic thromboembolic pulmonary hypertension (CTEPH) should be suspected.
  - The final diagnosis of CTEPH requires CT pulmonary angiography, right heart catheterization, and selective pulmonary angiography.

If a ventilation/perfusion scan is normal, or shows only subsegmental patchy perfusion defects, a tentative diagnosis of Group 1 (pulmonary hypertension) or the rarer condition of Group 5 PH is made.

- A CT pulmonary angiography may also show signs suggestive of Group 1′ pulmonary veno-occlusive disease (PVOD).
- Additional specific diagnostic tests including hematology, biochemistry, immunology, serology, and ultrasonography will allow the final diagnosis to be refined:
  - Cardiac magnetic resonance (CMR) imaging provides a direct evaluation of RV size, morphology, and function, and allows noninvasive assessment of blood flow including stroke volume, cardiac output (CO), distensibility of pulmonary artery, and RV mass; CMR is also used to distinguish pulmonary hypertension associated with congenital heart disease.
  - Blood, immunology, and serological tests are important to detect underlying connective tissue disease, human immunodeficiency virus (HIV) infection, and hepatitis; liver function tests and hepatitis serology should be examined, if clinical abnormalities are noted.
  - An abdominal ultrasound scan can reliably exclude liver cirrhosis and/or portal hypertension.
  - Right heart catheterization (RHC) represents the diagnostic gold standard for the confirmation of a diagnosis of pulmonary hypertension, and usually includes vasoreactivity testing.

Table 2.5 Functional classification for pulmonary hypertension

Functional class	*Symptomatic profile*
I	Patients with pulmonary hypertension but without resulting limitation of physical activity. Ordinary physical activity does not cause dyspnea or fatigue, chest pain, or near syncope
II	Patients with pulmonary hypertension resulting in slight limitation of physical activity. They are comfortable at rest. Ordinary physical activity causes undue dyspnea or fatigue, chest pain, or near syncope
III	Patients with pulmonary hypertension resulting in marked limitation of physical activity. They are comfortable at rest. Less than ordinary activity causes undue dyspnea or fatigue, chest pain, or near syncope
IV	Patients with pulmonary hypertension with inability to carry out any physical activity without symptoms. These patients manifest signs of right heart failure. Dyspnea and/or fatigue may even be present at rest. Discomfort is increased by any physical activity

Cardiopulmonary Exercise Testing (CPET)[15-20]

It has become the gold standard for assessing a patient's exercise capacity and maximal cardiovascular response. It is a maximal stress test—the patient exercises at a workload that progressively increases to their symptom tolerance (i.e. the maximum workload the patient can tolerate). As such, it is difficult to perform in patients with severe disease.

Pulmonary hypertension patients show reduced peak Vo_2 and this measurement correlates with a patient's prognosis. Cardiopulmonary exercise testing with measuring of the $VO_{2\ max}$ offers some advantages over the 6-minute walk test (6MWT) in terms of sensitivity, but these tests are more difficult to perform and require specialist equipment. As they are a maximal stress test, they are not suitable for more severe patients who may not be able to tolerate the exercise and may be exposed to risk of syncope and discomfort. Routine tredmill test with Naughton protocol in less symptomatic patients and 6 MWT in symptomatic patients may be used.

Biochemical Markers

Serum levels of N-terminal pro-hormone brain-type natriuretic peptide (NT-pro BNP) have been shown to be associated with prognosis in PH.[1] A level of serum NT-pro BNP below 1,400 pg/mL seems to identify patients with good prognosis.

Primary therapy is initiated after determining the severity of the disease; however, RHC is often deferred until advanced therapy is indicated because it is an invasive procedure.[24,25]

Primary therapy: It refers to treatment directed at the underlying cause of the PH. The disease severity should be reassessed following primary therapy in order to determine whether advanced therapy is indicated:

- *Group 1 PH*: There are no effective primary therapies for most types of group 1 PH. As a result, advanced therapy is often needed.
- *Group 2 PH*: These have PH secondary to left heart disease and hence treatment is aimed at treatment of the underlying heart disease, which is discussed in detail separately.
- *Group 3 PH*: Patients in group 3 have PH secondary to various pulmonary causes and the management consist of treatment of the underlying cause of hypoxemia and correction of the hypoxemia with supplemental oxygen. Oxygen is the only modality with proven mortality benefit in some patients with group 3 PH.
- *Group 4 PH*: In the patients with thromboembolic occlusion. Anticoagulation is primary medical therapy.
- Surgical thromboendarterectomy is primary surgical therapy for selected patients with thromboembolic obstruction of the proximal pulmonary arteries.[8] Perioperative mortality for this procedure is <10%, and hemodynamic response may be dramatic and sustained. Prior to proceeding with this invasive approach, a 3-month period of anticoagulation is required.
- *Group 5 PH*: Group 5 PH is uncommon and includes PH with unclear multifactorial mechanisms (Table 2.1). Primary therapy is directed at the underlying cause.

General Care

This includes care in all patients such as avoiding pregnancy, prevention and prompt treatment of chest infections, and awareness of the potential effects of altitude.[1,5,6]

Supportive Care

They include oxygen, diuretic, anticoagulant, and digoxin therapy, as well as exercise.

Oxygen therapy: Continuous oxygen administration remains the corner stone of therapy in patients with group 3.[1,9,10] The flow of oxygen needed to correct hypoxemia should be determined by measurement of the oxygen saturation. Oxygen is administered at 1–4 L/min generally via nasal prongs and adjusted to maintain the oxygen saturation above 90% at rest and, if possible, with exercise and sleep.[11]

Supplemental oxygen will not significantly improve the oxygen saturation of patients who have congenital heart disease with a right-to-left shunt (Eisenmenger physiology).

Diuretics: It will diminish hepatic congestion and peripheral edema.[9] But overuse can decreased cardiac output (due to decreased RV and/or LV preload), arrhythmias induced by hypokalemia, and metabolic alkalosis. Fluid can also be removed by dialysis or ultrafiltration if necessary.

Anticoagulation:[21,22] Patients with PH are at increased risk for intrapulmonary thrombosis and thromboembolism due to sluggish pulmonary blood flow, dilated right heart chambers, venous stasis, and a sedentary lifestyle. Even a small thrombus can produce hemodynamic deterioration in a patient with a compromised pulmonary vascular bed that is unable to dilate or recruit unused vasculature.

It is generally accepted that anticoagulation is indicated in patients with idiopathic PH, hereditary PAH, drug-induced PH, or group 4. Limited experience with newer anticoagulants makes *warfarin* the anticoagulant of choice, with a therapeutic goal of an international normalized ratio (INR) of approximately two.

The risk of bleeding on vitamin K antagonists may differ among patients with different types of PH. A retrospective study of 198 patients with PH receiving anticoagulation reported major bleeding events in 23%. Patients with PH frequently have other risk factors for thromboembolism (e.g. atrial fibrillation, severe left heart failure) that may warrant anticoagulation.

***Digoxin*:**[23] Digoxin therapy has been shown to have both beneficial effects and drawbacks:

- *Digoxin* improves the RV ejection fraction of patients with group 3. This group of patient may be more sensitive to digitalis toxicity and thus require close monitoring.
- *Digoxin* helps control the heart rate of patients who have supraventricular tachycardias associated with RV dysfunction. *Verapamil* may be used for multifocal atrial tachycardia, unless there is concurrent LV failure.

***Exercise*:** Exercise training appears to be beneficial for patients with PH. Exercise training does not improve hemodynamic abnormalities, but there is data to suggest that skeletal muscle training may play a major role in the treatment of patients with PH. Exercise is known to elevate PA pressures so graded exercises such as bike riding in which patients can gradually increase their workload are considered safer then isometric exercises.[15-20]

Pregnancy Issues

Changes occurring during pregnancy may be detrimental to mother and the fetus. The changes in blood volume, increased oxygen consumption, circulating procoagulant factors and risk of pulmonary embolism from deep veins and amniotic fluid are additional risk factors. Thus, the subject needs to be discussed with women of childbearing age with appropriate contraceptive advice.

Advanced Therapy

Advanced therapy is directed at the PH irrespective of the underlying cause. It includes treatment with prostanoids, endothelin receptor antagonists, phosphodiesterase type 5 inhibitors, or, rarely, certain calcium channel blockers (CCB).

***Patient selection*:** Advanced therapy is considered for patients who have evidence of persistent PH and a functional class II, III, or IV despite adequate primary therapy.[24-26] There are special considerations for each group of PH.

- *Group 1 PH*: There are no effective primary therapies, so advanced therapy is often needed for patients with group 1 PAH.
- *Group 2 PAH*: Treatment is directed toward the primary cause, yet there are a few conditions where advanced therapy may be considered:
  - Patients with persistent PH due to mitral stenosis who have undergone mitral valve replacement.
  - However, for most patients with group 2 PH, advanced therapy should be avoided because it may be harmful.[3,4]
- *Group 3 PH*: Advanced therapy is occasionally considered for patients in group 3, who remain WHO functional class III or IV despite correction of hypoxemia and optimization of the underlying disease, especially if the severity of PH is out of proportion to the severity of the parenchymal lung disease. The tendency of advanced therapy to worsen ventilation-perfusion mismatch and increase hypoxemia in patients with group 3 PH may be formulation- and disease-specific.
- *Formulation-specific effect*:
  - *Epoprostenol* may increase hypoxemia in patients who have pulmonary fibrosis. Inhaled nitric oxide, inhaled *Iloprost*, and oral *Sildenafil* may be used as they do not appear to have this effect.[26,27] All of these agents decrease the pulmonary vascular resistance.
- *Evidence of a disease-specific effect*: Oral *Sildenafil* did not appear to worsen hypoxemia in pulmonary fibrosis,[26] but was associated with worsened hypoxemia due to chronic obstructive pulmonary disease.[28] In both diseases, oral Sildenafil decreased the PA pressure.
- *Group 4 PH*: Advanced therapy can be considered for patients with group 4 who remain WHO functional class III or IV even after anticoagulation or thromboendarterectomy. Pharmacologic therapy can also act as a bridge to surgical intervention.
- *Group 5 PH*: Few studies have shown role of advanced therapy related to sarcoidosis. A series of eight patients described a favorable response to intravenous *Epoprostenol* in most patients,[29] while another study reported that carefully selected patients can be transitioned from prostanoid infusion to oral *Bosentan*.[30]

General Approach

Patients with PH who are selected for advanced therapy should undergo an invasive hemodynamic assessment and should undergo a vasoreactivity test (detailed below). Patients with positive vasoreactivity test are candidates of oral CCB therapy with a dihydropyridine or *diltiazem*. Patients with a negative vasoreactivity test require advanced therapy with a prostanoid, endothelin receptor antagonist, or phosphodiesterase type 5 inhibitor. Combination therapy may be appropriate in refractory cases. In patients with treatment refractory to medical therapy lung transplantation or creation of a right to left shunt by atrial septostomy may be considered.[8] An algorithm for advanced therapy is shown in Flow chart 2.1.

***Vasoreactivity test*:** Patients of group 1 PAH should undergo a vasoreactivity test with *Epoprostenol*, adenosine, or inhaled nitric oxide[31]:

- *Epoprostenol*: Infusion is started at 1–2 ng/kg per minutes, increased gradually by 2 ng/kg per minute every 5–10 minutes until a clinically significant fall in blood pressure, an increase in heart rate, or adverse symptoms (e.g. nausea, vomiting, and headache) develop.
- Adenosine is administered intravenously at 50 µg/kg per minute and increased every 2 minutes to a maximal dose of 200–350 µg/kg per minute. As a practical guide starting

Flow chart 2.1 An algorithm for advanced therapy

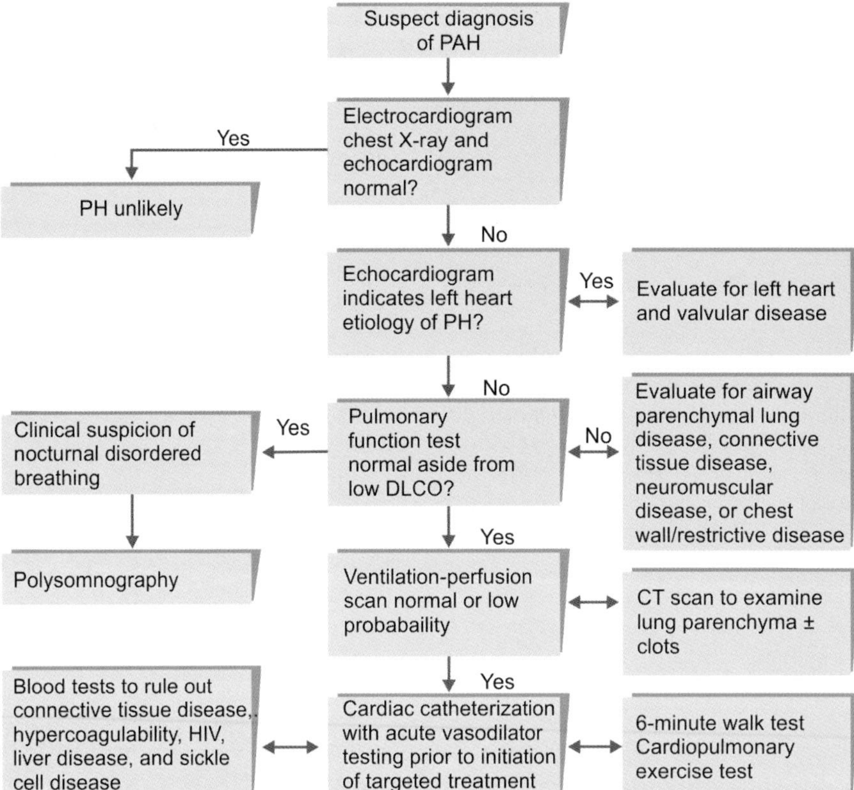

the undiluted adenosine (1 mL = 3 mg) at the body weight per mL gives the requisite dose at 50 µg/kg per minute, e.g. for a 60 kg adult 60 mL/h of adenosine (strength 1 mL = 3 mg) gives 50 µg/kg per minute. This starting dose can be appropriately increased.

- Inhaled nitric oxide is administered at 10–20 ppm may be used.[31-36]
- Vasoreactivity test is considered positive if mean PA pressure decreases at least 10 mm Hg and to a value <40 mm Hg, with an increased or unchanged cardiac output, and a minimally reduced or unchanged systemic blood pressure. Patients with porto-PH should not undergo vasoreactivity testing, as they are at increased risk of adverse sequelae from pure vasodilator therapy.

Calcium-channel blockers (CCB):[37-42] Patients with reactive vasodilator response may be considered for treatment with CCBs like dihydropyridine or *diltiazem.*[12,37-39] The CCB therapy can be initiated with either long-acting *nifedipine* (30 mg/day) or *diltiazem* (120 mg/day), and gradually increased to maximal dose. Systemic blood pressure, heart rate, and oxygen saturation should be carefully monitored during titration. Long-acting dihydropyridine like *amlodipine* is a useful alternative for patients who are intolerant of the other agents. Patients who respond to CCB therapy with a dihydropyridine or *diltiazem* (defined as asymptomatic or minimal symptoms) should be reassessed after 3–6 months of treatment. Patients on CCB have been shown to have better quality of life with improved functional class and survival than nonresponders.

Prostanoids: Prostanoid formulations include intravenous *Epoprostenol* (prostacyclin), intravenous *treprostinil,* subcutaneous treprostinil, inhaled treprostinil, and inhaled Iloprost.[43,44] All of the prostanoid formulations have the limitations of a short half-life and a heterogeneous response to therapy.

Epoprostenol (Flolan): It is available for intravenous use. It improves hemodynamic parameters, functional capacity, and survival in patients with idiopathic pulmonary arterial hypertension (IPAH).[45-49] It is delivered continuously through an implanted central venous catheter using a portable infusion pump, usually initiated at doses of 1–2 ng/kg per minute and increased as per tolerance by 1–2 ng/kg per minute every 1–2 days. Once an initial level of 6–10 ng/kg per minute is achieved (usually within 1–2 weeks), most patients require dose increases of 1–2 ng/kg per minute every 2–4 weeks to sustain the clinical effect. In children, the maintenance dosage is higher than in adults. A maximal dose has not been established.[50-54] Side effects include jaw pain, foot pain, poorly defined gastropathy, diarrhea, and arthralgias. Also are the side effects of the delivery systems including thrombosis, pump malfunction, and interruption of the infusion. Central venous catheter infection can also contribute to the morbidity and mortality of continuous *Epoprostenol* therapy.[55,56]

Treprostinil (Remodulin):[57-63] It is administered intravenously, subcutaneously and recently inhaled. Subcutaneous administration is uncommon due to severe pain at the injection site. It improves hemodynamic parameters, symptoms, exercise capacity, and possibly survival in patients with group 1.[44,57-59] It has not been evaluated in patients with other types of PH.

There are no available trials comparing *Epoprostenol* to *treprostinil.* Advantages of parenteral treprostinil, compared to Epoprostenol, include the option of continuous subcutaneous delivery, a longer half-life (4 hours) that may make interruption of the infusion less immediately life-threatening, and no need for refrigeration. All of these advantages allow more flexibility and easier administration. For patients who desire the advantages associated with treprostinil administration, it can be offered as first-line therapy. Based upon preliminary results, patients who are already receiving Epoprostenol generally can be transitioned to treprostinil (subcutaneous or intravenous) without a significant loss of clinical efficacy.[60,61] Reciprocally, Epoprostenol can be given if the desired effect is not achieved with treprostinil.

Iloprost (Ventavis)[64] is administered via inhalational route. It is thus selective to lung vasculature without systemic side effects, but it requires frequent administration (6–9 up to 12 times per day).

Beraprost: It is orally active prostacyclin analog. In a large European trial (ALPHABET), it improved exercise capacity over 12 weeks period, but large scale trials are needed especially for children.

Endothelin Receptor Antagonists

Endothelin-1 is a smooth muscle mitogen and a potent vasoconstrictor.[65-67] The endothelin receptor antagonists improved exercise capacity, dyspnea, and hemodynamic measures (PA pressure, pulmonary vascular resistance, and cardiac index).

Bosentan (Bosentas) is a nonselective endothelin receptor antagonist.[68-71] It is administered orally. In BREATHE-1 trial, Bosentan improved symptoms, the 6-minute walking distance, and the WHO functional class.

Selective agents include type A endothelin-1 receptor antagonists administered orally including *ambrisentan* (Volibris, Endobloc) and Sitaxsentan. The ARIES-1 and ARIES-2 trials suggest that ambrisentan[72-74] and sitaxsentan[75-78] improve exercise tolerance, WHO functional class, hemodynamics, and quality of life in patients with PH. Hepatotoxicity is the main adverse effect of some endothelin receptor antagonists. It was for this reason the sitaxsentan was withdrawn from the market.[79-81] Liver function tests should be monitored monthly during treatment with Bosentan, but monitoring of LFTs is no longer required for patients treated with ambrisentan. Side effects include peripheral edema. Mild cases of edema can be managed with diuretics, but more severe cases warrant discontinuation of the medication. Endothelin receptor antagonists are also potent teratogens hence requiring meticulous contraception in childbearing age group.[82]

PDE5 inhibitors: *Sildenafil* (Assurans, Viagra, Revatio), *Tadalafil* (Cialis, Adcirca), and *Vardenafil (*Levitra) are orally administered cyclic GMP phosphodiesterase type 5 (PDE5) inhibitors.

- *Sildenafil* improves pulmonary hemodynamics and exercise capacity in patients with group 1.[83-86] In SUPER-1 trial the Sildenafil demonstrated significant improvement in hemodynamics and 6-minute walk distances, which persisted during 1 year of follow-up.[85] Mortality was not reported. In SUPER-2 trial,[87] there was persistent improvement in the 6-minute walk distance and WHO functional class of 46% and 29% of patients, respectively, compared with the baseline values measured prior to the SUPER-1 trial. The estimated 3-year survival rate was 79%. *Tadalafil* and *Vardenafil* also appear to improve outcomes in patients with group 1. The PHIRST done with Tadalafil (40 mg) showed significantly increased the 6-minute walk distance and the time to clinical worsening, while decreasing the incidence of clinical worsening and improving health-related quality of life. This improvement of the 6-minute walk distance was sustained for an additional 52 weeks in the PHIRST-2 trial, an uncontrolled extension trial. Similar response has been shown with Vardenafil.[88-90]

Guanylate cyclase stimulant: Stimulators of the nitric oxide receptor, soluble guanylate cyclase (sGC) have dual mode of action. They increase the sensitivity of sGC to endogenous nitric oxide (NO), a pulmonary vasodilator, and they also directly stimulate the receptor to mimic the action of NO.

Riociguat[91] had a favorable safety profile and was well tolerated, with dyspepsia, headache, and hypotension as the most frequent side effects. Preliminary results from phase III randomized placebo-controlled trials of riociguat in patients with PAH (PATENT-1) and inoperable CTEPH (CHEST-1), also suggest similar benefit.[92-94]

Dosage of various drugs is tabulated in Table 2.6.

Combination Therapy

Combining pharmacologic agents with different mechanisms of action may produce an additive effect as under:

Table 2.6 Pulmonary vasodilators with appropriate dosages

	Mode of administration	Starting dose	Maximal dose
Diltiazem	PO	240–720 mg/day	960 mg/day
Nifedipine	PO	90–180 mg/day	240 mg/day
Epoprostenol	IV	2–4 ng/kg/min	25–40 ng/kg/min
Treprostinil	IV/SC	1–2 ng/kg/min	75–150 ng/kg/min
Beraprost	Oral	20–100 μ BID to QID	
Iloprost	Nebulizer system	6–9 times/day (2.5–5 μg/inhalation)	
Bosentan	Oral	62.5 mg BID (1–2 mg/kg twice daily) increased to 2–4 mg/kg after 4 weeks	125 mg BID
Sildenafil	Oral	20 mg TID (1–5 mg/kg in 4 divided dosages)	80 mg TID
Tadalafil	Oral	10 mg OD	40 mg OD

- *Bosentan added to either Epoprostenol or treprostinil*: Bosentan can be used safely, and effectively added to Epoprostenol or subcutaneous treprostinil therapy.[59,95] BREATHE-2 trial showed improved hemodynamic parameters, exercise capacity, and functional class, compared to baseline.
- *Treprostinil* added to either *Bosentan* or *Sildenafil*: The addition of inhaled treprostinil may improve the exercise capacity and quality of life of patients with persistent symptoms despite Bosentan or Sildenafil therapy. In TRIUMPH trial,[96] patients on Bosentan or Sildenafil therapy were randomly assigned to receive either inhaled treprostinil or placebo for 12 weeks. The treprostinil group had a larger improvement in their 6-minute walking distance and quality of life, but there were no differences in the time to clinical worsening, dyspnea, or WHO functional class.
- Oral *treprostinil* added to an endothelin receptor antagonist and/or a phosphodiesterase type 5 inhibitor: The addition of oral treprostinil in patients with group 1 PAH already on an endothelin receptor antagonist and/or a phosphodiesterase type 5 inhibitor did not improve the 6MWD at 16 weeks in the FREEDOM-C Study.[62]
- *Sildenafil* added to *Epoprostenol*: The addition of Sildenafil to long-term Epoprostenol therapy improves clinical outcomes.[97]
- *Sildenafil* added to *Bosentan*: The benefits of adding Sildenafil to Bosentan therapy are more certain among patients with IPAH than those with scleroderma-associated PAH.[98]
- *Sildenafil* added to *Iloprost*: The combination of Iloprost plus Sildenafil may improve outcomes compared to either agent alone.[99,100]

Selection of an agent:[101,102] In general the usage of the agents (when available) can be guided by the following suggestion:

- *WHO functional class II*: Preferred agents include ambrisentan, Bosentan, Sildenafil, or *Tadalafil.*
- *WHO functional class III*: Preferred agents include *ambrisentan, Bosentan,* intravenous *Epoprostenol,* intravenous or subcutaneous *treprostinil,* inhaled *Iloprost, Sildenafil,* or *Tadalafil.*
- *WHO functional class IV*: Patients with severe PH who are WHO functional class IV should be treated with an intravenous prostanoid. Most clinicians consider intravenous *Epoprostenol* to be the preferred agent. Intravenous *treprostinil* is considered a reasonable alternative by some. Inhaled *Iloprost* can be considered for patients who refuse or cannot receive intravenous therapy.

Combination therapy is appropriate in cases refractory to monotherapy.[1,9] It should consist of two agents with different mechanisms of action. In other words, it should consist of agents from any two of the following three classes: prostanoids, endothelin receptor antagonists, and PDE5 inhibitors.

The randomized, double-blind, multicenter, "AMBITION" trial showed that first-line treatment of PAH with the combination of ambrisentan 10 mg and Tadalafil 40 mg decreased the risk of clinical failure by 50% compared to pooled ambrisentan and Tadalafil monotherapy arm.

Most therapy as per the available recomendation above gets limited by the non availability of drugs in various centers around the globe.

Follow-up: Patients on parental or combination therapy and those who have advanced right heart failure should ideally be seen every 3 months (or more frequently). Less ill patients should be seen every 3–6 months. Follow-up visits should include a thorough clinical examination for signs of right heart failure; and resting and ambulatory oximetry. Investigations that can be done include brain natriuretic peptide (BNP), 6MWT, echocardiogram, and invasive hemodynamic assessment (RHC), which is determined on a case-by-case basis.

INTERVENTIONAL THERAPY

Right-to-Left Shunt[103-114]

Creation of a right-to-left shunt may be considered in adults with severe symptomatic PH. These include atrial septostomy and Potts shunt.[103-113] The purpose of right-to-left shunting is to divert blood flow to bypass the pulmonary vascular bed and enter the systemic circulation, thereby elevating systemic blood flow and maintaining tissue perfusion, albeit with less oxygenated blood.

TRANSPLANTATION

Transplantation has been performed in patients with IPAH.[8,115,116] Bilateral lung or heart-lung transplantation is the procedure of choice.[8] The 3-year survival of patients who had a lung or heart-lung transplant for IPAH is approximately 50%.[110,117] Guidelines for when to refer a patient for transplant evaluation are as follows:[118]

- WHO functional class III or IV
- Mean RAP >10 mm Hg
- Mean pulmonary arterial pressure >50 mm Hg
- Cardiac index <2.5 L/min per m^2
- Failure to improve functionally despite medical therapy
- Rapidly progressive disease.

ACKNOWLEDGMENT

I thank Dr Prashant Bhopate, Clinical Research Fellow, Division of pulmonary hypertension and Paediatric cardiology, Department of Paediatrics, University of Alberta, Canada for giving valuable comments on the manuscript enabling us to improve upon it.

REFERENCES

1. Barst RJ, Gibbs JS, Ghofrani HA, et al. Updated evidence-based treatment algorithm in pulmonary arterial hypertension. J Am Coll Cardiol. 2009;54:S78.
2. Galiè N, Rubin Lj, Hoeper M, et al. Treatment of patients with mildly symptomatic pulmonary arterial hypertension with Bosentan (EARLY study): a double-blind, randomised controlled trial. Lancet. 2008;371:2093.
3. McLaughlin VV, Archer SL, Badesch DB, et al. ACCF/AHA 2009 expert consensus document on pulmonary hypertension a report of the American College of Cardiology Foundation Task Force on Expert Consensus Documents and the American Heart Association developed in collaboration with the American College of Chest Physicians; American Thoracic Society, Inc; and the Pulmonary hypertension Association. J Am Coll Cardiol. 2009;53:1573.
4. Badesch DB, Champion HC, Sanchez MA, et al. Diagnosis and assessment of pulmonary arterial hypertension. J Am Coll Cardiol. 2009;54:S55.
5. Long term domiciliary oxygen therapy in chronic hypoxic cor pulmonale complicating chronic bronchitis and emphysema. Report of the Medical Research Council Working Party. Lancet. 1981;1:681.
6. Continuous or nocturnal oxygen therapy in hypoxemic chronic obstructive lung disease: a clinical trial. Nocturnal Oxygen Therapy Trial Group. Ann Intern Med. 1980;93:391.
7. Ashutosh K, Dunsky M. Noninvasive tests for responsiveness of pulmonary hypertension to oxygen. Prediction of survival in patients with chronic obstructive lung disease and cor pulmonale. Chest. 1987;92:393.
8. Keogh AM, Mayer E, Benza RL, et al. Interventional and surgical modalities of treatment in pulmonary hypertension. J Am Coll Cardiol. 2009;54:S67.
9. Galiè N, Hoeper MM, Humbert M, et al. Guidelines for the diagnosis and treatment of pulmonary hypertension: the Task Force for the Diagnosis and Treatment of Pulmonary hypertension of the European Society of Cardiology (ESC) and the European Respiratory Society (ERS), endorsed by the International Society of Heart and Lung Transplantation (ISHLT). Eur Heart J. 2009;30:2493.
10. McLaughlin VV, Archer SL, Badesch DB, et al. ACCF/AHA 2009 expert consensus document on pulmonary hypertension: a report of the American College of Cardiology Foundation Task Force on Expert Consensus Documents and the American Heart Association: developed in collaboration with the American College of Chest Physicians, American Thoracic Society, Inc., and the Pulmonary hypertension Association. Circulation. 2009;119:2250.
11. Hildenbrand FF, Bloch KE, Speich R, et al. Daytime measurements underestimate nocturnal oxygen desaturations in pulmonary arterial and chronic thromboembolic pulmonary hypertension. Respiration. 2012;84:477.
12. Rich S, Kaufmann E, Levy PS. The effect of high doses of calcium-channel blockers on survival in primary pulmonary hypertension. N Engl J Med. 1992;327:76.
13. Fuster V, Steele PM, Edwards WD, et al. Primary pulmonary hypertension: natural history and the importance of thrombosis. Circulation. 1984;70:580.
14. Kawut SM, Horn EM, Berekashvili KK, et al. New predictors of outcome in idiopathic pulmonary arterial hypertension. Am J Cardiol. 2005;95:199.
15. Paraskos JA. Pulmonary heart disease including pulmonary embolism. In: Cardiology, Parmley WW, Chatterjee K (Eds). Philadelphia, PA: JB Lippincott; 1987.
16. Mereles D, Ehlken N, Kreuscher S, et al. Exercise and respiratory training improve exercise capacity and quality of life in patients with severe chronic pulmonary hypertension. Circulation. 2006;114:1482.
17. de Man FS, Handoko ML, Groepenhoff H, et al. Effects of exercise training in patients with idiopathic pulmonary arterial hypertension. Eur Respir J. 2009;34:669.
18. Grünig E, Lichtblau M, Ehlken N, et al. Safety and efficacy of exercise training in various forms of pulmonary hypertension. Eur Respir J. 2012;40:84.

19. Chan L, Chin LM, Kennedy M, et al. Benefits of intensive treadmill exercise training on cardiorespiratory function and quality of life in patients with pulmonary hypertension. Chest. 2013;143:333.
20. Weinstein AA, Chin LM, Keyser RE, et al. Effect of aerobic exercise training on fatigue and physical activity in patients with pulmonary arterial hypertension. Respir Med. 2013;107:778.
21. Johnson SR, Mehta S, Granton JT. Anticoagulation in pulmonary arterial hypertension: a qualitative systematic review. Eur Respir J. 2006;28:999.
22. Henkens IR, Hazenoot T, Boonstra A, et al. Major bleeding with vitamin K antagonist anticoagulants in pulmonary hypertension. Eur Respir J. 2013;41:872.
23. Mathur PN, Powles P, Pugsley SO, et al. Effect of digoxin on right ventricular function in severe chronic airflow obstruction. A controlled clinical trial. Ann Intern Med. 1981;95:283.
24. Badesch DB, Abman SH, Simonneau G, et al. Medical therapy for pulmonary arterial hypertension: updated ACCP evidence-based clinical practice guidelines. Chest. 2007;131:1917.
25. Hoeper MM, Barberà JA, Channick RN, et al. Diagnosis, assessment, and treatment of non-pulmonary arterial hypertension pulmonary hypertension. J Am Coll Cardiol. 2009;54:S85.
26. Ghofrani HA, Wiedemann R, Rose F, et al. Sildenafil for treatment of lung fibrosis and pulmonary hypertension: a randomised controlled trial. Lancet. 2002;360:895.
27. Olschewski H, Ghofrani HA, Walmrath D, et al. Inhaled prostacyclin and Iloprost in severe pulmonary hypertension secondary to lung fibrosis. Am J Respir Crit Care Med. 1999;160:600.
28. Blanco I, Gimeno E, Munoz PA, et al. Hemodynamic and gas exchange effects of Sildenafil in patients with chronic obstructive pulmonary disease and pulmonary hypertension. Am J Respir Crit Care Med. 2010;181:270.
29. Fisher KA, Serlin DM, Wilson KC, et al. Sarcoidosis-associated pulmonary hypertension: outcome with long-term Epoprostenol treatment. Chest. 2006;130:1481.
30. Steiner MK, Preston IR, Klinger JR, et al. Conversion to Bosentan from prostacyclin infusion therapy in pulmonary arterial hypertension: a pilot study. Chest. 2006;130:1471.
31. Badesch DB, Abman SH, Ahearn GS, et al. Medical therapy for pulmonary arterial hypertension: ACCP evidence-based clinical practice guidelines. Chest. 2004;126:35S.
32. Pepke-Zaba J, Higenbottam TW, Dinh-Xuan AT, et al. Inhaled nitric oxide as a cause of selective pulmonary vasodilatation in pulmonary hypertension. Lancet. 1991;338:1173.
33. Morales-Blanhir J, Santos S, de Jover L, et al. Clinical value of vasodilator test with inhaled nitric oxide for predicting long-term response to oral vasodilators in pulmonary hypertension. Respir Med. 2004;98:225.
34. Sitbon O, Humbert M, Jagot JL, et al. Inhaled nitric oxide as a screening agent for safely identifying responders to oral calcium-channel blockers in primary pulmonary hypertension. Eur Respir J. 1998;12:265.
35. Ricciardi MJ, Knight BP, Martinez FJ, et al. Inhaled nitric oxide in primary pulmonary hypertension: a safe and effective agent for predicting response to nifedipine. J Am Coll Cardiol. 1998;32:1068.
36. Atz AM, Adatia I, Lock JE, et al. Combined effects of nitric oxide and oxygen during acute pulmonary vasodilator testing. J Am Coll Cardiol. 1999;33:813.
37. Rich S, Brundage BH. High-dose calcium channel-blocking therapy for primary pulmonary hypertension: evidence for long-term reduction in pulmonary arterial pressure and regression of right ventricular hypertrophy. Circulation. 1987;76:135.
38. Humbert M, Sitbon O, Simonneau G. Treatment of pulmonary arterial hypertension. N Engl J Med. 2004;351:1425.
39. Sitbon O, Humbert M, Jaïs X, et al. Long-term response to calcium channel blockers in idiopathic pulmonary arterial hypertension. Circulation. 2005;111:3105.
40. Packer M, Medina N, Yushak M. Adverse hemodynamic and clinical effects of calcium channel blockade in pulmonary hypertension secondary to obliterative pulmonary vascular disease. J Am Coll Cardiol. 1984;4:890.
41. Palevsky HI, Fishman AP. Chronic cor pulmonale: etiology and management. JAMA. 1990;263:2347.
42. Melot C, Hallemans R, Naeije R, et al. Deleterious effect of nifedipine on pulmonary gas exchange in chronic obstructive pulmonary disease. Am Rev Respir Dis. 1984;130:612.
43. Badesch DB, McLaughlin VV, Delcroix M, et al. Prostanoid therapy for pulmonary arterial hypertension. J Am Coll Cardiol. 2004;43:56S.
44. Tapson VF, Gomberg-Maitland M, McLaughlin VV, et al. Safety and efficacy of IV Treprostinil for pulmonary arterial hypertension: a prospective, multicenter, open-label, 12-week trial. Chest. 2006;129:683.
45. Barst RJ, Rubin LJ, McGoon MD, et al. Survival in primary pulmonary hypertension with long-term continuous intravenous prostacyclin. Ann Intern Med. 1994;121:409.
46. Rubin LJ, Mendoza J, Hood M, et al. Treatment of primary pulmonary hypertension with continuous intravenous prostacyclin (Epoprostenol). Results of a randomized trial. Ann Intern Med. 1990;112:485.
47. Barst RJ, Rubin LJ, Long WA, et al. A comparison of continuous intravenous Epoprostenol (prostacyclin) with conventional therapy for primary pulmonary hypertension. N Engl J Med. 1996;334:296.
48. Shapiro SM, Oudiz RJ, Cao T, et al. Primary pulmonary hypertension: improved long-term effects and survival with continuous intravenous Epoprostenol infusion. J Am Coll Cardiol. 1997;30:343.
49. Higenbottam T, Butt AY, McMahon A, et al. Long-term intravenous prostaglandin (Epoprostenol or Iloprost) for treatment of severe pulmonary hypertension. Heart. 1998; 80:151.
50. Tuder RM, Cool CD, Geraci MW, et al. Prostacyclin synthase expression is decreased in lungs from patients with severe pulmonary hypertension. Am J Respir Crit Care Med. 1999;159:1925.
51. McLaughlin VV, Genthner DE, Panella MM, et al. Compassionate use of continuous prostacyclin in the management of secondary pulmonary hypertension: a case series. Ann Intern Med. 1999;130:740.
52. Rosenzweig EB, Kerstein D, Barst RJ. Long-term prostacyclin for pulmonary hypertension with associated congenital heart defects. Circulation. 1999;99:1858.
53. Humbert M, Sanchez O, Fartoukh M, et al. Short-term and long-term Epoprostenol (prostacyclin) therapy in pulmonary hypertension secondary to connective tissue diseases: results of a pilot study. Eur Respir J. 1999;13:1351.

54. Rich S, McLaughlin VV. The effects of chronic prostacyclin therapy on cardiac output and symptoms in primary pulmonary hypertension. J Am Coll Cardiol. 1999;34:1184.
55. Oudiz RJ, Widlitz A, Beckmann XJ, et al. Micrococcus-associated central venous catheter infection in patients with pulmonary arterial hypertension. Chest. 2004;126:90.
56. Kitterman N, Poms A, Miller DP, et al. Bloodstream infections in patients with pulmonary arterial hypertension treated with intravenous prostanoids: insights from the REVEAL REGISTRY®. Mayo Clin Proc. 2012;87:825.
57. Simonneau G, Barst RJ, Galie N, et al. Continuous subcutaneous infusion of Treprostinil, a prostacyclin analogue, in patients with pulmonary arterial hypertension: a double-blind, randomized, placebo-controlled trial. Am J Respir Crit Care Med. 2002;165:800.
58. Barst RJ, Galie N, Naeije R, et al. Long-term outcome in pulmonary arterial hypertension patients treated with subcutaneous Treprostinil. Eur Respir J. 2006;28:1195.
59. Benza RL, Rayburn BK, Tallaj JA, et al. Treprostinil-based therapy in the treatment of moderate-to-severe pulmonary arterial hypertension: long-term efficacy and combination with Bosentan. Chest. 2008;134:139.
60. Vachiéry JL, Hill N, Zwicke D, et al. Transitioning from i.v. Epoprostenol to subcutaneous Treprostinil in pulmonary arterial hypertension. Chest. 2002;121:1561.
61. Gomberg-Maitland M, Tapson VF, Benza RL, et al. Transition from intravenous Epoprostenol to intravenous Treprostinil in pulmonary hypertension. Am J Respir Crit Care Med. 2005;172:1586.
62. Tapson VF, Torres F, Kermeen F, et al. Oral Treprostinil for the treatment of pulmonary arterial hypertension in patients on background endothelin receptor antagonist and/or phosphodiesterase type 5 inhibitor therapy (the FREEDOM-C study): a randomized controlled trial. Chest. 2012;142:1383.
63. Jing ZC, Parikh K, Pulido T, et al. Efficacy and safety of oral Treprostinil monotherapy for the treatment of pulmonary arterial hypertension: a randomized, controlled trial. Circulation. 2013;127:624.
64. Olschewski H, Simonneau G, Galiè N, et al. Inhaled Iloprost for severe pulmonary hypertension. N Engl J Med. 2002;347:322.
65. Channick RN, Sitbon O, Barst RJ, et al. Endothelin receptor antagonists in pulmonary arterial hypertension. J Am Coll Cardiol. 2004;43:62S.
66. Liu C, Chen J, Gao Y, et al. Endothelin receptor antagonists for pulmonary arterial hypertension. Cochrane Database Syst Rev. 2013;2:CD004434.
67. Gabler NB, French B, Strom BL, et al. Race and sex differences in response to endothelin receptor antagonists for pulmonary arterial hypertension. Chest. 2012;141:20.
68. Channick RN, Simonneau G, Sitbon O, et al. Effects of the dual endothelin-receptor antagonist Bosentan in patients with pulmonary hypertension: a randomised placebo-controlled study. Lancet. 2001;358:1119.
69. Rubin LJ, Badesch DB, Barst RJ, et al. Bosentan therapy for pulmonary arterial hypertension. N Engl J Med. 2002;346:896.
70. McLaughlin VV, Sitbon O, Badesch DB, et al. Survival with first-line Bosentan in patients with primary pulmonary hypertension. Eur Respir J. 2005;25:244.
71. Sitbon O, Badesch DB, Channick RN, et al. Effects of the dual endothelin receptor antagonist Bosentan in patients with pulmonary arterial hypertension: a 1-year follow-up study. Chest. 2003;124:247.
72. Galié N, Badesch D, Oudiz R, et al. Ambrisentan therapy for pulmonary arterial hypertension. J Am Coll Cardiol. 2005;46:529.
73. Galiè N, Olschewski H, Oudiz RJ, et al. Ambrisentan for the treatment of pulmonary arterial hypertension: results of the Ambrisentan in pulmonary arterial hypertension, randomized, double-blind, placebo-controlled, multicenter, efficacy (ARIES) study 1 and 2. Circulation. 2008;117:3010.
74. Oudiz RJ, Galiè N, Olschewski H, et al. Long-term Ambrisentan therapy for the treatment of pulmonary arterial hypertension. J Am Coll Cardiol. 2009;54:1971.
75. Barst RJ, Langleben D, Badesch D, et al. Treatment of pulmonary arterial hypertension with the selective endothelin-A receptor antagonist Sitaxsentan. J Am Coll Cardiol. 2006;47:2049.
76. Wittbrodt ET, Abubakar A. Sitaxsentan for treatment of pulmonary hypertension. Ann Pharmacother. 2007;41:100.
77. Seligman BG, Ribeiro RA, Kuchenbecker Rde S, et al. Critical steps in fluoroquinolones and carbapenems prescriptions: results from a prospective clinical audit. Int J Clin Pract. 2007;61:147.
78. Benza RL, Barst RJ, Galie N, et al. Sitaxsentan for the treatment of pulmonary arterial hypertension: a 1-year, prospective, open-label observation of outcome and survival. Chest. 2008;134:775.
79. Thelin (sitaxentan) to be withdrawn due to cases of unpredictable serious liver injury. European Medicines Agency. Available from *http://www.ema.europa.eu/docs/en_GB/document_library/Press_release/2010/12/WC500099707.pdf. [Accessed on December 15, 2010].*
80. McGoon MD, Frost AE, Oudiz RJ, et al. Ambrisentan therapy in patients with pulmonary arterial hypertension who discontinued Bosentan or Sitaxsentan due to liver function test abnormalities. Chest. 2009;135:122.
81. D'Alto M. An update on the use of Ambrisentan in pulmonary arterial hypertension. Ther Adv Respir Dis. 2012;6:331.
82. Raghu G, Behr J, Brown KK, et al. Treatment of idiopathic pulmonary fibrosis with Ambrisentan: a parallel, randomized trial. Ann Intern Med. 2013;158:641.
83. Abrams D, Schulze-Neick I, Magee AG. Sildenafil as a selective pulmonary vasodilator in childhood primary pulmonary hypertension. Heart. 2000;84:E4.
84. Prasad S, Wilkinson J, Gatzoulis MA. Sildenafil in primary pulmonary hypertension. N Engl J Med. 2000;343:1342.
85. Galiè N, Ghofrani HA, Torbicki A, et al. Sildenafil citrate therapy for pulmonary arterial hypertension. N Engl J Med. 2005;353:2148.
86. Pepke-Zaba J, Gilbert C, Collings L, et al. Sildenafil improves health-related quality of life in patients with pulmonary arterial hypertension. Chest. 2008;133:183.
87. Rubin LJ, Badesch DB, Fleming TR, et al. Long-term treatment with Sildenafil citrate in pulmonary arterial hypertension: the SUPER-2 study. Chest. 2011;140:1274.
88. Galiè N, Brundage BH, Ghofrani HA, et al. Tadalafil therapy for pulmonary arterial hypertension. Circulation. 2009;119:2894.
89. Oudiz RJ, Brundage BH, Galie N. Tadalafil for the treatment of pulmonary arterial hypertension. J Am Coll Cardiol. 2012. [Epub ahead of print].

90. Jing ZC, Yu ZX, Shen JY, et al. Vardenafil in pulmonary arterial hypertension: a randomized, double-blind, placebo-controlled study. Am J Respir Crit Care Med. 2011;183:1723.
91. Ghofrani HA, Hoeper MM, Halank M, et al. Riociguat for chronic thromboembolic pulmonary hypertension and pulmonary arterial hypertension: a phase II study. Eur Respir J. 2010;36:792.
92. Frey R, Mück W, Unger S, et al. Single-dose pharmacokinetics, pharmacodynamics, tolerability, and safety of the soluble guanylate cyclase stimulator BAY 63-2521: an ascending-dose study in healthy male volunteers. J Clin Pharmacol. 2008;48:926.
93. Ghofrani HA, Grimminger F, Hoeper MM, et al. Riociguat for the treatment of inoperable chronic thromboembolic pulmonary hyptertension: A randomised, double-blind, placebo-controlled study (CHEST-1) (abstract). Chest. 2012;142:1023A.
94. Ghofrani HA, Galie N, Grimminger F, et al. Riociguat for the treatment of pulmonary arterial hyptertension: A randomised, double-blind, placebo-controlled study (PATENT-1) (abstract). Chest. 2012;142:1027A.
95. Humbert M, Barst RJ, Robbins IM, et al. Combination of Bosentan with Epoprostenol in pulmonary arterial hypertension: BREATHE-2. Eur Respir J. 2004;24:353.
96. McLaughlin VV, Benza RL, Rubin LJ, et al. Addition of inhaled Treprostinil to oral therapy for pulmonary arterial hypertension: a randomized controlled clinical trial. J Am Coll Cardiol. 2010;55:1915.
97. Simonneau G, Rubin LJ, Galiè N, et al. Addition of Sildenafil to long-term intravenous Epoprostenol therapy in patients with pulmonary arterial hypertension: a randomized trial. Ann Intern Med. 2008;149:521.
98. Mathai SC, Girgis RE, Fisher MR, et al. Addition of Sildenafil to Bosentan monotherapy in pulmonary arterial hypertension. Eur Respir J. 2007;29:469.
99. Ghofrani HA, Rose F, Schermuly RT, et al. Oral Sildenafil as long-term adjunct therapy to inhaled Iloprost in severe pulmonary arterial hypertension. J Am Coll Cardiol. 2003;42:158.
100. Ghofrani HA, Wiedemann R, Rose F, et al. Combination therapy with oral Sildenafil and inhaled Iloprost for severe pulmonary hypertension. Ann Intern Med. 2002;136:515.
101. Hoeper MM, Taha N, Bekjarova A, et al. Bosentan treatment in patients with primary pulmonary hypertension receiving nonparenteral prostanoids. Eur Respir J. 2003;22:330.
102. Hoeper MM, Leuchte H, Halank M, et al. Combining inhaled Iloprost with Bosentan in patients with idiopathic pulmonary arterial hypertension. Eur Respir J. 2006;28:691.
103. Reichenberger F, Pepke-Zaba J, McNeil K, et al. Atrial septostomy in the treatment of severe pulmonary arterial hypertension. Thorax. 2003;58:797.
104. Kerstein D, Levy PS, Hsu DT, et al. Blade balloon atrial septostomy in patients with severe primary pulmonary hypertension. Circulation. 1995;91:2028.
105. Nihill MR, O'Laughlin MP, Mullins CE. Effects of atrial septostomy in patients with terminal cor pulmonale due to pulmonary vascular disease. Cathet Cardiovasc Diagn. 1991;24:166.
106. Rich S, Dodin E, McLaughlin VV. Usefulness of atrial septostomy as a treatment for primary pulmonary hypertension and guidelines for its application. Am J Cardiol. 1997;80:369.
107. Sandoval J, Gaspar J, Pulido T, et al. Graded balloon dilation atrial septostomy in severe primary pulmonary hypertension. A therapeutic alternative for patients nonresponsive to vasodilator treatment. J Am Coll Cardiol. 1998;32:297.
108. Rothman A, Sklansky MS, Lucas VW, et al. Atrial septostomy as a bridge to lung transplantation in patients with severe pulmonary hypertension. Am J Cardiol. 1999; 84:682.
109. Sandoval J, Rothman A, Pulido T. Atrial septostomy for pulmonary hypertension. Clin Chest Med. 2001;22:547.
110. Doyle RL, McCrory D, Channick RN, et al. Surgical treatments/interventions for pulmonary arterial hypertension: ACCP evidence-based clinical practice guidelines. Chest. 2004; 126:63S.
111. Kurzyna M, Dabrowski M, Bielecki D, et al. Atrial septostomy in treatment of end-stage right heart failure in patients with pulmonary hypertension. Chest. 2007;131:977.
112. Sandoval J, Gaspar J, Peña H, et al. Effect of atrial septostomy on the survival of patients with severe pulmonary arterial hypertension. Eur Respir J. 2011;38:1343.
113. Esch JJ, Shah PB, Cockrill BA, et al. Transcatheter Potts shunt creation in patients with severe pulmonary arterial hypertension: initial clinical experience. J Heart Lung Transplant. 2013;32:381.
114. Barst RJ. Role of atrial septostomy in the treatment of pulmonary vascular disease. Thorax. 2000;55:95.
115. Pasque MK, Trulock EP, Kaiser LR, et al. Single-lung transplantation for pulmonary hypertension. Three-month hemodynamic follow-up. Circulation. 1991;84:2275.
116. Schaffer JM, Singh SK, Joyce DL, et al. Transplantation for idiopathic pulmonary arterial hypertension: improvement in the lung allocation score era. Circulation. 2013;127:2503.
117. Christie JD, Edwards LB, Kucheryavaya AY, et al. The Registry of the International Society for Heart and Lung Transplantation: 29th adult lung and heart-lung transplant report-2012. J Heart Lung Transplant. 2012;31:1073.
118. Orens JB, Estenne M, Arcasoy S, et al. International guidelines for the selection of lung transplant candidates: 2006 update—a consensus report from the Pulmonary Scientific Council of the International Society for Heart and Lung Transplantation. J Heart Lung Transplant. 2006;25:745.

3

Pulmonary Embolism: Anticoagulation/ Lytics or Intervention for Whom?

AK Khera, Rajeev Dhalwani

INTRODUCTION

Pulmonary embolism (PE) is quite a common occurrence, often under diagnosed, but a potentially fatal disease. Of the patients who develop PE, approximately 10% die within the first hour and 30% die from recurrent embolism. Massive PE is one of the most common causes of sudden death.

DIAGNOSTIC APPROACH

Pulmonary embolism should be high on the list of suspicion in all the patients who present with new onset or worsening of pre-existing dyspnea, chest pain, or hypotension when no alternative cause is obvious. The diagnostic approach to the patient should be based on hemodynamic status of the patient.

In *hemodynamically stable patients*, the patient should undergo a clinical probability assessment, multidetector computed tomography (CT) or ventilation-perfusion scanning, and D-dimer testing,[1,2] but one must remember that in patients who have a high clinical probability of PE, the D-dimer analysis has a limited value.[3]

In *hemodynamically unstable patients*, multidetector CT, because of its high sensitivity for detecting pulmonary emboli, should be performed immediately.[4] If this facility is not available, at least echocardiography should be performed by an experienced operator to determine whether or not right ventricular dysfunction is present. Transesophageal echocardiography is a useful tool as it can delineate emboli in the pulmonary artery clearly.

In *critically ill patients*, if unmistakable signs of right ventricular overload are present on echocardiography, thrombolytic therapy is indicated. CT scan can be performed after patient's condition stabilizes. Currently, use of conventional pulmonary angiography is confined to cases in whom catheter-based treatment is being contemplated.

THERAPEUTIC CONSIDERATIONS

The patient may be asymptomatic or may present with only mild dyspnea, while a few may present with severe shock and sustained hypotension. In patients who are at low-risk, *anticoagulation alone* may be sufficient, but high-risk patients may need *thrombolysis* or *embolectomy along with anticoagulation*. A selected few may require insertion of *vena caval filters*.

MANAGEMENT OF ACUTE PULMONARY EMBOLISM (FLOW CHARTS 3.1 AND 3.2)

- In patients who have a *high probability of PE*, *anticoagulation* with low-molecular-weight heparin (LMWH), unfractionated heparin (UFH) or fondaparinux[5,6] should be initiated even before diagnosis is confirmed.
- *Hemodynamically unstable patients* should be treated more aggressively with *thrombolysis* as there is a high incidence of death among such unstable patients. Thrombolysis also causes faster resolution of the occluding thrombus. Prompt and aggressive approach is justified as mortality may be as high as 60% in untreated patients but can be reduced by half with immediate action. A recent meta-analysis has shown that among hemodynamically unstable patients with PE thrombolysis was associated with a reduction in mortality,[7] but at the same time more patients had bleeding with intravenous (IV) thrombolysis than with anticoagulant therapy.

Thrombolytic regimens with short infusion time of 2 hours or less are recommended over prolonged infusion times, since with short regimes thrombolysis is more rapid and bleeding is less. IV UFH is the only anticoagulant that has been used in combination with thrombolytic therapy. Thus, if thrombolytic therapy is being considered, initial anticoagulation with IV UFH is a reasonable option.

Flow chart 3.1 Diagnostic work-up for pulmonary embolism (Ref: N Engl J Med 2010;363:267)

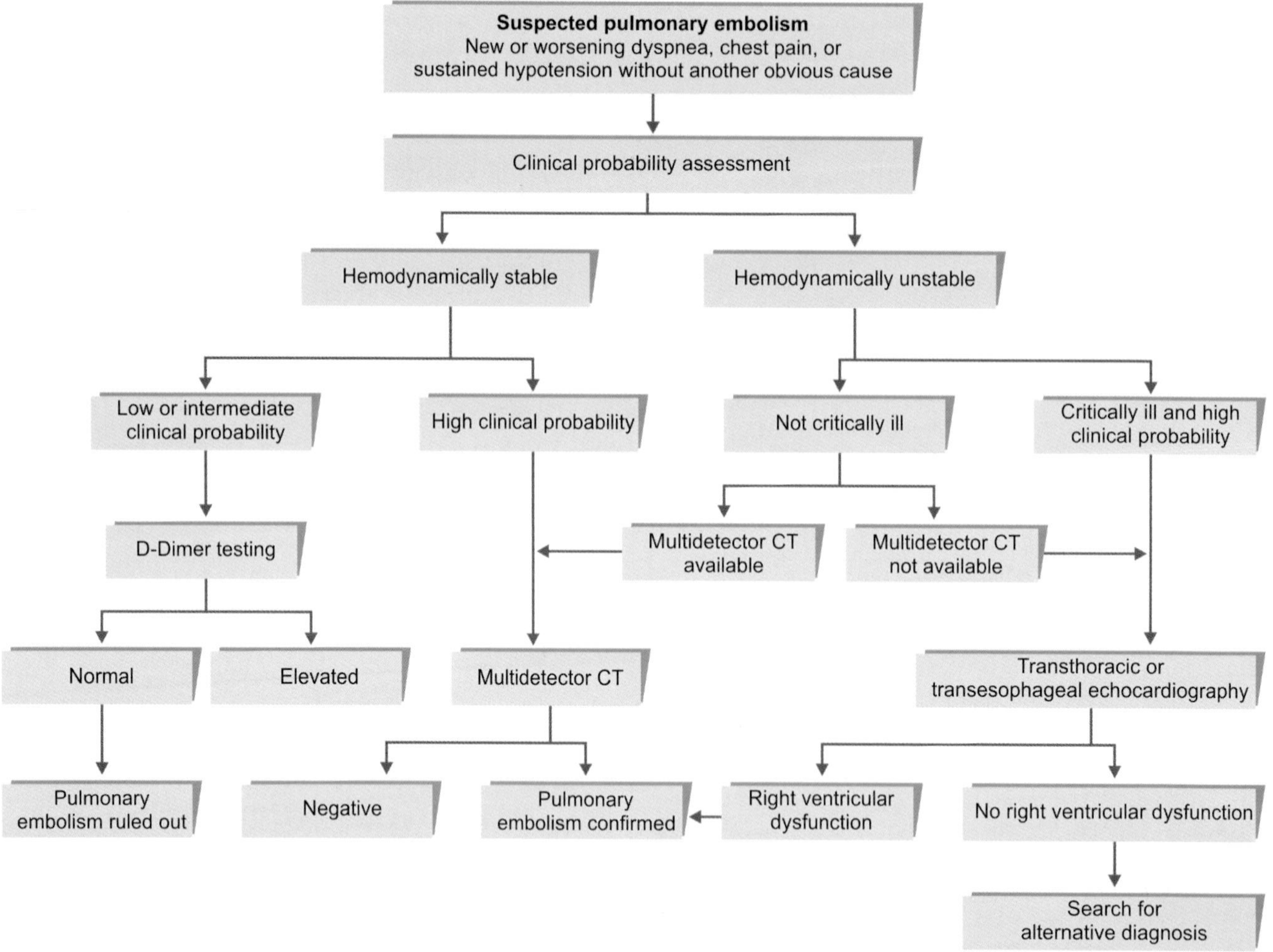

- The initial assessment of the clinical probability of pulmonary embolism is based on either clinical judgment or clinical decision rules (Wells and Revised Geneva Scores).
- Patients are considered to be hemodynamically unstable if they are in shock or have a systolic blood pressure of <90 mm Hg or a drop in pressure of more than 40 mm Hg for >15 minutes (in the absence of new onset arrhythmia, hypovolemia, and sepsis).
- In cases in which multidetector computed tomography (CT) is not available or in patients with renal failure or allergy to contrast dye, the use of ventilation–perfusion scanning is an alternative.
- In patients with a high clinical probability and an elevated D-dimer level but with negative findings on multidetector CT, venous ultrasonography should be considered.
- Among critically ill patients with right ventricular dysfunction, thrombolysis is an option; multidetector CT should be performed when the patient's condition has been stabilized if doubts remain about clinical management.
- In patients who are candidates for percutaneous embolectomy, conventional pulmonary angiography can be performed to confirm the diagnosis of pulmonary embolism immediately before the procedure, after the finding of right ventricular dysfunction.

Flow chart 3.2 Clinical management of confirmed acute pulmonary embolism (Ref: N Engl J Med. 2010;363:269)

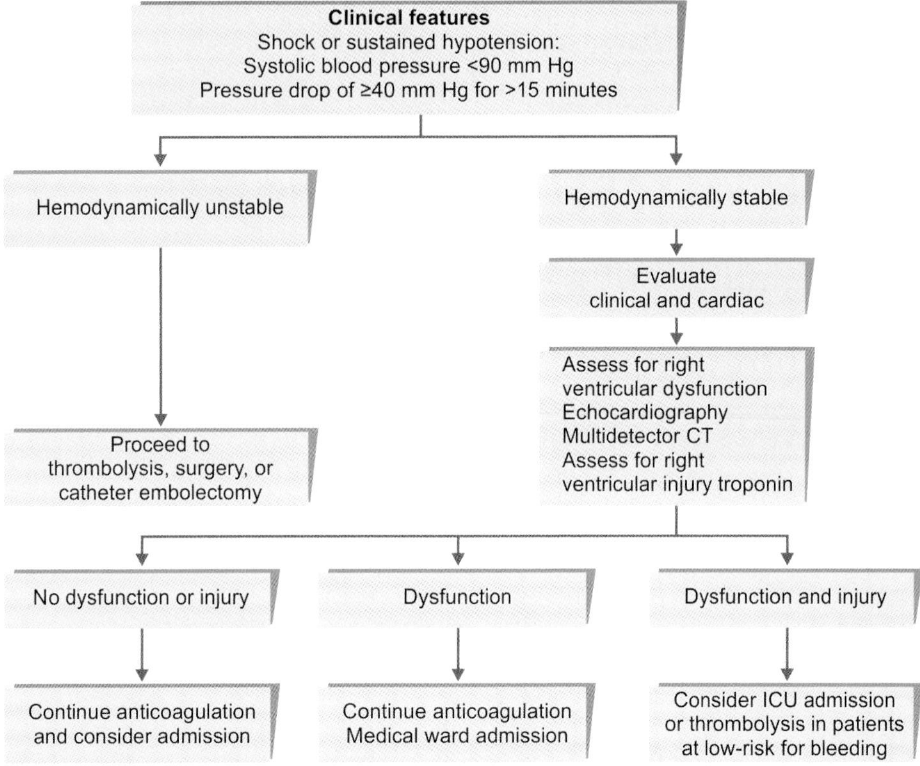

- Patients who are at high-risk and who have an absolute contraindication to thrombolytic treatment should undergo either *percutaneous thrombectomy* or *surgical embolectomy.*
- If immediate access to cardiopulmonary bypass is unavailable, percutaneous mechanical thrombectomy is an alternative to surgical embolectomy.
- Patients with contraindications to anticoagulant treatment and recurrent thromboembolism should have *vena cava filters* inserted after a conventional course of anticoagulation.
- *Vitamin K antagonists* should be started as soon as possible, but in patients with cancer and in pregnant women LMWH is preferred to vitamin K antagonists.[8]

Cues for Management

- Patients with acute PE are at *risk of recurrent thromboembolism.*[9] Risk factors for recurrences include male sex, advanced age, idiopathic PE, and patients with cancer. The risk is <1% per year in patients on anticoagulant therapy but the risk may increase up to 10% per year after discontinuing the use of anticoagulants.
- After an acute event *warfarin therapy* with international normalized ration (INR) optimized in the range 2.0 to 3.0 is recommended. In patients with *PE secondary to reversible risk factors,* vitamin K antagonists should be prescribed for at least 3 months.
- *Low-intensity warfarin therapy with INR optimized between 1.5 and 1.9* is advised in patients having idiopathic PE or recurrent venous thromboembolism.
- Dabigatran has been shown to be as effective and safe as warfarin for the treatment of venous thromboembolism.
- Since the incidence of chronic thromboembolic pulmonary hypertension 2 years after the acute event is around 4%, patients should be monitored during this period.

THERAPEUTIC OPTIONS: INDICATIONS, CONTRAINDICATIONS, AND RATIONALE FOR USE (TABLE 3.1)

- Anticoagulant therapy
- Thrombolytics
- Embolectomy
- Vena caval filters.

Anticoagulant Therapy

In all patients of acute PE, anticoagulant therapy should be initiated since anticoagulation therapy reduces mortality rates markedly. Without optimal anticoagulant therapy, there is a 25% risk of developing recurrent PE,[9] whereas the risk of major bleed with anticoagulant therapy is barely

Table 3.1 Treatment of acute pulmonary embolism (Ref: N Engl J Med 2010;363:271)

- Low-molecular-weight heparin (administered either intravenously or subcutaneously) should be the treatment of choice in hemodynamically stable patients.
- Thrombolysis should be administered to patients whose condition is unstable and should be considered for high-risk, hemodynamically stable patients.
- Percutaneous mechanical thrombectomy should be restricted to high-risk patients with absolute contraindications to thrombolytic treatment and those in whom thrombolytic treatment has failed to improve hemodynamic status.
- Low-molecular-weight heparin is preferable to vitamin K antagonists in patients with cancer and in pregnant women.
- For patients receiving vitamin K antagonists, the international normalized ratio (INR) should be maintained within a therapeutic range (2.0–3.0) during long-term therapy (≥3 months).
- A low-intensity INR target of 1.5–1.9 is an option for extended (indefinite) anticoagulant therapy. Extended treatment should be considered for patients with active cancer, unprovoked pulmonary embolism, or recurrent venous thromboembolism. Extended treatment requires a reassessment of the patient's risk—benefit ratio at periodic intervals. Indefinite treatment refers to anticoagulation that is continued without a scheduled stop date but that may be stopped because of an increase in the risk of bleeding or a change in the patient's preference.

Initial treatment	*Long-term treatment*	*Extended treatment*
• Unfractionated heparin • Low-molecular-weight heparin • Fondaparinux • Thrombolysis • Percutaneous mechanical embolectomy • Surgery • Vitamin K antagonists	Vitamin K antagonists (INR target, 2.0–3.0)	Vitamin K antagonists (INR target, 2.0–3.0 or 1.5–1.9)
≥5 days	**≥3 months**	**Indefinite**

3%.[10] Patients who are over 65 years are at risk of bleeding. The other risk factors for bleeding are thrombocytopenia, antiplatelet therapy, and poor anticoagulant control. One must be vigilant for bleeding risk in patients who have had recent surgery, frequent falls, or previous stroke. Diabetes, liver failure, anemia, cancer, renal failure, and alcohol abuse are other risk factors of bleed that one must keep in mind.

Indications for Anticoagulant Therapy

- Anticoagulation is a must for all patients suspected of having deep vein thrombosis (DVT) or PE. Wells criteria are often used for predicting probability of acute PE.
- One must not delay starting anticoagulant therapy while awaiting results of diagnostic investigations in patients in whom there is a high clinical suspicion of acute PE or in patients with moderate clinical suspicion of acute PE in whom the result of diagnostic tests is expected to take over 4 hours.[10] In contrast, in patients in whom there is a low clinical suspicion of acute PE, it is suggested NOT to employ anticoagulation empirically. Achieving a therapeutic level of anticoagulation within the first 24 hours of treatment regulates the effectiveness of anticoagulation therapy.[9]

Anticoagulants

A. Parenteral:
   I. UFH
   II. LMWH
   III. Fondaparinux .

B. Oral:
   I. Vitamin K antagonists
      1. Warfarin
   II. Newer oral anticoagulants
      1. Dabigatran
      2. Rivaroxaban
      3. Apixaban
      4. Edoxaban.

A. *Parenteral*
   I. *UFH*: Though heparin does not dissolve the existing clot, it slows as well as prevents the progression of

DVT. Heparin also reduces the size of pulmonary embolus.

When is UFH preferred to LMWH and fondaparinux?

- In cases of acute massive PE and hypotension, IV UFH has been recommended most widely, in clinical practice as well as in clinical trials.
- In patients with severe renal insufficiency, UFH is preferred over LMWH and fondaparinux because renal insufficiency alters the pharmacokinetics of the anticoagulants requiring their activity to be monitored and since activated partial thromboplastin time (aPTT) is more commonly available than anti-Xa assays, it is easier to monitor UFH. Moreover, the effectiveness of LMWH and subcutaneous fondaparinux in patients with severe renal failure has not been well studied.
- IV UFH is preferred in morbid obesity as subcutaneous absorption is unpredictable in presence of excessive fat.
- As UFH has a shorter half-life than LMWH, it is advantageous for patients who might require intervention at a later date in the form of an inferior vena cava (IVC) filter, thrombolysis or embolectomy.
- One advantage of using IV UFH is that it is shortest-acting anticoagulant and if major bleeding occurs its activity can be reversed by protamine sulfate.

Dose: If IV UFH is chosen, an initial bolus of 80 U/kg or 5000 U followed by an infusion of 18 U/kg/hour or 1300 Units/hour should be given. Target aPTT should be between 1.5 and 2.5 times control value.

II. *LMWH*

Advantages of LMWH over UFH

- Greater bioavailability
- Predictable dose response
- Longer half-life
- Decreased frequency of administration
- Fixed dosing
- Decreased likelihood of thrombocytopenia

When is LMWH or subcutaneous fondaparinux preferred over UFH?

Current guidelines recommend LMWH over UFH in patients with nonmassive PE because trials have shown that vis-à-vis UFH, LMWH reduces mortality, incidence of bleeding, and thromboembolism.[10-12] This was documented in three meta-analyses[10,11] that compared LMWH and IV UFH in patients with acute PE or DVT.

Dose:

- *Enoxaparin*: 1 mg/kg twice daily
- *Dalteparin*: 100 units/kg once daily
- *Reviparin*: 3500 units twice daily (weight 35–45 kg); 4200 units twice daily (weight 46–60 kg) and 6300 units twice daily (weight >60 kg)
- *Nadoparin*: 4100 units twice daily (weight <50 kg); 6150 units twice daily (weight 50–70 kg) and 9200 units twice daily (weight >70 kg).

Patients who are above 90 kg should receive enoxaparin or tinzaparin, rather than dalteparin. In one trial, comparing tinzaparin and dalteparin,[13] it was noted that there was no difference in the incidence of side effects like major bleeding and the incidence of recurrent PE and recurrent DVT was almost the same in both tinzaparin and dalteparin suggesting that both are equally safe and effective in the management of acute PE; but trials comparing various different types of LMWH are far and few.

In patients being treated with LMWH, monitoring of anti-Xa levels is necessary in a few cases like pregnant women, obese patients, or patients with extremely low body weight and in patients with renal insufficiency. It must be kept in mind that patients with severe renal insufficiency are not treated with LMWH; however, in patients with mild or moderate renal insufficiency LMWH may be used and that too with no specific dose adjustment.

III. *Fondaparinux*: It is preferred in most of the hemodynamically stable patients with acute PE.

Fondaparinux v/s UFH: Fondaparinux has several advantages over UFH—it is not only given in fixed dose but also the frequency of dose is decreased. Incidence of thrombocytopenia is also decreased.[10] But in renal insufficiency, UFH, instead of fondaparinux is recommended as fondaparinux may accumulate in the body and increase the risk of hemorrhage.

Fondaparinux v/s LMWH: In patients with acute PE, there have not been many trials comparing fondaparinux and LMWH. However, they have been a few comparative studies in patients with DVT. In one trial, it was found that there is no difference in mortality, recurrent thromboembolic disease, or major bleeding.[14] For most *hemodynamically stable patients with acute non-massive PE,*[10] the choice between LMWH and subcutaneous fondaparinux is left to clinician since effectiveness and side effects in both are similar.

B. *Oral anticoagulants*: In most cases of acute PE, heparin is administered initially and then overlapped with an oral anticoagulant.

I. *Vitamin K antagonists*

- *Warfarin*: Long-term treatment with warfarin is commonly used for preventing recurrent PE.[10,15-18]

Initiation: Warfarin should be overlapped with heparin or subcutaneous fondaparinux for a minimum of 5 days, until the INR has been optimized to 2.0–3.0 for at least 24 hours.[10] Warfarin should NOT be started prior to heparin because warfarin alone is associated with a three-fold increase in the incidence of recurrent PE or DVT.

Dose: Warfarin is started with an initial dose of 5 mg per day for the first 2 days and then the daily dose is adjusted according to the INR. Since the dose of warfarin is influenced by age, concomitant medications, diet, and because the rate at which individuals metabolize warfarin varies greatly, the maintenance dose needs to be monitored regularly.

Monitoring: In hospitalized patients, INR is measured daily until the therapeutic range has been achieved. Following discharge, INR is monitored once every few days, and once the dose has been stabilized, the frequency of INR measurement is reduced to once every 4 weeks.

Precaution: If anticoagulation is less intense with INR <2.0, there is an increased likelihood of recurrent PE or DVT. However, risk of bleeding should be borne in mind with a more intense anticoagulation.

II. *Newer oral anticoagulants*

- *Dabigatran*: Dabigatran is an oral anticoagulant. Its efficacy has been studied mostly in patients with DVT rather than PE.[19] It is recommended that dabigatran should NOT be used routinely following acute PE until more trials have been conducted.
- *Rivaroxaban*: Rivaroxaban, an oral factor Xa inhibitor, has been approved by the US FDA for treatment of acute PE.

  Dose: 15 mg twice daily for a few weeks that is then followed by 20 mg once daily.

  Efficacy: Data from EINSTEIN-PE and EINSTEIN-DVT studies in the treatment of DVT or PE suggest that rivaroxaban is as effective as standard therapy (enoxaparin followed by a vitamin K antagonist) in preventing venous thromboembolism recurrence. It has a good safety profile as it is associated with less bleeding, especially in elderly and in patients with moderate renal impairment. As compared with current management strategies of anticoagulation rivaroxaban is a safe and effective regimen and has the advantage of simple dosage and is cost effective.

  Contraindications: Rivaroxaban should not be used during pregnancy, in patients with renal insufficiency or significant hepatic disorder. Although a specific antidote to rivaroxaban is presently unavailable, discontinuance of drug or use of oral charcoal may be good enough to control bleeding.
- *Apixaban*: It is a factor Xa inhibitor. AMPLIFY trial comparing apixaban and conventional anticoagulation and another trial AMPLIFY-EXT comparing apixaban and placebo in patients who had already completed 6–12 months of conventional anticoagulation concluded that as an initial anticoagulation drug for DVT and PE, efficacy of apixaban is comparable to conventional anticoagulation and at the same time is associated with fewer bleeding events. In addition, extended treatment with apixaban for prophylaxis or treatment was found to be quite effective. Though use of apixaban has not yet been universally accepted, this drug holds a bright promise.
- *Edoxaban*: It is an oral factor Xa inhibitor. Compared with conventional anticoagulation for the initial treatment of DVT and PE, edoxaban was reported to be as effective with the benefit of lower risk of bleeding. But the efficacy and safety profile of edoxaban beyond the initial therapy has not been studied in detail.

Thrombolysis

Mechanism of Action

Thrombolytic agents act mainly by converting plasminogen to plasmin. Plasmin causes the thrombus to lyse. Thrombolytic agents are used in a variety of disorders including acute myocardial infarction, acute PE, and DVT where accelerated lysis of thrombus is required. Whether or not thrombolytic therapy should be started is decided mainly after assessing severity of PE and risk of bleeding besides other factors.

Advantages of Using Thrombolytic Therapy

- Thrombolysis dissolves the obstructing thrombus in pulmonary artery as well as in deep leg veins, thereby reversing right heart failure leading to reduction of right ventricular pressure overload.
- Prevents persistent release of serotonin and various other neurohumoral factors that may worsen patient's condition.
- Thrombolysis has a role in increasing pulmonary capillary blood flow, thereby reducing the probability of developing chronic pulmonary hypertension.

American College of Clinical Pharmacology Recommendations for Thrombolytic Therapy

According to American College of Clinical Pharmacology (ACCP) recommendations, thrombolytic therapy is indicated in patients with PE who are hemodynamically unstable and have no major bleeding risks (class IB). Thrombolysis should be initiated as soon as possible because these patients are likely to develop irreversible cardiogenic shock. For patients with PE who are hemodynamically stable, recommendation is against thrombolytic therapy (class 1C).

Outcomes

The effects of thrombolytic therapy followed by anticoagulant therapy have been compared with those of anticoagulant therapy alone. The evidence indicates that thrombolytic therapy leads to early hemodynamic improvement, but at a cost of increased major bleeding. Thrombolytic therapy has not been proven to improve mortality or reduce the frequency of recurrent thromboembolism.

Complications

Bleeding occurs mostly at sites where invasive procedures, such as pulmonary arteriography or arterial puncture, have been performed. It is advisable to reduce invasive procedures as far as possible when thrombolytic therapy is being contemplated as well as during its administration. In cases when bleeding does occur, manual compression followed by pressure dressing should be undertaken. Intracranial hemorrhage occurs in around 3% of patients receiving systemic thrombolytic therapy and is considered by far the most disturbing complication associated with this form of therapy.[20]

Contraindications to Systemic Thrombolytic Therapy in Acute PE (Flow chart 3.3)

- Intracranial neoplasm
- Active bleeding or recent internal bleeding during the prior 6 months
- Hemorrhagic stroke or nonhemorrhagic stroke within the prior 2 months
- Severe uncontrolled hypertension
- Bleeding diathesis
- Intracranial surgery or trauma within last 2 months or surgery within the previous 10 days
- Thrombocytopenia.

Dose

Patients with PE receiving thrombolysis have a wide "window" as is evidenced by the fact that those who receive thrombolysis even up to 2 weeks after the event have an effectual response. The reason for this is possibly because of the presence of bronchial collateral circulation.

***Alteplase*:** 100 mg within 2 hours as continuous infusion.

***Streptokinase*:** Two lacs fifty thousand units are administered intravenously over the initial 30 minutes, followed by 1 lac units/hour for 24 hours. Hypotension, anaphylaxis, and allergic reactions are the known side effects associated with streptokinase. In case of mild adverse reactions, decreasing rate of infusion is a good option. Thrombolytic agents can be infused directly into the pulmonary artery but whether it confers additional benefit as compared with peripheral venous infusion remains to be evidenced.

Use of Heparin Before and After Thrombolysis

- Discontinue the continuous infusion of IV UFH as soon as decision has been made to administer thrombolysis.
- At 2-hour infusion of alteplase, thrombolyse with 100 mg.
- Do not delay the thrombolysis infusion by obtaining an aPTT.
- At conclusion of 2-hour infusion, obtain a stat aPTT.
- If aPTT is 80 seconds or less, resume UFH as a continuous infusion.
- If aPTT exceeds 80 seconds, hold off resuming heparin for 4 hours and repeat the aPTT. If aPTT is now 80 seconds or less, resume UFH as a continuous infusion.

Pros and Cons of Using Thrombolysis

Fear of risk of bleeding complications in normotensive high-risk patients outweighs any potential benefit accrued with thrombolysis, but improved survival is considered a reasonable justification for the use of thrombolytics.

Embolectomy

Types

1. *Catheter embolectomy and fragmentation*
   - Mechanical fragmentation of thrombus, pigtail rotational catheter embolectomy, clot pulverization and percutaneous rheolytic. thrombectomy are the commonly used interventional catheterization techniques for massive PE.
   - Mechanical clot fragmentation combined with thrombolysis is another option.
   - Sometimes use of pulmonary artery balloon dilation and stenting is also employed.

   Effect of catheter embolectomy: Successful catheter embolectomy rapidly restores normal blood pressure and decrease hypoxemia.

   Limitations: Catheter techniques have been limited by poor maneuverability, mechanical hemolysis, macroembolization, and microembolization.
2. *Surgical embolectomy*: Patient selection for surgical embolectomy:
   - Massive PE in whom thrombolysis is contraindicated or patients who are refractory to thrombolysis.
   - Acute PE patients who require surgical excision of a right atrial thrombus.

Indications for Embolectomy

- American Heart Association (AHA) guidelines recommend embolectomy as a reasonable option for patients with massive PE in whom fibrinolysis is contraindicated or who remain unstable after receiving fibrinolysis.
- In patients with submassive acute PE with hemodynamic instability, worsening respiratory failure, severe right ventricular dysfunction, or major myocardial necrosis should be subjected to catheter or surgical embolectomy.
- Embolectomy is not recommended for patients with low risk or submassive acute PE who are clinically stable.

Flow chart 3.3 Contraindications

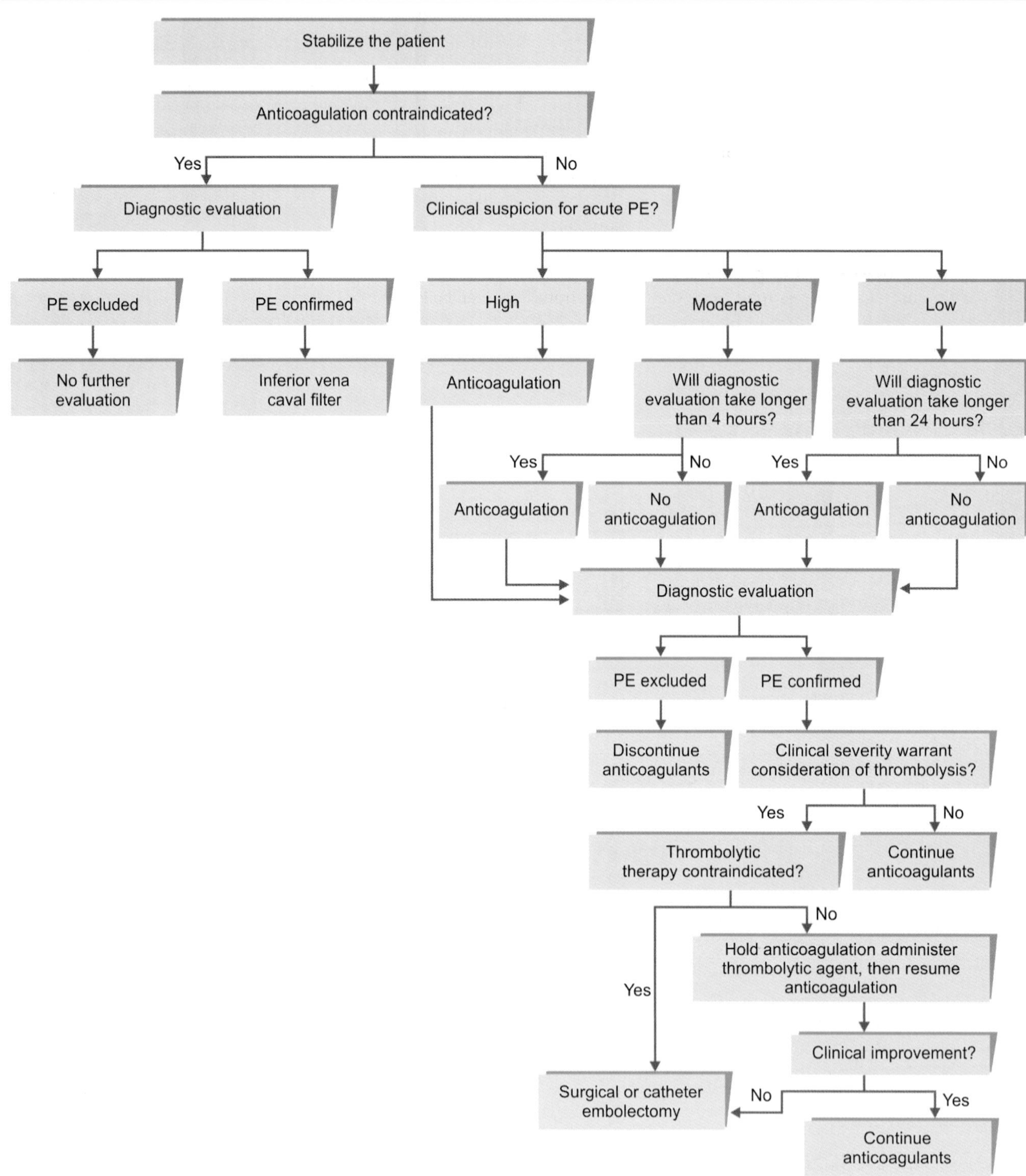

Vena Cava Filters

Indications for IVC Filter

- Patients having an absolute contraindication to anticoagulant therapy.
- Survivors of massive PE in whom it is important to prevent recurrence of embolism as it may prove detrimental to life.
- Patients who have recurrent venous thromboembolism despite adequate anticoagulant therapy.
- In patients who have a short-term contraindication to anticoagulation, it is logical to choose a retrievable IVC filter and evaluate the patient from time-to-time. Anticoagulation can be resumed once contraindications to anticoagulation or active bleeding complications have resolved.[21]
- The current grade 1A recommendation is that patients with acute PE *vena cava filters should not be used routinely.*

Potential complications of IVC filter insertion

- Bleeding from the site of insertion of IVC filter
- Filter erosion through the wall of IVC
- Hematoma or deep venous thrombosis at the site of insertion
- Filter migration
- Filter fracture and embolization of ensuing fragments
- Thrombosis of IVC

Because patients with IVC filters are at risk for above mentioned complications it is recommended that anticoagulants be used concomitantly.

PROGNOSIS

Most of the patients treated with anticoagulants do not develop any long-term complications. In a small proportion of patients, PE does not resolve, resulting in chronic thromboembolic pulmonary arterial hypertension. Anticoagulant treatment decreases mortality to <5%, whereas in patients with undiagnosed PE, mortality rises to almost 30%. In the Prospective Investigation of Pulmonary Embolism Diagnosis (PIOPED) study, the 1-year mortality rate was 24%.[22] It was seen that recurrent PE, infection, cardiac disease, and cancer were important causes of mortality. Presence of proximal venous thrombosis increases the risk of recurrent PE; approximately one-sixth of the patients with recurrent PE have proximal DVT. Higher mortality has also been seen with elevated levels of natriuretic peptides.

FUTURE RESEARCH

Significant advances over the past several decades have led to impressive treatment of PE. However, a lot of work needs to be done and there is a definite need for clear guidelines on several issues, specially the role of LMWH and the optimal duration of anticoagulant therapy in different subgroups of patients. Because warfarin often causes bleeding, other drugs need to be studied that are safer and more effective. Future research should also focus on safety profile and effectiveness of drugs that inhibit the action of thrombin directly.

REFERENCES

1. Wells PS, Ginsberg JS, Anderson DR, et al. Use of a clinical model for safe management of patients with suspected pulmonary embolism. Ann Intern Med. 1998;129:997-1005.
2. Le Gal G, Righini M, Roy PM, et al. Prediction of pulmonary embolism in the emergency department: the revised Geneva score. Ann Intern Med. 2006;144:165-71.
3. Gupta RT, Kakarla RK, Kirshenbaum KJ, et al. D-dimers and efficacy of clinical risk estimation algorithms: sensitivity in evaluation of acute pulmonary embolism. AJR Am J Roentgenol. 2009;193:425-30.
4. van Belle A, Büller HR, Huisman MV, et al. Effectiveness of managing suspected pulmonary embolism using an algorithm combining clinical probability, D-dimer testing, and computed tomography. JAMA. 2006;295:172-9.
5. Kearon C, Kahn SR, Agnelli G, et al. Antithrombotic therapy for venous thromboembolic disease: American College of Chest Physicians Evidence-Based Clinical Practice Guidelines (8th edition). Chest. 2008;133(Suppl):454S-545S.
6. Torbicki A, Perrier A, Konstantinides S, et al. Guidelines on the diagnosis and management of acute pulmonary embolism. Eur Heart J. 2008;29:2276-315.
7. Wan S, Quinlan DJ, Agnelli G, et al. Thrombolysis compared with heparin for the initial treatment of pulmonary embolism: a meta-analysis of the randomized controlled trials. Circulation. 2004;110:744-9.
8. Marik PE, Plante LA. Venous thromboembolic disease and pregnancy. N Engl J Med. 2008;359:2025-33.
9. Raschke RA, Reilly BM, Guidry JR, et al. The weight-based heparin dosing nomogram compared with a "standard care" nomogram. A randomized controlled trial. Ann Intern Med. 1993;119:874.
10. Kearon C, Akl EA, Comerota AJ, et al. Antithrombotic therapy for VTE disease: Antithrombotic Therapy and Prevention of Thrombosis, 9th ed: American College of Chest Physicians Evidence-Based Clinical Practice Guidelines. Chest. 2012;141: e419S.
11. van Dongen CJ, van den Belt AG, Prins MH, et al. Fixed dose subcutaneous low molecular weight heparins versus adjusted dose unfractionated heparin for venous thromboembolism. Cochrane Database Syst Rev. 2004;CD001100.
12. Quinlan DJ, McQuillan A, Eikelboom JW. Low-molecular-weight heparin compared with intravenous unfractionated heparin for treatment of pulmonary embolism: a meta-analysis of randomized, controlled trials. Ann Intern Med. 2004;140:175.
13. Wells PS, Anderson DR, Rodger MA, et al. A randomized trial comparing 2 low-molecular-weight heparins for the outpatient treatment of deep vein thrombosis and pulmonary embolism. Arch Intern Med. 2005;165:733.
14. Büller HR, Davidson BL, Decousus H, et al. Fondaparinux or enoxaparin for the initial treatment of symptomatic deep

venous thrombosis: a randomized trial. Ann Intern Med. 2004; 140:867.
15. Hull R, Delmore T, Genton E, et al. Warfarin sodium versus low-dose heparin in the long-term treatment of venous thrombosis. N Engl J Med. 1979;301:855.
16. Hull R, Delmore T, Carter C, et al. Adjusted subcutaneous heparin versus warfarin sodium in the long-term treatment of venous thrombosis. N Engl J Med. 1982;306:189.
17. Ridker PM, Goldhaber SZ, Danielson E, et al. Long-term, low-intensity warfarin therapy for the prevention of recurrent venous thromboembolism. N Engl J Med. 2003;348:1425.
18. Hutten BA, Prins MH. Duration of treatment with vitamin K antagonists in symptomatic venous thromboembolism. Cochrane Database Syst Rev. 2006;CD001367.
19. Schulman S, Kearon C, Kakkar AK, et al. Dabigatran versus warfarin in the treatment of acute venous thromboembolism. N Engl J Med. 2009;361:2342.
20. Meyer G, Gisselbrecht M, Diehl JL, et al. Incidence and predictors of major hemorrhagic complications from thrombolytic therapy in patients with massive pulmonary embolism. Am J Med. 1998;105:472.
21. Campbell IA, Bentley DP, Prescott RJ, et al. Anticoagulation for three versus six months in patients with deep vein thrombosis or pulmonary embolism, or both: randomised trial. BMJ. 2007;334(7595):674.
22. Worsley DF, Alavi A. Comprehensive analysis of the results of the PIOPED Study. Prospective investigation of pulmonary embolism diagnosis study. J Nucl Med. 1995;36(12):2380-7.

4

Sleep Apnea and Cardiovascular Disease

RS Chatterji, V Nangia, N Dalal, AK Singh

INTRODUCTION[1-5]

Obstructive sleep apnea (OSA) is a sleep-related breathing disorder (SRBD) causing a myriad of health effects. It is a risk factor for cardiac, neurologic, and perioperative morbidities. The disorder is elusive and remains undiagnosed until complications appear. The disease remains undiagnosed in majority of population.

Obstructive sleep apnea activates pathways resulting in insulin resistance, atherosclerosis, and hypertension (HT). Sleep apnea and obesity activate similar pathways. OSA is risk factor for HT, heart failure (HF), arrhythmias, and stroke, especially in men. Many epidemiological studies and randomized clinical trials show that OSA is a modifiable risk factor and treatment of OSA may prevent cardiovascular diseases (CVDs) and complications. In susceptible individuals, HT and HF, by stimulating the sympathetic, renin-angiotensin-aldosterone systems to induce renal sodium retention, probably initiate or exacerbate sleep apnea through nocturnal fluid shifts. Nocturnal and daytime sympathetic activation promotes HT that further causes ventricular hypertrophy, dilatation, and failure, exacerbating sleep apnea.

Sleep apneas, OSA, central sleep apnea (CSA), and complex sleep apnea affect cardiovascular function and diseases. OSA is caused by repeated pharyngeal airway closure during sleep leading to cessation of respiration for 10 seconds or more. Obstructive hypopneas are decreased in flow for 10 seconds or more associated with oxygen desaturation or arousal. Both obstructive apneas and hypopneas are associated with fall in oropharyngeal flow with ongoing respiratory efforts. Apnea-hypopnea index (AHI) is defined as number of apneas and hypopneas occurring per hour during sleep. A diagnosis of OSA is reached if AHI is more than five and the person has symptoms of daytime sleepiness.

Central sleep apnea (CSA) is seen in HF, stroke, and elderly patients. The exact cause is still not completely understood. There is a cessation of airflow for 10 seconds or more resulting from lack of respiratory impulses from respiratory center. This is recorded as cessation of airflow with no ventilatory efforts. It is associated with disrupted sleep and/or excessive daytime sleepiness. Positive airway pressure is the gold standard treatment for OSA and is proven to be of benefit in CVDs.

EXTENT OF THE PROBLEM[6-11]

In Delhi, India, Sharma et al found a prevalence rate of OSA to be 13.74% in habitual snorers and 3.57% among nonsnorers in the age group of 30–60 years. In another study, Sharma et al observed OSA in 32.4% among habitual snorers and 4% among nonhabitual snorers. The estimated prevalence of OSA in India is 9.3% and of OSA hypopnea syndrome (OSAHS) is 2.8%. OSA was diagnosed in 12 (28.6%) of the 44 patients of myocardial infarction in a study from South India.

The prevalence of SRBDs is higher in CVD patients. The estimated prevalence of OSA in adult Americans is about 15 million, and large proportion of them have cardiovascular disorders such as HT, coronary artery disease (CAD), atrial fibrillation (AF), and stroke. About 2–4% of the middle-aged population of world is affected with OSA and OSAHS. Many studies have shown a correlation between CVDs and SRBDs. OSA is still not considered as a specific risk factor for CAD by the clinical guidelines for the management of CAD, though the Sleep Heart Health Study (SHHS) shows that OSA with an AHI ≥30 may increase the risk of CAD in men in middle-age group.

HOW OBSTRUCTIVE SLEEP APNEA AFFECTS CARDIOVASCULAR SYSTEM?[12-15]

Obstructive sleep apnea leads to repeated inspiratory efforts against the closed pharyngeal airway, in turn leading to increase in negative intrathoracic pressure, which increases both preload and afterload. The hypoxemia due to OSA causes pulmonary vasoconstriction and thus increases right ventricular afterload. This may cause right ventricular distension and leftward displacement of interventricular septum during diastole impairs left ventricular (LV) filling. Increase in LV afterload and decrease in LV preload during obstructive apneas causes a drop in stroke volume and cardiac output. It is more marked in LV systolic dysfunction patients than with normal LV function.

Myocardial oxygen demand increases by increased LV transmural pressure that also causes a fall in coronary blood flow. At the same time, apnea-related hypoxia reduces oxygen supply and increases efferent sympathetic outflow. All these mechanisms together can precipitate myocardial ischemia in those with pre-existing coronary disease. If uncorrected, ventricular remodeling occurs, causing asymmetrical septal or concentric LV hypertrophy, or ventricular dilatation. Negative intrathoracic pressure also increases atrial and intrathoracic aortic wall stress, increasing the likelihood of nocturnal atrial arrhythmias and thoracic aortic dissection.

SYMPATHETIC AND PARASYMPATHETIC EFFECTS OF OBSTRUCTIVE SLEEP APNEA[16-18]

Obstructive sleep apnea immediately causes increased sympathetic nerve activity (SNA) and decreases parasympathetic activity. Sympathetic overactivity is caused by apnea-induced hypoxia and CO_2 retention and apnea-induced cessation of pulmonary stretch receptor-mediated inhibition of central sympathetic outflow. The fall in stroke volume and blood pressure (BP) during obstructive apneas causes a decrease in sympathoinhibitory inputs from carotid sinus baroreceptors, leading to further sympathomimetic activity.

A rise in heart rate (HR) and BP is observed during arousals due to increased SNA and decreased vagal activity. Patients with OSA and cardiac dysfunction also have elevated SNA and depressed cardiac vagal activity when awake. Reduced cardiac vagal activity increases HR and reduces respiratory sinus arrhythmia, which is a marker of adverse outcomes, including malignant arrhythmias. Increased sympathetic activity augments HR, arrhythmias, adrenergic receptor desensitization, injury, and necrosis of myocytes and peripheral vasoconstriction, leading to increased afterload and BP, and promoting renal sodium retention, both directly and by activation of the renin–angiotensin-aldosterone axis. This adversely affects cardiovascular system (CVS) prognosis. Treating OSA by continuous positive airway pressure (CPAP) decreases SNA and increases cardiac vagal modulation of HR variability both at night and during wakefulness.

OBSTRUCTIVE SLEEP APNEA AS AN INFLAMMATORY CONDITION[19-22]

Obstructive sleep apnea causes oxidative stress injury by repetitive episodes of hypoxia and reoxygenation. Reactive oxygen and inflammatory mediators impair vascular endothelial function and promote atherogenesis. Sporadic hypoxia also leads to activation of nuclear transcriptional factors, like nuclear factor B, which augments the production of inflammatory mediators and adhesion molecules causing more endothelial damage and atherogenesis. There are low plasma concentrations of nitrite and nitrates and high concentration of stress markers in OSA. Studies suggest that these derangements are reversed by CPAP therapy.

Endothelium-dependent vasodilatation is impaired in OSA patients who are otherwise healthy, and, in randomized trials, treating OSA by CPAP improved both endothelium-dependent and/or independent vasodilatation without reducing plasma biomarkers of inflammation. Butt et al recently reported that even healthy patients with OSA had deranged myocardial perfusion and that improved with CPAP. OSA patients have increased endothelial cells apoptosis and paucity of endothelial progenitor cells in circulation.

HYPERCOAGULABILITY[23-25]

The risk of thrombosis increases during sleep in OSA patients. CPAP reduces this risk as brought out by platelet marker studies in nonrandomized studies. Morning fibrinogen concentration and plasminogen activator inhibitor type-1 level also are increased in OSA patients. In an epidemiological study done by Mehra et al revealed that both fibrinogen and plasminogen activator inhibitor type-1 are directly related with AHI and increase in AHI leads to increase in concentration of both. These indicate less fibrinolytic potential and a hypercoagulable state.

In a nonrandomized study, morning fibrinogen concentration was shown to decrease after 1 night of CPAP. One randomized study showed that CPAP therapy for just 2 weeks led to considerable decrease in plasminogen activator inhibitor type-1. These observations suggest that increased platelet activation and hypercoagulability together could increase susceptibility of OSA patients to thromboembolic phenomena such as stroke. Figure 4.1 summarizes the pathogenesis of CVD in OSA.

CENTRAL SLEEP APNEA AND CARDIOVASCULAR SYSTEM[26,27]

Heart failure (HF) causes CSA. CSA also initiates a vicious cycle that could cause further deterioration in cardiovascular function. Daytime muscle SNA and cardiac SNA are higher in HF patients with CSA compared for HF without CSA, or those with OSA, possibly because of greater HF severity. There are associated changes in BP and HR in sinus rhythm patients. Cycles of CSA entrain, rhythmically, low-frequency oscillations in BP and HR in sinus rhythm patient, and the ventricular response to AF, as well.

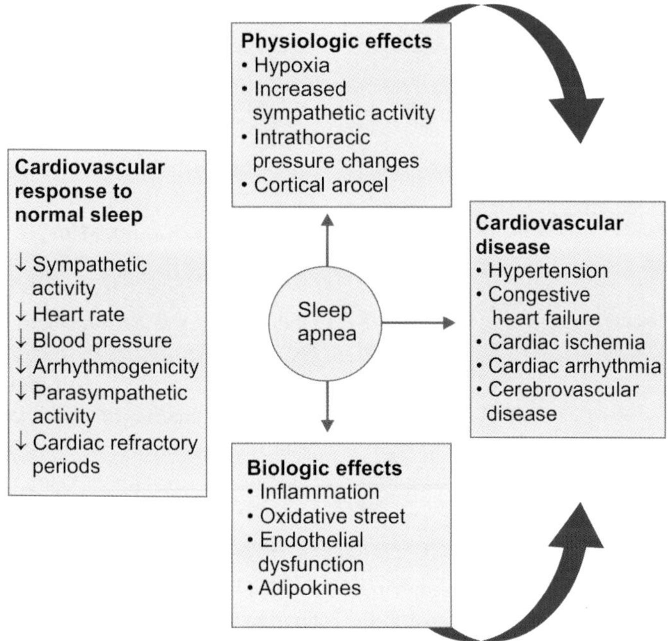

Fig. 4.1 Pathogenesis of cardiovascular system disease in obstructive sleep apnea

HYPERTENSION[28-31]

Obstructive sleep apnea is not considered as an independent risk factor for HT, but prevalence of OSA in primary HT is about 35%. In the Wisconsin Sleep Cohort, subjects with an AHI ≥15 had a 2.89 or greater likelihood of developing HT than those with an AHI of 0.77. In contrast, in the more recent 5-year follow-up from the SHHS, O'Connor et al reported that there is an increased risk of HT in unison with AHI when not adjusted for body mass index (BMI) but became nonsignificant after adjustment.

No association was found between OSA and incidence of HT when potential confounding variables were adjusted in the Vitoria Sleep Cohort. Though the findings may be due to different study designs, it was seen that in patients with drug-resistant HT, OSA, present in about 65–80%, was by far the most common secondary causes identified, and that its treatment may lower BP in such patients. This suggests that OSA plays a provocative role in HT. HT may be a particularly potent yet reversible stimulus to LV hypertrophy and failure.

Suppression of OSA by CPAP immediately reduces nocturnal SNA and BP. Although one meta-analysis showed no significant effect of CPAP on BP, while two others reported a modest effect of CPAP of about 2 mm Hg in mean BP reduction. So, treating OSA with CPAP can reduce BP in hypertensive patients.

CORONARY ARTERY DISEASE[32-34]

In CAD patients, prevalence of OSA is about 30%. OSA increases the risk of CAD modestly in subjects with relatively higher AHI in comparison with those with lower AHI. In patients with CAD, OSA can provoke ischemic changes in the electrocardiogram (ECG), and nocturnal angina as well predisposes to serious cardiac events and chances of restenosis after coronary angioplasties for acute coronary syndromes.

Myocardial infarction (MI) occurring during the night is more likely to be associated with OSA than those whose infarct occurred during daytime hours, suggesting that OSA can trigger plaque rupture or myocardial ischemia. After acute MI, those patients with OSA as comorbidity have higher death rates, myocardial infarction, stroke, and impaired recovery of LV systolic function.

Continuous positive airway pressure (CPAP) can immediately alleviate ischemic changes in the ECG and nocturnal angina. In an observational study, patients with both CAD and OSA (AHI ≥15) who were treated had fewer cardiovascular events than those who were not treated. In another observational study, Cassar et al reported similar findings in OSA patients (AHI ≥15) who underwent percutaneous coronary intervention in comparison with untreated OSA patients; the cardiovascular death rate was reduced significantly ($P = 0.027$) and there was less all-cause mortality ($P = 0.058$). More data from randomized trials are required to assess the benefits of CPAP treatment in such patients.

HEART FAILURE[35-38]

Repeated LV wall stress, hypoxia, and sympathetic activation in susceptible individuals may lead to LV hypertrophy, dilatation, and a decline in systolic function. Data from a cross-sectional study (SHHS) showed that patients having an AHI of ≥11 have 2.38 times increased chances of having HF irrespective of other factors.

In patients of HF, the incidence of OSA has been reported from 12% to 53%, more than the general population. CSA is considered as an independent predictor of mortality in patients with HF. The prevalence of CSA in HF patient as reported in different studies ranges from 21% to 37%.

The mechanical, autonomic, and oxidative stresses imposed by sleep apnea can aggravate myocardial ischemia and contribute to increased mortality, perhaps through the generation of malignant ventricular arrhythmias. These observations, in addition to those described above, that fluid retention related to the HF state can contribute to the pathogenesis of sleep apnea, suggest a bidirectional relationship between HF and sleep apnea. The precipitation and progression of HF are always linked to the presence and severity of the OSA and CSA.

Data from three trials demonstrate consistently that systolic HF patients with OSA showed increase in left ventricular ejection fraction (LVEF) and reduction in SNA when treated with CPAP therapy. The effect of CPAP on morbidity and mortality in HF patients with OSA has not been investigated by any randomized trials, but two observational studies comparing CPAP-treated and untreated HF patients have been performed, which showed greater hospitalization-free survival (mean 2.1 years) in patients who were treated for OSA with a CPAP.

Total 258 HF patients with CSA were enrolled in CANPAP (Canadian Continuous Positive Airway Pressure for Patients With Central Sleep Apnea and Heart Failure Trial) trial which showed that in patients who were treated with CPAP there was improvement in LV function and reduction in plasma norepinephrine concentration initially, but, after a mean follow-up of 2 years, the difference between the two groups was nonsignificant.

The effect of adaptive servo ventilation (ASV) was better in HF patients with CSA, even in those whose CSA was found resistant to CPAP or to bilevel-positive airway pressure. In a randomized trial, brain natriuretic peptide and nocturnal urinary metadrenaline concentrations were reduced by ASV, but there was no improvement in LVEF. In two other short-term randomized trials involving HF patients with either CSA or with coexisting OSA and CSA, LVEF increased more in ASV than in CPAP-treated patients. Data from these trials suggest that ASV may be more effective in suppressing CSA than CPAP.

ARRHYTHMIAS[39-41]

In OSA, arrhythmias have many causes. These factors include myocardial wall stretch due to abrupt decreases in intrathoracic pressure, decreased cell-to-cell communication through remodeling, myocardial ischemia secondary to apnea-induced intermittent hypoxia, increased wall tension and cardiac inflammatory pathways getting activated. Hypoxia is induced with the apneas that in turn provoke parasympathetically mediated atrioventricular. Individuals with severe forms of OSA and CSA have two to four times higher chances of developing complex arrhythmias (AF, NSVT, and complex ventricular ectopy) than those without sleep disorders even after treating other confounding factors. OSA predicts a greater risk of new onset AF or its recurrence following treatment of sinus rhythm. Two studies have reported a strong relationship between AF and CSA, in patients with and without HF.

In an analysis, involving 71 patients followed for 6 months after implantable cardioverter-defibrillator implantation, sleep apnea patients had fourfold appropriate device discharge more frequently than those without sleep apnea, with most of the events between midnight and 6 AM. A more recent study involving 283 patients followed for 54 months after implantation of an implantable cardioverter-defibrillator in conjunction with biventricular pacing, discharge risk doubled, and the time to first appropriate discharge was 25 months earlier in patients of CSA, and 17 months earlier in patients of OSA, in comparison with patients who did not have sleep apnea.

Several reports indicate that effective treatment of OSA can reduce cardiac arrhythmias. In an observational study, there was reversal of sinus bradyarrhythmias and second-degree heart block. Another study reported that in patients of OSA in which tracheostomy was done, there was marked reduction in frequency of tachyarrhythmias. CPAP-treated OSA patients were found to be reduced rate of recurrence of AF 1 year post-cardioversion than nontreated patients (42% vs. 82%). In a small, 1-month randomized trial involving HF patients with OSA and frequent ventricular ectopy during sleep, Ryan et al found a significant reduction in the ectopic frequency in those treated with CPAP. These data therefore suggest a causal role for OSA as an initiator of ventricular arrhythmias.

STROKE[42,43]

The prevalence of OSA in patients who had a stroke is about 60%, and of CSA about 12%. Data from cross-sectional study (SHHS) revealed that there are 1.58 times greater chances for stroke in the patients with highest AHI quarter than in the lowest AHI, more significant in men but not in women. Impaired neurological function related to OSA may result from decrease in cerebral blood flow, intermittent hypoxia, and hampered cerebral autoregulation. OSA patients had 1.76 times greater mortality due to CVA than controls.

Three randomized studies on OSA and stroke were studied. Only one found a substantial benefit with respect to overall stroke recovery, functional and motor outcomes, and severity of depression, but no improvement in cognitive performance after treatment of OSA with CPAP. Protocol differences likely account for the superior outcomes involving patients having ischemic cerebrovascular disease and patients with an AHI ≥20 treated with CPAP. This study suggested that CPAP treatment of OSA can reduce the mortality and morbidity rate in patients who have already experienced an ischemic cerebrovascular event but randomized trials are needed to verify this observation.

PULMONARY HYPERTENSION[44-46]

The World Health Organization (WHO) conference on pulmonary arterial HT in the year 1998 recognized sleep disordered breathing as a secondary cause of PH. In patients with sleep disordered breathing, the pulmonary hypertension (PH) varies considerably, from 15% to 70%. This variation in part depends on inclusion in studies of patients with COPD, which contributes to increased frequency, prevalence, and severity of PH in OSA. Meanwhile, in patients with OSA without comorbid disorders, PH is usually mild, but can be severe in advanced OSA, resulting in cor pulmonale (Pickwickian syndrome).

A small study involving OSA patients underwent right heart catheterization that showed marked changes in pulmonary artery pressures, which coincided with apnea cycles. These hemodynamical abnormalities were also found to be associated with episodes of hypoxemia and hypercapnia. This study indicated that there is a strong correlation between the degree of impairment of normal physiological process by OSA especially in pulmonary circulation. A French study involving 220 OSA patients with an AHI > 20, around 17% patients mean pulmonary artery pressure of at least 20 mm Hg in resting state, and around 8% patients had the mean pressure was 25 mm Hg or higher. Patients with PH had more severe OSA, a low level of arterial oxygen, a higher level of arterial carbon dioxide, and higher BMI, than patients without PH.

However, there is still a debate as to whether sustained PAH can be a primarily caused by OSA, but it has been observed that patients of OSA who are treated with CPAP have lower PA pressures. This is recently being supported by many studies.

CARDIOVASCULAR MORTALITY[47,48]

Eighteen-year follow-up in the Wisconsin Sleep Cohort showed that patients without sleep apnea had 5.2 times for lower cardiovascular mortality than the patients with severe untreated OSA. Gami et al reported that, in OSA patients, the relative risk of sudden cardiac death during the nighttime was 2.57-fold greater than the non-OSA population, whose peak for sudden cardiac death was in the morning after awakening. The SHHS showed that men with an AHI ≥15 had a 1.69 times higher risk of fatal cardiovascular events as compared to the patients with an AHI <5.

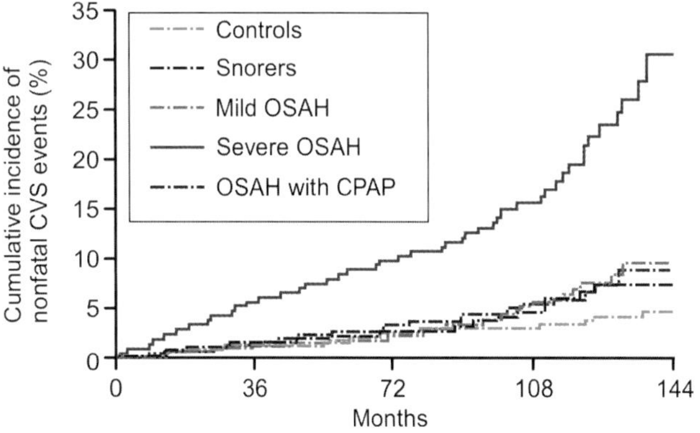

Fig. 4.2 Cardiovascular nonfatal events related to various groups of obstructive sleep apnea and improvement with continuous positive airway pressure therapy

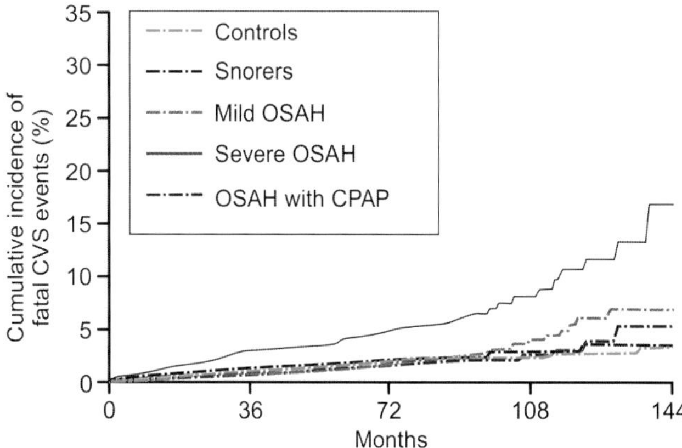

Fig. 4.3 Cardiovascular fatal events related to various groups of obstructive sleep apnea and improvement with continuous positive airway pressure therapy

A study with 264 healthy control men matched for age, sex, and weight, 235 men with untreated OSA (AHI ≥30) had 3.5 times more fatal and 4.7 times more nonfatal cardiovascular events in a mean follow-up period of 10 years. Figures 4.2 and 4.3 show the cardiovascular mortality and morbidity related to OSA compared to those treated with CPAP.

CONCLUSION[49]

Obstructive sleep apnea is an important risk factor for CVD that has been supported by many studies from time to time. A vital issue to address optimal management of OSA may be an important approach to reduce further cardiovascular morbidity and mortality, particularly in obese subjects in whom both OSA and cardiovascular consequences are highly prevalent. The current evidence is highly suggestive, but there are still counterarguments that can be advanced. This can only be proven by data from randomized trials, but results are likely years away. Given that the treatment of OSA, i.e. nasal CPAP, is effective and essentially totally safe, many workers agree that all patients with OSA should be treated with CPAP. ASV may be more effective in suppressing CSA than CPAP.

REFERENCES

1. Park JG, Ramar K, Olson EJ. Updates on definition, consequences, and management of obstructive sleep apnea. Mayo Clin Proc. 2011;86(6):549-55.
2. Kasai T, Floras JS, Bradley TD. Sleep apnea and cardiovascular disease: a bidirectional relationship. Circulation. 2012;126: 1495-510.
3. Somers Virend K. Sleep apnea and cardiovascular disease. In: Bonow RO, Mann DL, Zipes DP, Libby P. Braunwald's Heart Disease: A Textbook of Cardiovascular Medicine, 9th edition. Philadelphia: Saunders. 2012;79:1719-25.
4. The Report of an American Academy of Sleep Medicine Task Force. Sleep-related breathing disorders in adults: recommendations for syndrome definition and measurement techniques in clinical research. Sleep. 1999;22:667-9.
5. Somers VK, White DP, Amin R, et al. Sleep apnea and cardiovascular disease: an American Heart Association/ American College of Cardiology Foundation scientific statement from the American Heart Association Council for High Blood Pressure Research Professional Education Committee, Council on Clinical Cardiology, Stroke Council, and Council on Cardiovascular Nursing Council. J Am Coll Cardiol. 2008;52:686-717.
6. Epstein LJ, Kristo D, Strollo PJ Jr, et al. Adult Obstructive Sleep Apnea Task Force of the American Academy of Sleep Medicine. Clinical guideline for the evaluation, management and long-term care of obstructive sleep apnea in adults. J Clin Sleep Med. 2009;5(3):263-76.
7. Sharma SK, Kumpawat S, Banga A, et al. Prevalence and risk factors of obstructive sleep apnea syndrome in a population of Delhi, India Chest. 2006;130(1):149-56.
8. Sharma SK, Reddy TS, Mohan A, et al. Sleep disordered breathing in chronic obstructive pulmonary disease. Indian J Chest Dis Allied Sci. 2002;44(2):99-105.
9. Devaraj U, Ramachandran P, D'souza GA. Obstructive sleep apnea in patients with myocardial infarction: experience from a tertiary care hospital in South India. Heart India. 2013;1:12-6.
10. Lattimore JD, Celermajer DS, Wilcox I. Obstructive sleep apnea and cardiovascular disease. J Am Coll Cardiol. 2003;41:1429-37.
11. Gottlieb DJ, Yenokyan G, Newman AB, et al. Prospective study of obstructive sleep apnea and incident coronary heart disease and heart failure: the sleep heart health study. Circulation. 2010;122(4):352-60.
12. Bradley TD, Floras JS. Obstructive sleep apnoea and its cardiovascular consequences. Lancet. 2009;373:82-93.
13. Balfors EM, Franklin KA. Impairment of cerebral perfusion during obstructive sleep apneas. Am J Respir Crit Care Med. 1994;150:1587-91.
14. Usui K, Parker JD, Newton GE, et al. Left ventricular structural adaptations to obstructive sleep apnea in dilated cardiomyopathy. Am J Respir Crit Care Med. 2006;173:1170-75.
15. Franz MR, Cima R, Wang D, et al. Electrophysiological effects of myocardial stretch and mechanical determinants of stretch-activated arrhythmias. Circulation. 1992;86:968-78.
16. Floras JS. Sympathetic nervous system activation in human heart failure: clinical implications of an updated model. J Am Coll Cardiol. 2009;54:375-85.
17. Spaak J, Egri ZJ, Kubo T, et al. Muscle sympathetic nerve activity during wakefulness in heart failure patients with and without sleep apnea. Hypertension. 2005;46:1327-32.
18. Nauman J, Janszky I, Vatten LJ, Wisloff U. Temporal changes in resting heart rate and deaths from ischemic heart disease. JAMA. 2011;306:2579-87.
19. Kohler M, Stradling JR. Mechanisms of vascular damage in obstructive sleep apnea. Nat Rev Cardiol. 2010;7:677-85.
20. Butt M, Khair OA, Dwivedi G, et al. Myocardial perfusion by myocardial contrast echocardiography and endothelial dysfunction in obstructive sleep apnea. Hypertension. 2011;58:417-24.
21. Berger S, Lavie L. Endothelial progenitor cells in cardiovascular disease and hypoxia-potential implications to obstructive sleep apnea. Transl Res. 2011;158:1-13.
22. Drager LF, Bortolotto LA, Figueiredo AC, et al. Effects of continuous positive airway pressure on early signs of atherosclerosis in obstructive sleep apnea. Am J Respir Crit Care Med. 2007;176:706-12.
23. Chin K, Ohi M, Kita H, et al. Effects of NCPAP therapy on fibrinogen levels in obstructive sleep apnea syndrome. Am J Respir Crit Care Med. 1996;153:1972-6.
24. Mehra R, Xu F, Babineau DC, et al. Sleep-disordered breathing and prothrombotic biomarkers: cross-sectional results of the Cleveland Family Study. Am J Respir Crit Care Med. 2010;182:826-33.
25. Minoguchi K, Yokoe T, Tazaki T, et al. Silent brain infarction and platelet activation in obstructive sleep apnea. Am J Respir Crit Care Med. 2007;175:612-7.
26. Spaak J, Egri ZJ, Kubo T, et al. Muscle sympathetic nerve activity during wakefulness in heart failure patients with and without sleep apnea. Hypertension. 2005;46:1327-32.
27. Leung RS, Bowman ME, Diep TM, et al. Influence of Cheyne-Stokes respiration on ventricular response to atrial fibrillation in heart failure. J Appl Physiol. 2005;99:1689-96.
28. Sjostrom C, Lindberg E, Elmasry A, et al. Prevalence of sleep apnoea and snoring in hypertensive men: a population based study. Thorax. 2002;57:602-7.
29. O'Connor GT, Caffo B, Newman AB, et al. Prospective study of sleep-disordered breathing and hypertension: the Sleep Heart Health Study. Am J Respir Crit Care Med. 2009;179(12):1159-64.
30. Pedrosa RP, Drager LF, Gonzaga CC, et al. Obstructive sleep apnea: the most common secondary cause of hypertension associated with resistant hypertension. Hypertension. 2011;58: 811-7.
31. Haentjens P, Van Meerhaeghe A, Moscariello A, et al. The impact of continuous positive airway pressure on blood pressure in patients with obstructive sleep apnea syndrome: evidence from a meta-analysis of placebo-controlled randomized trials. Arch Intern Med. 2007;167:757-64.
32. Yumino D, Tsurumi Y, Takagi A, Suzuki K, Kasanuki H. Impact of obstructive sleep apnea on clinical and angiographic outcomes following percutaneous coronary intervention in patients with acute coronary syndrome. Am J Cardiol. 2007;99:26-30.
33. Milleron O, Pilliere R, Foucher A, et al. Benefits of obstructive sleep apnoea treatment in coronary artery disease: a long-term follow-up study. Eur Heart J. 2004;25:728-34.
34. Cassar A, Morgenthaler TI, Lennon RJ, et al. Treatment of obstructive sleep apnea is associated with decreased cardiac death after percutaneous coronary intervention. J Am Coll Cardiol. 2007;50:1310-14.

35. Vazir A, Hastings PC, Dayer M, et al. A high prevalence of sleep disordered breathing in men with mild symptomatic chronic heart failure due to left ventricular systolic dysfunction. Eur J Heart Fail. 2007;9:243-50.
36. Yumino D, Wang H, Floras JS, et al. Relationship between sleep apnoea and mortality in patients with ischaemic heart failure. Heart. 2009;95:819-24.
37. Arzt M, Floras JS, Logan AG, et al. Suppression of central sleep apnea by continuous positive airway pressure and transplant-free survival in heart failure: a post hoc analysis of the Canadian Continuous Positive Airway Pressure for Patients with Central Sleep Apnea and Heart Failure Trial (CANPAP). Circulation. 2007;115:3173-80.
38. Philippe C, Stoica-Herman M, Drouot X, et al. Compliance with and effectiveness of adaptive servo ventilation versus continuous positive airway pressure in the treatment of Cheyne-Stokes respiration in heart failure over a six month period. Heart. 2006;92:337-42.
39. Becker H, Brandenburg U, Peter JH, Von Wichert P. Reversal of sinus arrest and atrioventricular conduction block in patients with sleep apnea during nasal continuous posit positive airway pressure. Am J Respir Crit Care Med. 1995;151:215-8.
40. Kanagala R, Murali NS, Friedman PA, et al. Obstructive sleep apnea and the recurrence of atrial fibrillation. Circulation. 2003;107:2589-94.
41. Serizawa N, Yumino D, Kajimoto K, et al. Impact of sleep-disordered breathing on life-threatening ventricular arrhythmia in heart failure patients with implantable cardioverter-defibrillator. Am J Cardiol. 2008;102:1064-8.
42. Sahlin C, Sandberg O, Gustafson Y, et al. Obstructive sleep apnea is a risk factor for death in patients with stroke: a 10-year follow-up. Arch Intern Med. 2008;168:297-301.
43. Martinez-Garcia MA, Soler-Cataluna JJ, Ejarque-Martinez L, et al. Continuous positive airway pressure treatment reduces mortality in patients with ischemic stroke and obstructive sleep apnea: a 5-year follow-up study. Am J Respir Crit Care Med. 2009;180:36-41.
44. Bady E, Achkar A, Pascal S,et al. Pulmonary arterial hypertension in patients with sleep apnea syndrome. Thorax. 2000; 55:934-9.
45. Sajkov D, Wang T, Saunders NA, et al. Continuous positive airway pressure treatment improves pulmonary hemodynamics in patients with obstructive sleep apnea. Am J Respir Crit Care Med. 2002;165:152-8.
46. Arias MA, Garcia-Rio F, Alonso-Fernandez A, et al. Pulmonary hypertension in obstructive sleep apnoea: effects of continuous positive airway pressure: a randomized, controlled cross-over study. Eur Heart J. 2006;27:1106-13.
47. Young T, Finn L, Peppard PE, et al. Sleep disordered breathing and mortality: eighteen-year follow-up of the Wisconsin sleep cohort. Sleep. 2008;31:1071-8.
48. Marin JM, Carrizo SJ, Vicente E, Agusti AG. Long-term cardiovascular outcomes in men with obstructive sleep apnoea-hypopnoea with or without treatment with continuous positive airway pressure: an observational study. Lancet. 2005;365:1046-53.
49. Pack AI, Gislason T. Obstructive sleep apnea and cardiovascular disease: a perspective and future directions. Prog Cardiovasc Dis. 2009;51:434-51.

5

Syncope: An Update

TS Kler, Niti Chadha

DEFINITION

Syncope is a transient loss of consciousness (T-LOC) due to transient global cerebral hypoperfusion. The Task Force for the Diagnosis and Management of Syncope of the European Society of Cardiology (2009)[1] have provided a pathophysiological classification of the principal causes of syncope. Broadly, an episode of syncope is classified into reflex-mediated, orthostatic, or cardiac syncope. Identification of the specific trigger of a syncopal episode is important as it gives clue to its classification into one of the above-mentioned types and is also instrumental in the further management of the patient.

Classification of Syncope (as per ESC 2009 Update)

- *Reflex (neurally mediated) syncope*
  - Vasovagal, mainly mediated by emotional or orthostatic stresses as in fear, pain, instrumentation, hot-humid environment.
  - Situational, as associated with cough, sneeze, swallowing, defecation, micturition, postprandial, etc.
  - Carotid sinus syncope.
- *Syncope due to orthostatic hypotension*
  - Primary autonomic failure
  - Secondary autonomic failure
    - Diabetes, amyloidosis, uremia, spinal cord injuries.
  - Drug-induced
    - Alcohol, vasodilators, diuretics, phenothiazines, antidepressants.
  - d. Volume depletion, as in hemorrhage, diarrhea, vomiting, etc.
- *Cardiac syncope*
  - Arrhythmic
    - Bradyarrhythmias
    - Tachyarrhythmias
  - Structural heart disease
    - Cardiac, as in coronary artery diseases, hypertrophic obstructive cardiomyopathy (HOCM), cardiac masses, valvular stenosis, valve prolapse, pericardial tamponade.
    - Others, as in aortic dissections, pulmonary hypertension, pulmonary embolism.

IMPACT ON THE QUALITY OF LIFE OF PATIENTS WITH SYNCOPE

The impact on the quality of life for patients can be huge, especially for those with recurrent syncope. The threat of recurrence can loom on in the minds of patients though out their life especially in cases of syncope associated with physical trauma.

APPROACH TO EVALUATION OF A PATIENT OF SYNCOPE

A number of patients presenting with circumstances suggestive of a T-LOC spell may not actually have a T-LOC. A T-LOC[1] is defined by presence of four features: transient, with rapid onset, short duration, and spontaneous recovery. If the medical history and eyewitness reports are carefully assessed, the patient may never have lost consciousness at all.

Conditions that Mimic T-LOC

- Cataplexy
- Drop-attacks
- Psychogenic pseudosyncope
- Simple falls.

Conditions with Partial or Complete LOC but Without Global Cerebral Hypoperfusion

- Epilepsy
- Metabolic disorders including hypoglycemia, hypoxia, hyperventilation with hypocapnia
- Intoxication
- Vertebrobasilar transient ischemic attack.

Some of these conditions may be episodes of abnormal responsiveness, but are not T-LOC (and therefore are not syncope). Once it is established that a T-LOC has actually occurred, the clinician must differentiate between syncopal and nonsyncopal causes of T-LOC. According to the latest

European Society of Cardiology (ESC) 2009 guidelines on the management of syncope, only those circumstances where the T-LOC has occurred due to transient cerebral hypoperfusion should be considered 'syncope'. Disorders such as cerebrovascular diseases should be ruled out in patients presenting with loss of consciousness.

EVALUATION OF A PATIENT OF SYNCOPE

In the absence of underlying heart disease, syncope is not associated with excess mortality. The main risk of syncope is related to physical injury to the patient and concern for public well-being in patients with high-risk occupation (aeroplane pilots or professional drivers). For patients not in such high-risk occupations, the intensity of work-up to establish a diagnosis is determined by the "malignancy" of the episode. *The 2006 AHA/ACCF Scientific Statement on the Evaluation of Syncope*[2] defines malignant syncope as an episode that occurs with little or no warning and results in a significant injury or property damage (e.g. car accident).

Patients with syncope usually present in emergency department accompanied by panicky family associates; however, outdoor presentations of such patients are not rare. An immediate hemodynamic assessment of the patient is essential to rule out any cause that might be acutely life-threatening. An electrocardiogram (ECG) should be obtained as part of the initial assessment. Malignant ventricular arrhythmias or critical pulmonary emboli are a few causes that might lead to an acute threat to life.

Once an immediately life-threatening cause is ruled out, concentration and efforts should then be directed toward a detailed historical evaluation. For a patient presenting with a syncopal episode, the key to finding the cause of an episode lies in a carefully taken history. Several pointers in the history can help reach a reliable etiological diagnosis in these patients. Directed history should include a detailed analysis of the present episode including factors associated with environmental, physical, and emotional stresses to the patient at and around the period of syncope. History regarding posture of the patient at the time of the episode, possible predisposing factors, and eyewitness accounts should be obtained in as much details as is reasonably possible.

Historical evaluation should preferably include the following details:

- Position of the patient just prior to the attack (supine, sitting, or standing)
- Activity just prior to the attack (during or after exercise, during or immediately after urination, defecation, cough or swallowing)
- Environmental stress (prolonged exposure to hot/humid environment, crowded places, sun exposure)
- Precipitating events (fear, intense pain, neck movements)
- Eyewitness account (skin color during episode pallor, cyanosis, flushing, tonic-clonic movements, duration of syncope, etc.)
- Past history of similar episodes, previous cardiac diseases, drug history
- Family history of sudden death.

DETAILED PHYSICAL EXAMINATION AND ELECTROCARDIOGRAM

A detailed physical examination should include a hemodynamic assessment including supine and upright blood pressure (BP), BP in all four limbs. An ECG should also be obtained at this point.

MAKE A PROVISIONAL DIAGNOSIS

Once through with history, physical examination, and ECG, a provisional diagnosis should be made. Further assessment should be directed toward proving the definitive diagnosis based on suspected type of syncope: *neurally mediated, orthostatic, or cardiac.* The stress of this chapter will mainly be on the evaluation of patients with a probable reflex (neurally mediated) syncope, vasovagal being the most common form. Those patients where a specific orthostatic or cardiac cause of syncopal episode is present should be evaluated and treated based on the established guidelines for the same.

ECHOCARDIOGRAM

Evaluation of cardiac structure and function should be done by an echocardiogram to rule out probable cardiac causes of syncope. Exercise stress test for those suspected of cardiac ischemic etiology should be undertaken as per guidelines.

CARDIAC RHYTHM MONITORING

Cardiac arrhythmias are an important cause of cardiac syncope, one of the lethal forms of syncope. Hence, cardiac rhythm monitoring is an integral part of evaluation for syncope. Monitoring of arrhythmias can be done by a stat ECG or by prolonged rhythm recorders as detailed below:

- A 12-lead ECG is the most valuable tool to catch several causes of cardiac syncope. Arrhythmias related to acute myocardial infarction (MI), Wolff-Parkinson-White syndrome, long QT, and Brugada disease are diagnosed using 12-lead ECG. The diagnostic yield of ECG in such cases is excellent.
- A 24-hour recording of ECG in the form of Holter monitoring helps in cases of syncope who may have symptomatic or asymptomatic recurrence of arrhythmias during the day similar in nature, though may be less intense than the one that caused the index event.

These monitors are attached to the body with a strap belt and 10-leads on and patient instructed to carry on his routine activities. Hospital admission is usually not required during this period of 24-hour monitoring. The yield of Holter monitoring for the evaluation of a cause of syncope is low (about 1–2% in unselected population).

- Event monitors or external loop recorders are available for loop recordings for a maximum period of 12 weeks. They are noninvasive recording instruments available as cutaneous patches that allow patients to continue their routine activity, while their heart rhythm is being continuously monitored. Utility of such devices in the diagnosis of patients with syncope is less, as manual activation by the patient is required for the device to store the recording for a preset time. These recorders are more often useful for the diagnostic evaluation of palpitations rather than for syncope.
- Implantable loop recorders (ILRs) are devices meant for prolonged periods of rhythm monitoring, as required for patients with infrequent recurrence of symptoms. As the name indicates, these devices are implanted into the body subcutaneously through a small incision usually in a parasternal pocket. These loop recorders allow a maximum monitoring for a period of 3 years before there battery wears out.

TILT-TABLE TESTING

Tilt-table test is meant to reproduce a neurally mediated reflex in laboratory settings. Blood pooling in lower limb veins due to orthostasis and immobilization trigger the reflex. Head-up tilt-table testing is an accepted test to evaluate patients presenting with syncopal symptoms. Substantial evidence suggests that tilt-table test is an effective technique for providing direct diagnostic evidence indicating susceptibility to vasovagal syncope.

The main indication for upright tilt testing is to confirm a diagnosis of neurally mediated syncope when the initial evaluation is insufficient to establish this diagnosis. Upright tilt testing is generally not recommended in patients in whom the diagnosis can be established by the initial history and physical examination. In patients without structural heart disease, the induction of reflex hypotension or bradycardia with reproduction of symptoms is considered diagnostic of neurally mediated syncope. The induction of reflex hypotension or bradycardia without reproduction of syncope points toward a diagnosis of neurally mediated syncope but is a less specific response. If a patient has structural heart disease, other cardiovascular causes of syncope should be excluded before a positive response to upright tilt testing is considered to be diagnostic of neurally mediated syncope.

Upright tilt testing is generally performed for 30–45 minutes after a 20-minute horizontal pretilt stabilization phase, at an angle between 60° and 80° (with 70° the most common). A positive response during a head-up tilt test is indicative of a neurocardiogenic cause for syncopal episode.

Who should Undergo Tilt-table Testing?

The ACC expert consensus document for tilt-table testing was published in 1996 that has provided general indication as to who should undergo tilt-table testing.[3]

Tilt-table Testing is Warranted

- If recurrent syncope or single syncopal episode in a high-risk patient has occurred, whether or not the medical history is suggestive of neurally mediated (vasovagal) origin, and
  - No evidence of structural cardiovascular disease.
  - Structural cardiovascular disease is present, but other causes of syncope have been excluded by appropriate testing.
- For further evaluation of patients in whom an apparent cause has been established (e.g. asystole, atrioventricular block), but in whom demonstration of susceptibility to neurally mediated syncope would affect treatment plans.
- Parts of the evaluation of exercise-induced or exercise-associated syncope.

Tilt-table Test is not Warranted After

1. Single syncopal episode, without injury and not in a high-risk setting with clear-cut vasovagal clinical features.
2. Syncope in which an alternative specific cause has been established and in which additional demonstration of a neurally mediated susceptibility would not alter treatment plans.

Classification of Positive Responses to Tilt Testing

- Type 1 (Mixed)
- Type 2 (Cardioinhibitory)
- Type 3 (Vasodepressor).

Complications of Head-up Tilt Test (HUTT)

The tilt-table test is a safe procedure, and the occurrence of complications is very low. Side effects are infrequent and include tachycardia (45%), nausea (35%), chest pain (2.2%), arrhythmias (6%), and other effects (10.3%).

ELECTROPHYSIOLOGY STUDY

In recent years, several options for noninvasive monitoring of cardiac rhythm have decreased the use of electrophysiology studies in the evaluation of patients with syncope and a normal ECG and normal left ventricular functions. However, this remains a useful tool for diagnosis in patients with suspected bradycardias or tachycardias in patients with suggestive but nondiagnostic ECGs.

MANAGEMENT OF PATIENTS WITH VASOVAGAL SYNCOPE

Physical Counterpressure Maneuvers Trial (PC Trial)[4]

The PC Trial was a multicenter, prospective, randomized clinical trial, which included 223 patients aged 38.6 (±15.4) years with recurrent vasovagal syncope and recognizable prodromal symptoms. The physical counter-pressure maneuvers included leg crossing, hand-grip, and arm-tensing. This trial concluded that physical counter-pressure maneuvers are a risk-free, effective, and low-cost treatment method in patients with vasovagal syncope and recognizable prodromal symptoms, and should be advised as first-line treatment in patients presenting with vasovagal syncope with prodromal symptoms.

Role of Cardiac Pacing

Pacing for reflex syncope has been a subject of five major multicenter randomized controlled trials. In all these trials, the preimplant selection was based on tilt-table test responses. The ISSUE-3 trial[5] is a double-blind randomized placebo-controlled study conducted in 29 centers. This study was based on ILR-documented asystolic syncope where patients were randomized to two groups: dual chamber pacemaker with rate drop response 'on' versus dual chamber pacemaker in sensing only mode. The observed 32% absolute and 57% relative reduction in syncope recurrence supports pacing for prolonged documented episodes of asystole during neurally mediated syncope. The results of this trial were published in 2012, hence awaiting induction into syncope management guidelines that have not been refreshed since 2009.

Do All Patients Presenting with Syncope Need Hospitalization?

The decision to hospitalize a patient with syncope for diagnostic evaluation depends primarily on the immediate perceived mortality risk to the patient should similar circumstances recur. A near-term morbidity risk is also considered especially in elderly or frail individuals presenting with ongoing hypotension.

Who Requires Hospitalization?

- Severe structural heart disease (low ejection fraction, prior MI, heart failure)
- Clinical or electrocardiographic features suggesting arrhythmic syncope
- Syncope during exertion or while supine
- Palpitations at the time of syncope
- Family history of sudden death
- Nonsustained ventricular tachycardia
- Bifascicular block or QRS >120 ms
- Severe sinus bradycardia (<50 beats/min) in absence of medications or physical training
- Pre-excitation
- Prolonged or very short QT interval
- Brugada electrocardiographic pattern (RBBB with ST elevation in leads V1–V3)
- Arrhythmogenic right ventricular dysplasia electrocardiographic pattern (T wave inversion in leads V1–V3 with or without epsilon waves)
- ECG suggestive of hypertrophic cardiomyopathy
- Clinical evidence or suspicion of a pulmonary embolus
- Severe anemia
- Important comorbidities
- Significant electrolyte abnormalities
- Severe anemia.

MANAGEMENT RECOMMENDATIONS OF NEURALLY MEDIATED SYNCOPE (EUROPEAN SOCIETY OF CARDIOLOGY/ 2009 RECOMMENDATIONS)

Class I Recommendation

- Reassurance of the benign prognosis of the condition
- Physical counter-pressure maneuver exercises.

Class IIA Recommendation

- Cardiac pacing should be considered in patients with dominant cardioinhibitory carotid sinus syncope
- Cardiac pacing should be considered in patients with recurrent reflex syncope, age >40 years, and dominant spontaneous cardioinhibitory response during monitoring.

Class IIB Recommendation

- Midodrine indicated for patients with vasovagal syncope (VVS) refractory to lifestyle measures
- Tilt training may be useful, but long-term result is based on compliance
- Cardiac pacing may be indicated in patients with tilt-induced cardioinhibitory syncope, age >40 years, and recurrent spontaneous syncope, when other measures have failed.

Class III Recommendation

- Cardiac pacing not indicated when dominant cardioinhibitory component for syncope not documented
- Beta-blockers not indicated.

Driving Recommendations for Patients with Syncope

The 2004 European Society of Cardiology (ESC) guidelines on syncope[6] have recommended *no restrictions* for drivers of self/private vehicles. For professional drivers, permanent restriction for driving is recommended for 'severe' vasovagal syncope. Neurally mediated syncope is defined as severe if it is very frequent, or occurring during the prosecution of a 'high-risk' activity, or recurrent or unpredictable in 'high-risk' patients. No change in recommendation is made in the 2009 guidelines on driving.

CONCLUSION

Syncope is a relatively common clinical presentation in day-to-day practice of physicians, cardiologists, as well as neurologists. Careful history taking, physical examination, and judicious use of tests increase the diagnostic yield of tests, increase patient safety, and reduce overall health cost.

REFERENCES

1. Moya A, Sutton R, Ammirati F, et al. Guidelines for the diagnosis and management of syncope (version 2009). Eur Heart J. 2009;30:2631-71.
2. Strickberger SA, Benson DW Jr, Biaggioni I, et al. AHA/ACCF scientific statement on the evaluation of syncope. Circulation. 2006;113:316-27.
3. Benditt DG, Ferguson DW, Grubb BP, et al. Tilt table testing for assessing syncope. J Am Coll Cardiol. 1996;28:263-75.
4. Van Dijk, Quartieri F, Blanc JJ, et al. Effectiveness of physical counterpressure maneuvers in preventing vasovagal syncope: the Physical Counterpressure Manoevers Trial (PC Trial). J Am Coll Cardiol. 2006;48(8):1652-7.
5. Brignole M, Menozzi C, Moya A, et al. Pacemaker therapy in patients with neurally mediated syncope and documented asystole. Third International Study on Syncope of Uncertain Etiology (ISSUE-3) Trial. Circulation. 2012;125:2566-71.
6. Bringnole M, Alboni P, Benditt DG, et al. Guidelines on management (diagnosis and treatment) of syncope—update 2004. Europace. 2004;6:467-537.

6

Infective Endocarditis Update: What is the Difference Now?

Vivek Kumar, Lal C Daga

INTRODUCTION

Infective endocarditis (IE) is an uncommon but life-threatening infection. While developments in cardiac imaging, therapeutics, and surgical techniques as well as potent therapeutic agents have led to improved outcomes in individual patients, the overall incidence of IE has remained relatively stable despite the varying incidence of predisposing conditions (e.g. rheumatic heart disease and injection drug use) over time among different areas. The incidence of IE in women increased from 1.4 cases to 6.7 cases/100,000 person-years.[1,2] Other studies have reported incidence rates ranging from 0.6 to 6.0 cases per 100,000 person-years.[3-6] One review of 15 population-based epidemiologic studies of IE found that crude incidence rates ranged from 1.4 to 6.2 per 100,000.[7] Sex and age have an impact on the incidence of IE. Men predominate in most case series, with male-to-female ratios ranging from 3:2 to 9:1.[6,8,9] New trends in the epidemiology of IE have occurred during the past 30 years. Most of these changes relate to the numbers and types of susceptible hosts, rather than to shifts in the virulence of the infecting micro-organisms. Endocarditis is becoming more common in older adults.[6,10,11] This is probably because of decreasing rheumatic valvular heart disease cases and increasing survival. The frequent use of intravenous (IV) route for diagnosis, treatment, and drug abuse as catheters, devices, valves, percutaneous devices, shunts, and pacemaker leads has led to increase in cases of IE. Despite advances in diagnostis and therapeutics, IE still has high morbidity and mortality rates and that makes us to follow and upgrade infection prevention strategies more religiously.

ETIOLOGY

A variety of micro-organisms can cause IE; staphylococci and streptococci account for the majority of cases.[12] Staphylococcal IE is substantially more common in healthcare-associated cases of IE. Streptococci remain common causes of community-acquired IE.[12] The International Collaboration on Endocarditis-Prospective Cohort Study identified the microbiologic etiology in 2781 patients from 58 sites in 25 countries with definite endocarditis as defined by Duke criteria.[13,14] Most patients had native valve IE (72%), while 23% patients were healthcare associated. Various etiological micro-organisms are illustrated in Figure 6.1.

PATHOGENESIS

The initial step in formation of vegetation is injury to the endocardium that is followed by focal adherence of platelets and fibrin. The initially sterile platelet–fibrin nidus then becomes infected by micro-organisms circulating in the bloodstream, either from a distant source of focal infection or as a result of transient bacteremia from a mucosal or skin source. Following colonization of the platelet–fibrin aggregate, microbial growth results in the secondary accumulation

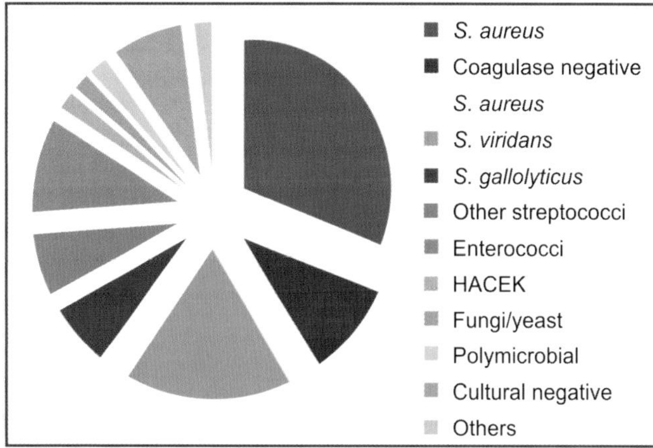

Fig. 6.1 Microbiologic etiology of endocarditis. Modified from Murdoch DR, Corey CR, Hoen B, et al. Clinical presentation, etiology, and outcome of infective endocarditis in the 21st century. Arch Intern Med. 2009;169:463.

of more platelets and fibrin and the further activation of the coagulation system via the extrinsic clotting pathway, until a macroscopic excrescence or vegetation is present. Intrinsic binding affinity to fibronectin also appears to be a contributing pathogenic factor. Glucosyltransferases (GTFs), which are proteins made by various members of the viridians group of streptococci, have the ability to convert sucrose into polysaccharides that in turn may act as "modulins" to express various cytokines (such as interleukin-6) or adhesions that in turn further recruit leukocytes into the vegetations.[15-19] Fibrinogen, type 4 collagen, and laminin found in damaged endothelium and platelet-fibrin aggregates mediate adherence. After colonization of a platelet-fibrin nidus, the bacterial-platelet interactions are responsible for the vegetation induction and its enlargement. In some patients with IE, the source of bacteria is obvious (like the infected skin lesion, dental infection or an infected vascular access), while in others a history of an infection cannot be elicited. In such patients, the source is like a minor injury to genitourinary, oropharyngeal, or gastrointestinal mucosa. In IV drug users, the pre-existing cardiac disease may not be known, and in these cases, the seeding of infection occurs from bacterial skin at the injection site, infected needle, or syringe. These patients commonly develop endocarditis of the tricuspid valve, while some may only have left-sided vegetations and others may have bilateral—left and right heart—endocarditis. Pre-existing antibodies to certain bacteria is a risk factor for the development of IE. Horses, who are administered repetitive injections of live pneumonia, develop pneumococcal endocarditis.[20-24]

In some animal models, pre-existing high antibody titers increase the median infective dose to induce endocarditis. The highest concentration of bacteria is located in the low pressure area immediately distal to a narrowed opening, i.e. vegetations occur when blood moves from an area of high pressure through a narrow orifice into an area of low pressure. In patients with pre-existing valvular disease, the vegetations are usually found on the atrial surface of the regurgitant A-V valves or the ventricular surface of regurgitant semilunar valves. Patients with mitral regurgitation may develop vegetations on the left-atrial wall where the regurgitant jet strikes the left atrial wall. In patient with ventricular septal defects, the vegetations develop on the right ventricular side of the defect and secondarily on the tricuspid and pulmonary valves. Similarly in aortic regurgitation, the patient may develop vegetation on the chordae tendineae—of the anterior mitral leaflet—where the AR jet strikes. There is a decrease in lateral pressure downstream a regurgitant flow, resulting in decreased perfusion of the intima; this might explain the propensity of vegetations to form at certain specific sites.[20-24]

CLASSIFICATION[25] AND DIAGNOSIS

IE should be regarded as a set of clinical situations that are sometimes very different from each other. In an attempt to avoid overlap, the following four categories of IE must be separated.

1. IE according to localization of infection and presence or absence of intracardiac material
   a. Left-sided native valve IE
   b. Left-sided prosthetic valve IE (PVE). Early PVE ≤ 1 year after surgery, late PVE ≥ 1 year after surgery
   c. Right-sided IE
   d. Device-related IE (PPI/ICD)
2. IE according to mode of acquisition
   a. Healthcare-associated IE.
      i. Nosocomial—IE developing in hospitalized patient for >48 hours prior to onset of symptoms and signs consistent with IE
      ii. Non nosocomial—-Signs and/or symptoms of IE started <48 hours after admission of a patient with healthcare contact.
   b. Community-acquired IE—Signs and/or symptoms of IE started <48 hours after admission not fitting in to healthcare-related IE.
   c. IV drug abuse-associated IE—IE in an active injection drug user without alternative source of infection
3. Active IE
   a. IE with persistent fever and positive cultures
   b. Active inflammatory morphology found at surgery
   c. Patient still under antibiotic therapy
   d. Histopathological evidence of active IE
4. Recurrence
   a. Relapse—Repeat episode of IE within 6 months after initial episode by same micro-organism
   b. Reinfection—Infection with a different micro-organism or repeat infection with same micro-organism after 6 months

To establish a diagnosis of IE sometimes requires a clinical wisdom and early suspicion (Table 6.1) because most of manifestations are constitutional, and early in the course of disease, the classic signs may not be present, as post bacteremia, the onset of symptoms of IE occurs in <2 weeks in >80% of patients with native valve endocarditis. The physician should analyze clinical manifestations, microbiologic results, and echocardiographic findings. Bacteremia leading to septicemia and predisposing valves (i.e. an active endocardial process proven by echocardiography) and an embolic event confirm the diagnosis of IE. Various clinical pathways have been derived to provide a diagnosis in cases with subclinical presentations; the Duke criteria are the most accepted one.

We should suspect IE in the presence of new regurgitant murmur, embolic events, sepsis of unknown cause, and fever in special situations:

1. Intracardiac prosthetic valves, devices, leads, conduits, and devices
2. Previous IE
3. Congenital heart defects and valvular heart diseases
4. Recent interventions, surgeries, and associated bacteremia
5. New onset congestive heart failure (CHF)

Table 6.1 Diagnosis of IE based on the modified Duke criteria[26]

Definitive IE	Possible IE	Rejected
Micro-organisms demonstrated by culture or histology in an intracardiac vegetation, in a vegetation that has embolized, or in an intracardiac abscess or Pathological lesions: Vegetation or intracardiac abscess present and confirmed by histology showing active endocarditis or Two major criteria are met or One major and three minor criteria are met or Five minor criteria are met	Findings consistent with IE that fall short of "definitive" but not "rejected" One major and one minor criteria are met or Three minor criteria are met	No pathological evidence of IE at surgery or autopsy after antibiotic therapy for 4 days or less Firm alternative diagnosis for manifestations of endocarditis or Resolution of manifestations of endocarditis with antibiotic therapy for 4 days or less

IE, infective endocarditis.

6. Positive blood cultures by typical IE organisms
7. Vascular and immunological phenomenon
8. New conduction defects
9. Focal neurological defects
10. Peripheral abscess of unknown cause
11. Immunocompromised situation
12. Valvulopathy in transplanted heart
13. Hypertrophic cardiomyopathy.

Many diseases that mimic the signs and symptoms of IE can be differentiated from IE by incorporating epidemiologic, historical, clinical, and diagnostic laboratory or imaging data. None of the differential diagnoses is characterized by positive blood cultures that are a distinguishing feature of endocarditis in most of cases. Clinical mimickers are acute rheumatic fever, SLE, Lyme disease, acute glomerulonephritis, reactive endocarditis, and cardiac tumors. The Duke criteria include microbiologic evidence, clinical manifestations, and echocardiographic findings into the diagnosis, and are divided into major and minor criteria.

Major Criteria

- *Positive blood cultures*: Positive for micro-organisms typical for IE from two separate blood cultures or Persistently positive for micro-organisms typical for IE:
  - Blood cultures drawn >12 hours apart
  - All of three, or a majority when four or more cultures are drawn; the first and last must be at least 1 hour apart

  Typical micro-organisms are considered to be viridians streptococci, *Streptococcus bovis*, *Streptococcus aureus*, enterococci (without a primary focus), and HACEK species.

  A single positive blood culture for *Coxiella burnetii* (or anti-phase 1 IgG antibody titer >1:800)
- *Evidence of endocardial involvement*
  Positive echocardiogram:
  - Oscillating intracardiac mass on valve or supporting structures, in the path of regurgitant jets, or on implanted material, in the absence of an alternative explanation
  - Abscess or new partial dehiscence of prosthetic valve
  - New valvular regurgitation (increase or change in pre-existing murmur not sufficient).

Minor Criteria

- *Fever*
  - 38°C (100.4°F)
- *Predisposition*
  - Predisposing heart condition or IV drug use
- *Vascular phenomenon*
  - Major arterial embolus
  - Septic pulmonary infarct
  - Mycotic aneurysm
  - Intracranial hemorrhage
  - Conjunctival hemorrhages
  - Janeway lesions
- *Immunologic phenomenon*
  - Glomerulonephritis
  - Osler nodes
  - Roth spots
  - Rheumatoid factor
- Microbiologic evidence
- Positive blood culture, but does not meet major criterion or provide serologic evidence of active infection with organisms consistent with IE
- *PCR*: Broad-range PCR of 16S
- *ECHO*: Consistent with IE but do not meet a major criterion as noted above.

CLINICAL PRESENTATION

Most common symptoms of IE are following:

Fever is the most common symptom of IE; it may be absent in patients with severe debility, in elderly patients, in those who have had prior antibiotic treatment, in cases in which the organism involved is less virulent, and if the causative organism is coagulase-negative *Staphylococcus*. Fever is frequently intermittent. The constitutional symptoms are weight loss, fatigue, and anorexia. Respiratory symptoms are dyspnea and chest pain, which may result from CHF or from septic pulmonary emboli. Renal manifestations are hematuria and flank pain may be present. Rheumatologic symptoms joint pain, lower back pain, and myalgia are commonly seen in IE patients. Musculoskeletal complaints may occur in many patients. Neurologic manifestations are confusion, lethargy, or psychosis due to the toxic effects of infection. Meningoencephalitis and frank hemiparesis, which can result from embolization of infective material, can also occur. A history of IV drug user, cardiac surgeries/devices, other predisposing factors, and a previous episode of endocarditis is important in the diagnosis and management of IE.

EXAMINATION

General and systemic examination:

- *Physical examination:* Includes signs of infective endocarditis
- *Cardiac manifestations:*
  - *CHF*: It may result acutely from the rupture of infected mitral chordae, valve obstruction by large vegetations, perforation of a bioprosthetic or native valve leaflet, or sudden intracardiac shunts from fistulous tracts or dehiscence of a prosthetic valve. The classic signs and symptoms, which are observed, include dyspnea, orthopnea, rales, a third heart sound (S_3), hepatomegaly, and edema of the extremities.
  - *New heart murmur (or changes in the characteristics of a pre-existing murmur)*: The most prominent murmurs are those of acute aortic and mitral regurgitation. The physical signs of acute aortic regurgitation are different from those of chronic aortic regurgitation. There is a softening of the first heart sound and shortening of the regurgitant murmur brought by rapid filling of the ventricles. A narrow pulse pressure is also found, rather than the wide pulse pressure present in chronic aortic regurgitation. In mitral regurgitation, the murmur may be truncated, and a fourth heart sound may be auscultated due to high filling pressures in the left ventricle.

Peripheral or cutaneous manifestations are as follows:

- *Roth spots*: These are round, boat-, or flame-shaped hemorrhages in the retina that result from septic emboli to the eye. White centers may or may not be present.
- *Splenomegaly*: This is seen in up to 50% of patients and may be caused by an accompanying embolism or vasculitis.
- *Petechial rash*: Rash may either be isolated or in crops and may recur.
- *Splinter hemorrhages*: These are minute petechiae found under the fingernails caused by damage to the capillary wall.
- *Janeway lesions*: These are nontender pink or purple, irregular, macular lesions occurring mostly in the palmar and plantar surfaces.
- *Osler nodes/Osler spots*: These are tender erythematous nodules on the hands and feet. The most commonly affected sites are the fingertips, but the side of the fingers, palms, soles, and toes may also be affected.

INVESTIGATIONS

Blood cultures and echocardiography are specific. Other modalities especially in combination provide supportive evidence of infection. The main diagnostic procedures for IE are blood culture, echocardiography, and histologic analysis. Ancillary procedures include hematology studies, urinalysis, immunologic studies, determination of C-reactive protein and cardiac troponin levels, molecular techniques, electrocardiography, chest radiography, and computed tomography (CT), and magnetic resonance imaging (MRI) scans (Figs 6.2 to 6.4).

TREATMENT—ANTIMICROBIAL THERAPY[29]

Host defenses are of little help, and bactericidal regimens are more effective than bacteriostatic therapy, both in animal experiments and in humans.[27-28] Surgery contributes by removing infected material and draining abscesses. Successful treatment of IE relies on eradication of etiological

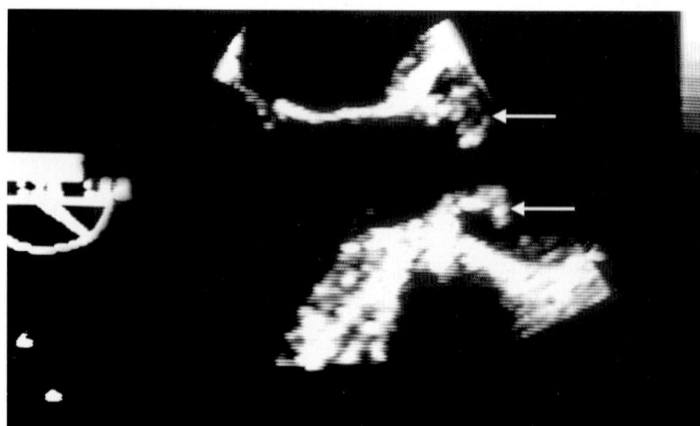

Fig. 6.2 Transesophageal echocardiography image showing vegetations on native valve

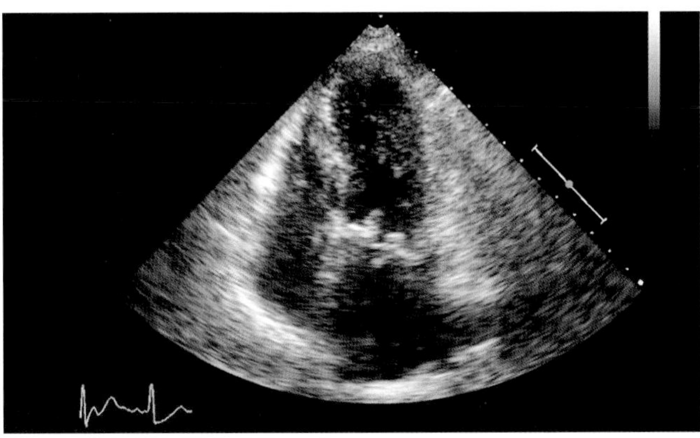

Fig. 6.3 Transthoracic echocardiography four-chamber view shows vegetation on bioprosthetic mitral valve

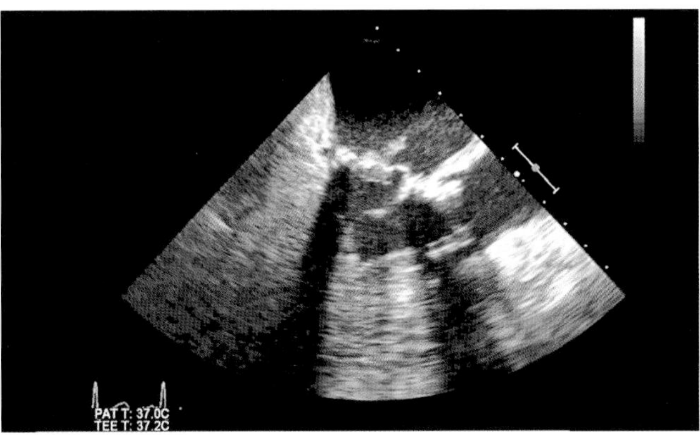

Fig. 6.4 Transesophageal echocardiography image shows vegetation on bioprosthetic mitral valve

microorganism by antimicrobial drugs. Empirical therapy is offered till the blood culture results are pending (Table 6.2).

TREATMENT OPTIONS FOR STREPTOCOCCI (PENICILLIN MIC ≤0.125 MG/L)

1. Benzyl penicillin monotherapy—1.2 g q4h IV 4–6 weeks preferred narrow-spectrum regimen, particularly for patients at risk of *Clostridium difficile* or at high risk of nephrotoxicity.
2. Ceftriaxone monotherapy—2 g once a day IV/IM 4–6 weeks not advised for patients at risk of *C. difficile* infection; suitable for OPAT monotherapy.
3. Benzyl penicillin and 1.2 g q4h IV 2 weeks and gentamicin 1 mg/kg q12h IV 2 weeks—not advised for patients with PVE, extra-cardiac foci of infection, any indications for surgery, high risk of nephrotoxicity or at risk of *C. difficile*.
4. Ceftriaxone—2 g once a day IV/IM 2 weeks and gentamicin 1 mg/kg q12h IV 2 weeks not advised for patients with PVE, extracardiac foci of infection, any indications for surgery, high risk of nephrotoxicity, or at risk of *C. difficile*.

TREATMENT OF STREPTOCOCCI (PENICILLIN MIC >0.125 TO ≤0.5 MG/L)

5. Benzyl penicillin 2.4 g q4h IV 4–6 weeks and gentamicin 1 mg/kg q12h IV 2 weeks—preferred regimen, particularly for patients at risk of *C. difficile*.

TREATMENT OF *ABIOTROPHIA* AND *GRANULICATELLA* SPP.

6. Benzyl penicillin 2.4 g q4h IV 4–6 weeks and gentamicin 1 mg/kg q12h IV 4–6 weeks preferred regimen, particularly for patients at risk of *C. difficile*.

TREATMENT OF STREPTOCOCCI IN PATIENTS WITH SIGNIFICANT PENICILLIN ALLERGY (PENICILLIN MIC >0.5 MG/L)

7. Vancomycin 1 g q12h 4–6 weeks and gentamicin 1 mg/kg q12h IV ≥2 weeks or dosed according to local guidelines.
8. Teicoplanin and gentamicin 1 mg/kg IV q12h ≥2 weeks preferred option when high risk of nephrotoxicity.

Native Valve Endocarditis, Methicillin-Susceptible *Staphylococcus* spp.

1. Flucloxacillin 2 g every 4–6 h IV 4 weeks. Use q4h regimen if weight is 85 kg.

Native Valve Endocarditis, Methicillin-Resistant, Vancomycin-Susceptible (MIC ≤2 mg/L) Rifampicin-Susceptible *Staphylococcus* or Penicillin Allergy

2. Vancomycin 1 g IV q 12h 4 weeks and rifampicin 300–600 mg q12h po 4 weeks or dose according to local guidelines. Modify dose according to renal function and maintain predose level 15–20 mg/L. Use lower dose of rifampicin if creatinine clearance <30 mL/min.

   Native Valve Endocarditis, Methicillin-Resistant, Vancomycin-Resistant (MIC >2 mg/L), Daptomycin-Susceptible (MIC ≤1 mg/L) *Staphylococcus* spp. or Patient Unable to Tolerate Vancomycin
3. Daptomycin 6 mg/kg q24h IV 4 weeks and rifampicin 300–600 mg q12h po 4 weeks or gentamicin 1 mg/kg IV,

Table 6.2 Empirical treatment regimens for endocarditis

1. Native valve endocarditis—indolent presentation	Amoxicillin—2 g q4h IV and gentamicin (optional)—1 mg/kg	If patient is stable, ideally await blood cultures. Better activity against enterococci and many HACEK micro-organisms compared with benzyl penicillin. Use regimen 2 (mentioned below) if genuine penicillin allergy. *The role of gentamicin is controversial before culture results are available*
2. Native valve endocarditis—severe sepsis (no risk factors for enterobacteriaceae, *Pseudomonas*)	Vancomycin and gentamicin—1 mg/kg	In severe sepsis, staphylococci (including methicillin-resistant staphylococci) need to be covered If allergic to vancomycin, replace with daptomycin 6 mg/kg q 24h IV If there are concerns about acute kidney injury, use ciprofloxacin in place of gentamicin
3. Native valve endocarditis, severe sepsis, and risk factors for multiresistant enterobacteriaceae, *Pseudomonas*	Vancomycin and meropenem—2 g q8h IV	Will provide cover against staphylococci (including methicillin-resistant staphylococci), streptococci, enterococci, and HACEK, enterobacteriaceae and *P. aeruginosa*
4. Prosthetic valve endocarditis pending blood cultures or with negative blood cultures	Vancomycin—1 g q12h IV and gentamicin—1 mg/kg q12h IV and rifampicin—300–600 mg q12h pop/IV	Use lower dose of rifampicin in severe renal impairment

Doses require adjustment according to renal function.

q12h 4 weeks. Monitor creatine phosphokinase weekly. Adjust dose according to renal function. Use lower dose of rifampicin if creatinine clearance <30 mL/min.

Prosthetic Valve Endocarditis, Methicillin, Rifampicin-Susceptible *Staphylococcus* spp.

4. Flucloxacillin 2 g every 4–6 h IV 6 weeks and rifampicin and 300–600 mg q12h po 6 weeks and gentamicin 1 mg/kg IV, q12h 6 weeks. Use q4h regimen if weight >85 kg. Use lower dose of rifampicin if creatinine clearance <30 mL/min.

Prosthetic Valve Endocarditis, Methicillin-Resistant, Vancomycin-Susceptible (MIC ≤2 mg/L), *Staphylococcus* spp. or Penicillin Allergy

5. Vancomycin 1 g IV q12h 6 weeks and rifampicin 300–600 mg q12h po 6 weeks and gentamicin 1 mg/kg q12h IV ≥2 weeks or dose according to local guidelines. Modify dose according to renal function and maintain predose level 15–20 mg/L. Use lower dose of rifampicin if creatinine clearance <30 mL/min. Continue gentamicin for the full course if there are no signs or symptoms of toxicity.

Prosthetic Valve Endocarditis, Methicillin-Resistant, Vancomycin-Resistant (MIC >2 mg/L), Daptomycin-Susceptible (MIC ≤1 mg/L) *Staphylococcus* spp. or Patient Unable to Tolerate Vancomycin

6. Daptomycin 6 mg/kg q24h IV 6 weeks and rifampicin 300–600 mg q12h po 6 weeks and gentamicin 1 mg/kg q12h IV ≥2 weeks—Increase daptomycin dosing interval to 48 hourly if creatinine clearance <30 mL/min. Use lower dose of rifampicin if creatinine clearance <30 mL/min. Continue gentamicin for the full course if there are no signs or symptoms of toxicity.

RECOMMENDATIONS FOR ENTEROCOCCAL ENDOCARDITIS

1. Amoxicillin 2 g q4h IV 4–6 weeks for amoxicillin-susceptible (MIC ≤4 mg/L) or penicillin 2.4 g q4h IV 4–6 duration 6 weeks for PVE and gentamicin 1 mg/kg q12h IV 4–6 weeks for gentamicin-susceptible (MIC ≤128 mg/L).
2. Vancomycinl g q12h IV or dose according to local guidelines for 4–6 weeks for penicillin-allergic patient or amoxicillin or penicillin-resistant isolate; ensure vancomycin MIC ≤4 mg/L and gentamicin 1 mg/kg IBW q12h IV 4–6 duration 6 weeks for PVE.

3. Teicoplanin 10 mg/kg q24h IV 4–6 weeks and gentamicin 1 mg/kg q12h IV 4–6 weeks (as alternative to Regimen 2, ensure teicoplanin MIC ≤2 mg/L).
4. Amoxicillin 2 g q4h IV ≥6 for amoxicillin-susceptible (MIC ≤4 mg/L) and high-level gentamicin resistant (MIC 128 mg/L) isolates.

TREATMENT RECOMMENDATIONS FOR Q FEVER

1. Doxycycline100 mg q12h po and hydroxyl chloroquine 200 mg q8h po both antibiotics for ≥18 months and <4 years.
2. Doxycycline100 mg po and ciprofloxacin 200 mg q12h po for ≥3 years.

TREATMENT RECOMMENDATIONS FOR *BARTONELLA INFECTIVE ENDOCARDITIS*

1. Amoxicillin 2 g q4h IV 6 weeks, if penicillin allergic use tetracycline and gentamicin 1 mg/kg q8h IV 4 weeks regular serum levels are needed to guide maintenance dose.
2. Doxycycline 200 mg q24h po and gentamicin 1 mg/kg q8h IV.

OTHER GRAM-NEGATIVE BACTERIA

A range of other gram-negative bacteria continues to cause a small proportion (<5%) of IE.[30] Risk factors include IV drug use, end-stage liver disease, central venous catheters, and old age. Members of the enterobacteriaceae, *Acinetobacter* spp., and *P. aeruginosa* have all been implicated. Ever-changing resistance patterns, such as the spread of extended spectrum β-lactamases-producing isolates and multidrug- or pan-drug-resistant strains, complicate therapy and preclude clear evidence-based recommendations for therapy. Because a combination of an aminoglycoside and β-lactam (carbopenem, amoxicillin or a cephalosporin) might be synergetic and prevent resistance. It would be prudent to use β-lactam antibiotic in therapeutic once daily dosing regimen of gentamicin (e.g. 7 mg/Kg) for treating these infections, instead of lower combination dose recommended for use in gram-positive IE, as the recommended post-dose levels (3–5 mg/Kg) for gram-positive bacteria might not be reliable for gram-negative septicemia, in which case, high-dose therapy based on sensitivity testing and early surgery is recommended. For an antibiotic course of >2 weeks, of an aminoglycoside like gentamicin, in view of high risk of nephrotoxicity, careful monitoring for toxicity, including an audiometry, should be undertaken. For this reason only, addition of an aminoglycoside might not always be an appropriate reason.

FUNGAL ENDOCARDITIS

Incidence of fungal endocarditis is 2–4% of all cases of IE[31], of which 50% is caused by *Candida* spp. (a half of these by *Candida albicans*), another 25% is caused by *Aspergillus* spp. (e.g. *A. flavus*, *A. kerreus*, and *A. fumigatus*), and rest 25% is caused by other fungi.[32] Almost all cases of *Aspergillus* endocarditis occur in adults. Preterm neonates with candidaemia may also develop *Candida* endocarditis. Endocarditis due to fungus mostly occurs in patients with prosthetic valves, but immunocompromised patients, neonates, and IV drug abusers may also be affected. IE due to *Candida* is commonly a healthcare-associated infection (87%).[31] About three-fourth cases of *Aspergillus* endocarditis occurs after some form of cardiac surgery and may be related to high spore counts in the ward environment[34] or contaminated operating room air.[33] Antifungal agents are described in Table 6.3.

SURGICAL MANAGEMENT

Early surgery is recommended in about 50% of all patients with IE, because of severe complications.[35] It should be considered even while the patient is receiving antibiotic therapy. This is to prevent systemic embolism, structural damage due to severe infection and progressive heart failure,[36,37-40] but it should be kept in mind that an early surgery is associated with significantly high risk of mortality. The surgery is indicated in patients who do not have complications or co-morbid conditions and have high-risk features that make the post-op recovery eventful. In such patients with mere antibiotic therapy, the chances of cure are very remote. Age alone is not a contraindication of surgery.[41] Indication and time of surgery as per evidence is described in Tables 6.4 and 6.5.

SUMMARY

IE is an infection affecting endovascular structures as well as shunts, conduits, valves, and newer devices. New trends in the epidemiology of IE are related to the numbers (Table 6.6), types of susceptible hosts, and frequency of etiological organisms, rather than shifts in the virulence of the micro-organisms. IE is not so uncommon disease mostly affecting the elderly patients with prosthetic valves and congenital heart defects, and IV drug users. IE affects men more commonly than women.

The diagnosis of IE is based on criteria including clinical manifestations, microbiology, and echo findings. Advances in echocardiography including three-dimensional echo and transesophageal echocardiography have improved the diagnostic yield particularly in a scenario where numbers of culture negative cases have increased. Management primarily consists of antimicrobial therapy based on causative

Table 6.3 Antifungal agents

Antifungal agent	*Dose/route*	*Serum levels required?*	*Role in treating Candida endocarditis*	*Role in treating Aspergillus endocarditis*
Fluconazole	400 mg daily	No	Long-term suppressive therapy	None
Voriconazole	IV therapy preferred initially	Yes, with dose modification important	Long-term suppressive therapy for fluconazole-resistant, voriconazole-susceptible isolates	First-line therapy with long-term suppression
Amphotericin B	3 mg/kg/24h (AmBisome) 5 mg/kg/day (Abelcet) 1 mg/kg/day (Fungizone)	No	Second-line therapy	Second-line therapy, or first line if azole resistance; should not be used for *A. terreus* or *A. nidulans* infection
Micafungin	200 mg daily	No	First-line therapy	Third- or fourth-line therapy
Caspofungin	70 mg loading, 50–100 mg daily	No	First-line therapy	No role
Flucytosine	100 mg/kg/day in three doses, reduced with renal dysfunction	Yes, with dose modification important	As combination therapy with amphotericin B	As combination therapy with amphotericin B

Table 6.4 Indication and timing of surgical treatment in native valve endocarditis[25]

Indication for surgery in native valve endocarditis	*Timing*	*Class*	*Level*
Heart failure (HF)			
Aortic or mitral infective endocarditis (IE) with severe AR or valve obstruction causing refractory pulmonary edema and cardiogenic shock	Emergency	I	B
Aortic or mitral IE with fistula in to a cardiac chamber or pericardium causing refractory pulmonary edema or shock	Emergency	I	B
Mitral or aortic IE with stuck valve or significant regurgitation, persistent HF, or echo evidence of poor hemodynamics	Urgent	I	B
Mitral or aortic IE with significant regurgitation and no HF	Elective	IIa	B
Persistent infection			
Persistent local infection (fistula, enlarging vegetation, abscess, pseudoaneurysm)	Urgent	I	B
Positive blood cultures with continuous fever of >7–10 days	Urgent	I	B
Fungal infection or multi-infection by persistent organism	Urgent/Elective	I	B
Embolism prevention			
Mitral or aortic IE with >1 cm vegetations, with one or more episode of embolism, in spite of appropriate antibiotic therapy	Urgent	I	B
Mitral or aortic IE with large (>1 cm) vegetations with HF/abscess/persistent infection	Urgent	I	C
Very large vegetations (>1 cm)	Urgent	IIb	C

Emergency cardiac surgery: Cardiac surgery done within 24 hours.

Urgent cardiac surgery: Cardiac surgery performed within a few days.

Elective cardiac surgery: Cardiac surgery performed 1–2 weeks after initializing antibiotic therapy.

Table 6.5 Indication and timing of surgical treatment in prosthetic valve endocarditis[25]

Indication for surgery in prosthetic valve endocarditis	*Timing*	*Class*	*Level*
Heart failure (HF)			
Prosthetic heart valve (PHV) endocarditis causing dehiscence or obstruction, resulting in refractory pulmonary edema and cardiogenic shock	Emergency	I	B
PHV endocarditis causing perforation in cardiac chamber or pericardial perforation causing refractory pulmonary edema and shock	Emergency	I	B
PHV endocarditis with severe PHV dysfunction and persisting HF	Urgent	I	B
PHV deliscence without HF	Elective	I	B
Persistent infection			
Local uncontrolled infection (enlarging vegetation, pseudoaneurysm, abscess, fistula)	Urgent	I	B
Fungal or multiresistant organism PVE	Urgent/Elective	I	B
PVE with positive blood cultures (>7–10 days) and persisting fever	Urgent	I	B
PHV endocarditis by gram negative or staphylococci (majority of early PHV endocarditis	Urgent/Elective	IIa	C
Embolism prevention			
Prosthetic valve endocarditis on appropriate antibiotic treatment with recurrent emboli	Urgent	I	B
Prosthetic valve endocarditis with >10 mm vegetations and HF/abscess/persistent infection	Urgent	I	C
Prosthetic valve endocarditis with isolated >15 mm vegetations	Urgent	IIb	C

Emergency cardiac surgery: Cardiac surgery done within 24 hours.
Urgent cardiac surgery: Cardiac surgery performed within a few days.
Elective Cardiac Surgery: Cardiac surgery performed 1–2 weeks after initializing antibiotic therapy.

Table 6.6 Cardiac device-related infective endocarditis (CDRIE): treatment and prevention[25]

Recommendation	Class	Level
Prolonged antibiotic therapy and device removal are recommended in definite CDRIE	I	B
Device removal should be considered when CDRIE is suspected on the basis of occult infection without other apparent source of infection	IIa	C
In patient with native or PVE and an intracardiac device with no evidence of associated device infection, device extraction may be considered	IIb	C
Percutaneous extraction is recommended in most patients with CDRIE, even those with large vegetations (>10 mm)	I	B
Surgical extraction should be considered if percutaneous extract action is incomplete or impossible or when there is associated severe destructed tricuspid infective endocarditis (IE)	IIa	C
Surgical extraction may be considered in patients with very large vegetations (25 mm)	IIb	C
After device extraction, reassessment of the need for reimplantation is recommended	I	B
Routine antibiotic prophylaxis is recommended before device implantation	I	B

Recommendation for IE on pacemakers and intracardiac defibrillators.

Table 6.7 Prophylaxis[25]

	Class	Level
Antibiotic prophylaxis should be considered for patients at highest risk of infective endocarditis (IE)	IIa	C
1. Patient with a prosthetic valve or a prosthetic material used for cardiac valve repair 2. Patient with previous IE 3. Patient with congenital heart disease a. Cyanotic congenital heart disease, without surgical repair, or with residual defects, palliative shunts or conduits b. Congenital heart disease with complete repair with prosthetic material whether placed by surgery or by percutaneous technique, up to 6 months after the procedure c. When a residual defect persists at the site of implantation of a prosthetic material or device by cardiac surgery or percutaneous technique		
Antibiotic prophylaxis is no longer recommended in other forms of valvular or congenital heart disease	III	C
Dental procedure		
Antibiotic prophylaxis should be considered for dental procedures requiring manipulations of gingival or peripheral region of the teeth or perforation of the oral mucosa	IIa	C
Antibiotic prophylaxis is not recommended for local anesthetic injections in noninfected tissue, removal of sutures, dental X-rays, placement or readjustment of prosthodontics or orthodontic appliances or braces Prophylaxis is also not recommended following the shedding of deciduous teeth or trauma to lips and oral mucosa	III	C
Antibiotic prophylaxis is not recommended for bronchoscopy or laryngoscopy, transnasal, or endotracheal intubation Antibiotic prophylaxis is not recommended for gastroscopy, colonoscopy, cystoscopy, and transesophageal echocardiography Antibiotic prophylaxis is not recommended for any skin and soft tissue procedure	III	C

1. Cardiac conditions at highest risk of infective endocarditis for which prophylaxis is recommended when a high-risk procedure is performed.
2. Recommendations for prophylaxis of infective endocarditis in highest risk patients according to the type of procedure at risk.

organism, and in some cases it is surgical intervention. Despite advances in diagnostic and therapeutics, IE still has high morbidity and mortality rates and that makes us to follow and upgrade infection prevention strategies more religiously (Table 6.7).

REFERENCES

1. Griffin MR, et al. Infective endocarditis. Olmsted County, Minnesota, 1950 through1981. JAMA. 1985;254:1199.
2. Correa de Sa DD, et al. Epidemiological trends of infective endocarditis: a population-based study in Olmsted County, Minnesota. Mayo Clin Proc. 2010;85:422.
3. Smith RH, et al. Infective endocarditis: a survey of cases in the South-East region of Scotland, 1969-72. Thorax. 1976;31:373.
4. Hickey AJ, et al. Mitral valve prolapse and bacterial endocarditis: when is antibiotic prophylaxis necessary? Am Heart J. 1985; 109:431.
5. Williams RC, Kunkel HG. Rheumatoid factors and their disappearance following therapy in patients with sub acute bacterial endocarditis. Arthritis Rheum. 1962;5:126.
6. Hill EE, et al. Infective endocarditis: changing epidemiology and predictors of 6-month mortality: a prospective cohort study. Eur Heart J. 2007;28:196.
7. Tleyjeh IM, et al. A systematic review of population-based studies of infective endocarditis. Chest. 2007;132:1025.
8. Lerner PI, Weinstein L. Infective endocarditis in the antibiotic era. N Engl J Med 1966;274:199.
9. Watanakunakorn C. Changing epidemiology and newer aspects of infective endocarditis. Adv Intern Med. 1977;22:21.
10. Cantrell M, Yoshikawa TT. Infective endocarditis in the aging patient. Gerontology. 1984;30:316.
11. Durante ME, et al. Current features of infective endocarditis in elderly patients: results of the International Collaboration on Endocarditis Prospective Cohort Study. Arch Intern Med. 2008;168:2095.
12. Selton SC, et al. Preeminence of Staphylococcus aureus in infective endocarditis: a 1-year population-based survey. Clin Infect Dis. 2012;54:1230.
13. Fowler VG Jr, et al. *Staphylococcus aureus* endocarditis: a consequence of medical progress. JAMA. 2005;293:3012.
14. Murdoch DR, et al. Clinical presentation, etiology, and outcome of infective endocarditis in the 21st century: the International Collaboration on Endocarditis-Prospective Cohort Study. Arch Intern Med. 2009;169:463.
15. Garrison PK, Freedman LR. Experimental endocarditis I. Staphylococcal endocarditis in rabbits resulting from placement of a polyethylene catheter in the right side of the heart. Yale J Biol Med. 1970;42:394.

16. Durack DT, Beeson PB. Experimental bacterial endocarditis. I. Colonization of a sterile vegetation. Br J Exp Pathol. 1972;53:44.
17. Scheld WM, et al. Bacterial adherence in the pathogenesis of endocarditis. Interaction of bacterial dextran, platelets, and fibrin. J Clin Invest. 1978;61:1394.
18. Kuypers JM, Proctor RA. Reduced adherence to traumatized rat heart valves by a low-fibronectin-binding mutant of *Staphylococcus aureus*. Infect Immun. 1989;57:2306.
19. Yeh CY, et al. Glucosyltransferases of viridians group streptococci modulate interleukin-6 and adhesion molecule expression in endothelial cells and augment monocytic cell adherence. Infect Immun. 2006;74:1273.
20. Mair W. Pneumococcal endocarditis in rabbits. J Pathol Bacteriol. 1923;26:426.
21. Durack DT, et al. Effect of immunization on susceptibility to experimental *Streptococcus mutans* and *Streptococcus sanguis* endocarditis. Infect Immun. 1978;22:52.
22. Rodbard S. Blood velocity and endocarditis. Circulation. 1963; 27:18.
23. Bansal RC. Infective endocarditis. Med Clin North Am. 1995; 79:1205.
24. Freedman LR, Valone J Jr. Experimental infective endocarditis. Prog Cardiovasc Dis. 1979;22:169.
25. Gilbert Habib, et al. Guidelines on the prevention, diagnosis, and treatment of infective endocarditis (new version 2009). Eur Heart J. 2009;30:2369-2413.
26. Li JS, et al. Proposed modifications to the Duke criteria for the diagnosis of infective endocarditis. Clin Infect Dis. 2000;30: 633-8.
27. Durack DT, et al. Chemotherapy of experimental streptococcal endocarditis. II. Synergism between penicillin and streptomycin against penicillin-sensitive streptococci. J Clin Invest. 1974;53: 829-33.
28. Wilson WR, et al. 2nd. Short-term intramuscular therapy with procaine penicillin plus streptomycin for infective endocarditis due to viridans streptococci. Circulation. 1978;57:1158-61.
29. Gould FK, et al. Guidelines for the diagnosis and antibiotic treatment of endocarditis in adults: a report of the Working Party of the British Society for Antimicrobial Chemotherapy. J Anti Microb Chemother. 2012;67:269-89.
30. Reyes MP, Reyes KC. Gram-negative endocarditis. Curr Infect Dis Rep. 2008;10:267-74.
31. Falcone M, et al. Italian Study on Endocarditis. *Candida* infective endocarditis: report of 15 cases from a prospective multicenter study. Medicine. 2009;88:160-8.
32. Ellis ME, et al. Fungal endocarditis: evidence in the world literature, 1965–1995. Clin Infect Dis. 2001;32:50-62.
33. McCormack J, Pollard J. Aspergillus endocarditis 2003–2009. Med Mycol. 2011;49(Suppl 1):S30-4.
34. Jensen J, et al. Post-surgical invasive aspergillosis: an uncommon and under-appreciated entity. J Infect. 2010;60:162-7.
35. Tornos P, et al. Infective endocarditis in Europe: lessons from the Euro heart survey. Heart. 2005;91:571-5.
36. Baddour LM, et al. Infective endocarditis: diagnosis, antimicrobial therapy, and management of complications: a statement for healthcare professionals from the Committee on Rheumatic Fever, Endocarditis, and Kawasaki disease, Council on Cardiovascular Disease in the Young, and the Councils on Clinical Cardiology, Stroke, and Cardiovascular Surgery and Anesthesia, American Heart Association: endorsed by the Infectious Diseases Society of America. Circulation. 2005;111:e394-e434.
37. Hasbun R, et al. Complicated left-sided native valve endocarditis in adults: risk classification for mortality. JAMA. 2003;289: 1933-40.
38. Aksoy O, et al. Early surgery in patients with infective endocarditis: a propensity score analysis. Clin Infect Dis. 2007;44:364-72.
39. Vikram HR, et al. Impact of valve surgery on 6-month mortality in adults with complicated, left-sided native valve endocarditis: a propensity analysis. JAMA. 2003;290:3207-14.
40. Delahaye F, et al. Indications and optimal timing for surgery in infective endocarditis. Heart. 2004;90:618-20.
41. Di Salvo G, et al. Endocarditis in the elderly: clinical, echo-cardiographic, and prognostic features. Eur Heart J. 2003;24: 1576-83.

7

Hypertension: Controversies in Newer Guidelines

Ankush Sachdeva

INTRODUCTION

This discussion intends to take you through various different guidelines and controversies in newer guidelines, to improve our understanding on the subject of hypertension (HT) and to best we can offer our patients in day-to-day practice. HT is prevalent in more than a quarter of world adult population and is projected to increase to 29%, i.e. 1.56 billion by 2025.[1] In developing countries where infectious diseases and natural calamities take the bulk of the finances, it is predicted that almost three-quarters of worldwide hypertensive population will be from developing countries because of urbanization. The possible ways to stop this is widely understood by reduction in dietary sodium, exercise, and avoiding obesity. In spite of cost and pains taking effort to control HT, less than a third of patients with BP above 140/90 mm Hg are adequately treated.[2,3] This and also because HT being a complex and multifactorial disease leaves the patient vulnerable to stroke and heart attacks.[4,5]

UNDERSTANDING THE CONTROVERSY

As more and more data from newer trials are emerging, there has been modification of practice guidelines, giving rise to changes in the management of patients with systemic arterial HT. The guidelines provided by World Health Organization (WHO) and International Society of Hypertension (ISH) in 2003 were targeted toward a global audience including developing countries with limited resources. So, in low-resource situation WHO recommended lower priority for low-risk population and diuretics as the cheapest and most cost-effective drug. WHO had surveyed 167 countries and documented that 61% had no available guidelines, 45% health professionals had no training to manage HT, and 25% antihypertensive therapy was not affordable. The basic equipment for managing HT was unavailable in 8% of countries and antihypertensive drugs were missing in 12% countries.

The seventh report of Joint National Committee on Prevention, Detection, Evaluation, and Treatment of high BP (JNC 7) published by the US national heart, lung, and blood was to simplify the classification of BP and are regulated according to American and African Americans population who show a less BP response to monotherapy with beta-blockers (BBs), angiotensin-converting enzyme (ACE) inhibitors, or angiotensin receptor blockers (ARBs) compared to diuretics or calcium channel blockers (CCBs). Thiazide-type diuretics should be initial drug therapy either alone or in combination with other drugs. Systolic BP (SBP) between 120 and 139 mm Hg or diastolic BP (DBP) between 80 and 89 mm Hg should be considered prehypertensive and need a change in lifestyle. Essential HT accounts for 90–95% and secondary HT for 2–10% of the patients.

Therefore, according to JNC 7, the BP classification offered is shown in Table 7.1.[6]

European Society of Cardiology (ESC) and European Society of Hypertension (ESH) initially in 2003 endorsed WHO/ISH guidelines but later decided to have their own guidelines suitable to the European population. After number of important studies on HT, e.g. action in diabetes and vascular disease (*ADVANCE*) trial,[7] Losartan intervention for end point reduction in HT (*LIFE*) trial,[8] and ongoing telmisartan alone and in combination with ramipril global end point (*ONTARGET*) trial,[9] a reappraisal of 2007 guidelines was published in the year 2009.

Table 7.1 Classification for BP-JNC 7

BP classification (mm Hg)	*SBP (mm Hg)*		*DBP (mm Hg)*
Normal	<120	and	<80
Prehypertension	120–139	or	80–89
Stage 1 HT	140–159	or	90–99
Stage 2 HT	≥160	or	≥100

Table 7.2 ESH/ESC guidelines for definition and classification of hypertension

Category	SBP (mm Hg)		DBP (mm Hg)
Optimal	<120	and	<80
Normal	120–129	and/or	80–84
High normal	130–139	and/or	85–89
Grade 1 HT	140–159	and/or	90–99
Grade 2 HT	160–179	and/or	100–109
Grade 3 HT	≥180	and/or	≥110
Isolated systolic HT	≥140	and	<90

The 2013 ESH and ESC guidelines approve ambulatory blood pressure monitoring (ABPM) to be used in the assessment of cardiovascular (CV) risk factors and HT.[10] HT diagnosis should be based on elevated BP on three separate occasions and a detailed history about end-organ damage for heart, kidney, eyes, and brain; exclusion of secondary causes of HT and assessment of patient CV risk status need to be looked into.

The classification and definition of HT as per ESH/ESC guidelines remain unchanged as shown in Table 7.2.

The 2011 guidelines from National Institute for Health and Clinical Excellence (NICE) in UK advise the use of ambulatory and home measurement of BP to confirm the diagnosis of HT. The AB/CD algorithm, i.e. ACE inhibitor or BBs/Calcium channel antagonist or Diuretic was updated to ACD in patients under 55 years of age and patients over 55 years are recommended to start on CCBs. These guidelines went under lot of criticism for lack of evidence and being overcomplicated.[11] The JNC 8 guidelines were expected to be paired after the declaration of latest NICE guidelines.

BASIC WORKUP AND MANAGEMENT OF HYPERTENSION

The baseline workup includes accurate measurement of BP, history, physical examination, and biochemical parameters to determine any end-organ damage, any CV risk factors, and to find out other causes of HT beyond essential HT.[12] This includes a 12-lead electrocardiogram (ECG), complete blood count (CBC), evidence of target organ damage, chest X-ray, urine for microalbumin, and serum uric acid levels.[13]

The management is based on lifestyle modification and pharmacologic therapy: Lifestyle modifications are the initial step to achieve HT control. JNC 7 recommends the following lifestyle modifications:

- Weight loss (approximate SBP, 5–20 mm Hg per 10 kg)
- Limit alcohol intake to 1 oz (30 mL) of ethanol per day for men or 0.5 oz (15 mL) of ethanol per day for women
- Reduce sodium intake to 100 mmol/day (2.4 g sodium or 6 g sodium chloride; approximate SBP reduction, 2–8 mm Hg)
- Adequate intake of dietary potassium (approximately 90 mmol/day)
- Adequate intake of dietary calcium and magnesium for general health
- Quit smoking and reduce intake of dietary saturated fat and cholesterol
- Aerobic exercise at least 30 minutes daily for most days (approximate SBP reduction, 4–9 mm Hg).

The 2013 ESH/ESC guidelines recommend a low salt diet (5–6 g/day) and a body mass index (BMI) of 25 kg/m^2 and waist circumference of <102 cm for men and <88 cm for women.[14]

The AHA/ASA promotes the consumption of fruits, vegetables, low-fat dairy products for BP and stroke reduction. Other important steps are increase in physical activity (30 minutes or more on a daily basis) and weight reduction. Pharmacological therapy is needed in cases that are not well controlled in spite of lifestyle modification. The thiazide diuretic is first-line therapy, but the treatment needs to be modified as per the clinical setting, examples of which are as follows:

- *Post-myocardial infarction (MI)*: BBs, ACE inhibitor, aldosterone antagonist
- *Diabetes*: Diuretic, BB, ACE inhibitor, ARB, CCB
- *Chronic kidney disease (CKD)*: ACE inhibitor, ARB
- *Congestive heart failure*: Diuretic, BB, ACE inhibitor, ARB, aldosterone antagonist
- *Stable angina*: BBs, long-acting CCBs.

TRIALS INFLUENCING THE GUIDELINES

ALLHAT (Antihypertensive and Lipid-Lowering Treatment to Prevent Heart Attack Trial) included over 40,000 patients aged 55 years or older follow-up for 5 years. About 33,357 patients were randomized to treatment with chlorthalidone 12.5–25 mg/day, amlodipine 2.5–10 mg/day, and lisinopril 10–40 mg/day. Doses of these drugs were increased until BP <140/90 mm Hg was achieved. Also atenolol (25–100 mg/day), reserpine (0.1–0.2 mg/day), or clonidine (0.1–0.3 mg bid) could be added at discretion of investigator and hydralazine could be added as step 3 drug. Primary outcome was fatal coronary artery disease (CAD) or nonfatal MI combined. Secondary outcomes included all-cause mortality, fatal or nonfatal stroke, CAD, peripheral vascular disease, heart failure, end-stage renal disease (ESRD), and cancer. The result showed that thiazide-type diuretics should be considered first line therapy in HT and for patient unable to take a diuretic, first choice could be a CCB or ACE inhibitor.[15]

ACCOMPLISH (Avoiding Cardiovascular Events in Combination Therapy in Patients Living with Systolic Hypertension) trial included 11,454 high-risk older hypertensive patients of mean age 68 years out of which 46%

patients had prior CV events and 13% had history of stroke. About 60% patients had diabetes mellitus and had a baseline mean BP of 145/80 mm Hg. The primary end point was a composite of major fatal and nonfatal CV events. The trial was prematurely stopped as results indicated that patients treated with an ACE inhibitor/CCB (A+C) had a 20% lower risk of major CV events as compared with patients treated with ACE inhibitor/diuretic combination (A+D).[16]

ACCORD (Action to Control Cardiovascular Risk in Diabetes) blood pressure trial (ACCORD BP) had 4733 participants assigned to standard or intensive BP control and hypothesized that SBP <120 mm Hg improves CV outcomes <140 mm Hg in type 2 diabetics. The results showed no benefits of primary outcome, i.e. first nonfatal MI, nonfatal stroke, CV events/death but showed benefits for fatal stroke. Moreover, patients in intensive group are more likely for complications like increased potassium levels or abnormally low BP.[17]

AASK (African American Study on Kidney Disease and Hypertension) trial was done as there is no evidence that the current guideline of BP <130 mm Hg in presence of CKD improves CV or renal outcomes. About 1094 patients received intensive or standard BP control according to the level of urinary protein excretion with a baseline protein to creatinine ratio of ≤0.22 versus >0.22. The primary outcome, i.e. a doubling of serum creatinine level, ESRD, or death occurred in 328 patients during the trial phase and in 239 patients during the cohort phase. The result showed no difference in renal disease or death in intensive BP control versus standard BP control; however, subgroup analysis showed a lower BP may retard disease process in patients with hypertensive CKD in patients with protein to creatinine ratio of >0.22 at baseline.[18]

VALISH (Valsartan in Elderly Isolated Systolic Hypertension) study compared strict BP control (SBP <140 mm Hg) with moderate (140–149 mm Hg) SBP for ≥2 years in 3260 patients (aged 70–84 years) on valsartan. The result showed no difference in primary end point between moderate and strict control and also lower BP can lead to syncope and increases the risk of injury. Moderate control of <150 mm Hg may be sufficient to decrease CV events in elderly HT patients.[19]

SHEP (Systolic Hypertension in Elderly Patient) trial was a randomized, double-blind multisite trial in which 4763 participants over 60 years were randomized to active treatment or placebo. The step 1 drug was chlorthalidone (dose 1:12.5 mg/day and dose 2:25 mg/day). The step 2 drug was atenolol (dose 1:25 mg/day and dose 2:50 mg/day). The average SBP was 170 mm Hg and DBP was 77 mm Hg. The result showed that 5-year average SBP was 155 mm Hg for placebo group and 143 mm Hg for active group, while average DBP was 72 and 68 mm Hg. It concluded that lowering SBP reduced the combined rate of fatal and nonfatal stroke by 36% in male and females above 60 years of age.[20]

HYVET (Hypertension in Very Elderly Trial) randomized 3845 patients to either indapamide 1.5 mg sustained release (SR) plus perindopril 2–4 mg if required or placebo for a target BP of <150/80 mm Hg. A 2-year follow-up compared to placebo reduced all-cause mortality by 21%. Nonfatal stroke was reduced by 30%, fatal stroke by 39%, heart failure by 64%, and CV death by 23%.[21]

CAMELOT (Effect of Antihypertensive Agents and CV Events in Patients with Coronary Disease and Normal Blood Pressure Trial) was a randomized, double-blind multicenter 24-month trial in 1991 patients comparing 10 mg amlodipine or 20 mg enalapril with placebo in angiographically documented CAD (>20% stenosis) and DBP <100 mm Hg. Intravascular ultrasound (IVUS) was performed at baseline and study completion. The result showed that amlodipine in CAD patients reduced adverse CV events with slowing of atherosclerosis on IVUS and comparatively smaller and no significant effects were observed with enalapril.[22]

HOPE (Heart Outcomes Prevention Evaluation) trial had 9297 women and men of 55 years and above at high risk of MI and stroke who were recruited over 18 months. It was a large randomized trial in which patients were randomly assigned to 10 mg/day ramipril or placebo for 5 years. In addition, all patients were randomly assigned to receive vitamin E 400 IU/day or placebo. The results showed significant reduction in MI, stroke, and death by 16% in ramipril group.[23]

INVEST (International Verapamil SR/Trandolapril Study) was a randomized trial including 22,576 patients who were mostly elderly and were followed up for average 2.7 years. It compared verapamil SR plus trandolapril with atenolol plus hydrochlorothiazide (HCTZ) for HT and prevention of CV events. The result signifies that BP reduction is important to prevent CV mortality and morbidity and selection of drug needs to be based on comorbidities and risk factors and one drug may not be suitable for everyone.[24]

ROADMAP (Randomized Olmesartan and Diabetes Microalbuminuria Prevention) study showed that strict BP control (<130/80 mm Hg) was achieved in 80% of patients with olmesartan compared to placebo along with significant reduction in microalbuminuria; however, there were more fatal CV events that might be because of excessive BP lowering.[25]

ACCELERATE (Aliskiren and the CCB Amlodipine Combination as Initial Treatment Strategy for Hypertension Control): a randomized parallel group trial. Patients above 18 years or older had a SBP between 150 and 180 mm Hg. About 318 patients were assigned to aliskiren, 316 to amlodipine, and 620 to aliskiren plus amlodipine. Patients given initial combination therapy had a 6.5 mm Hg or greater reduction in mean BP compared to monotherapy groups. Therefore, for initial reduction of SBP >150 mm Hg, combination therapy of aliskiren and amlodipine can be given.[26]

HOT (Hypertension Optimal Treatment) trial in which 18,790 hypertensive patients were treated with long-acting dihydropyridine CCBs felodipine for mean 3.8 years and showed that aggressive BP control in hypertensive diabetics is required that is not possible by monotherapy and suggested ACE inhibitor and CCBs as rational choice in such patients.[27]

ASPIRANT (Addition of Spironolactone in Patients with Resistant Arterial Hypertension) trial in which 25 mg spironolactone was studied in patients with resistant arterial HT. A double-blind, placebo controlled, multicenter trial in which patients with office SBP >140 mm Hg or diastolic BP >90 mm Hg despite treatment with 3 antihypertensives including a diuretic were enrolled. About 117 patients were randomly assigned to receive placebo or spironolactone. The ABPM nighttime systolic, 24 hour ABPM and office SBP were significantly (difference of -8.6, -9.8, -6.5 mm Hg) decreased, while the fall in respective DBP was not significant (-3.0, -1.0, -2.5 mm Hg). Therefore, SBP can be effectively controlled with spironolactone in resistant arterial HT.[28]

SYMPLICITY (Renal Denervation in Patients with Uncontrolled Hypertension) trials include a following series:

***Symplicity HTN-1*:** Series of pilot studies (*n* = 153)

***Symplicity HTN-2*:** Randomized controlled study (*n* = 106)

***Symplicity HTN-3*:** US randomized controlled study (*n* = 530)

***Symplicity HF*:** Pilot study evaluating heart failure patients (*n* = 40)

***Global Symplicity Registry*:** Open label multi-indication registry (*n* = 5000).

Symplicity HTN-1 was a multicenter trial of 153 patients with resistant HT in which endovascular catheter-based renal denervation (RD) was done using Symplicity catheter.[29] Inclusion criteria had patients above 18 years on >3 antihypertensive medications including 1 diuretic with still a office SBP ≥ 160 mm Hg and patients with estimated glomerular filtration rate (eGFR) of <45 mL/min/1.73 m^2 were excluded. Results after 6 months showed a BP reduction of 25/11 mm Hg and 32/14 mm Hg at 2 years that were reconfirmed on Symplicity HTN-2, which was a randomized controlled study.[30] Symplicity HTN-3 has a primary end point office of BP after 6 months of denervation. The data was very positive and RD is already approved in Europe for management of resistant HT. However, the results of SYMPLICITY 3 HTN were pretty shocking as it showed no significant difference between sham control and patients with drug resistant hypertension and it came to an halt. Similarly *EnligHTN* multielectrode RD has following trials:

EnligHTN I trial is a multicenter prospective study including 46 patients using EnligHTN RD system and results have shown an average SBP reduction of 27 mm Hg 1 year after RD.[31]

EnligHTN II trial and *EnligHTN III* trials will further expand on this research and simultaneous ablations with touch screen generator that was shown to reduce the procedure time from 24 minutes to 4 minutes.

EnligHTN IV trial will be conducted by US FDA under an Investigational Device Exemption (IDE).

With this basic understanding of the above trials, we will try and understand how the upcoming JNC 8 guidelines are influenced and what changes one expected to see in the newer guidelines which will make things more crystal clear.

UNDERSTANDING JOINT NATIONAL COMMITTEE (JNC) 8 GUIDELINES

The treating physician wants to understand:

- Latest recommendations in BP measurement
- BP goals in elderly and in presence of co morbidities
- Initial drug therapy options in HT
- Role of compelling indications in choice for management of HT.

Treatment goals are set in HT to reduce the risk of stroke, MI, renal disease, and overall CV disease. Even for patients who are normotensive at the age of 55 years, 90% will develop HT as they age. Guidelines are meant to treat most patients while improving care for all. Currently, JNC 7 recommends BP <130/80 mm Hg for diabetes and CKD and <140/90 mm Hg for elderly.

The expected changes to JNC were as follows:

- Change in BP goals
- Change in methods of measurement
- Priority of getting chosen BP goal rather than choice of first antihypertensive drug
- Salt intake decrease from current recommendation of 2400 mg/day to 1500 mg/day.

The use of automated oscillometric device for BP monitoring will be validated as no trials use stethoscope and sphygmomanometers and oscillometric BP monitors have shown that central aortic pressure can be estimated by noninvasive brachial pressure wave alone.[32] Home BP monitoring (HBPM) recommendation is preferred as it is more truly associated with CV outcomes and target organ damage, improves BP medication compliance, helps to differentiate from white coat HT. HBPM ideally should be done at different times of the day, i.e. am and pm and a note of readings can be made that can be followed up.

ABPM recommendation gives a 24-hour monitoring that can assist in the evaluation of newly diagnosed HT patients, effect of treatment, white coat HT, and drug-resistant HT. Current American Diabetes Association (ADA)/JNC guidelines recommend SBP <130 mm Hg in diabetics that may be different based on patients characteristic and response to therapy and higher or lower BP may be appropriate. The DBP of <80 mm Hg is a good evidence-based goal. The *HOT* trial proved that 81 mm Hg DBP was better than <90 mm Hg. So, new evidence may show BP <140/80 mm Hg in these subset of patients may be the best.

The *ACCORD-BP* trial showed that there is no conclusive evidence that targeting a normal SBP compared with targeting <140 mm Hg lowers the overall risk of CV events in high-risk adults with type 2 diabetes; however, it may reduce the risk of stroke. In CKD patients, there is no evidence to suggest that the guideline of SBP <130 mm Hg improves CV risk or renal outcomes. The *AASK* trial showed no difference in intensive BP control versus standard BP control in these patients. The optimal BP control in patients with CKD remains unclear that may have influenced JNC 8 guidelines.

In elderly patient population, the *VALISH* study showed no difference in primary end point between moderate and strict control. So, a moderate control, i.e. <150 mm Hg may be sufficient to decrease CV risk in elderly HT patients. The debate regarding the initial therapy needs to be sorted out. The BP reduction is more important than the specific agent. Choice of initial therapy will be broadened to include thiazide diuretic, ACE inhibitor, ARB, CCB, or combination therapy as shown by data put forward by *ACCELERATE* and *ACCOMPLISH* trials. Thiazide diuretic is still a good option. Chlorthalidone is more evidence based than HCTZ. Chlorthalidone is one to two times more potent than HCTZ has a longer half life and is good for resistant HT as it can be used with lower GFR as compared to HCTZ.

BBs are not a good choice in elderly patients until there is a compelling indication. The treatment of resistant HT requires screening for identifiable cause like CKD, coarctation of aorta, Cushing disease, drugs like chronic steroid therapy, pheochromocytoma, obstructive sleep apnea (OSA), renovascular HT, thyroid and parathyroid disease, and mineralocorticoid excess states.

Therefore, the preferred combinations for uncomplicated HT are as follows:

- ACE inhibitor with diuretic
- ARB with diuretic
- ACE inhibitor with CCB
- ARB with CCB.

The combinations that are not preferred are as follows:

- ACE inhibitor with ARB as it increases syncope, hypotension, and renal disease.
- Direct rennin inhibitor with ACE inhibitor or ARB.
- BB with sympatholytic (reserpine and clonidine) as it has additive effect and work by similar mechanisms.
- ACE inhibitor or ARB with BBs as it provides little benefit but is appropriate in post MI and systolic heart failure patients.
- Nondihydropyridine CCB (verapamil and diltiazem) with BB as it can cause heart block, bradycardia, and abrupt discontinuation can lead to hypertensive crisis.

Adding spironolactone 12.5–25 mg as add-on therapy to previous treatment is highly effective in patients with resistant HT as proven by *ASPIRANT* trial.

The recommendations for compelling indication to use a drug or combination were unlikely to change in JNC 8 guidelines. The choice of anti-HT drug in the presence of stable angina will be BB, long-acting CCB. In cases of acute coronary syndrome, the choice is BB and ACE inhibitor and addition of other classes to control BP. In post-MI patients, BB and ACE inhibitor decrease in pathological remodeling of heart, lower BP, and prevent myocardial damage. Similarly, in patients with heart failure heart who are asymptomatic; ACE inhibitor and BBs are useful and in symptomatic end stage heart disease ACE inhibitor, BBs, ARBs, aldosterone blockers, and loop diuretics are drugs of choice.

In last 15–20 years when HCTZ was dominant, metolazone, indapamide and role of aldosterone antagonist like spironolactone was being developed. The main issue was the metabolic parameters in patients with chlorthalidone and fixed-dose combinations contained HCTZ. The *MRFIT* (Multiple Risk Factor Intervention Trial) that contained about 6400 patients out of which 60% were originally on HCTZ and remaining on chlorthalidone compared with the results in patients who were on HCTZ at the same time.[33] It showed that the BP was better controlled with chlorthalidone and uric acid and low-density lipoprotein (LDL) levels were higher in HCTZ group. There was a 20% reduction in soft end points like angina, heart failure, and stroke.[32]

The *ACHIEVE-ONE* [Ambulatory Blood Pressure Control and Home Blood Pressure (Morning and Evening) Lowering By N-Channel Blocker cilnidipine] trial is a large scale study on BP and pulse rate (PR) by use of L/N-type CCB cilnidipine for 12 weeks. Clinical SBP decreased 19.6 mm Hg from 155 mm Hg and morning SBP and PR (–3.2 mm Hg and –1.3 beats/minute in first quartile and –30.9 mm Hg and –3.2 beats/minute in fourth quartile) in hypertensive patients at clinic and home with use of clinidipine.[34] HT complicates one in ten pregnancies. It is important to distinguish between a pre-existing HT (chronic) from pregnancy induced (gestational HT) and syndrome of preeclampsia. The norms and treatment are discussed in Tables 7.3 and 7.4.[35]

None of the anti-HT drugs have been proven to be safe in first trimester of pregnancy. Table 7.4 highlights the management of HT in pregnancy along with the recommendations.[36,37]

The management of acute HT in pregnancy is shown in Table 7.5.

Intravenous and intramuscular formulations are needed in severe uncontrolled HT in pregnancy. Drugs that are compatible with breastfeeding are captopril, diltiazem, enalapril, hydralazine, HCTZ, labetalol, methyldopa, minoxidil, nadolol, nifedipine, oxprenolol, propranolol, spironolactone, timolol, and verapamil. In cerebrovascular disease as in acute stroke, the risk and benefit of lowering BP are unclear. Therefore, control of BP to intermediate levels (160/100 mm Hg) is preferable. In case of recurrent stroke, combination of ACE inhibitor and thiazide type diuretic is useful.

The *Rheos Pivotal trial* evaluated BAT (Baroreflex Activation Therapy) on SBP in patients with resistant HT.

Table 7.3 NHBPEP (National High Blood Pressure Education Program Working Group Report on High Blood Pressure in Pregnancy) classification

NHBPEP classification (pregnant) mm Hg	*SBP*	*DBP*
Normal/acceptable	≤140	≤90
Mild HT	140–150	90–109
Severe HT	≥160	≥110

Table 7.4 Drugs for gestational or chronic HT in pregnancy

Drugs	Dose	Comments
Preferred agent		
Methyldopa	0.5–3 g/day in two divided doses	Drug of choice according to NHBPEP, safety in 1st trimester not documented
Second-line agents		
Labetalol	200–1200 mg/day in two to three divided doses	May be associated with fetal growth restriction
Nifedipine	30–120 mg/day slow release preparation	May inhibit labor; have synergistic action with magnesium sulfate in BP lowering
Hydralazine	50–300 mg/day in two-four divided doses	Useful in combination with sympatholytic agent, may cause neonatal thrombocytopenia
β-receptor blockers	Depends on agent	May decrease uteroplacental blood flow, may impair fetal response to hypoxic stress; risk of growth restriction when started in first or second trimester (atenolol); may be associated with neonatal hypoglycemia at higher doses
Hydrochlorothiazide	12.5–25 mg/day	Controlled studies in normotensive pregnant women rather than hypertensive patients; can cause volume contraction and electrolyte disorders; may be useful in combination with methyldopa and vasodilator
Contraindicated		
ACE inhibitor and ARB		Fetal loss, cardiac defects and renal agenesis

Table 7.5 Management of acute severe HT in pregnancy

Agent	Dosage
Hydralazine (preferred)	5 mg IV bolus, then 10 mg every 20–30 minutes (maximum –25 mg); repeat in several hours if needed
Labetalol (second line)	20 mg IV bolus, 40 mg 10 minutes later, 80 mg every 10 minutes for two additional doses (maximum –220 mg)
Nifedipine (controversial)	10 mg orally, repeat every 20 minutes (maximum –30 mg), can precipitate BP drop with magnesium sufate; short acting not FDA approved
Sodium nitroprusside (when other agent fail)	0.5 µg/kg/min to maximum 5 µg/kg/min. Fetal cyanide poisoning may occur if used >4 hours

Resistant HT is defined as failure to achieve target BP (<140/90 mm Hg and <130/80 mm Hg in diabetics and CKD) in patients on three appropriate antihypertensives including a diuretic that is mostly seen in metabolic syndrome, CKD, or diabetics. The Rheos system consists of a device with bilateral leads that are tunneled subcutaneously to attach to carotid sinus and a pulse generator. Programming is accomplished via an external programming system. It showed that BAT can significantly reduce SBP in resistant HT. However, it did not meet end points for acute responders and procedural safety will be addressed in future trials.[38] Other, important trials in resistant HT have been shown in *SYMPLICITY* and *EnligHTN* trials with catheter based radiofrequency ablation known as RD. It will be interesting to see how this data eventually influences the JNC 8 guidelines.

There is strong evidence for J-shaped relationship between DBP and SBP and outcomes in HT, high-risk hypertensives, CAD, diabetes mellitus, elderly and in left ventricular hypertrophy (LVH) but further studies need to clarify the issue. This is because most of the studies are observational. The Systolic Blood Pressure Interventional Trial (*SPRINT*)[39] in 2018 and Optimal Blood Pressure and Cholesterol Targets for Preventing Recurrent Stroke in Hypertensives (*ESH-CHL-SHOT*)[40] will be finally able to answer the questions. As per current knowledge, it may be reasonable to suggest BP levels of 130–135/80–85 mm Hg in HT patients and one has to be careful while lowering BP further in high-risk HT patients (Table 7.6). In pediatric age group, the recommendations are as follows:

- HT is average SBP and/or DBP ≥95th percentile for gender, age, and height on three or more occasions.
- Prehypertension is defined as average SBP or DBP levels that are ≥90th percentile but <95th percentile.

Table 7.6 Recommended dimensions for BP cuff bladders

Age range	Width (cm)	Length (cm)	Maximum arm circumference (cm)
Newborn	4	8	10
Infant	6	12	15
Child	9	18	22
Small adult	10	24	26
Adult	13	30	34
Large adult	16	38	44

- In both adults and adolescents, BP ≥120/80 mm Hg is prehypertension.
- BP >95th percentile in doctor's office and normal outside is white-coat HT and needs ABPM.

Randomized controlled trials of yoga and biofeedback in management of HT have shown a highly significant reduction in HT compared to control groups. Similar results have been shown in pregnant women, decreasing the hospital admissions for HT.[41,42]

Vaccines in HT are injected every 4–6 months and are an innovative treatment. The disruption of rennin-angiotensin-aldosterone system is the most common etiology; therefore, the first vaccine study was carried against rennin. The vaccines reduced BP in animals but also produced an autoimmune disease. Vaccines against angiotensin 1, angiotensin II, angiotensin II type-1 have shown good safety profiles in both animals and humans. CYT006-AngQb (angiotensin-II vaccine) reduced BP in humans, but the result was not reproducible. The RAAS may be an important target for the development of vaccines for the treatment and prevention of HT and hypertensive complications in future.[43]

The BP goals as per JNC 8 for patients < 60 years, diabetes, CKD patients is <140/90 mm Hg and for patients >60 years is <150/90 mm Hg.

CONCLUSION

Based on the available data, one expects to see certain changes in the current guidelines that can sort out these controversies. First, use of oscillometric method of measuring BP and home monitoring helps in achieving target BP goals in a better way. Second, recent evidence may change the current BP goals in diabetes mellitus and CKD patients. JNC 8 has considered a BP goal of < 140/90 mm Hg for both diabetes and CKD patients. It does not make much difference which agent is first used to achieve target BP unless there is a compelling indication as discussed. So, what matters the most is that BP is appropriately reduced to the chosen goal. Last, most patients will require combination therapy with two or more agents at diagnosis.

REFERENCES

1. Kaerney PM, Whelton M, Reynolds K, et al. Global burden of hypertension: analysis of worldwide data. Lancet. 2005;365:217-23.
2. Whelton PK, He J, Munter P. Prevalence, awareness, treatment and control of hypertension in North America, North Africa and Asia. J Hum Hypertens. 2004;18:545-51.
3. Wolf-Maier K, Cooper RS, Kramer H, et al. Hypertension treatment and control in five European countries, Canada and United States. Hypertension. 2004;43:10-17.
4. Blood Pressure Lowering Treatment Trialist's collaboration. Effects of different blood pressure-lowering regimens on major cardiovascular events: results of prospectively-designed overviews of randomized trials. Lancet. 2003;362:1527-35.
5. Staessen JA, Wang JG, Thijs L. Cardiovascular prevention and blood pressure reduction: a quantitative overview updated until March 1 2003. J Hypertens. 2003;21:1055-76.
6. Chobanian AV, Bakris GL, Black HR, et al. Seventh report of Joint National Committee on Prevention, Detection, Evaluation and Treatment of High Blood Pressure. Hypertension. 2003;42(6): 1206-52.
7. Dluhy RG, McMohan GT. Intensive glycemic control in ACCORD and advance trials. N Engl J Med. 2008;358:2630-33.
8. Lindholm LH, Ibsen H, Dahlof B, et al. Cardiovascular morbidity and mortality in patients with diabetes in Losartan Intervention for Endpoint reduction in hypertension study (LIFE): a randomized trial against atenolol. Lancet. 2002;359:1004-10.
9. The ONTARGET/TRANSCEND Investigators. Rationale, design, and baseline characteristics of 2 large, simple, randomized trials evaluating telmisartan, ramipril, and ramipril and their combination in high-risk patients: The Ongoing Telmisartan Alone and in Combination with Ramipril Global Endpoint Trial/Telmisartan Randomized AssessmeNT Study in ACE iNtolerant subjects with cardiovascular Disease (ONTARGET/TRANSCEND) trials. Am Heart J. 2004;148(1):52-61.
10. The Task Force for management of arterial hypertension of the European Society of Hypertension (ESH) and the European Society of Cardiology (ESC). 2013 ESH/ESC Guidelines for management of arterial hypertension. Eur Heart J. 2013:i:10.1093/eurheartj/eht151.
11. Godlee F. Controversies over hypertension guidelines. BMJ. 2012;344:e653.
12. Katakam R, Brukamp K, Townsend RR. What is the proper workup of a patient with hypertension? Cleve Clin J Med. 2008; 75(9):663-72.
13. Bianchi S, Bigazzi R, Campese VM. Microalbuminuria in essential hypertension: significance, pathophysiology and therapeutic implications. Am J Kidney Dis. 1999;34(6):973-95.
14. Mancia G, Fagard R, Narkiewicz K, et al. 2013 ESH/ESC Guidelines for the management of arterial hypertension. 23rd European Meeting on Hypertension and Cardiovascular Protection.
15. The ALLHAT officers and coordinators for the ALLHAT Collaborative Research Group. Major outcomes in high-risk hypertensive patients randomized for angiotensin-converting enzyme inhibitor or calcium channel blockers vs. diuretic.

The Antihypertensive and Lipid-Lowering Treatment to Prevent Heart Attack Trial (ALLHAT). JAMA 2002;288:2981-97.
16. Weber MA, Bakris GL, Dalhöf B, et al. Baseline characteristics in Avoiding Cardiovascular events through Combination therapy in Patients Living with Systolic Hypertension (ACCOMPLISH) trial: a hypertensive population at high cardiovascular risk. Blood Press. 2007;16:13-9.
17. Gerstein HC, Riddle MC, Kendall DM, et al. Glycemic treatment strategies in the Action to Control Cardiovascular Risk in Diabetes (ACCORD) trial. AM J Cardiol. 2007;99:34i-43i.
18. Wright JT, Jr, Bakris G, Greene T, et al. Effect of blood pressure lowering and antihypertensive drug class on progression of hypertensive kidney disease: results from the AASK trial. JAMA. 2002;288(19):2421-31.
19. Ogihara T, Saruta T, Rakugi H, et al., for the Valsartan in Elderly Isolated Systolic Hypertension Study Group. Target blood pressure for treatment of isolated systolic hypertension in the elderly: Valsartan in Elderly Isolated Systolic Hypertension study. Hypertension. 2010;56:196-202.
20. SHEP Cooperative Research Group. Prevention of stroke by antihypertensive drug treatment in older persons with isolated systolic hypertension: final results of Systolic Hypertension in the Elderly program (SHEP). JAMA.1991;265:3255-64.
21. Beckett NS, Peters R, Fletcher AE, et al. Treatment of hypertension in patients 80 years of age or older. N Engl J Med. 2008;358: 1887-98.
22. Nissen SE,Tuzcu EM, Libby P, et al. Effect of antihypertensive agents on cardiovascular events in patients with coronary disease and blood pressure: the CAMELOT study: a randomized control trial. JAMA. 2004;292:2217-25.
23. Svensson P, de Faire U, Sleight P, et al. Comparative effects of ramipril on ambulatory and office blood pressures: a HOPE substudy. Hypertension. 2001;38:E28-32.
24. Pepine CJ, Handberg EM, Cooper-DeHoff RM, et al. A calcium antagonist vs. a non-calcium antagonist hypertension strategy for patients with coronary artery disease. The International Verapamil-Trandolapril Study (INVEST): a randomized controlled trial. JAMA. 2003;290:2805-16.
25. Haller, H, Ito, S Izzo JL, et al. Olmesartan for the delay or prevention of microalbuminuria in type 2 diabetes. N Engl J Med. 2011;365:907-17.
26. Brown MJ, McInnes GT, Papst CC, et al. Aliskiren and calcium channel blocker amlodipine combination as an initial treatment strategy for hypertension control (ACCELERATE): a randomized, parallel-group trial. Lancet. 2011;377:312-20.
27. Hansson L, Zanchetti A, Carruthers SG, et al. The HOT study group. Effects of intensive blood-pressure lowering and the low-dose aspirin in patients with hypertension: principal results of the Hypertension Optimal Treatment (HOT) randomized trial. Lancet. 1998;351:1755-62.
28. Vaclavik J, Sedlak R, Plachy M, et al. Addition of Spironolactone in Patient with Resistant Arterial Hypertension (ASPIRANT). A randomized, double-blind, placebo-controlled trial. Hypertension. 2011; 57:1069-75.
29. Symplicity HTN-1 Investigators. Catheter-based renal sympathetic denervation for resistant hypertension durability of blood pressure reduction out to 24 months Symplicity HTN-1 investigators. Hypertension. 2011;57:911-7.
30. Symplicity HTN-2 Investigators. Renal sympathetic denervation in patients with treatment-resistant hypertension (the Symplicity HTN-2 Trial): a randomized controlled trial. Lancet. 2010;376: 1903-09.
31. Worthley SG, Tsioufis CP, Worthley MI, et al. Safety and efficacy of multielectrode renal sympathetic denervation system in resistant hypertension: the EnligHTN1trial. Eur Heart J. 2013 doi:10.1093/eurheartj/eht197. Europeon heart journal Advance Access published June 19, 2013.
32. Chenq HM, Wanq KL, Chen YH, et al. Estimation of central systolic blood pressure using an oscillometric blood pressure monitor. Hypertens Res. 2010;33(6):592-9.
33. Dorsch MP, Gillespie BW, Erickson SR, et al. Chlorthalidone reduces cardiovascular events compared with hydrochlorothiazide: a retrospective cohort analysis. Hypertension. 2011;57:689-94.
34. Kario K, Nariyama J, Kido H, et al. Effect of a novel calcium blocker on abnormal nocturnal blood pressure in hypertensive patients. J Clin Hypertens (Greenwich). 2013;15(7):465-72.
35. Report of the National High Blood Pressure Education Program Working Group on high blood pressure in pregnancy. Am J Obstet Gynecol. 2000;183:S1-S22.
36. Sibai BM. Treatment of hypertension in pregnancy. N Eng J Med. 1996;335:257-65.
37. Walker JJ. Pre-eclampsia. Lancet. 2000;356:1260-5.
38. Bisognano JD, Bakris G, Nadim MK, et al. Baroreflex activation therapy lowers blood pressure in patients with resistant hypertension. Results from the double-blind, randomized, placebo-controlled Rheos Pivotal Trial. J Am Coll Cordiol. 2011;58(7):763-73.
39. Systolic Blood Pressure Intervention Trial (SPRINT). Clinical Trials.gov Identifier: NCT0120606.
40. Optimal Blood Pressure and Cholesterol Targets for Preventing Recurrent Stroke in Hypertensives (ESH-CHL-SHOT).Clinical Trials.gov Identifier:NCT01563731.
41. Little BC, Benson P, Beard RW, et al. Treatment of hypertension in pregnancy by relaxation and biofeedback. Lancet. 1984; 323(8832):865.
42. Patel C, North WR. Randomized controlled trial of yoga and biofeedback in management of hypertension. Lancet. 1975; 306(7925):93-5.
43. DO TH, Chen Y, Nquyen VT, et al. Vaccines in the management of hypertension. Expert Opin Biol Ther. 2010;10(7):1077-87.

8

Statin-induced Myopathy

Peeyush Jain

INTRODUCTION

Statins [3-hydroxy-3-methylglutaryl coenzyme A (HMG-CoA) reductase inhibitors] reduce cardiovascular (CV) morbidity and mortality in various populations at risk and are safe in majority of patients.[1] These agents have been in clinical use for more than two decades and concerns about their side effects continue to be raised.[2,3] Some patients on statin therapy report varying degrees of muscle-related symptoms. Though muscle symptoms are reversible in majority of cases after statin withdrawal, CV risk reduction in severe statin intolerance remains challenging.

STATIN-INDUCED MUSCLE SYMPTOMS

Statin-induced muscle symptoms may manifest as muscle pain, tenderness, or weakness. Pain is typically aching or cramping, widespread or generalized, and may be exacerbated by exercise. Muscle weakness is usually proximal. Nocturnal leg cramps may occur. Subjective variations in symptoms may lead to description of discomfort as backache or proximal limb or localized pain that may prompt some clinicians to overlook the possibility of statin myopathy.[3-5] Rhabdomyolysis occurs rarely.

For descriptive purposes, muscle symptoms may be broadly classified into myalgia [muscle symptoms without creatine phosphokinase (CK) elevation], myositis [muscle symptoms with CK elevation], and rhabdomyolysis [muscle symptoms with marked CK elevations (>10 times upper limit of normal, ULN) with an elevated serum creatinine and occasional myoglobinuria]. Myopathy is a general term for any of these.

INCIDENCE

A meta-analysis of 71,108 subjects in 18 randomized placebo-controlled primary and secondary prevention trials of statin monotherapy with 3,01,374 person-years of follow-up concluded that the numbers needed to harm (NNH) with statin therapy were 197 for any adverse event against the number needed to treat (NNT) of 27 to prevent one CV event. NNH for CK >10 times of ULN or rhabdomyolysis was 3,400 and NNH for rhabdomyolysis was 7,428. The adverse event rate was highest with atorvastatin and lowest with fluvastatin.[6]

In another systematic review of 20 randomized clinical trials, voluntary notifications, and case reports with 1,80,000 person-years of follow-up, the incidence of muscle symptoms in cohort studies and randomized controlled trials was 11/1,00,000 patient years, while the incidence of muscle symptoms and CK elevation >10-fold above ULN was 5/1,00,000 person-years.[7] The incidence of rhabdomyolysis (CK elevation >10,000 IU/L, elevation of serum creatinine, or need for hydration) was 3.4/1,00,000 patient years. Incidence was higher with lovastatin, simvastatin, and atorvastatin [statins metabolized by cytochrome P450 3A4 (CYP3A4)] than pravastatin and fluvastatin.

The incidence of statin-induced myopathy in real-world practice is higher than reported in randomized clinical trials as in the latter, high-risk patients like elderly, and those with renal and hepatic impairment are generally excluded.[8] In the United States Food and Drug Administration (US FDA) Adverse Event Reporting System Database, recorded till 2002, myopathy was reported in 0.38 cases per million statin prescriptions with rhabdomyolysis in 1.07 cases per million statin prescriptions.[9] However, these findings are likely an underestimation due to voluntary nature of reporting in such databases. Prediction of Muscular Risk in Observational Conditions (PRIMO), a managed care database in France, found that 832 of 7924 (10.5%) unselected patients treated with high-dose statin therapy reported myalgias during 1 year follow-up. The number of patients reporting muscle symptoms was highest in those receiving simvastatin (18.2%), followed by atorvastatin (14.9%), pravastatin (10.9%), and fluvastatin (5.1%).[10]

MECHANISM OF STATIN MYOPATHY

Despite several hypotheses, the mechanism of statin myopathy is not known. Cholesterol plays an important role in cell membrane fluidity. Therefore, it has been suggested that cholesterol reduction with statins may affect membrane integrity. However, if statin myopathy is due to changes in skeletal muscle membrane fluidity, every other cholesterol-lowering agent should also have the same effect.

Another set of hypotheses have suggested that reduced synthesis of mevalonate following inhibition of HMG-CoA reductase reduces a number of isoprenoids besides inhibition of cholesterol synthesis. Isoprenoid deficiency may have varied effects including impairment of synthesis of ubiquinone [Coenzyme Q10 (CoQ10)]. Depletion of CoQ10 has been proposed to predispose to myopathy. As CoQ10 participates in electron transport chain, its deficiency may result in abnormal mitochondrial energy production.[11] CoQ10 may also have antioxidant function at the level of mitochondria and lipid membranes.[12] Though statin treatment does reduce circulating CoQ10 levels, its effect on muscle CoQ10 content is not clear, and there are few studies of muscle CoQ10 content in patients with statin myopathy.[13,14] CoQ10 supplementation can raise its circulating levels but whether it prevents or improves myopathy is also not clear.[15] Besides reduction in CoQ10 generation, in vivo and in vitro studies support that statins-induced reduction in isoprenoid levels may induce skeletal muscle apoptosis and myopathy in a dose-dependent manner.[16,17] Statins block the production of farnesyl pyrophosphate and this prevents the prenylation of GTP-binding proteins RacI, and RhoA and their translocation from cytosol to the membrane.[17] A reduction in the levels of the prenylated forms of these proteins leads to increased cytosolic calcium levels with subsequent activation of the proteolytic enzymes capase-3 and capase-9, which play a central role in cell death.[18] This is supported by an in-vitro study that demonstrated that statin-induced apoptosis of muscle cells is prevented by supplementation with the isoprenoids farnesyl pyrophosphate and geranylgeranyl pyrophosphate.[17] Statins may also affect intracellular calcium homeostasis by other mechanisms. In animal models, statins increase cytosplasmic calcium by increasing mitochondrial calcium permeability. It also increases calcium release from the sarcoplasmic reticulum by reducing calcium ATPase activity.[12,19] Increased cytoplasmic calcium levels have been shown to cause cramps, myalgias, and apoptosis.[20,21]

Statin myopathy may have genetic determinants. Study of the Effectiveness of Additional Reductions in Cholesterol and Homocysteine (SEARCH) trial hypothesized that genetic variants may affect statin blood levels.[22] In this trial, a genome-wide analysis demonstrated that myopathy was strongly associated with a single nucleotide polymorphism within intron 11 of *SLCO1B1* gene on chromosome 12. *SLCO1B1* encodes the organ anion transporting polypeptide responsible for hepatic uptake of statins. In SEARCH trial, 60% of myopathy cases were associated with *SLCO1B1* variants. As many as 31 candidate genes have been associated with statin-induced myalgia. A recent investigation of genetic variants predictive of muscle side effects in statin-treated patients utilizing a physiogenomic approach validated three previously hypothesized candidate genes: CoQ2 encoding para-hydroxybenzoate-polyprenyl-transferase, which participates in the biosynthesis of CoQ10; ATP2B1 that encodes a calcium transporting ATPase involved in calcium homeostasis; and DMPK that encodes a protein kinase implicated in myotonic dystrophy.[23] Further understanding of such genetic markers could help in prediction of statin myopathy.

PREDISPOSING FACTORS (TABLE 8.1)

While mechanism of statin myopathy is not known, there is a better understanding of factors that predispose to it (Table 8.1). Major risk factors for rhabdomyolysis include concomitant therapy with gemfibrozil and chronic kidney disease (CKD). Statins metabolized by CYP3A4 (lovastatin, simvastatin, and atorvastatin) are four times more likely to cause rhabdomyolysis than fluvastatin and pravastatin [FDA Adverse Effects Reporting System (FAERS)].[9] Adverse drug interaction of statins with fusidic acid has also been reported.[24]

Table 8.1 Risk factors for statin myopathy

Demographic features	*Concomitant disorders (Contd.)*
Elderly	Uncontrolled hypothyroidism
Personal or family history of muscular symptoms or cramps	Major recent surgery
Female gender	Elevated CK levels
Caribbean and black Africans	Hypoalbuminemia
Anthropometric characteristics	Renal insufficiency
Low body mass index	*Medication affecting statin metabolism*
Lifestyles	Amiodarone
Excessive physical activity	Cyclosporin
Excessive alcohol consumption	Diltiazem
Genetic factors	Gemfibrozil
Statin-related factors	Macrolide antibiotics
High dose	Protease inhibitors
Statins metabolized by CYP3A4	Systemic azole antifungals
Lipophilic statins	Verapamil
Concomitant disorders	*Other concomitant medication*
Hepatic dysfunction	Corticosteroids

DETERMINANTS OF STATIN MYOPATHY

***Duration of statin therapy*:** Most cases of myopathy manifest within first 3 months of initiation of statin treatment but may be delayed as much as 1 year.[25] In one study of 45 subjects with statin-induced myopathy, symptoms developed after a mean of 6.3 ± 9.8 months and persisted up to 2.3 ± 3.0 months after discontinuation of therapy.[26]

***Statin dosage*:** It is generally believed that an increase in statin exposure increases the risk of myopathy[3] but some studies have found no such correlation. In a review of atorvastatin trials, the reported frequency of myalgias was identical with low versus high doses (1.4% with 10 mg/day and 1.5% with 80 mg/day).[27] Nevertheless, some high-dose statins may be more risky than others. The rate of myopathy and rhabdomyolysis for simvastatin 80 mg/day has been reported to be about four times higher than that for atorvastatin 80 mg/day.[28]

***Achieved low-density lipoprotein cholesterol (LDL-C)*:** Retrospective analysis of Pravastatin or Atorvastatin Evaluation and Infection Therapy (PROVE-IT) study and another meta-analysis suggested that adverse effects of statins are not related to achieved LDL-C.[29] In one meta-analysis, with 3,09,506 person-years of follow-up, there was no significant relationship between percent LDL-C lowering and rates of rhabdomyolysis. Similar results were obtained when absolute LDL-C reduction or achieved LDL-C levels were considered.[30]

***Combination lipid-lowering drug therapy*:** While the combination of ezetimibe, bile-acid sequestering agents, niacin, and fenofibrate with moderate doses of statins appears to be reasonably safe, there is paucity of data related to long-term safety of combination therapy with high-dose statins.

LOW-DENSITY LIPOPROTEIN CHOLESTEROL LOWERING IN STATIN INTOLERANT PATIENTS

Statin intolerance should be considered in patients with muscle-related symptoms after elimination of other causes. Those with tolerable symptoms and CK elevation less than five times ULN may be followed clinically. Patients with severe myalgia and those with CK elevation more than five times ULN should stop statin. After CK has fallen in normal range, the same statin may be reintroduced to confirm statin intolerance. LDL-C reduction in such cases is difficult and there are no established rules to follow in such a situation but the following may be tried:

Reduce the Statin Dose

Though practiced commonly, no clinical trial has been addressed to the feasibility and efficacy of such a strategy.

Switch to Another Statin

There are scarce data documenting the safety of another statin if a patient has not been able tolerate one statin. The available evidence indicates that this is unsuccessful in more than half of the instances. In one study of 45 patients with confirmed statin myopathy, 37 were given another statin. Twenty one (57%) had recurrence of myalgia and sixteen (43%) tolerated the new statin without myalgia.[26] To minimize recurrence of statin myopathy with another statin, it may be worthwhile to switch over from (i) a lipophilic statin to a hydrophilic statin or (ii) a CYPP450 dependent on a non-CYP450-dependent statin, or (iii) a high dose of a less potent statin to a lower dose of a more potent statin. A prospective open-label pilot study of 9 months duration in 61 hypercholesterolemic patients found that small doses of rosuvastatin (5 or 10 mg/day) were generally well tolerated by statin-intolerant patients. Of the 61 subjects, only one discontinued rosuvastatin after 4 weeks due to myalgia without CK elevation,[31] (iv) switch over to fluvastatin, the statin that is least likely to cause myopathy. A 12-week double-blinded, double-dummy trial of 199 statin intolerant patients found that fluvastatin 80 mg/day lowered LDL-C by 32.8% compared with 15.6% with ezetimibe ($P < 0.0001$) and the fluvastatin XL/ezetimibe combination lowered LDL-C by 46.1%. The incidence of muscle related symptoms was 24% (ezetimibe group), 17% (fluvastatin group), and 14% (the combination group) with no instances of CK increases ≥10 times ULN. Thus, fluvastatin alone or in combination with ezetimibe may offer an effective and well-tolerated lipid-lowering option in patients with a history of statin myopathy.[32]

Intermittent Statin Dosing

Statins with long half-life like atorvastatin and rosuvastatin may have lipid-lowering effect beyond 24 hours. The rationale is that the adverse effects of statins may be related to the cumulative amount of drug ingested over time, and if so, the adverse effects may be attenuated by alternate-day dosing.[33] Thus, intermittent dosing, ranging from alternate day to once a week dosing, may be justified for atorvastatin with a mean half-life of 14 hours that also has active metabolites with a half-life of 20–30 hours that contribute to 70% of its HMG CoA reductase activity.[34] Rosuvastatin also has a long half-life of 18 hours.[35]

Studies with Alternate Day Atorvastatin

Uncontrolled studies

- In one study, 61 hypercholesterolemic patients received 10 mg atorvastatin every alternate days for 8 weeks that resulted in 23% reduction in LDL-C.[36]
- In another study, 25 patients given alternate day atorvastatin (mean dose 18.8 mg) or rosuvastatin (mean dose 9.7 mg) had 43% reduction in LDL-C with atorvastatin and 28% reduction with rosuvastatin ($P < 0.05$ for both).[37]

Controlled studies

- Alternate Day versus Daily Dosing of Atorvastatin Study (ADDAS) reported equal efficacy of 10 mg daily or alternate day 20 mg of atorvastatin.[38]
- In another study of 61 patients, there was an equal improvement in lipids after 3 months of 20 mg atorvastatin every day or every alternate day.[39]

Studies with Alternate Day Rosuvastatin

- Rosuvastatin 2.5 mg and 5 mg on alternate days for 6 weeks in two atorvastatin intolerant patients resulted in LDL-C reduction of 38% and 20%, respectively, without further myalgias.[40]
- In a retrospective analysis, 37 of 51 (72.5%) patients with statin intolerance were able to tolerate alternate day rosuvastatin, mean dose 5.6 mg, for 4 months that led to 34.5% reduction in mean LDL-C in patients who were able to tolerate rosuvastatin ($P < 0.001$), enabling approximately 50% to achieve their LDL-C goal.[41]
- Thirty-seven Chinese patients who were randomly given rosuvastatin 10 mg every other day ($n = 19$) or once-daily ($n = 18$) for 6 weeks had identical reduction in LDL-C (37.5% vs. 36.9%, $P > 0.05$).[42]

Studies with Twice Weekly Rosuvastatin

In one study, 80% (32 of 40) patients intolerant to daily statins were able to tolerate 5–10 mg of rosuvastatin twice weekly for a mean of 8 weeks with 26% reduction in mean LDL-C.[43]

Studies with Once a Week Rosuvastatin

In one study, eight patients intolerant to daily statin given 5–20 mg of rosuvastatin once a week registered 29% reduction in mean LDL-C.[44]

Combination Therapy with Intermittent Statin Dosing

Fifty-six statin intolerant patients were given ezetimibe 10 mg/day and atorvastatin 10 mg twice weekly was added after evaluating patients' response. By this strategy, there was 34% reduction in the mean LDL-C levels and 84% of the subjects were able to achieve target LDL-C.[45]

A recent review of 10 studies of varying regimens with atorvastatin and/or rosuvastatin concluded that at least 70% of statin intolerant patients were able to tolerate an intermittent dosing strategy without recurrence of previous treatment-limiting adverse effects. The LDL-C lowering varied from 12% to 38%, which is lower than daily dosing.[46] Another review of 17 studies (14 prospective and 3 retrospective) involving alternate-day statin dosing concluded that alternate-day statin therapy may limit adverse reactions and potentially increase compliance and positively affecting the lipids concurrently.[47] Yet, these conclusions are based on uncontrolled or small studies with brief follow-up. The efficacy of CV risk reduction cannot be determined from such trials; therefore, large-scale randomized trials are necessary to define the role of this strategy and an optimal regimen.

Nonstatin Lipid-lowering Therapy

Nonstatin drugs like a bile acid sequestrant, ezetimibe, or nicotinic acid may be considered if the patient remains intolerant to alternative statin(s), dose reduction, or intermittent dosing.

***Bile acid sequestrants*:** Colesevelam, a nonabsorbable water-soluble hydrogel, reduces LDL-C by 15–19%, but there is no clinical trial data demonstrating its efficacy in statin intolerant patients.[48]

***Ezetimibe*:** It is a specific inhibitor of intestinal cholesterol absorption, reduces LDL-C by 15–20% with monotherapy.[49] In a series of 27 statin intolerant patients, ezetimibe was well-tolerated over 3 months and resulted in 26% reduction in LDL-C ($P < 0.001$).[50]

***Colesevelam and ezetimibe*:** In a retrospective analysis of 16 statin intolerant patients, a combination of colesevelam and ezetimibe reduced LDL-C by 42.2% and was well tolerated.[51]

***Nicotinic acid (Niacin)*:** In addition to increasing HDL-C and decreasing triglyceride levels, nicotinic acid leads to a modest reduction in LDL-C.[52] Even though there are no published data on its safety and efficacy in statin-intolerant patients, coronary drug project, a large randomized controlled trial in prestatin era, reported a significant decrease in coronary events.[53] Angiographic trials in the 80^{S} also demonstrated that a combination of niacin and colestipol slowed angiographic progression of coronary atherosclerosis.[54,55]

Alternative Therapies

Chinese red yeast rice, made by fermenting the yeast, *Monascus purpureus*, over rice contains monacolin K, a natural form of lovastatin that reduces LDL-C by inhibiting HMG CoA reductase.[56] In a randomized placebo-controlled trial of 62 statin-intolerant dyslipidemic patients (mean baseline LDL-C 163 mg/dL), red yeast rice reduced LDL-C by 21.3% after 6 months without increase in CK levels or myalgias.[57] LDL-C reduction was maintained up to 1 year in a study of 48 statin-intolerant patients with a combination of monacoline K, phytostanols, and benerine.[58] A community-based trial compared the tolerability of red yeast rice and pravastatin in patients unable to tolerate other statins. A total of 43 adults were randomly assigned to red yeast rice

2400 mg twice daily (group 1) or pravastatin 20 mg twice daily (group 2) for 12 weeks. The incidence of treatment discontinuation due to myalgia was 5% in group 1 versus 9% in group 2 ($P = 0.99$). No difference was found in pain severity or muscle strength between the two groups. Thus, red yeast rice was as well tolerated as pravastatin in patients intolerant to other statins.[59] Another retrospective study identified 25 patients treated with red yeast rice for ≥4 weeks who had discontinued lipid-lowering drug therapy due to myalgias (68%), gastrointestinal intolerance (16%), and/or elevated alanine aminotransferase levels (8%). In statin-intolerant patients, red yeast rice was found to reduce LDL-C by 19% during 74 ± 39 days of treatment and was well tolerated by 92% of the patients.[60] Monacolin K contents of various formulations of red yeast rice may vary substantially from brand to brand and batch to batch. The long-term effects of red yeast rice on CV events are also not known.

MANAGEMENT OF STATIN MYOPATHY

Few options are available for management of statin myopathy, given a lack of understanding of its pathogenesis. Limited data are available on the role of CoQ10 or vitamin D supplementation.

Coenzyme Q10

In a double-blinded study in patients with myopathic symptoms ($n = 18$), 100 mg/day of CoQ10 for 4 weeks reduced myalgias by 40% ($P < 0.001$).[61] Another double-blinded study of 60 patients also found significant improvement in symptoms of statin-induced myopathy with CoQ10 supplementation ($P < 0.001$).[62] In another open-label study of 28 patients, administration of CQ10 for 6 months led to about 50% reduction in muscle pain and weakness ($P < 0.0001$).[63] These findings have not been substantiated by other studies and systematic reviews.[64-67] An ongoing placebo-controlled cross over trial of CoQ10 in patients with history of myalgia during statin treatment is currently underway to examine the extent and intensity of muscle pain during treatment with simvastatin.[68]

Vitamin D

An association between statin-related myopathy and vitamin D deficiency has been reported. It has been proposed that low CYP enzyme activity related to vitamin D deficiency may increase blood levels, and hence, toxicity of CYP metabolized statins. As vitamin D deficiency has been proposed to predispose to toxicity of CYP metabolized statins, concurrent vitamin D may reduce dosage requirements, thereby reducing toxicity. A case series report suggested an association between vitamin D insufficiency and statin-induced myalgia that may be reversed with vitamin D supplementation while continuing statin therapy; 92% (35/38) of the patients with statin-induced myalgias and low vitamin D levels were rendered myalgia free after vitamin D supplementation for 3 months.[69] In a recent prospective study, 150 hypercholesterolemic patients with low serum 25-hydroxy (25-OH) vitamin D, unable to tolerate statin(s) because of myopathy, were restarted on statin therapy after 3 weeks of vitamin D supplementation. After a median of 8.1 months, 87% of previously intolerant patients were able to continue statins without myalgia.[70] However, in a recent pilot study of 93 statin-treated patients, 33% of whom reported myopathy, serum 25-OH vitamin D was not found to be a predictor of myopathy.[71] In another retrospective study of electronic database of 6808 patients to whom statins were dispensed, no association was found between low 25-OH vitamin D levels and statin-induced myalgia or CK elevation.[72] Given the paucity of studies, their suboptimal quality, and contradictory findings, further study is needed to define the role of vitamin D deficiency in statin myopathy.[73]

PERSISTENCE OF MYOPATHY AFTER STATIN WITHDRAWAL

Persistence of neuromuscular symptoms and elevated CK levels after withdrawal of statin therapy is not uncommon and may be the result of statin-related myotoxicity or an underlying neuromuscular disorder. In a series of 52 consecutive patients with muscle weakness, myalgia, or both, along with elevated CK levels (mean 1000 U/L) that had persisted for more than 3 months after discontinuation of statin therapy, 47 (90%) were found to have possible statin-induced myotoxicity with a good prognosis at the 6-month follow-up. Five patients (10%) presented with abnormalities on electromyography and muscle biopsy and received the diagnoses of paraneoplastic polymyositis, amyotrophic lateral sclerosis, Kennedy's disease, muscle phosphorylase *b* kinase deficiency, and necrotic myopathy of uncertain cause. It was suggested that patients with neuromuscular symptoms and elevated CK levels that persist after statin withdrawal should be systematically evaluated for an underlying neuromuscular disease. Electromyography was an excellent screening test to determine whether a muscle biopsy was needed. As some patients who are believed to have a statin-induced myopathy may have pre-existing myopathies, routine measurement of CK before the initiation of statin therapy should be helpful in making an earlier diagnosis of a neuromuscular disease.[74]

REFERENCES

1. Baigent C, Keech A, Kearney PM, et al. Cholesterol Treatment Trialists' (CTT) Collaborators. Efficacy and safety of cholesterol-lowering treatment: prospective meta-analysis of data from 90,056 participants in 14 randomised trials of statins. Lancet. 2005;366:1267-78.

2. Gotto AM Jr. Statins, cardiovascular disease, and drug safety. Am J Cardiol. 2006;97(8A):3C-5C.
3. Armitage J. The safety of statins in clinical practice. Lancet. 2007; 370:1781-90.
4. Harper CR, Jacobson TA. The broad spectrum of statin myopathy: from myalgia to rhabdomyolysis. Curr Opin Lipidol. 2007;18:401-8.
5. Phillips PS, Haas RH. Statin myopathy as a metabolic muscle disease. Exp Rev Cardiovasc Ther. 2008;6:955-69.
6. Silva MA, Swanson AC, Gandhi PJ, et al. Statin-related adverse events: a meta-analysis. Clin Ther. 2006;28:26-35.
7. Law M, Rudnicka AR. Statin safety: a systematic review. Am J Cardiol. 2006;97(8A):52C-60C.
8. Jacobson TA. Toward "pain-free" statin prescribing: clinical algorithm for diagnosis and management of myalgia. Mayo Clin Proc. 2008;83:687-700.
9. Davidson MH, Clark JA, Glass LM, et al. Statin safety: an appraisal from the adverse event reporting system. Am J Cardiol. 2006; 97(8A):32C-43C.
10. Bruckert E, Hayem G, Dejager S, et al. Mild to moderate muscular symptoms with high-dosage statin therapy in hyperlipidemic patients—the PRIMO study. Cardiovasc Drugs Ther. 2005;19:403-14.
11. Klopstock T. Drug-induced myopathies. Curr Opin Neurol. 2008; 21:590-5.
12. Owczarek J, Jasiñska M, Orszulak-Michalak D. Drug-induced myopathies. An overview of the possible mechanisms. Pharmacol Reports. 2005;57:23-4.
13. Lamperti C, Naini AB, Lucchini V, et al. Muscle coenzyme Q10 level in statin-related myopathy. Arch Neurol. 2005;62(11):1709-12.
14. Laaksonen R, Jokelainen K, Sahi T, et al. Decreases in serum ubiquinone concentrations do not result in reduced levels in muscle tissue during short-term simvastatin treatment in humans. Clin Pharmacol Ther. 1995;57:62-6.
15. Marcoff L, Thompson PD. The role of coenzyme Q10 in statin-associated myopathy: a systematic review. J Am Coll Cardiol. 2007;49:2231-7.
16. Dirks AJ, Jones KM. Statin-induced apoptosis and skeletal myopathy. Am J Physiol Cell Physiol. 2006;291:C1208-C12.
17. Guijarro C, Blanco-Colio LM, Ortego M, et al. 3-Hydroxy-3-methylglutaryl coenzyme a reductase and isoprenylation inhibitors induce apoptosis of vascular smooth muscle cells in culture. Circ Res. 1998;83:490-500.
18. Mammen AL, Amato AA. Statin myopathy: a review of recent progress. Curr Opin Rheumatol. 2010;22:644-50.
19. Liantonio A, Giannuzzi V, Cippone V, et al. Fluvastatin and atorvastatin affect calcium homeostasis of rat skeletal muscle fibers in vivo and in vitro by impairing the sarcoplasmic reticulum/mitochondria Ca2+-release system. J Pharmacol Exp Ther. 2007;321:626-34.
20. Mohaupt MG, Karas RH, Babiychuk EB, et al. Association between statin-associated myopathy and skeletal muscle damage. CMAJ. 2009;181:E11-E18.
21. Sirvent P, Mercier J, Vassort G, et al. Simvastatin triggers mitochondria-induced Ca2+ signaling alteration in skeletal muscle. Biochem Biophys Res Commun. 2005;329:1067-75.
22. SEARCH Collaborative Group, Link E, Parish S, Armitage J, et al. SLCO1B1 variants and statin-induced myopathy—a genome wide study. N Engl J Med. 2008;359:789-99.
23. Ruaño G, Windemuth A, Wu AH, et al. Mechanisms of statin-induced myalgia assessed by physiogenomic associations. Atherosclerosis. 2011;218:451-6.
24. Magee CN, Medani SA, Leavey SF, et al. Severe rhabdomyolysis as a consequence of the interaction of fusidic acid and atorvastatin. Am J Kidney Dis. 2010;56:e11-5.
25. Molokhia M, McKeigue P, Curcin V, et al. Statin induced myopathy and myalgia: time trend analysis and comparison of risk associated with statin class from 1991-2006. PLoS One. 2008;3:e2522.
26. Hansen KE, Hildebrand JP, Ferguson EE. Outcomes in 45 patients with statin-associated myopathy. Arch Intern Med. 2005;165: 2671-6.
27. Newman C, Tsai J, Szarek M, et al. Comparative safety of atorvastatin 80 mg versus 10 mg derived from analysis of 49 completed trials in 14,236 patients. Am J Cardiol. 2006;97:61-7.
28. Davidson MH, Robinson JG. Safety of aggressive lipid management. J Am Coll Cardiol. 2007;49:1753-62.
29. Wiviott SD, Cannon CP, Morrow DA, et al. PROVE IT-TIMI 22 Investigators. Can low-density lipoprotein be too low? The safety and efficacy of achieving very low low-density lipoprotein with intensive statin therapy: a PROVE IT-TIMI 22 substudy. J Am Coll Cardiol. 2005;46:1411-6.
30. Alsheikh-Ali AA, Maddukuri PV, Han H, et al. Effect of the magnitude of lipid lowering on risk of elevated liver enzymes, rhabdomyolysis, and cancer: insights from large randomized statin trials. J Am Coll Cardiol. 2007;50:409-18.
31. Glueck CJ, Aregawi D, Agloria M, et al. Rosuvastatin 5 and 10 mg/d: A pilot study of the effects in hypercholesterolemic adults unable to tolerate other statins and reach LDL cholesterol goals with nonstatin lipid-lowering therapies. Clin Ther. 2006;28:933-42.
32. Stein EA, Ballantyne CM, Windler E, et al. Efficacy and tolerability of fluvastatin XL 80 mg alone, ezetimibe alone, and the combination of fluvastatin XL 80 mg with ezetimibe in patients with a history of muscle-related side effects with other statins. Am J Cardiol. 2008;101:490-6.
33. Marcus FI, Baumgarten AJ, Fritz WL, et al. Alternative-day dosing with statins Am J Med. 2013;126:99-104.
34. Lennernäs H. Clinical pharmacokinetics of atorvastatin. Clin Pharmacokinet. 2003;42:1141-60.
35. Martin PD, Mitchell PD, Schneck DW. Pharmacodynamic effects and pharmacokinetics of a new HMG CoA reductase inhibitor, rosuvastatin after morning or evening administration in healthy volunteers. Br J Clin Pharmacol. 2002;54:472-7.
36. Piamsomboon C, Laothavorn P, Saguanwong S, et al. Efficacy and safety of atorvastatin 10 mg every other day in hypercholesterolemia. J Med Assoc Thai. 2002;85:297-300.
37. Juszczyk MA, Seip RL, Thompson PD. Decreasing LDL cholesterol and medication cost with every-other-day statin therapy. Prev Cardiol. 2005;8:197-9.
38. Matalka MS, Ravnan MC, Deedwania PC. Is alternate daily dose of atorvastatin effective in treating patients with hyperlipidemia? The Alternate Day Versus Daily Dosing of Atorvastatin Study (ADDAS). Am Heart J. 2002;144:674-7.
39. Keleş T, Akar Bayram N, Kayhan T, et al. The comparison of the effects of standard 20 mg atorvastatin daily and 20 mg atorvastatin every other day on serum LDL-cholesterol and high sensitive C-reactive protein levels. Anadolu Kardiyol Derg. 2008;8:407-12.
40. Mackie BD, Satija S, Nell C, et al. Monday, Wednesday, and Friday dosing of rosuvastatin in patients previously intolerant to statin therapy. Am J Cardiol. 2007;99:291.
41. Backes JM, Venero CV, Gibson CA, et al. Effectiveness and tolerability of every-other-day rosuvastatin dosing in patients with prior statin intolerance. Ann Pharmacother. 2008;42:341-6.

42. Jian-Jun Li, Ping Yang, Jun Liu, et al. Impact of 10 mg rosuvastatin daily or alternate-day on lipid profile and inflammatory markers. Clin Chim Acta. 2012;413:139-42.
43. Gadaria M, Kearns AK, Thompson PD. Efficacy of rosuvastatin (5 mg and 10 mg) twice a week in patients intolerant to daily statins. Am J Cardiol. 2008;101:1747-8.
44. Backes JM, Moriarty PM, Ruisinger JF, Gibson CA. Effects of once weekly rosuvastatin among patients with a prior statin intolerance. Am J Cardiol. 2007;100:554-5.
45. Athyros VG, Tziomalos K, Kakafika AI, et al. Effectiveness of ezetimibe alone or in combination with twice a week Atorvastatin (10 mg) for statin intolerant high-risk patients. Am J Cardiol. 2008;101:483-5.
46. Keating AJ, Campbell KB, Guyton JR. Intermittent nondaily dosing strategies in patients with previous statin-induced myopathy. Ann Pharmacother. 2013;47:398-404.
47. Reindl EK, Wright BM, Wargo KA. Alternate-day statin therapy for the treatment of hyperlipidemia. Ann Pharmacother. 2010;44: 1459-70.
48. Davidson MH, Donovan JM, Misir S, et al. A 50-week extension study on the safety and efficacy of colesevelam in adults with primary hypercholesterolemia. Am J Cardiovasc Drugs. 2010;10:305-14.
49. Pandor A, Ara RM, Tumur I, et al. Ezetimibe monotherapy for cholesterol lowering in 2,722 people: systematic review and meta-analysis of randomized controlled trials. J Intern Med. 2009;265:568-80.
50. Gazi IF, Daskalopoulou SS, Nair DR, et al. Effect of ezetimibe in patients who cannot tolerate statins or cannot get to the low density lipoprotein cholesterol target despite taking a statin. Curr Med Res Opin. 2007;23:2183-92.
51. Rivers SM, Kane MP, Busch RS, et al. Colesevelam hydrochloride-ezetimibe combination lipid-lowering therapy in patients with diabetes or metabolic syndrome and a history of statin intolerance. Endocr Pract. 2007;13:11-6.
52. Brooks EL, Kuvin JT, Karas RH. Niacin's role in the statin era. Expert Opin Pharmacother. 2010;11:2291-300.
53. Canner PL, Berge KG, Wenger NK, et al. Fifteen year mortality in Coronary Drug Project patients: long-term benefit with niacin. J Am Coll Cardiol. 1986;8:1245-55.
54. Blankenhorn DH, Nessim SA, Johnson RL, et al. Beneficial effects of combined colestipol-niacin therapy on coronary atherosclerosis and coronary venous bypass grafts. JAMA. 1987; 257:3233-40.
55. Brown G, Albers JJ, Fisher LD, et al. Regression of coronary artery disease as a result of intensive lipid-lowering therapy in men with high levels of apolipoprotein B. N Engl J Med. 1990;323: 1289-98.
56. Jiyuan Ma, Yongguo Li, Qing Ye, et al. Constituents of red yeast rice, a traditional Chinese food and medicine. J Agri Food Chem. 2000;48:5220-25.
57. Becker DJ, Gordon RY, Halbert SC, et al. Red yeast rice for dyslipidemia in statin-intolerant patients: a randomized trial. Ann Intern Med. 2009;150:830-9.
58. Cicero AFG, Derosa G, Bove M, et al. Long-term effectiveness and safety of a nutraceutical based approach to reduce cholesterolemia in statin intolerant subjects with or without metabolic syndrome. Curr Top Nutraceut Res. 2009;7:121-6.
59. Halbert SC, French B, Gordon RY, et al. Tolerability of red yeast rice (2,400 mg twice daily) versus pravastatin (20 mg twice daily) in patients with previous statin intolerance. Am J Cardiol. 2010;105:198-204.
60. Venero CV, Venero JV, Wortham DC, Thompson PD. Lipid-lowering efficacy of red yeast rice in a population intolerant to statins. Am J Cardiol. 2010;105:664-6.
61. Caso G, Kelly P, McNurlan MA, Lawson WE. Effect of coenzyme q10 on myopathic symptoms in patients treated with statins. Am J Cardiol. 2007;99:1409-12.
62. Fedacko J, Pella D, Fedackova P, et al. Coenzyme Q(10) and selenium in statin-associated myopathy treatment. Can J Physiol Pharmacol. 2013;91:165-70.
63. Zlatohlavek L, Vrablik M, Grauova B, et al. The effect of coenzyme Q10 in statin myopathy. Neuro Endocrinol Lett. 2012;33(Suppl 2):98-101.
64. Marcoff L, Thompson PD. The role of coenzyme Q10 in statin-associated myopathy: a systematic review. J Am Coll Cardiol. 2007;49:2231-7.
65. Young JM, Florkowski CM, Molyneux SL, et al. Effect of coenzyme Q(10) supplementation on simvastatin-induced myalgia. Am J Cardiol. 2007;100:1400-3.
66. Bookstaver DA, Burkhalter NA, Hatzigeorgiou C. Effect of coenzyme Q10 supplementation on statin-induced myalgias. Am J Cardiol. 2012;110:526-9.
67. Bogsrud MP, Langslet G, Ose L, et al. No effect of combined coenzyme Q10 and selenium supplementation on atorvastatin-induced myopathy. Scand Cardiovasc J. 2013;47:80-7.
68. Parker BA, Gregory SM, Lorson L, et al. A randomized trial of coenzyme Q10 in patients with statin myopathy: rationale and study design. J Clin Lipidol. 2013;7:187-93.
69. Ahmed W, Khan N, Glueck CJ, et al. Low serum 25 (OH) vitamin D levels (<32 ng/mL) are associated with reversible myositis-myalgia in statin-treated patients. Transl Res. 2009;153:11-6.
70. Glueck CJ, Budhani SB, Masineni SS, et al. Vitamin D deficiency, myositis-myalgia, and reversible statin intolerance. Curr Med Res Opin. 2011;27:1683-90.
71. Riphagen IJ, van der Veer E, Muskiet FA, et al. Myopathy during statin therapy in the daily practice of an outpatient cardiology clinic: prevalence, predictors and relation with vitamin D. Curr Med Res Opin. 2012;28:1247-52
72. Kurnik D, Hochman I, Vesterman-Landes J, et al. Muscle pain and serum creatine kinase are not associated with low serum 25(OH) vitamin D levels in patients receiving statins. Clin Endocrinol (Oxf). 2012;77:36-41.
73. Gupta A, Thompson PD. The relationship of vitamin D deficiency to statin myopathy. Atherosclerosis. 2011;215:23-9.
74. Echaniz-Laguna A, Mohr M, Tranchant C. Neuromuscular symptoms and elevated creatine kinase after statin withdrawal. N Engl J Med. 2010;362:564-5.

9

Atrial Fibrillation Update, 2014

Sanjiv Bharadwaj, Sujeet Narain

INTRODUCTION

Atrial fibrillation (AF) is defined as a supraventricular tachyarrhythmia characterized by uncoordinated atrial activation and mechanical function with consequent deterioration of ventricular mechanical function.

It is characterized electrocardiographically by:

1. Low-amplitude baseline oscillations (fibrillatory or "f" waves) and an irregularly irregular ventricular rhythm. The "f" waves have a rate of 300–600 beats/min and are variable in amplitude, shape, and timing
2. Irregular RR intervals
3. There are no distinct P waves on the surface electrocardiography (ECG). Some apparently regular atrial electrical activity may be seen in some ECG leads, most often in lead V1.

GENETICS PREDISPOSITION

Atrial fibrillation is also seen in family members especially AF of early onset.[1] Numerous inherited cardiac syndromes that are associated with AF have been identified. For example, both short and long QT syndromes, Brugada syndrome, hypertrophic cardiomyopathy, a familial form of ventricular pre-excitation, and abnormal LV hypertrophy associated with mutations in the *PRKAG* gene. Atrial fibrillation is also associated with mutations in the gene coding for atrial natriuretic peptide, loss-of-function mutations in the cardiac sodium channel gene *SCN5A*, or gain of function in a cardiac potassium channel.[2-4] Furthermore, several genetic loci close to the *PITX2* and *ZFHX3* genes are associated with AF and cardioembolic stroke in population-wide studies.[5] The pathophysiological role of other genetic defects in the initiation and perpetuation of AF is currently unknown (Table 9.1).

CLASSIFICATION

1. *First diagnosed AF*: A patient who presented with AF for the first time is the first diagnosed AF. After two or more episodes, AF is considered recurrent. First detected AF may be either paroxysmal or persistent.
2. *Paroxysmal*: Atrial fibrillation that terminates spontaneously within 7 days of occurrence (usually ≤48 hours) without cardioversion is paroxysmal AF.
3. *Persistent*: Atrial fibrillation that presents continuously for >7 days and that requires cardioversion for normal sinus rhythm.
4. *Long-standing persistent AF*: Presented for ≥1 year and can be cardioverted.
5. *Permanent*: Atrial fibrillation when persist for more than 1 year and refractory to cardioversion.
6. *Lone AF*: Atrial fibrillation that occurs in patients younger than 60 years and who do not have hypertension or any evidence of structural heart disease.
7. *Silent AF (asymptomatic)*: The patients may manifest as an AF-related complication (ischemic stroke or tachycardiomyopathy) or may be diagnosed by an opportunistic ECG.

Table 9.1 Condition predisposing to, or encouraging progression of AF

Common	Uncommon
• Hypertension • Ischemic heart disease • Mitral valve disease (RHD) • Hypertrophic cardiomyopathy and dilated cardiomyopathy • Thyrotoxicosis • COPD • Obesity and obstructive sleep apnea	• Restrictive cardiomyopathies • Constrictive pericarditis • Cardiac tumors • Severe pulmonary hypertension • Excessive alcohol intake (holiday heart) • Open heart or thoracic surgery • Myocarditis • Pulmonary embolism • Congenital heart disease

NATURAL HISTORY

The incidence of AF depends on age and gender of patients, occurring in 1–2% of the general population, ranging from 0.1% per year before the age of 40 years to >1.5% per year in women and >2% per year in men older than 80 years.[6] The Framingham Study estimated the lifetime risk for development of AF after the age of 40 years to be 26% for men and 23% for women. The Natural time course of AF is it progresses from short, rare episodes, to longer and more frequent attacks. Over time (years), many patients will develop sustained forms of AF. Only a small proportion of patients without AF-promoting conditions will remain in paroxysmal AF over several decades (2–3% of AF patients).

HATCH score is the best independent predictors of AF progression (Table 9.2).

This scoring system was developed to help identify patients who are likely to progress from paroxysmal to persistent AF within 1 year. About 50% of the patients of HATCH score >5 progressed to persistent AF, while AF progression was observed in only 6% of patients with a HATCH score of 0.[7] Atrial fibrillation progression is of clinical and prognostic relevance, as it makes it more challenging to restore and maintain sinus rhythm and it could contribute to the occurrence of AF-related events.

Table 9.2 HATCH score

HATCH	*Score*
H—Hypertension	1
A—Age older than 75 years	1
T—Previous transient ischemic attack or stroke	1
C—Chronic obstructive pulmonary disease	1
H—Heart failure	1

Table 9.3 EHRA score of AF-related symptoms

EHRA	*Symptom severity*	*Definition*
I	No symptoms	
II	Mild symptoms	Normal daily activity not affected
III	Severe symptoms	Normal daily activity affected
IV	Disabling symptoms	Normal daily activity discontinued

CLINICAL PRESENTATION

Many patients with paroxysmal AF also have asymptomatic episodes, and some patients with persistent AF have symptoms only intermittently.

Most common are as follows:

1. Palpitations
2. Fatigue
3. Dyspnea
4. Effort intolerance
5. Light headedness
6. Polyuria

Assessment of symptoms is very important in the management of AF. Nowadays a symptom score for AF is in use that is EHRA score, which is comparable to the New York Heart Association (NYHA) scores for heart failure and angina (Table 9.3).

DIAGNOSIS

An irregular pulse should always raise the suspicion of AF, but an ECG recording is necessary to diagnose AF. Any arrhythmia that has the ECG characteristics of AF and lasts sufficiently long for a 12-lead ECG to be recorded, or at least 30 sec on a rhythm strip, should be considered as AF (Fig. 9.1).

Diagnostic evaluation is especially done in paroxysmal AF. Ambulatory monitoring is useful to document AF in this case. If the symptoms occur on a daily basis, a 24-hour Holter recording is appropriate, and if sporadic then extended monitoring for 2–4 weeks with an event monitor or by mobile cardiac outpatient telemetry is appropriate.

MANAGEMENT

It comprises of the following:

1. Acute management
2. Chronic management
   a. Rate control
   b. Correction of the rhythm disturbance
3. Prevention of thromboembolism
4. New treatment option

When the patients who present to the emergency department because of AF for the first time generally have a rapid ventricular rate, and in this case, control of the ventricular rate is priority and this is achieved rapidly with intravenous diltiazem or Beta-blockers like esmolol. And an immediate cardioversion is usually appropriate for patient who had symptoms like hypotension, HF, and angina pectoris. If cardioversion is planned than duration of AF is most important. If the AF has been present for >48 hours or if the duration is unclear and the patient is not anticoagulated, cardioversion ideally should be preceded by transesophageal echocardiography to rule out a left atrial thrombus. The decision to restore sinus rhythm by cardioversion is based on several factors, including symptoms, prior AF episodes, age, left atrial size, and current antiarrhythmic drug therapy.

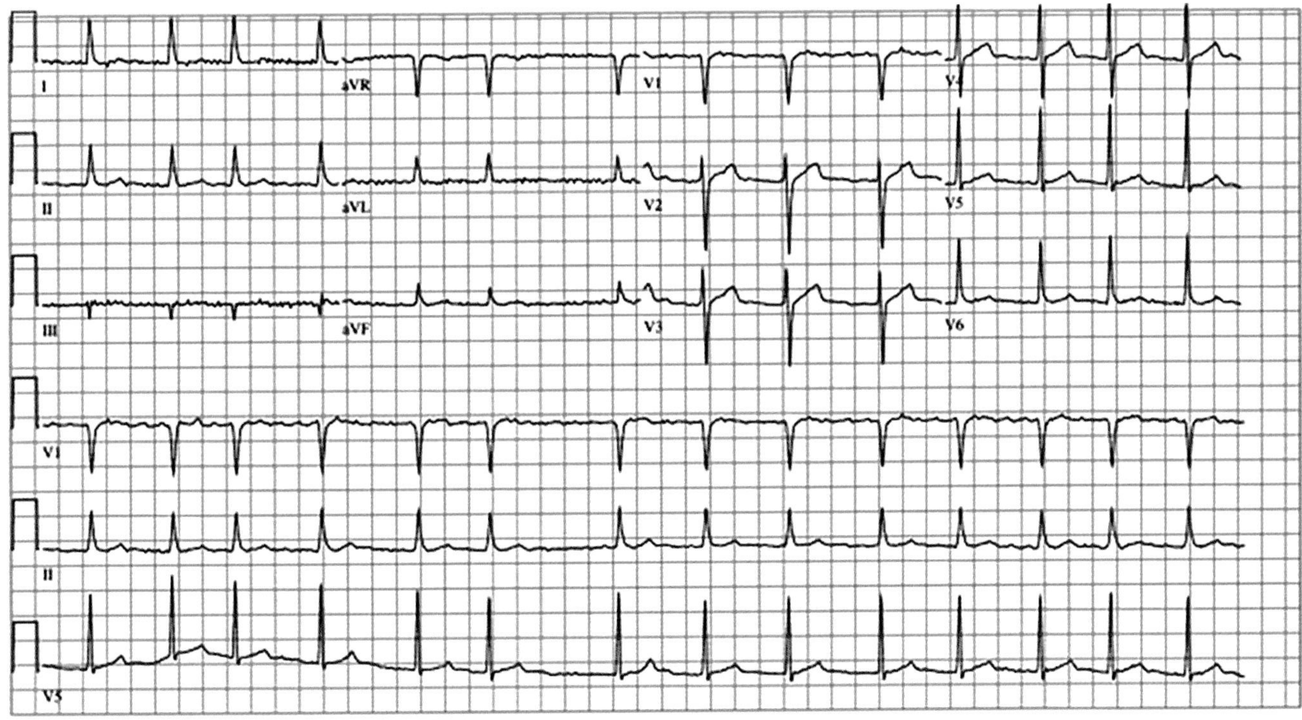

Fig. 9.1 ECG of atrial fibrillation

If it is accepted as permanent AF then only rate control and anticoagulant is appropriate.

Two management decisions are to be made during acute persistent AF: early versus delayed cardioversion and pharmacological versus electrical cardioversion. The advantages of early cardioversion are rapid relief of symptoms, avoidance of the need for transesophageal echocardiography or therapeutic anticoagulation for 3–4 weeks before cardioversion. If cardioversion is performed within 48 hours of AF onset, there is possibly a lower risk of early AF recurrence because of less atrial remodeling. Possible reasons to defer cardioversion include an AF duration longer than 48 hours or duration unclear in a patient who is not anticoagulated and for whom transesophageal echocardiography is not available. When cardioversion is performed early in the course of an episode of AF, there is the option of either pharmacological or electrical cardioversion. Pharmacological cardioversion has the advantage of not requiring general anesthesia or deep sedation. In addition, the probability of an immediate recurrence of AF may be lower with pharmacological cardioversion than with electrical cardioversion. However, pharmacological cardioversion is associated with the risk of adverse drug effects and is not as effective as electrical cardioversion. Pharmacological cardioversion is very unlikely to be effective, if the duration of AF is longer than 7 days.

The efficacy of transthoracic direct current cardioversion is approximately 95%. Biphasic waveform shocks convert AF more effectively than monophasic waveform shocks and allow the use of lower energy shocks, resulting in a lower risk of skin irritation. An appropriate first-shock strength using a biphasic waveform is 150–200 J followed by higher output shocks if needed. If a 360-J biphasic shock is unsuccessful, ibutilide should be infused before another shock is delivered because it lowers the defibrillation energy requirement and improves the success rate of transthoracic cardioversion.

There are two types of failure of transthoracic cardioversion in patients with AF. The first type is a complete failure to restore sinus rhythm. For this situation, an increase in shock strength or infusion of ibutilide often results in successful cardioversion. The second type of failure is an immediate recurrence of AF within a few seconds of successful conversion to sinus rhythm. The incidence of an immediate recurrence of AF is approximately 25% for episodes <24 hours in duration and approximately 10% for episodes >24 hours in duration. For this type of failure of cardioversion, an increase in shock strength is of no value. If the patient has not been receiving an oral rhythm-control agent, infusion of ibutilide may be helpful for prevention of an immediate recurrence of AF.

In patients with symptomatic recurrent paroxysmal AF, the aggressiveness with which a rhythm-control strategy is pursued should be dictated by the frequency and severity of symptoms and how well antiarrhythmic drug therapy is tolerated. Drug therapy is said to be successful when the goal of therapy is not complete suppression of AF but a clinically meaningful reduction in frequency, duration, and severity of episodes.

A pharmacological rhythm-control strategy is not necessarily consisting of daily drug therapy especially in recurrent paroxysmal AF. In this patient, episodic drug therapy (the "pill-in-the-pocket" approach) is useful for patients whose episodes of AF are relatively infrequent. Episodic drug therapy is a reasonable option for patients who are clearly aware of the onset and termination of AF episodes and who have lone AF or only minimal structural heart disease. This therapy consists of a class IC drug (flecainide or propafenone) plus a short-acting b-blocker (e.g. propranolol) or calcium channel blocker (e.g. verapamil). Many patients with infrequent episodes prefer this approach because it eliminates the inconvenience, cost, and possible side effects of daily prophylactic therapy (Flow chart 9.1).

However, patients who are disabled by severe symptoms during AF may prefer daily prophylactic therapy even if episodes are infrequent. Daily antithrombotic therapy to prevent thromboembolic events is appropriate for all patients being treated for recurrent AF, whether it is persistent or paroxysmal and whether a rhythm-control or rate-control strategy is employed (Flow charts 9.2 and 9.3; Tables 9.4 and 9.5).

Chronic management comprises of the following:
1. Pharmacological approach
2. Nonpharmacological approach
3. Pharmacological approach—it comprises of either:
   a. Sinus rhythm maintenance
   b. Heart rate control

Flow chart 9.1 Pharmacological management of patients with newly discovered atrial fibrillation

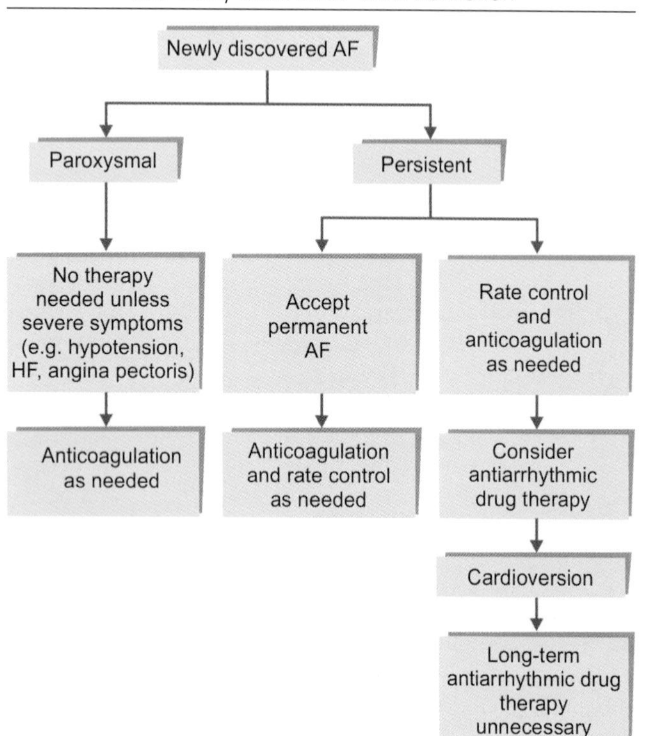

Flow chart 9.2 Pharmacological management of patients with recurrent paroxysmal atrial fibrillation

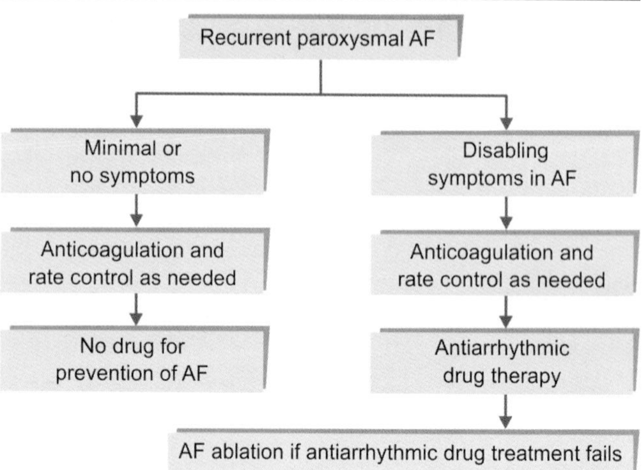

Flow chart 9.3 Pharmacological management of patients with recurrent persistent or permanent atrial fibrillation

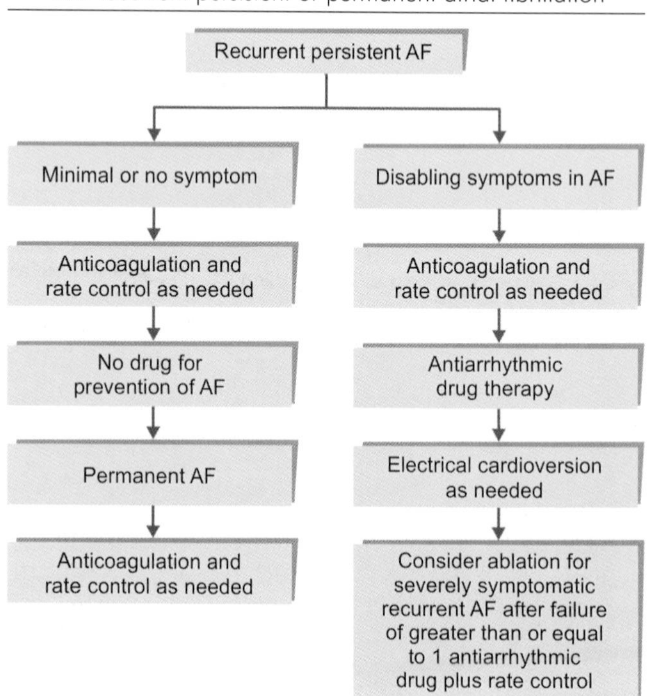

Table 9.4 Recommendations for pharmacological cardioversion of atrial fibrillation of up to 7-days duration

Drug	Route of administration	Recommendation evidence	Class of level
Dofetilide	Oral	I	A
Flecainide, Propafenone	Oral or intravenous	I	A
Ibutilide	Intravenous I	I	A
Amiodarone	Oral or intravenous	IIa	A

Table 9.5 Recommendations for pharmacological cardioversion of atrial fibrillation present for >7 days duration

Drug	Route of administration	Recommended evidence	Class of level
Dofetilide	Oral	I	A
Amiodarone	Oral or intravenous	IIa	A
Ibutilide	Intravenous	IIa	A

Several randomized studies have compared a rate-control strategy with a rhythm-control strategy in patients with AF. The largest study by far was the atrial fibrillation follow-up investigation of rhythm management (AFFIRM) study, which consisted of 4,060 patients with a mean age of 70 years who had AF for 6 hours to 6 months. At 5 years of follow-up, the prevalence of sinus rhythm was 35% in the rate-control arm and 63% in the rhythm-control arm. There was no significant difference between the two study arms in total mortality, stroke rate, or quality of life. The percentage of patients requiring hospitalization was significantly lower in the rate-control arm (73%) than in the rhythm-control arm (80%), and the incidence of adverse drug effects such as torsades de pointes was also significantly lower in the rate-control arm (0.2% vs. 0.8%). The authors of the AFFIRM study concluded that there is no survival advantage of a rhythm-control strategy over a rate-control strategy and that a rate-control strategy has advantages such as a lower probability of hospitalization and of adverse drug effects.

The results of the AFFIRM study should not be applied routinely to all patients with AF. The decision to pursue a rhythm-control strategy versus a rate-control strategy should be individualized, with several factors taken into account such as the nature, frequency, and severity of symptoms; the length of time that AF has been present continuously in patients with persistent AF; left atrial size; comorbidities; the response to prior cardioversion; and age.

If the AF has been continuous for >1 year or if the left atrial diameter is very large (>5.0 cm), in this patients there is a high probability of an early recurrence of AF, and this should be taken into account in deciding on the best strategy. After cardioversion, the decision to maintain the patient on antiarrhythmic drug therapy to delay the next episode of AF is based on the patient's preference, the perceived risk of an early recurrence of AF, and the duration of sinus rhythm between prior cardioversion. Treatment by cardioversion without daily antiarrhythmic drug therapy is acceptable if episodes of AF are separated by at least 6 months. Treatment with a rhythm-control drug usually is appropriate when AF recurs within a few months of cardioversion.

The studies AFFIRM RACE and AF-CHF trials have shown no mortality benefit to a rhythm control strategy compared to a rate control strategy. Therefore, a rate control strategy, without attempts at restoration or maintenance of sinus rhythm (SR), is reasonable in some patients with AF, especially those who are elderly and asymptomatic. If rate control offers inadequate symptomatic relief, restoration of sinus rhythm may become a long-term goal. Restoration and maintenance of SR continues to be a reasonable treatment approach in many patients with AF especially in patients of low left ventricular (LV) ejection fraction.

The goals of rate control strategy are to adequately control the ventricular response during AF that can significantly improve symptoms and also to prevent development of tachycardia-mediated cardiomyopathy. Most patients managed using a rhythm-control strategy also requires medications for rate control. Control of the ventricular rate during AF is important both at rest and with exertion. Criteria for adequate rate control vary. In AFFIRM trial, adequate control was defined as an average heart rate <80 bpm at rest and either an average rate <100 bpm during Holter monitoring with no rate above 100% of the maximum age-adjusted predicted exercise HR, or a maximum HR of 110 bpm during a 6-minute walk test. In the RACE II trial, lenient HR control (target <110 bpm) was seen noninferior to strict HR control (resting rate <80 bpm and rate during moderate exercise <110 bpm).[8,9]

The agents available for long-term heart rate control in patients with AF are digitalis, beta-blockers, calcium channel antagonists, and amiodarone. The first-line agents for rate control are beta-blockers and the calcium channel antagonists like verapamil and diltiazem. A combination is often used to improve efficacy or to limit side effects by allowing the use of smaller dosages of the individual drugs. Digitalis may adequately control the rate at rest but often does not provide adequate rate control during exertion. Its use is appropriate in patients with systolic heart failure, in whom digitalis has been shown to improve outcomes such as heart failure hospitalizations and mortality. Furthermore, in patients without systolic heart failure, the use of a digitalis glycoside may have a deleterious effect on survival in AFFIRM study; digitalis was found to be independently associated with a 50% higher risk of all-cause mortality. Amiodarone may be an appropriate choice for rate control if the other agents are not tolerated or are ineffective (Flow chart 9.4 and Table 9.6).

NEWER ANTIARRHYTHMIC DRUG

Dronedarone

It is an amiodarone analog. As compared to amiodarone, it is less lipophilic and without iodine moieties that cause thyroid

Flow chart 9.4 Antiarrhythmic drug therapy to maintain sinus rhythm in patients with recurrent paroxysmal or persistent atrial fibrillation (updated)

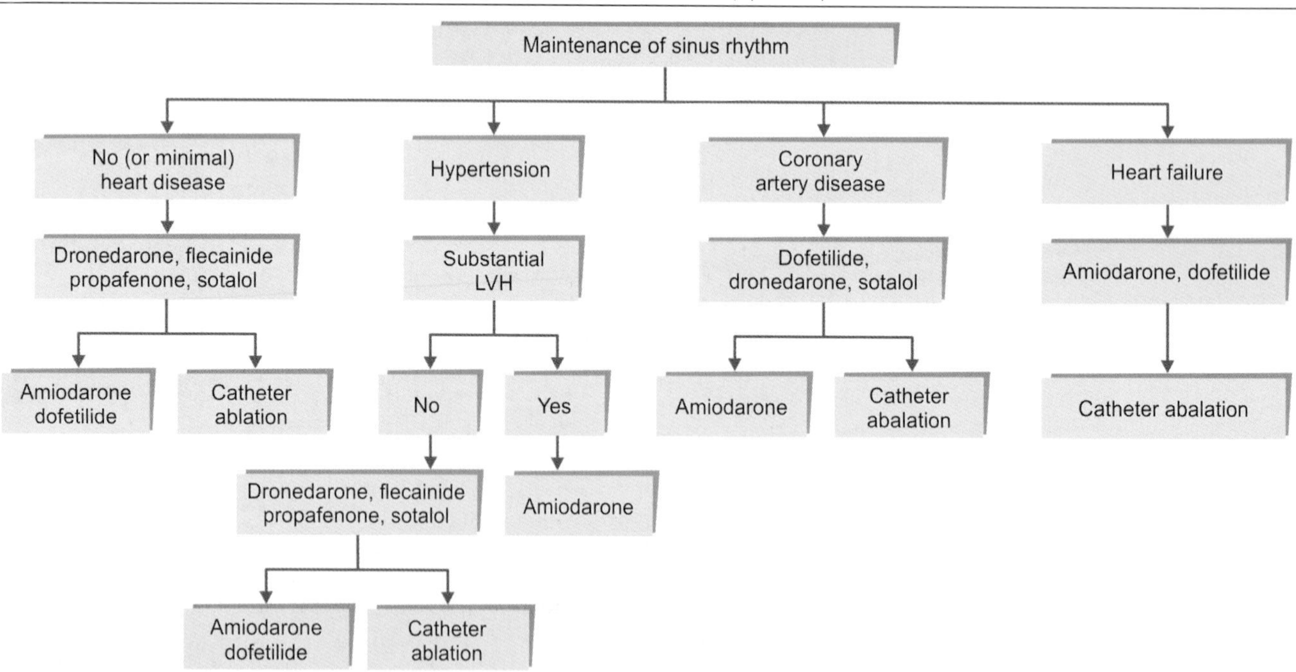

Table 9.6 Daily doses and common adverse effect of commonly used antiarrhythmics

Drug	Dosage (mg/day)	Adverse effects
Amiodarone	100–400 mg	Eye complications, photosensitivity, pulmonary toxicity, polyneuropathy, GI upset, bradycardia, torsades de pointes (rare), hepatic toxicity, thyroid dysfunction like hypothyroidism, or hyperthyroidism
Disopyramide	400–750 mg	Torsades de pointes, heart failure, glaucoma, urinary retention
Dofetilide	500–1000 mcg	Torsades de pointes, gastrointestinal upset
Flecainide	200–300 mg	Ventricular tachycardia, atrial flutter, heart failure
Procainamide	1,000–4,000 mg	Torsades de pointes, lupus-like syndrome, gastrointestinal upset
Propafenone	450–900 mg	Ventricular tachycardia, heart failure, atrial flutter
Quinidine	600–1500 mg	Torsades de pointes, gastrointestinal upset
Sotalol	160–320 mg	Torsades de pointes, heart failure, bradycardia, exacerbation of chronic obstructive pulmonary disease (COPD) or bronchial asthma

dysfunction. Like amiodarone, dronedarone is having multi-channel blocker and antiadrenergic properties. It prolongs action potential duration and decreases heart rate, while lower potential of polymorphic ventricular tachycardia. Plasma level of dronedarone is reached to maximum within 1–4 hours and its plasma protein binding is around 98%, but oral bioavailability is about 15%. Mean concentrations of dronedarone are reached within 1 week of 400 mg twice daily. Dronedarone is metabolized by cytochrome P450 (CYP3A4) enzymes, with excretion of small amount of unchanged drug in bile and urine. The elimination half-life (about 24 hours) is shorter than that for the amiodarone. It is contraindicated in symptomatic heart failure.

A meta-analysis from various randomized controlled trials Efficacy and Safety of Dronedarone for the Control of Ventricular Rate during Atrial Fibrillation (ERATO), Dose Adjustment for Normal Eating (DAFNE), The American-Australian Trial with Dronedarone in Atrial Fibrillation or Flutter Patients for the Maintenance of Sinus Rhythm (ADONIS), European Trial in Atrial Fibrillation or Flutter Patients Receiving Dronedarone for the Maintenance of Sinus Rhythm (EURIDIS), and A placebo-controlled, double-blind, parallel arm (ATHENA) patients with AF showed reduced time to first cardiovascular mortality or admission to hospital and decreased incidence of cardiovascular or sudden death.[10]

Dronedarone versus amiodarone were compared in Efficacy and Safety of Dronedarone versus Amiodarone for the Maintenance of Sinus Rhythm in Patients with Atrial Fibrillation (DIONYSOS) study trial in patients with persistent AF[11] and results showed that, AF recurrence over period of 7 months after electrical cardioversion was more with dronedarone group (63.5%) than with amiodarone group (42.0%). Above data suggest higher compliance, but lesser efficacies for dronedarone as compared to amiodarone. A meta-analysis revealed that the patients treated with amiodarone maintained sinus rhythm over time than those treated with dronedarone. Subsequently, dronedarone was approved by the United States Food and Drug Administration (FDA) on March 18, 2009, for maintenance of sinus rhythm in patients with AF or atrial flutter, provided the ejection fraction is >35%.

Nonpharmacological Approach

The nonpharmacological strategy is basically a catheter ablation method. It is divided into two general strategies: rate control and rhythm control. Rate can be controlled through modifying the AV node or ablating the node and implanting a permanent pacemaker. Rhythm control can be done by targeting the triggers of AF, and restoring sinus rhythm.

Left Atrial Catheter Ablation

Pulmonary veins play a key role in initiating or maintaining the episodes of AF.[12] Pulmonary veins isolation using catheter ablation technique virtually eliminates AF in few patients. Catheter ablation requires trans-septal catheterization that attempts to target individual pulmonary veins (PVs) ectopic foci to circumferential electrical isolation of the entire PV musculature. Left atrial catheter ablation is usually undertaken in patients with symptomatic paroxysmal AF who have failed at least one ion channel antiarrhythmic drug. The choice for catheter ablation and its result depend on various factors that determine severity of AF (i.e. duration of AF, AF type, and atrial size), associated diseases, possibility of alternative strategy, and patient preference. Now the guidelines suggest that catheter ablation should be considered as one of the initial therapy in selected group of patients, like in those patients with symptomatic paroxysmal AF without structural heart disease.

Medical therapy remains the cornerstone in treatment of AF, but catheter ablation is a new horizon and gaining popularity while treating AF. Results of meta-analysis and randomized trials of antiarrhythmic medication versus ablation revealed 77% success rate for catheter ablation and 52% success for antiarrhythmics.

After catheter ablation, complication rate ranges from 2% to 12% and mortality rate is <0.1%. Atrial tachyarrhythmias have been reported within first few weeks after ablation. However, first medical therapy should be tried for these benign arrhythmias, if it persist a repeat ablation procedure can be considered. Postablation patients should be anticoagulated for at least 2 months. Long-term oral anticoagulation should be offered to high-risk patients. Left atrial thrombus remains a contraindication to catheter ablation for AF (Table 9.7).

Atrioventricular Node Ablation

Ablation of the atrioventricular node is a palliative but irreversible procedure and is therefore reasonable in patients in whom pharmacological rate control, including combination of drugs, has failed or rhythm control with drugs and/or LA ablation has failed. And it is followed by VVI, DDD, cardiac resynchronization therapy, and ICD depending on need. AV node ablation does not cure AF and requires placement of a permanent pacemaker to ensure adequate ventricular rates. Ideally, the most proximal portion of the AV node is targeted, leaving the distal portion intact, resulting in complete heart block. Success rates for AV node

Table 9.7 Complications of AF catheter ablation[13]

- Thromboembolism leading to TIA and stroke
- PV stenosis
- Atrioesophageal fistula
- Tamponade
- Mitral valve injury
- Air embolism
- Radiation injury
- Hematoma at puncture site
- Phrenic nerve injury
- Periesophageal injury
- Arteriovenous fistula
- Acute coronary syndrome
- Death

ablation are nearly 100%. The procedure improves quality of life and may improve LV ejection fraction modestly, probably from improved rate control. Patients who have a history of congestive heart failure benefit from biventricular pacing after AV node ablation. It is a class IIa indication.

Surgical Approaches to Atrial Fibrillation

The most effective surgical procedure for AF is the "cut-and-sew" maze procedure developed by Cox in 1987. This operation involves 12 atrial incisions to isolate the pulmonary veins and to create lines of block in the left atrium and right atrium. Long-term freedom from AF after the Cox maze procedure has been reported to range from 70% to 95%, but 10% to 35% of patients still require antiarrhythmic drug therapy. The efficacy of the Cox maze procedure is lower in patients with very large left atria or with persistent AF for many years. The Cox maze procedure has not been widely performed because it requires cardiopulmonary bypass, is technically difficult, and is associated with a mortality risk of approximately 1-2%.

A large variety of other surgical ablation tools like pulmonary vein isolation and left atrial ablation have been developed to simplify the classic Cox maze procedure. Several different types of energy have been used for surgical ablation: radiofrequency energy, cryoenergy, microwave, laser, and high-intensity focused ultrasound.[14] In patients who do not require concomitant coronary artery bypass grafting or valve repair or replacement, surgical ablation typically is performed by a nonsternotomy approach. The efficacy of these procedures generally has been reported to range from 70% to 85%. However, because of inadequate monitoring for recurrent AF during follow-up, it is likely that these success rates are overestimates.

At present, surgery for AF most commonly is performed as a concomitant procedure in patients with AF undergoing open heart surgery for coronary artery disease or valvular disease. A stand-alone surgical procedure for AF may be appropriate for patients who have not had a successful outcome from catheter ablation, who are not good candidates for catheter ablation, or who prefer a surgical procedure over catheter ablation.

Prevention of Thromboembolism

Pharmacological approach

Major goal is prevention of stroke especially in patients of paroxysmal AF. For this risk stratification is necessary to find out who will get benefit from this complication. It is well established that oral anticoagulant is more effective than antiplatelet for prevention of thromboembolic complications. However, because of the risk of hemorrhage during anticoagulant therapy, its use should be limited to patients whose risk of thromboembolic complications is greater than the risk of hemorrhage. Therefore, it is useful to risk-stratified patients with AF to identify appropriate candidates for warfarin therapy and other anticoagulant (Table 9.8).

Approach to thromboprophylaxis in patients with AF

It should be kept in mind that the classification of paroxysmal, persistent, or permanent AF is not relevant in thromboprophylaxis. Instead, risk stratification should be based on the presence of accompanying risk factors in the individual patient (Table 9.9).

RISK OF BLEEDING

Bleeding risk should also be considered in the individual patient and this risk is stratified by HAS-BLED (Table 9.10).[15]

Systolic blood pressure >160 mm Hg is defined as hypertension and abnormal kidney function means patients on chronic dialysis or serum creatinine ≥200 mmol/L or renal transplantation. Abnormal liver function is defined as

Table 9.8 The simple clinical methods of risk stratification is the CHA2DS2-VASc

Risk factor	*Score*
• Congestive heart failure/LV dysfunction LVEF <40%	1
• Hypertension	1
• Age >75	2
• Diabetes mellitus	1
• Stroke/TIA/ thromboembolism	2
• Vascular disease (myocardial infarction, CAD. PAD)	1
• Age 65–74	1
• Sex category (i.e. female sex)	1
• Maximum score	9

Table 9.9 Recommendation of anticoagulant and antiplatelet

CHA2DS2-VASc score	*Recommended antithrombotic therapy*
>2	OAC INR value in the range of 2.0–3.0, unless contraindicated
1	Either OAC or aspirin 75–325 mg daily. *Preferred*: OAC rather than aspirin
0	Either aspirin 75–325 mg daily or no antithrombotic therapy. *Preferred*: No antithrombotic therapy rather than aspirin

Table 9.10 HAS-BLED score

HAS-BLED	*Score*
H—Hypertension	1
A—Abnormal renal/liver function (1 point each)	1 or 2
S—Stroke	1
B—Bleeding history or predisposition	1
L—Labile international normalized ratio (INR)	1
E—Elderly (>65)	1
D—Drugs/alcohol (1 point each)	1 or 2

chronic liver disease and/or serum bilirubin is twice upper limit of normal, and aspartate aminotransferase/alanine aminotransferase/alkaline phosphatase thrice the upper limit normal. Bleeding refers to history of bleeding and/or tendency to bleed, e.g. bleeding diathesis and anemia. Labile international normalized ratios (INRs) refer to high INRs or poor time in therapeutic range (e.g. <60%). Drugs/alcohol use refers to simultaneous use of drugs, such as antiplatelets, nonsteroidal anti-inflammatory drugs, or alcohol abuse.

Increased risk of bleeding is anticipated when HAS-BLED score ≥3 which is not absolute contraindication while starting anticoagulation, but more caution should be taken when starting anticoagulation, and frequent INR testings. Only problem is that a high CHA2DS2-VASc score is sometimes accompanied by a high HAS-BLED score.

NEWER ANTITHROMBOTIC DRUGS

After introduction of two most important classes of new anticoagulants like direct thrombin inhibitors (e.g. dabigatran) and the oral factor Xa inhibitors (rivaroxaban, apixaban), decision making somewhat become more easy in patients having higher HAS-BLED scores or lower CHA_2DS_2-VASc scores for those patients who cannot tolerate vitamin K antagonists. Other advantage of these drugs is predictable and consistent anticoagulant effects. It means that coagulation monitoring is not necessary, and standard dosages can be prescribed to the patients.

Dabigatran Etexilate

Dabigatran etexilate is a prodrug that is converted to active molecule dabigatran. The FDA approved dabigatran etexilate 150 mg orally twice daily, on October 19, 2010, for the prevention of stroke and systemic embolism in nonvalvular AF. In fact, dabigatran was FDA approved after the RELY trial. In Randomized Evaluation of Long-term Anticoagulation Therapy (RELY) trial that was a randomized controlled and noninferiority trial, a total of 18,113 patients with AF and having risk of stroke received fixed doses of dabigatran—110 mg or 150 mg twice daily, and in unblinded fashion, adjusted-dose warfarin was given.[16] The mean follow-up was 2 years and primary outcome was stroke or systemic embolism. Finally, inference was that in AF dabigatran used at a dose of 110 mg had similar rates of stroke and systemic embolism as that of warfarin and lower rates of major bleed. Dabigatran given at a dose of 150 mg, when compared to warfarin, found to have lower rates of stroke and systemic embolism but similar rates of major bleed. Patients with severe renal disease (creatinine clearance <30 mL/min) were excluded from the study. The FDA approved dabigatran 75 mg twice daily for those patients who are having creatinine clearance 15–30 mL/min. Renal function should be assessed periodically, if renal dysfunction is anticipated such as in patients >75 years of age and with creatinine clearance <50 mL/min.

Rivaroxaban

The FDA approved rivaroxaban 20 mg orally once daily for stroke prevention in AF based on the results Rivaroxaban Once-daily Oral Direct Factor Xa Inhibition Compared with Vitamin K Antagonism for Prevention of Stroke and Embolism Trial in Atrial Fibrillation (ROCKET AF) study on July 1, 2011.[17] ROCKET AF was a large, double-blind, randomized trial of 14,264 patients comparing rivaroxaban 20 mg once daily or a reduced dose of 15 mg once daily with warfarin (goal INR 2.0–3.0) in nonvalvular AF. In ROCKET AF study, once-daily rivaroxaban was compared with dose-adjusted warfarin for the stroke and systemic embolism prevention in nonvalvular AF for those who were at moderately high risk for stroke and rivaroxaban was found to be noninferior to warfarin. When safety analysis was done, it was found that there is no significant difference between rivaroxaban and warfarin group while major or nonmajor clinically significant bleeding compared. Rivaroxaban should not be cautiously used if renal dysfunction is present especially if creatinine clearance <15 mL/min, and a dose reduction to 15 mg once daily is offered if creatinine clearance is between 15 and 50 mL/min. Dabigatran as well as rivaroxaban should be avoided in patients with acute kidney injury.

Apixaban

The Apixaban for Reduction in Stroke and Other Thromboembolic Events in Atrial Fibrillation (ARISTOTLE) trial randomized approximately 18,000 patients with chronic nonvalvular AF to apixaban 5 mg orally twice daily or warfarin, target international normalized ratio (INR) 2.0–3.0.[18] The primary outcome was ischemic or hemorrhagic stroke or systemic embolism. The trial was designed to test for noninferiority, with key secondary objectives of testing for superiority with respect to the primary outcome and to the rates of major bleeding and death from any cause. The investigators found that apixaban was not only noninferior to warfarin, but actually superior, reducing the risk of stroke or systemic embolism by 21% and the risk of major bleeding by 31%. In patients with AF, apixaban was superior to warfarin in preventing stroke or systemic embolism, caused less bleeding, and resulted in lower mortality. There is an increased risk of stroke following discontinuation of apixaban in patients with nonvalvular AF. If apixaban must be discontinued for a reason other than bleeding, coverage with another anticoagulant should be strongly considered (FDA box warning).

Nonpharmacological Approach

The left atrial appendage (LAA) is considered the main site of atrial thrombogenesis. Thus, occlusion of the LAA orifice may reduce the development of atrial thrombi and stroke in patients with AF. In particular, patients with contraindications to chronic anticoagulation therapy might be considered as candidates for LAA occlusion.

The PROTECT AF (WATCHMAN Left Atrial Appendage System for Embolic PROTECTion in Patients with Atrial Fibrillation) randomized trial in which percutaneous closure of the LAA (using a WATCHMAN device) was done and subsequent discontinuation of warfarin or to VKA treatment.[19] The primary efficacy event rate (a composite endpoint of stroke, cardiovascular death, and systemic embolism) of the WATCHMAN device was considered noninferior to that of VKA. There was only higher rate of adverse events in the intervention mainly to periprocedural complications.

NEW TREATMENT OPTION

Upstream Therapy

It is seen that upstream therapy is more effective in the primary prevention of AF and in patients in whom remodeling processes are less advanced and patients of AF with a shorter history. The results in secondary AF prevention had been disappointing. A possible means are the renin-angiotensin-aldosterone system the Renin-angiotensin-aldosterone system (RAAS) blockers [ACE inhibitors, angiotensin receptor blockers (ARBs), aldosterone receptor antagonists (ARAs)], statins, and omega-3 polyunsaturated fatty acids (i.e. fish oils and anti-inflammatory agent).

The Renin-angiotensin-aldosterone System Blockers

It may prevent or reduce atrial structural remodeling, especially by decreasing fibrosis, improving hemodynamics by lowering blood pressure, and reducing LV and atrial wall stress. By their pleiotropic effects including reduction of inflammation and oxidative stress, it reduces structural remodeling and fibrosis. Possible mechanism is that atrial angiotensin II concentration increases in AF and stimulation of its receptors activates NADPH oxidase to produce oxidative stress and inflammation. It also activates mitogen-activated protein kinase, causing myocyte hypertrophy, apoptosis, and fibriblast proliferation.[20] The retrospective analyses of several large randomized trials in LV dysfunction and heart failure have reported a lower incidence of new-onset AF in patients treated with ACEIs and ARBs compared with placebo. Hypertension meta-analyses study also favor the ACEI- or ARB-based therapy for prevention of AF. In LIFE study, there was marked 33% reduction in the incidence of new-onset AF observed with losartan compared with atenolol. And similar result was found in Valsartan Antihypertensive Long-term Use Evaluation (VALUE) trial.

Anti-inflammatory Agent

It is seen that atrial tissue inflammation causes atrial arrhythmogenic remodeling and AF. Glucocorticoid is a potent anti-inflammatory agent. Its uses show significant decrease in AF especially in inflammatory stage but uses are restricted by its toxicity.

Spironolactone

Increased aldosterone levels have been reported in patients with AF. The role of aldosterone antagonists has not been specifically studied in humans, but preliminary data suggest that spironolactone reduces the incidence of recurrent AF after electrical cardioversion in patients with hypertension and mild LV dysfunction. Several trials with spironolactone and eplerenone are ongoing.

Statins

Statins are pleiotropic in nature and affect the metallo-proteinases, which further regulates structural remodeling of atria, i.e. dilatation and fibrosis. Evidence is mostly seen from the observational studies and retrospective analyses for primary prevention of AF. Few studies, especially in LV dysfunction and heart failure, have revealed 20–50% reduction in the incidence of new-onset AF. ARMYDA-3 trial (Atorvastatin for Reduction of Myocardial Dysrhythmia After cardiac surgery) reported a lower incidence of postoperative AF in patients who were on statin therapy.[21] It has been seen that statins are more effective for secondary prevention of recent-onset AF than in patients with recurrent persistent AF or after catheter ablation. In conclusion, there is enough evidence for statins use as primary or secondary prevention of AF, except for postoperative AF.[22]

Currently, there is strong thinking for the use of upstream therapy that may improve the outcome in AF patients who are on rhythm control drugs. Probably this could postpone the use of channel specific antiarrhythmic drugs or catheter ablation, while having lesser side effects and adverse events as well. Current guidelines do not recommend upstream therapy as first line.

NEWER PHARMACOLOGICAL AGENTS

Vernakalant

It is an atrial-selective agent. It block atrial-selective Na^+ channel blockade that is more specific for atrial potential than for ventricular action potential. Vernakalant has been used intravenously for rhythm conversion of recently detected AF. A longer-acting oral preparation of vernakalant is underway to its development. A phase 2 and few phase 3 randomized, double-blind studies have shown good efficacy for rhythm control of AF—about 50%, with fewer side effects.[23,24] Drug was found to be more efficacious in cases of recent-onset AF (3 hours to 7 days), but not for long-standing AF.

Drug is metabolized by enzyme CYP2D6, and plasma levels are similar in poor and extensive metabolizers. The elimination half-life is 2 hours. Vernakalant is still awaiting approval by the FDA for intravenous conversion of recent-onset AF.

Ranolazine

It is an antianginal drug of unspecified mechanism of action and has been approved for use in chronic stable angina. Ranolazine was tested in MERLIN-TIMI 36 trial in which a total of 6,500 patients showed reduction in nonsustained ventricular tachycardia without ischemia and incidence of AF was reported less frequently in the ranolazine group. Ranolazine is Na^+ channel blocker and inhibits late INa-inhibiting channels. It can be concluded that oral ranolazine converts new onset or paroxysmal AF and maintains sinus rhythm over a period of time.

CONCLUSION

Atrial fibrillation is common problem that is difficult to treat. Underlying factors or causes of AF should be identified and if possible should be corrected. If it is not possible then we have to decide about rhythm or rate control. As we know there is no difference between rhythm and rate control in term of mortality. If we decide whether to control rate or rhythm, patient's specific factors such as type of AF, comorbidities, and patients preference should be considered. In addition, several other factors such as side effect of drugs, pills burden, and regular monitoring of coagulation profile are also important in prescribing therapy for AF. New pharmacological approaches are in active development and the new drugs, such as vernakalant, are likely to be widely available in the future. Newer therapeutic approaches will probably have a substantial effect on future management of this disorder.

REFERENCES

1. Fox CS, Parise H, D'Agostino RB Sr, et al. Parental atrial fibrillation as a risk factor for atrial fibrillation in offspring. JAMA. 2004;291:2851-5.
2. Hodgson-Zingman DM, Karst ML, Zingman LV, et al. Atrial natriuretic peptide frameshift mutation in familial atrial fibrillation. N Engl J Med. 2008;359:158-65.
3. Olson TM, Michels VV, Ballew JD, et al. Sodium channel mutations and susceptibility to heart failure and atrial fibrillation. JAMA. 2005;293:447-54.
4. Chen YH, Xu SJ, Bendahhou S, et al. KCNQ1 gain-of-function mutation in familial atrial fibrillation. Science. 2003;299:251-4.
5. Gudbjartsson DF, Holm H, Gretarsdottir S, et al. A sequence variant in ZFHX3 on 16q22 associates with atrial fibrillation and ischemic stroke. Nat Genet. 2009;41:876-8.
6. Lloyd-Jones DM, Wang TJ, Leip EP, et al. Lifetime risk for development of atrial fibrillation: the Framingham Heart Study. Circulation. 2004;110:1042-6.
7. De Vos CB, Pisters R, Nieuwlaat R, et al. Progression from paroxysmal to persistent atrial fibrillation clinical correlates and prognosis. J Am Coll Cardiol. 2010;55:725e31.
8. Van Gelder IC, Hagens VE, Bosker HA, et al. A comparison of rate control and rhythm control in patients with recurrent persistent atrial fibrillation. N Engl J Med. 2002;347:1834-40.
9. Carlsson J, Miketic S, Windeler J, et al.; and the STAF Investigators. Randomized trial of rate-control versus rhythm control in persistent atrial fibrillation. J Am Coll Cardiol. 2003;41:1690-96.
10. Hohnloser S, Connolly S, Van Eickels M, et al. Effect of dronedarone on cardiovascular outcomes: a meta-analysis of fi ve randomized controlled trials in 6157 patients with atrial fibrillation/flutter. J Am Coll Cardiol. 2009;53(suppl 1): A113.
11. Piccini JP, Hasselblad V, Peterson ED, et al. Comparative efficacy of dronedarone and amiodarone for the maintenance of sinus rhythm in patients with atrial fibrillation. J Am Coll Cardiol. 2009;54:1089-95.
12. Shah AN, Mittal S, Sichrovsky TC, et al. Long-term outcome following successful pulmonary vein isolation: pattern and prediction of very late recurrence. J Cardiovasc Electrophysiol. 2008;19:661-7.
13. Cappato R, Calkins H, Chen SA, et al. Prevalence and causes of fatal outcome in catheter ablation of atrial fibrillation. J Am Coll Cardiol. 2009;53:1798-1803.
14. Khargi K, Hutten BA, Lemke B, et al. Surgical treatment of atrial fibrillation; a systematic review. Eur J Cardiothorac Surg. 2005;27:258.
15. Pisters R, Lane DA, Nieuwlaat R, et al. A novel user friendly score (HAS-BLED) to assess one-year risk of major bleeding in atrial fibrillation patients: the Euro Heart Survey. Chest. 2010. pp. 201-02.
16. Connolly SJ, Ezekowitz MD, Yusuf S, et al. Dabigatran versus warfarin in patients with atrial fibrillation. N Engl J Med. 2009;361:1139-51.
17. Patel MR, Mahaffey KW, Garg J, et al. Rivaroxaban versus warfarin in nonvalvular atrial fibrillation. N Engl J Med. 2011;365(10): 883-91.

18. Granger CB, Alexander JH, McMurray JJV, et al. Apixaban versus warfarin in patients with atrial fibrillation. N Engl J Med. 2011;365(11):981-92.
19. Holmes DR, Reddy VY, Turi ZG, et al. Percutaneous closure of the left atrial appendage versus warfarin therapy for prevention of stroke in patients with atrial fibrillation: a randomised non inferiority trial. Lancet. 2009; 374:534–42.
20. Goette A, Staack T, Rocken C, et al. Increased expression of extracellular signal-regulated kinase and angiotensin-converting enzyme in human atria during atrial fibrillation. J Am Coll Cardiol. 2000;35:1669-77.
21. Patti G, Chello M, Candura D, et al. Randomized trial of atorvastatin for reduction of postoperative atrial fibrillation in patients undergoing cardiac surgery: results of the ARMYDA-3 (Atorvastatin for Reduction of Myocardial Dysrhythmia after cardiac surgery) study. Circulation. 2006;114:1455-61.
22. Fauchier L, Pierre B, de Labriolle A, et al. Antiarrhythmic effect of statin therapy and atrial fibrillation: a meta-analysis of randomized controlled trials. J Am Coll Cardiol. 2008;51:828-35.
23. Naccarelli GV, Wolbrette DL, Samii S, et al. Vernakalant—a promising therapy for conversion of recent-onset atrial fibrillation. Expert Opin Investig Drugs. 2008;17:805-10.
24. Roy D, Pratt CM, Torp-Pedersen C, et al. for the Atrial Arrhythmia Conversion Trial Investigators. Vernakalant hydrochloride for rapid conversion of atrial fibrillation: a phase 3, randomized, placebo-controlled trial. Circulation. 2008;117:1518-25.

10

Newer Antiplatelets and Anticoagulants: Filling it into Clinical Practices

Arvind Sethi, Upendra Kaul

INTRODUCTION

Hemostasis is the physiological host defense mechanism by which formation of platelet- and fibrin-rich plugs helps prevent bleeding from sites of injured vessels. On the contrary, when this process assumes pathological proportions and fills intravascular, arterial, and venous lumens with its consequent effects, it is known as thrombosis.

Arterial thrombosis occurs mostly on top of disrupted atherosclerotic plaques. Breakdown of regulatory mechanisms that limit platelet activation and inhibit coagulation augments thrombosis at these sites. Products of blood coagulation contribute to atherogenesis, as well as microscopic erosions in the vessel wall trigger the formation of tiny platelet-rich thrombi. This complex interplay of atherosclerosis and thrombosis has prompted the term *atherothrombosis*.

Venous thrombosis, however, occurs due to hypercoagulability, which can be genetic or acquired, and the additional main acquired risk factors, such as advanced age, obesity, or cancer, which are associated with immobility. Superimposed triggering factors, such as surgery, pregnancy, or hormonal therapy, modify this risk, and thrombosis occurs when the combination of genetic, acquired, and triggering forces exceeds a critical threshold.

ANTIPLATELET DRUGS

Antiplatelet drugs are used in the management of thrombotic conditions like angina, acute coronary syndrome (ACS), acute myocardial infarction (AMI), stroke, percutaneous coronary intervention (PCI), cardiac surgery, peripheral vascular disease, and cardiovascular disease prevention. These are also utilized in atrial fibrillation.

There are many antiplatelet drugs available for use in clinical practice and quite a few under investigation.

Drugs in Use for the Purpose

Aspirin has been the leading therapeutic drug for the prevention of thromboembolic complications of atherosclerotic disease.[1] It permanently inactivates the key platelet enzyme (COX). This effect can be reversed only by generation of new platelets. It is thus given as once-daily dosing.[2]

Clopidogrel has been found to be marginally more effective than aspirin especially for the secondary prevention of vascular events. It is used for primary prevention only in the ones allergic or intolerant to aspirin as also to provide enhanced protection when combined with aspirin[3] (albeit at a cost of increased risk of bleeding).

Cilostazol is a phosphodiesterase 3 inhibitor. It has vasodilator and antiplatelet aggregation properties, has been shown to be more effective in peripheral vascular disease, and is currently recommended for patients with moderate-to-severe disabling symptoms and who are ineligible for surgical or catheter-based interventions.[4]

Dipyridamole, a pyrimidopyrimidine derivative, has vasodilator and antiplatelet properties. Recent guidelines have accepted aspirin and extended-release dipyridamole as agents of choice for the prevention of cerebral ischemic events in patients with noncardioembolic transient ischemic attack (TIA) or stroke.[5] It is, however, inferior to clopidogrel for aspirin-intolerant patients undergoing intervention.

ANTIPLATELET DRUG RESISTANCE

Aspirin and Clopidogrel "Resistance"

None of the available antithrombotic drugs is 100% effective in the prevention of adverse thrombotic events. True aspirin "resistance," defined as the inability of aspirin to inhibit COX-1-dependant TXA2 production, has a very low (approximately 1–2%) incidence.[6] It is estimated that a much higher number of treated individuals may, however, have an inadequate response to aspirin treatment at doses <300 mg daily. Several reasons for this inadequate drug effect have been investigated of which patient noncompliance contributes as a major cause (3–40%).[7] Such inadequate response has been seen to aspirin treatment even in patients receiving doses considered adequate for the majority. These patients can be detected by using an in vitro test of platelet function and are labeled as having "biochemical resistance."[8] Clinical thromboses can occur as a very late sign of such a phenomenon.

Inflammatory response associated with conditions such as unstable angina, AMI, diabetes, and cardiac surgery may enhance resistance to aspirin.

Similarly, up to a third of patients[9] who receive clopidogrel in the usual doses are reported to have an inadequate response in terms of antiplatelet activity leading to adverse outcomes. It has been suggested to be due to genetic polymorphism involving the enzymes utilized in the activation of the drug.

Although dual antiplatelet drug resistance is known to occur resulting in very high risk for drug-eluting stent thrombosis or death,[10] resistance to one class of antiplatelet drugs does not necessarily confer resistance to other classes of antiplatelet drugs. Some nonresponders to conventional doses of clopidogrel can be converted to responders by increasing the doses. Drug responsiveness may differ depending on things like body mass index (BMI), stress, and the timing of drug administration in relation to the degree of platelet reactivity during the intervention. Diabetics have been seen to have a consistently high level of resistance when treated with thienopyridines.[11]

Treatment failure may be associated with significant adverse outcomes as a consequence of thrombosis including death, MI, cerebrovascular accident, and closure of grafts.

NEED FOR NEWER ANTIPLATELET DRUGS

The drugs in use are not without limitations of delayed onset of action and serious side effects including bleeding. Also in view of the devastating complications despite advances in stent design and drug delivery, there is need for development of drugs with better platelet activity suppression and prompt reversibility of action.

Prasugrel

Prasugrel is a thienopyridine class of drug. It is one of the new P2Y12 receptor blocker and is being used for the prevention of thrombosis after PCI.[12]

Its efficacy as an antithrombotic drug has been established in randomized clinical trials. In the setting of PCI, it was suggested to have produced a greater degree of platelet inhibition than clopidogrel and was associated with fewer incidences of MACE (major adverse cardiac events) (MI, recurrent ischemia, and clinical target vessel thrombosis).[13] In TRITON-TIMI 38, a phase III study, patients undergoing PCI were randomized to receive either prasugrel (loading with 60 mg and followed with 10 mg daily) or clopidogrel (loading with 300 mg dose and followed with 75 mg daily) as a second antiplatelet along with aspirin and were followed for 6–15 months.[14] Prasugrel administration was associated with a significant reduction in primary end point, i.e. death from cardiovascular causes, nonfatal MI, or nonfatal stroke (9.9% vs. 12.1%). In addition, rates of MI (7.4% vs. 9.7%), urgent target vessel revascularization (2.5% vs. 3.7%), and stent thrombosis (1.1% vs. 2.4%) were significantly reduced. However, an increased risk of bleeding was noticed, particularly in specific groups of patients, i.e. those older than 75 years of age, with a small BMI as well as those with a history of stroke or TIA, and/or in those undergoing coronary artery bypass graft (CABG) surgery. However, subgroup analysis of patients undergoing PCI for ACS or STEMI (ST elevation myocardial infarction) had improved protection from stent thrombosis with no additional risk of major bleeding complications. Other subgroup analyses showed that diabetics had specifically benefitted from prasugrel with greater protection in terms of efficacy.

In animal studies, prasugrel has been shown to be 10–100 times more potent than clopidogrel in antiplatelet effect.[15] Like clopidogrel, prasugrel is also a prodrug and needs to be metabolized to an active form to exhibit its antiplatelet effect. This conversion process involves only a single cytochrome P450-dependant step (CYP3A4 and to a lesser extent CYP2B6), resulting in increased levels of the active metabolite and hence increased clinical effect. It is thus less affected by genetic variations in cytochromes than clopidogrel and also less affected by drug interactions involving CYP3A4 for metabolism leading to less variation in formation of active metabolite. It is rapidly absorbed and metabolized with peak concentrations occurring at 0.5 hour after oral administration in healthy volunteers. Approximately 68% of a dose is excreted as metabolites in the urine and the remainder in the feces. Dose-finding studies have shown maximum effects with an acceptable safety profile with an initial loading dose of 40–60 mg, and maintenance dosing of 15 mg producing a sustained response. Prasugrel has been shown to generate 2.2 times more active metabolite after a loading dose than for clopidogrel, and it also may explain the faster onset of activity, higher levels of active compound, and reduced variability of platelet inhibition.

As with other thienopyridine derivatives, prasugrel's active metabolite binds to the P2Y12 receptor irreversibly by forming disulfide bridges between extracellular cysteine residues at positions Cys17 and Cys270 and prevents platelet activation. Similarly in patients with stable CAD (coronary artery disease), prasugrel produces a faster and more effective inhibition of platelet function than clopidogrel. Maximum antiplatelet effect has been seen to occur after 2 days and platelet function recovers over the next 2 days after discontinuation of the drug. In a comparative study, the incidence of poor platelet aggregation response after loading with 60 mg prasugrel was lower than for 300 mg of clopidogrel.[16] Healthy subjects on clopidogrel therapy when switched directly to prasugrel (with or without a loading dose), also showed greater inhibition of platelet aggregation without any increase in bleeding risk.

Bleeding is the major adverse effect of prasugrel. In TRITON-TIMI 38, a phase III trial, prasugrel administration was associated with a significantly increased major adverse bleeding events (2.4% vs. 1.8%) with higher incidence of life-threatening bleeding (1.4% vs. 0.9%) including nonfatal bleeding (1.1% vs. 0.9%) and fatal bleeding (0.4% vs. 0.1%). On risk/benefit analysis, every additional life saved by the use of prasugrel, it was expected that an additional death due to bleeding is likely to occur. Patients with a history of stroke or TIA especially were found to more likely experience adverse bleeding (2.3% vs. 0%). On long-term analysis, it was detected that most of the bleeding complications occurred during maintenance phase. These effects could be avoided by restricting its use or by reducing the maintenance dose in high-risk groups including those with age > 75 years and those weighing < 60 kg.[17]

Prasugrel Resistance

Compared with clopidogrel, use of prasugrel leads to better clinical response especially in diabetic patients with only a few nonresponders.[11] Reduced response to clopidogrel is attributed to reductions in the amount of available active metabolite to interact with platelets and not due to alterations in the platelet P2Y12 receptor.

Prasugrel was approved by US Food and Drug Administration (FDA) in 2009, with a cited contraindication to its use in patients with a history of TIA or stroke or with active bleeding.[18] The FDA labeling also includes a general warning against its use in elderly with age ≥75 years because of increased bleeding risk except in high-risk situations, i.e. patients with diabetes or those with a history of prior MI, where the net benefit is considered to be greater.[18]

Ticagrelor

Ticagrelor is a cyclopentyltriazolopyrimidine class of drug that is orally active. It is a reversible $P2Y_{12}$ receptor antagonist.[19] Ticagrelor rapidly and effectively inhibits platelet aggregation at doses ranging from 50 to 200 mg twice daily. On day 1, peak inhibition is seen to occur at 2–4 hours, whereas clopidogrel in the doses of 75 mg twice a day showed minimal effect. In a phase II dose-finding study of ACS patients,[20] subset of those requiring CABG within 24 hours of its administration showed fivefold increase in the incidence of major bleeding, whereas reduced tendency of bleeding for those requiring surgery between days 1 and 5 was observed. Slightly reduced incidence of MI was noticed in ticagrelor-treated patients with no difference in deaths being observed in the overall analysis of the study.

It was subsequently evaluated in PLATO (Study of Platelet Inhibition and Patient Outcomes), a large phase III, double-blind, randomized clinical trial.[21] Patients with ACS, including those ST segment elevation, were randomized to receive loading dose of ticagrelor (180 mg) followed by 90 mg twice daily or clopidogrel (300–600 mg) followed by 75 mg daily. Over a 12 months follow-up, the primary end point (a composite of MI, stroke, or death from vascular causes) occurred in significantly fewer patients, i.e. 9.8% versus 11.7% ($P < 0.001$). Stent thrombosis was noticed to be significantly less in the ticagrelor group, i.e. 1.3% versus 1.9% ($P = 0.009$). No difference was seen in major bleeding complications, 11.6% versus 11.2% ($P = 0.43$). Trend towards increased incidence of hemorrhagic strokes, i.e. 0.2% versus 0.1% was noticed. No significant difference in the rate of major bleeding was observed in those undergoing CABG (7.4% vs. 7.9%). Other observations of the study as a whole included higher incidence of major or minor bleeding (16.1% vs. 14.6%), dyspnea (0.9% vs. 0.1%), ventricular pause > 3 seconds within first week of therapy (5.8% vs. 3.6%), and discontinuing of the study drug (7.4% vs. 6.0%). It was also expressed that due to its reversible effects, ticagrelor may have utility in patients with unknown coronary anatomy and a probable candidature for CABG.[22] It was also advised that it may be used with caution in patients with stroke/TIA. In a randomized study,[23] patients considered nonresponsive to clopidogrel when crossed over to ticagrelor also were seen to become responsive with respect to platelet inhibition.

Although there is one known active metabolite, ticagrelor, when administered orally, does not require metabolic activation for its clinical effect. Peak effect on platelet inhibition is measurable at 2–4 hours after oral dosage in healthy volunteers. The drug shows linear kinetics after twice-daily dosing with no age- or gender-related differences.[24] The terminal half-life of ticagrelor is 7 hours approximately.

Ticagrelor reversibly binds to the P2Y12 receptor with almost complete inhibition of platelet aggregation.[24] It has a faster onset and offset of action than clopidogrel. Alterations in single nucleotide polymorphisms of the receptor gene do not affect its ability to interact with the P2Y12 receptor at doses ranging from 50 to 200 mg twice daily. More rapid and greater inhibition of platelet aggregation is seen with ticagrelor than with clopidogrel[24] and doses > 100 mg do not give additional benefit in terms of its efficacy.

Bleeding is the most common adverse effect with ticagrelor administration. Dyspnea requiring discontinuation of therapy was seem to occur in a larger proportion of patients, i.e. 0.9% versus 0.1% in the PLATO trial.[21] In the ONSET/OFFSET study[25] comparing ticagrelor, clopidogrel, or placebo in patients with stable CAD, the incidences of dyspnea and effect on pulmonary function were 38.6%, 9.3%, and 8.3% in ticagrelor, clopidogrel, and placebo treated patients. This side effect occurred more commonly within the first week of initiation of therapy and was found to be reversible.

Ticagrelor was approved by FDA in 2011.[26] A "Boxed Warning" was also issued indicating that daily maintenance doses of >100 mg of aspirin decrease the effectiveness of ticagrelor. Caution was suggested against its use in patients with high risk of bleeding. However, it was recommended to be used in situations where its benefits outweigh the risks.

Cangrelor

Cangrelor is an adenosine diphosphate (ADP) receptor antagonist. It has recently been investigated in clinical trials.[19] Upon intravenous (IV) administration, it has a quick and short lasting reversible inhibitory effect on platelet function. Thus it may have a significant role in the management of patients in the perioperative period.

Cangrelor was found to be effective in patients with ACS, unstable angina, or non-Q wave MI in small studies. In a randomized clinical trial of patients with acute STEMI receiving cangrelor and, alteplase either alone or in varying combinations, cangrelor was found to be an effective adjunct when added to alteplase for resolution of ST segment elevation.[27] Subsequently, Bhatt et al.[28] in CHAMPION PLATFORM Study randomized patients undergoing PCI to either cangrelor or placebo in addition to clopidogrel in over 5,000 patients. There was no difference in the primary end point of composite of death, MI, ischemia-driven revascularization at 48 hours in the two groups. However, in a subgroup analysis, cangrelor did produce significant difference in stent thrombosis and death from any cause. Groin hematomas were more in cangrelor group, although no difference in the requirement of transfusions was noticed. The trial was, however, terminated early due to non-superiority of the drug for the primary end point. In another trial, CHAMPION PCI Trial, they checked its efficacy against clopidogrel in over 8,000 patients. This also did not show any significant advantage and was also terminated early.

Cangrelor has a rapid onset and offset of action following IV administration. Steady state is reached at 30 minutes (even in the absence of a loading dose) and elimination half-time of <9 minutes. Platelet function thus returns to normal within an hour of discontinuation of the drug.[29]

Cangrelor reversibly binds to the P2Y12 receptor on the platelet surface. It has greater inhibitory effect on platelet aggregation than that of clopidogrel. Cangrelor was well tolerated in early clinical trials with no significant bleeding complications.[27] Similar profile was seen even when it was coadministered with aspirin and/or heparin. However, bleeding risk increased with concomitant use of abciximab before PCI. Higher rates of bleeding with cangrelor have although been noticed in phase III trials.

When given in combination, cangrelor inhibits the antiplatelet activity of clopidogrel due to its inhibition of the binding of active metabolite of clopidogrel to the P2Y12 receptor on the platelet surface. However, because of the advantage of short acting nature and IV administration, it may serve as an effective bridge in the perioperative period to tide over to definitive surgical intervention.

ANTICOAGULANTS

Heparin and Low Molecular Weight Heparin

Unfractionated heparin (UFH) and low molecular weight heparin (LMWH) have a rapid onset of action. These are the agents of choice in acute thrombotic states. They are clinically indicated in the treatment of ACS, treatment and/or prevention of thromboembolism, as bridge to oral therapy for atrial fibrillation (AF), and during cardioversion. Bleeding is the major complication of heparin therapy. Major bleeding is reported up to 7% with fatal bleeding up to 3%. Heparin-induced thrombocytopenia (HIT) is another complication that may be encountered in up to 5% of those receiving the drug.[30] Hemorrhage is also the major complication of LMWH, however, the rates of bleeding may be less as compared to UFH.

Fondaparinux

Fondaparinux, a synthetic analog of the naturally occurring pentasaccharide found in heparins selectively binds to antithrombin. This irreversible binding result in neutralization of factor Xa leading to obliteration of the thrombotic pathway and the ultimate thrombus generation.

Fondaparinux is rapidly and completely absorbed following subcutaneous administration. It is excreted primarily unchanged in the urine. Its half-life is 17 resulours in patients with preserved renal function. It has predictable pharmacokinetics similar to LMWH and thus monitoring for anti-Xa levels is not required during fondaparinux administration.

Like LMWH and heparin, fondaparinux has been proven to be equally efficacious in the treatment of deep venous thrombosis (DVT) and pulmonary embolism (PE) respectively.[31,32] Fondaparinux has been extensively studied in medically ill and surgical patients for thromboprophylaxis.[33] It showed better efficacy in reducing venous thromboembolic event (VTE) in patients undergoing hip arthroplasty, knee arthroplasty, and hip fracture surgery in different trials. Overall analysis of these trials showed that the incidence of major bleeding was significantly higher with fondaparinux, i.e. 2.7% versus 1.7% for LMWH,[34] although the incidence of clinically relevant bleeding did not differ between the agents. The differences noted in efficacy and safety outcomes could possibly be related to the timing as well as dose of perioperative drug administration. Those given fondaparinux <6 hours after surgery showed increased frequency of major bleeding. Hence it is recommended to withhold therapy postprocedure for at least 6 hours in patients at risk of bleeding. In the setting of HIT, it may possibly be a potential option for thromboprophylaxis, although no conclusive data is available.[35] While fondaparinux has been studied in ACS with reasonable effect, it has not yet received approval from FDA.

Fondaparinux is contraindicated in patients with marked renal dysfunction [estimated creatinine clearance (CrCl) <30 mL/min]. It is also not recommended for use in patients weighing <50 kg for VTE prophylaxis. Prolonged half-life further complicates reversal of its effect when required. Although no known specific antidote exists for this drug-related hemorrhage, recombinant activated factor VII (rFVIIa) administration has been shown to improve coagulation parameters and thrombin formation.[36]

Direct Thrombin Inhibitors

As the name suggests, these agents selectively and directly bind to the active site of thrombin leading to inhibition of thrombin. The three currently approved direct thrombin inhibitors (DTIs) include desirudin and bivalirudin (hirudin analogs), and argatroban.[37]

Of these bivalirudin has the shortest half-life, which makes it a particularly useful agent for prevention of thrombosis in the periprocedural period. Selection of DTI is often affected by patient-specific variables such as age, left ventricular dysfunction, hemodynamic instability, and hepatic or renal impairment. Effect of DTI is monitored using activated partial thromboplastin time (aPTT), which is required to be maintained between 1.5 and 3 times control for argatroban and 1.5–2.5 times control for bivalirudin. Desirudin is, however, exempt of this monitoring. The aPTT level is required to be measured every 6 hours until the patient has adequate therapeutic levels, following which the frequency of monitoring may be reduced.[38]

Direct thrombin inhibitors can be especially useful in conditions like HIT or HIT-T.[39] Argatroban and bivalirudin are the agents that have a role of an anticoagulant for the prevention of thrombosis in patients undergoing PCI. Bivalirudin is indicated for use in moderate to high-risk ACS, unstable angina/NSTEMI who are scheduled to undergo early invasive management.[40]

As with other agents, hemorrhage is the most common complication with DTIs with an additional drawback of non-availability of specific reversal agents. However, rFVIIa has been reported to be useful in such a situation as per anecdotal reports. It could be considered for immediate treatment of complications like life-threatening hemorrhage.[41]

Oral Anticoagulants

The oral agents available are classified as vitamin K antagonists (VKAs). These drugs produce their effects by inhibition of vitamin K epoxy reductase, an enzyme required for the conversion of vitamin K to its active form. Warfarin is one such agent that is effective in conditions like the primary and secondary prevention of VTE, prevention of systemic embolism in patients having atrial fibrillation and those with prosthetic heart valves, as well as in patients with acute MI for the prevention of stroke, recurrent MI, or death.[42]

Bleeding is an important concern with warfarin treatment also. The drug has a narrow therapeutic index due to the possible influence of environmental factors as also the various probable drug interactions. The risk of major bleeding increases to 0.3–0.5% per year and the risk of intracranial hemorrhage by approximately 0.2% per year with the use of VKAs as compared to controls. The most important risk factors for hemorrhage in VKA therapy include intensity of anticoagulant effect, time within therapeutic range, and patient characteristics. Higher required goals of international normalized ratio (INR) (INR~3) have been shown to be directly associated with increased rates of hemorrhagic complications and these patients at high risk of bleeding may even benefit from lower targets.[43]

Issues with Available Anticoagulants

For more than half a century, warfarin had been the only anticoagulant available for oral use. Its narrow therapeutic index and multiple drug and diet interactions affected its safety, compliance, and efficacy. A meta-analysis revealed that 44% of bleeding complications with warfarin were associated with supra therapeutic INRs and that 48% of thromboembolic events occurred with sub therapeutic readings.[44] Difficulties in achieving optimal anticoagulation with warfarin therapy are attributed to its slow onset of action and variable efficacy especially due to interaction with, and numerous food items and drugs. These common shortcomings prompted the development of newer agents (NOAs) that target factors such as factors Xa and IIa (thrombin), key steps, or the coagulation cascade.

NEW ORAL ANTICOAGULANTS

Dabigatran

Dabigatran etexilate (Pradaxa) is the first oral DTI to be approved by the FDA. Dabigatran etexilate is a prodrug that is rapidly converted to its active compound, dabigatran, by nonspecific esterases in the plasma and liver. This active compound competitively and reversibly binds to the active site of free and clot-bound thrombin, thereby blocking its procoagulant activity.

Dabigatran is approved for use in the prevention of stroke and systemic embolism in adult patients with nonvalvular atrial fibrillation (AF) [FDA, European Medicines Agency (EMA), and Canada's Health Products and Food Branch

(HPFB)] and in the primary prevention of VTEs in adult patients who have undergone elective total hip (THA) or knee (TKA) arthroplasty (EMA and HPFB). Dabigatran has been evaluated in several phase 3 clinical trials to assess its safety and efficacy in different clinical situations.

Prevention of Stroke and Systemic Embolism in Nonvalvular AF

The RE-LY (randomized evaluation of long-term anticoagulant therapy, warfarin, compared with dabigatran) study was a noninferiority trial that evaluated the efficacy and safety of dabigatran at 110 or 150 mg twice daily compared with dose-adjusted warfarin targeting an INR of 2–3 in patients with nonvalvular AF and an intermediate risk of thromboembolism.[45]

The stroke (including hemorrhagic stroke) or systemic embolism rate per year was lower with the 150-mg dabigatran dose (1.11%; $P < 0.001$ for superiority) and equivalent with the 110-mg dabigatran dose (1.53%; $P < 0.001$ for noninferiority) compared with warfarin (1.69%). The superiority of the 150-mg dose was seen only when compared with patients taking warfarin with moderate/poor regulation of their INRs (defined as the INR being in the target range <65% of the time).[46]

The annual rate of major bleeding with the 150-mg dabigatran dose was not different (3.11%; P¼0.31) compared with warfarin (3.36%) but was lower with the 110 mg dose (2.71%; P¼.003). The rates of hemorrhagic stroke with the 110- and 150-mg dabigatran doses were lower than with warfarin (0.12% and 0.10% vs. 0.38%; $P < 0.001$), as were the rates of intracranial hemorrhage (0.23% and 0.30% vs. 0.74%; $P < 0.001$).

Treatment of Acute VTE

The RE-COVER study evaluated patients with acute VTE and compared 6 months of treatment with either dabigatran, 150 mg twice daily, or dose-adjusted warfarin after initial UFH or LMWH anticoagulation.[47]

The 6-month incidence of recurrent symptomatic VTE and related deaths was 2.4% (2.3% VTE; 0.1% deaths) in patients treated with dabigatran versus 2.1% (1.9% VTE; 0.2% deaths) in those treated with warfarin ($P < 0.001$ for noninferiority).

The rates of major bleeding episodes were similar in the dabigatran and warfarin groups (1.6% vs. 1.9%). However, the incidence of all bleeding events was lower with dabigatran use (16.1% vs. 21.9%).

Postoperative VTE Prophylaxis for TKA

Dabigatran dosed at 220 or 150 mg/day starting with half a dose 1–4 hours after surgery was evaluated for the prevention of VTE after TKA compared with enoxaparin, 40 mg/day, starting the evening before surgery for 6–10 days in the European RE-MODEL study[48] and enoxaparin, 30 mg twice daily, starting the morning after surgery for 13 days in the North American RE-MOBILIZE study.[49]

There were conflicting results between the two trials. In RE-MODEL, the incidence of VTE or mortality was 37.7% (37.5% VTE; 0.2% deaths) in the enoxaparin arm compared with 36.4% (36.2% VTE; 0.2% deaths) in the dabigatran, 220-mg, arm ($P = 0.0003$ for noninferiority) and 40.5% (40.3% VTE; 0.2% deaths) in the dabigatran, 150-mg, arm ($P = 0.017$ for noninferiority). However, in RE-MOBILIZE, the composite of VTE and death occurred in 25.3% (all VTE; no deaths) of those in the enoxaparin arm compared with 31.1% (all VTE; no deaths) of those in the dabigatran, 220-mg, arm ($P = 0.02$) and 33.7% (33.5% VTE; 0.2% deaths) of those in the dabigatran, 150-mg, arm ($P<0.001$). The differences in efficacy between the two trials may be due to the different dosing schedules of enoxaparin because the primary outcomes in dabigatran-treated patients were the same for both studies. The RE-MOBILIZE used the standard North American dose, which is more dose intensive with a longer duration than that used in Europe (RE-MODEL); thus, dabigatran may not be an equally efficacious prophylaxis option in this setting.

Among the three arms, the incidence of major bleeding did not differ significantly in RE-MODEL (1.3% for enoxaparin vs. 1.5% for dabigatran, 220 mg, and 1.3% for dabigatran, 150 mg) or in RE-MOBILIZE (1.4% for enoxaparin vs. 0.6% for dabigatran, 220 mg, and 0.6% for dabigatran, 150 mg).

Postoperative VTE Prophylaxis for THA

The European RE-NOVATE I[50] and the North American RE-NOVATE II[51] studies evaluated dabigatran dosed at 220 or 150 mg/day (the 150-mg dose arm was present only in RE-NOVATE I) starting with half a dose 1–4 hours after surgery in preventing VTE after THA compared with enoxaparin, 40 mg/day, starting preoperatively the evening before surgery for 28–35 days of treatment.

In RE-NOVATE I, the incidence of VTE or death was 6.7% (all VTE; no deaths) in the enoxaparin arm versus 6.0% (5.7% VTE; 0.3% deaths) in the dabigatran, 220-mg, arm ($P < 0.0001$ for noninferiority) and 8.6% (8.3% VTE; 0.3% deaths) in the dabigatran, 150-mg, arm ($P < 0.0001$ for noninferiority). Furthermore, RE-NOVATE II detected total VTE and death in 7.7% (all VTE; no deaths) in the dabigatran, 220 mg, arm versus 8.8% (8.7% VTE; 0.1% deaths) in the enoxaparin arm ($P = 0.43$).

In both RE-NOVATE studies, there was no difference in major bleeding rates with either dose of dabigatran compared with enoxaparin ($P = 0.44$ for 220 mg, $P = 0.60$ for 150 mg in RENOVATE I and $P = 0.40$ for 220 mg in RENOVATE II).

Recommendations for Stroke Prevention in Patients with AF

In patients with CrCl > 30 mL/min per 1.73 m^2 (to convert to mL/s per m^2, multiply by 0.0167), the recommended dose is 150 mg orally twice daily.[52]

***Renal impairment*:** For patients with CrCl of 15–30 mL/min per 1.73 m^2, the recommended dose approved by FDA is 75 mg twice daily. Because patients with CrCl < 30 mL/min per 1.73 m^2 were excluded from the RE-LY trial, and because >80% of the drug is renally excreted, extreme caution should be used in this group of patients, and our recommendation is that dabigatran be avoided or discontinued.[52]

***Hepatic impairment*:** Patients with moderate hepatic impairment (Child-Pugh class B) demonstrated no consistent change in pharmacodynamics properties. However, in patients with advanced liver disease causing impaired coagulation, the use of dabigatran is not recommended.[52]

***Pregnancy and breastfeeding*:** At present, its use in pregnant and nursing mothers is not recommended.[52]

Adverse Events

Nonhemorrhagic Adverse Events

Across all the clinical trials, approximately 10% of patients experienced severe dyspepsia compared with 5.8% taking warfarin, leading to the discontinuation of dabigatran therapy in 21% of patients.[45,48] This is possibly due to dabigatran's tartaric acid core needed to create a low pH for the drug's absorption. In the RELY trial, approximately 0.8% of patients taking dabigatran experienced an MI compared with 0.64% taking warfarin [hazard ratio, 1.29; 95% confidence interval (CI), 0.96–1.75; P = 0.09 for dabigatran, 110 mg, and hazard ratio, 1.27; 95% CI, 0.94–1.71; P = .12 for dabigatran, 150 mg];[53] the pathogenesis for this is unclear. In a meta-analysis, dabigatran therapy increased the risk of MI, cardiac death, or unstable angina compared with the control group (odds ratio, 1.27; 95% CI, 1.00-1.61).[54] However, the magnitude of increase was small compared with the benefit of ischemic stroke prevention.

Hemorrhagic Adverse Events

There was a higher rate of major gastrointestinal (GI) bleeding in patients receiving dabigatran, 150 mg, than warfarin (1.5% vs. 1.0%; P < 0.001), with a trend toward a higher incidence in patients older than 75 years (5.10% vs. 4.37% per year; P = 0.07).[45] In the months after FDA approval, there were multiple reports in the community of increased bleeding events with dabigatran use. However, on reviewing insurance claims from community practices, the FDA concluded that the rate of bleeding with dabigatran use was not higher than with warfarin use in patients using either drug for the first time and was likely secondary to the underreporting of bleeding events related to warfarin use.

Rivaroxaban

Rivaroxaban (Xarelto) is the first oral direct coagulation factor Xa inhibitor approved for clinical use in the United States. It reversibly binds to the active site of coagulation factor Xa without antithrombin mediation affecting free and platelet-bound factor Xa.

Rivaroxaban is approved by the FDA, EMA, and HPFB for use in the primary prevention of VTE in adult patients who have undergone elective THA or TKA, the prevention of stroke and systemic embolism in patients with nonvalvular AF, the treatment of DVT and PE, and to reduce the risk of recurrent DVT and PE after initial treatment. The efficacy and safety of rivaroxaban have been evaluated in phase 3 clinical trials across different clinical situations.

Postoperative VTE Prophylaxis for THA

The Regulation of Coagulation in Orthopedic Surgery to Prevent Deep Venous Thrombosis and Pulmonary Embolism (RECORD) 1[55] and 2[56] trials compared rivaroxaban, 10 mg/day, initiated 6–8 hours after wound closure for approximately 35 days with enoxaparin, 40 mg/day, given 12 hours before surgery and restarted 6–8 hours after wound closure for either 31–39 days as in RECORD 1 or 10–14 days as in RECORD 2 for the prevention of VTE after THA.

In RECORD 1, the primary efficacy outcome of VTE and mortality occurred in 1.1% (1% VTE; 0.1% deaths) of patients in the rivaroxaban arm and in 3.7% (3.5% VTE; 0.2% deaths) of those in the enoxaparin arm (P < 0.001). In RECORD 2, the rates were 2.0% (1.8% VTE; 0.2% deaths) in the rivaroxaban arm compared with 9.3% (8.6% VTE; 0.7% deaths) in the enoxaparin arm (P < 0.0001). There was no difference in the incidence of major bleeding between rivaroxaban and enoxaparin in both trials (RECORD 1: 0.3% vs. 0.1%, Ps no difference in the incidence of major bleeding).

Postoperative VTE Prophylaxis for TKA

The RECORD 3[57] and 4[58] trials compared rivaroxaban, 10 mg/day, initiated 6–8 hours after wound closure with enoxaparin, 40 mg once daily, initiated 12 hours before surgery in RECORD 3 or enoxaparin, 30 mg every 12 hours, initiated 12–24 hours after surgery in RECORD 4 for the prevention of VTE after TKA.

In the RECORD 3 trial, the primary efficacy outcome of VTE and mortality within 17 days after surgery occurred in 9.6% (all VTE events; no deaths) of patients in the rivaroxaban arm and in 18.9% (18.7% VTE; 0.2% deaths) of those in the enoxaparin arm (P < 0.001). In RECORD 4, the primary efficacy outcome occurred in 6.9% (6.7% VTE; 0.2% deaths) of patients in the rivaroxaban arm and in 10.1% (9.8% VTE; 0.3% deaths) of patients in the enoxaparin arm ($P = 0.0118$).

In either study, there was no difference in the incidence of major bleeding between the rivaroxaban and enoxaparin arms (RECORD 3: 0.6% vs. 0.5%, $P = 0.77$ and RECORD 4: 0.7% vs. 0.3%, $P = 0.11$).

Treatment of Acute VTE

The EINSTEIN study[59] compared oral rivaroxaban (15 mg twice daily for 3 weeks followed by 20 mg once daily) with enoxaparin followed by a VKA for 3, 6, or 12 months in patients with acute, symptomatic DVT (initial treatment study). A parallel, double-blind, randomized study compared rivaroxaban (20 mg/day) with placebo for an additional 6 or 12 months in patients who had completed 6-12 months of treatment for VTE (continued-treatment study). The EINSTEIN-PE[60] was a similar study that evaluated the same dose of rivaroxaban versus enoxaparin/VKA in patients with an acute, symptomatic PE with or without DVT.

In EINSTEIN, rivaroxaban therapy was noninferior to enoxaparin/VKA therapy with respect to recurrent VTE (2.1% vs. 3.0%; $P < 0.001$). In the continued-treatment study, rivaroxaban therapy was superior to placebo use with respect to recurrent VTE (1.3% vs. 7.1%; $P < 0.001$). The rates of symptomatic recurrent VTE in the EINSTEIN-PE study were also similar between the rivaroxaban and enoxaparin/VKA groups (2.1% vs. 1.8%; $P < 0.001$). The rates of symptomatic recurrent VTE in the EINSTEIN-PE study were also similar between the rivaroxaban and enoxaparin/VKA groups (2.1% vs. 1.8%; $P = 0.003$ for noninferiority).

In both studies, EINSTEIN and EINSTEIN-PE, the principal safety outcome of major or clinically relevant nonmajor bleeding occurred at similar rates in both treatment arms. In the continued-treatment study, four patients taking rivaroxaban (0.7%) and no patients taking placebo had nonfatal major bleeding, which was not significant.

Prevention of Stroke and Systemic Embolism in Nonvalvular AF

The Rivaroxaban Once Daily Oral Direct Factor Xa Inhibition Compared with Vitamin K Antagonism for Prevention of Stroke and Embolism Trial in Atrial Fibrillation (ROCKET AF)[61] study evaluated rivaroxaban for prevention of stroke or systemic embolization in patients with nonvalvular AF (intermediate to high risk of stroke). Patients were randomly assigned to receive either rivaroxaban 20 mg/day (15 mg/day in patients with CrCl of 30-49 mL/min per 1.73 m^2) or warfarin (target INR, 2.0–3.0).

Rivaroxaban was noninferior to warfarin (2.1% vs. 2.4% per year; $P < 0.001$ for noninferiority) in the intention-to-treat analysis for the primary efficacy end point of stroke and systemic embolism. There was no difference between patients taking rivaroxaban and those taking warfarin in terms of all bleeding events (14.9% vs. 14.5% per 100 patient-years; $P = 0.44$) and major bleeding events (3.6% vs 3.4% per 100 patient-years; $P = 0.58$). In addition the rates of intracranial hemorrhage and fatal bleeding were less with rivaroxaban therapy (0.4% vs. 0.8%, $P = 0.003$ and 0.5% vs. 0.7%, $P = 0.02$, respectively).

Thromboprophylaxis in Medically Ill Patients

The MAGELLAN study[62] evaluated the efficacy of rivaroxaban versus enoxaparin for VTE prophylaxis in medically ill patients. Patients were randomized to receive either rivaroxaban (10 mg/day) or enoxaparin (40 mg/day) to be given for 10 days (to assess noninferiority) or for 35 days (to assess for superiority). At day 10, rivaroxaban therapy was noninferior to enoxaparin therapy in reducing the composite risk of VTE and VTE-related deaths (2.7% in each group; $P = 0.0025$ for noninferiority. At day 35, rivaroxaban therapy was superior to enoxaparin therapy in reducing the composite risk of VTE and VTE-related deaths (4.4% vs. 5.7%; $P = 0.0211$ for superiority). The incidence of clinically relevant bleeding was low but still higher with rivaroxaban therapy (day 10: 2.8% vs. 1.2%, $P < 0.001$ and day 35: 4.1% vs. 1.7%, $P < 0.001$).

Recommendations for Postoperative Thromboprophylaxis

For TKA, use 10 mg/day for 12–14 days and for THA, use 10 mg/day for 35 days. The use of rivaroxaban is cautioned in patients with CrCl of 30-49 mL/min per 1.73 m^2. It is not recommended for those with CrCl < 30 mL/min per 1.73 m^2.[63]

DVT/PE: For DVT/PE, use 15 mg twice daily for 3 weeks followed by 20 mg once daily for at least 3-6 months; this can be followed by 20 mg/day for an additional 6–12 months after initial treatment for further reduction in the risk of recurrent DVT/PE. It is not recommended for those with CrCl < 30 mL/min per 1.73 m^2 and is contraindicated if <15 mL/min per 1.73 m^2.[63]

Stroke prevention in nonvalvular AF: In the setting of preserved renal function (CrCl ≥ 50 mL/min per 1.73 m^2), the recommended dose is 20 mg once daily. The use of rivaroxaban is 15 mg/day in patients with CrCl of 30–49 mL/min per 1.73 m^2. It is not recommended for those with CrCl < 30 mL/min per 1.73 m^2.[63]

Hepatic impairment: With mild impairment, no dosage adjustment is required as data indicate that the pharmacokinetic response is unchanged. However, in moderate to severe hepatic dysfunction (Child-Pugh class B or C) or impaired coagulation, its use is not recommended.[63]

Pregnancy and breastfeeding: At present, its use in pregnant and nursing mothers is not recommended.[63]

Adverse Events

The most common adverse event noted with the use of either therapeutic or prophylactic doses of rivaroxaban was bleeding. The incidence rates for major and all clinical bleeding were 0.3% and 5.8%, respectively, in the combined analysis from the RECORD trials and 1% and 28%, respectively, in a pooled analysis from the EINSTEIN DVT and PE studies. Other nonhematologic events observed in the phase 3 trials included musculoskeletal pain, wound secretions, pruritus, blisters, upper abdominal pain, and syncope.

Apixaban

Apixaban (Eliquis) is an oral direct coagulation factor Xa inhibitor approved for clinical use in the United States. Apixaban selectively and reversibly inhibits free and clot-bound factor Xa as well as prothrombinase activity. Apixaban is approved for use in the prevention of stroke and systemic embolism in adult patients with nonvalvular AF (FDA, EMA, and HPFB) and in the primary prevention of VTE in adult patients who have undergone elective THA or TKA (EMA and HPFB). The efficacy and safety of apixaban have been evaluated in phase 3 clinical trials.

Postoperative VTE Prophylaxis for TKA

The Apixaban Dose Orally versus Anticoagulation with Enoxaparin (ADVANCE)-1[64] and ADVANCE-2[65] trials compared apixaban, 2.5 mg twice daily, initiated 12–24 hours after surgery with enoxaparin, 30 mg twice daily, initiated at the same time as apixaban in ADVANCE-1 or enoxaparin, 40 mg/day, initiated 12 hours before surgery in ADVANCE-2. All the treatments in either arm of the two trials were continued for 10–14 days.

In ADVANCE-1, the primary efficacy outcome of VTE and all-cause mortality was 9.0% (8.8% VTE; 0.2% deaths) with apixaban therapy compared with 8.8% (8.6% VTE; 0.2% deaths) with enoxaparin therapy ($P = 0.06$ for noninferiority). On the other hand, the ADVANCE 2 study found the incidence of VTE and all cause mortality to be lower with Apixaban therapy at 15% (14.9% VTE; 0.1% deaths) than with enoxaparin therapy at 24% (all VTE events; no deaths) ($P < 0.0001$ for noninferiority and superiority). This difference in efficacy between the two trials may be related to the differences in enoxaparin dosing in the two studies.

The combined incidence of major bleeding and clinically relevant nonmajor bleeding was less with apixaban use compared with enoxaparin use (2.9% vs. 4.3%; $P = 0.03$) in ADVANCE-1 but equivalent in ADVANCE-2 (3.5% vs. 4.8%; $P = .09$).

Postoperative VTE Prophylaxis for THA

The ADVANCE-3[66] trial compared apixaban, 2.5 mg twice daily, initiated 12–24 hours after surgery with enoxaparin, 40 mg/day, initiated 12 hours before surgery; both drugs were continued for 35 days after surgery. The primary efficacy outcome of VTE and all-cause mortality in the intended treatment period was 1.4% in the apixaban group and 3.9% in the enoxaparin group ($P < 0.001$ for noninferiority and superiority). The incidence of major and clinically relevant nonmajor bleeding was 4.8% in patients treated with apixaban compared with 5.0% in patients treated with enoxaparin ($P = .72$).

Prevention of Stroke and Systemic Embolism in Nonvalvular AF

Apixaban was evaluated for stroke prevention in two large randomized controlled trials enrolling patients with nonvalvular AF. The apixaban versus acetylsalicylic acid to prevent stroke in atrial fibrillation patients who have failed or are unsuitable for vitamin K antagonist treatment (AVERROES) trial[67] compared apixaban at a dose of 5 mg twice daily with aspirin (81–324 mg) daily in patients intolerant to a VKA, whereas the Apixaban for Reduction in Stroke and Other Thromboembolic Events in Atrial Fibrillation (ARISTOTLE)[68] trial compared a similar dose of apixaban with warfarin (target INR, 2.0–3.0) in patients with nonvalvular AF and at least one additional risk factor for stroke.

In the AVERROES trial, the primary efficacy outcome of any type of stroke or systemic embolism was significantly less with apixaban use than with aspirin use (1.6% vs. 3.7% per year; $P < 0.001$). This trial was terminated earlier than planned owing to the superiority of apixaban observed in the interim analyses. Similarly, compared with warfarin therapy in the ARISTOTLE trial, apixaban therapy was superior in preventing stroke or systemic embolism (1.27% vs. 1.60% per year; $P < 0.001$ for noninferiority and $P = 0.01$ for superiority). The rate of major bleeding per year with apixaban use was 1.4% compared with 1.2% with aspirin use in the AVERROES trial ($P = 0.57$) and 2.1% compared with 3.1% with warfarin use in the ARISTOTLE trial ($P < 0.001$).

Extended Treatment of Acute VTE

The Apixaban after the Initial Management of Pulmonary Embolism and Deep Vein Thrombosis with First Line Therapy-Extended treatment (AMPLIFY-EXT) trial[69] evaluated the efficacy and safety of two doses of apixaban (2.5 and 5.0 mg twice daily) compared with placebo use in patients with a recent VTE who had completed 6–12 months of anticoagulation therapy and for whom there was clinical equipoise regarding the continuation or cessation of anticoagulation therapy. The duration of this extended treatment was 12 months.

The incidence of recurrent VTE and VTE-related mortality was 1.7% in both the apixaban arms compared with 8.8% in the placebo arm ($P < 0.001$ for both doses of apixaban). The rates of major bleeding were not significantly different across the three treatment groups (placebo: 0.5%; 2.5 mg of apixaban: 0.2%; and 5 mg of apixaban: 0.1%).

Recommendations for Stroke Prevention in Nonvalvular AF

The recommended dose is 5 mg twice daily. A lower dose of 2.5 mg twice daily should be used if a patient has any two of the following three factors; age 80 years or older, body weight of 60 kg or less, or a serum creatinine level of at least 1.5 mg/dL (to convert to mmol/L, multiply by 88.4). Patients with CrCl < 25 mL/min per 1.73 m^2 or a serum creatinine level >2.5 mg/dL were excluded from the AF clinical trials and the extended treatment of acute VTE study, and hence, until further data are available, this drug should not be used in these patients.

***Hepatic impairment*:** With mild hepatic impairment, no dosage adjustment is needed. However, in moderate hepatic dysfunction (Child-Pugh class B), there is limited experience, and the intrinsic coagulation status should be assessed before using the drug. Apixaban should be avoided in the setting of severe hepatic impairment (Child-Pugh class C).

***Pregnancy and breastfeeding*:** At present, the use of apixaban in pregnant and nursing mothers is not recommended.

Adverse Effects

The most common adverse event noted with the use of either therapeutic or prophylactic doses of apixaban was bleeding. There was a low incidence of GI symptoms, such as nausea (<3%) and hepatic transaminitis (<1%). Other rare nonhematologic events (<1%) included syncope, drug hypersensitivity (rashes), and anaphylactic reactions.

DRUG INTERACTIONS WITH NEW ORAL ANTICOAGULANTS

The NOAs have a low potential for drug interactions. Dabigatran etexilate, the prodrug, is a substrate of the P-glycoprotein (P-gp) efflux transporter. Hence, its plasma concentration increases with strong P-gp inhibitors (amiodarone, verapamil, clarithromycin, and ketoconazole) and reduces with potent P-gp inducers (rifampicin, carbamazepine, or phenytoin);[70] although no significant influence on its efficacy or safety has been reported, dosage adjustment may be needed. No dabigatran dose adjustment is recommended when coadministered with amiodarone, quinidine, or clarithromycin; however, their concomitant use should be avoided in patients with severe renal impairment (CrCl, 15–30 mL/min per 1.73 m^2). Furthermore, administration of dabigatran 2 hours before verapamil ingestion is recommended, and when coadministered with ketoconazole, the dabigatran dose must be reduced to 75 mg twice daily in patients with moderate renal impairment (CrCl, 30–50 mL/min per 1.73 m^2) and avoided in those with severe renal impairment (CrCl, 15–30 mL/min per 1.73 m^2).[71] Coadministration with inducers of P-gp should be avoided. Proton pump inhibitors increase the gastric pH and reduce dabigatran absorption by 12.5%, a phenomenon that has not been shown to affect drug efficacy.[72]

Rivaroxaban is metabolized by the cytochrome (CYP) P450 (CYP3A4, CYP3A5, and CYP2J2) enzymes and is also a substrate of P-gp transporters.[70] Inhibitors or inducers of these CYP450 enzymes or P-gp transporters can alter the clearance of rivaroxaban, making its levels either too high or too low, respectively. Drugs that inhibit or induce either the CYP450 enzymes or P-gp transporters, as opposed to both, do not significantly alter rivaroxaban to plasma levels that require dose changes.[70]

Apixaban is a substrate of CYP3A4 and P-gp such that inhibitors or inducers of CYP3A4 and P-gp will increase or decrease exposure to apixaban, respectively. Coadministration with strong dual inhibitors of CYP3A4 and P-gp (e.g. ketoconazole, itraconazole, ritonavir, and clarithromycin) should preferably be avoided, but, if necessary, the apixaban dose should be decreased to 2.5 mg twice daily. Similarly, concomitant use of strong dual inducers of CYP3A4 and P-gp (e.g. rifampin, carbamazepine, phenytoin, and St Johns of CYP3A4 and P-gp (eerably be avoided, but, if necessary, the apixaban dose.[70]

LABORATORY TESTING AND MONITORING FOR THE NOAs

Given their rapid onset of action, stable pharmacokinetic properties, and lack of significant drug interactions, the NOAs do not require coagulation monitoring. However, overdoses, emergency perioperative settings, and bleeding events may warrant an assessment of the degree of anticoagulation.

Prothrombin time (PT) is relatively insensitive at therapeutic levels of dabigatran compared with rivaroxaban and apixaban, whereas aPTT is more sensitive to dabigatran.[73] However, different aPTT and PT reagents used in different laboratories have different responsiveness to these NOAs, making it difficult to standardize results. The thrombin clotting time assay shows linear effects with dabigatran plasma concentrations but no activity to rivaroxaban or apixaban.[74] Both these NOAs cause a dose-dependent spurious decrease in PT- and aPTT-based specific factor assays. These agents can also cause false-positives in lupus anticoagulant screening or confirmatory assays, incomplete corrections in mixing studies (PT and aPTT), and falsely elevated activated protein C ratio assays, thereby misclassifying patients with a factor V Leiden mutation as normal. Dabigatran yields a dose-dependent prolongation of the ecarin clotting time, which is a thrombin clotting time like assay, making it a feasible monitoring test; however, it is not widely used.[75] Rivaroxaban and apixaban can be monitored using modified chromogenic anti-Xa assays that use specific rivaroxaban and apixaban standards, respectively.

PERIOPERATIVE MANAGEMENT

Perioperative management of the NOAs is based on the urgency of the procedure, level of bleeding risk, and current renal function.[72,76] The decision to stop treatment in nonurgent or elective surgery should depend on the risk of bleeding versus thrombosis.

Elective Surgery

Standard Bleeding Risk Procedure

Standard bleeding risk procedures include colonoscopy, uncomplicated laparoscopic procedures, and any aspirations not involving the spinal canal. In patients with normal CrCl (≥50 mL/min per 1.73 m^2), dabigatran use should be stopped at least 48 hours before the procedure. Rivaroxaban and apixaban use should be stopped at least 24 hours before the procedure. In patients with impaired CrCl (<50 mL/min per 1.73 m^2), dabigatran therapy should be stopped at least 72 hours before the procedure if CrCl is 30 to <50 mL/min per 1.73 m^2 and at least 4 days earlier if CrCl is <30 mL/min per 1.73 m^2. Rivaroxaban and apixaban administration should be stopped at least 48 hours before the procedure.

High Bleeding Risk Procedure

High bleeding risk procedures include major cardiac surgery, insertion of pacemakers or defibrillators, neurosurgery, major cancer/urologic/vascular surgery, and spinal puncture. In patients with normal CrCl (≥ 50 mL/min per 1.73 m^2), dabigatran, rivaroxaban, and apixaban administration should be stopped at least 48 hours before the procedure. In patients with impaired CrCl (<50 mL/min per 1.73 m^2), dabigatran use should be stopped at least 4 days before the procedure if CrCl is 30 to <50 mL/min per 1.73 m^2 and at least 6 days earlier if CrCl is <30 mL/min per 1.73 m^2. Rivaroxaban and apixaban administration should be stopped at least 4 days before the procedure.

Emergency Surgery

Ideally, surgical intervention should be delayed for the estimated time that the drugs are cleared. If available, assays may provide information on the presence or absence of residual drug. However, if urgent surgery is needed within a few hours after the last dose, clinicians should anticipate bleeding complications.

Reinitiation of NOAs after the Procedure

This process depends on the nature of the surgery, the urgency for restarting thromboprophylaxis therapy, and the hemostatic state of the patient.[72,76] Given the rapid clearance of the NOAs from the circulation and the rapid onset of action when reintroduced, no bridging therapy with LMWH or UFH is necessary. For procedures in which good hemostasis is achieved, anticoagulation may be resumed the same evening, at least 4–6 hours after surgery with a reduced dose (dabigatran, 75 mg; rivaroxaban, 10 mg; or apixaban, 2.5 mg) for the first dose and, thereafter, the usual maintenance dose. For major abdominal surgery or urologic surgery with incomplete hemostasis, resumption should be delayed until there is adequate hemostasis.

COMPLEX CLINICAL SCENARIOS

Acute Stroke Requiring Thrombolytics

The safety of administration of thrombolytics in patients receiving concurrent NOAs is not established and poses a very high risk of bleeding. Anecdotal reports have documented the successful use of thrombolytics in patients taking dabigatran who were at least 7 hours past their last dose.[77,78] Similar reports with rivaroxaban and apixaban are lacking.

Cardioversion

For patients with AF of >48 hours' duration, therapeutic anticoagulation for at least 3 weeks before and 4 weeks after cardioversion is recommended.[79] In the RE-LY trial, the stroke and systemic embolism rates within 30 days of this procedure were 0.8% and 0.3% for the dabigatran, 150- and 110-mg doses, respectively, versus 0.6% with the warfarin arm; major bleeding rates were similar between the groups.[80] Hence, patients may continue taking dabigatran for cardioversion; similar efficacy and safety data with rivaroxaban and apixaban are lacking.

Mechanical Heart Valves

Currently, the use of NOAs in patients with mechanical heart valves cannot be recommended owing to the lack of clinical evidence. A phase 2 study (the RE-ALIGN trial) investigated the use of dabigatran in patients with mechanical heart valves;[81] however, it was terminated early owing to excess thrombotic complications in the dabigatran group. This has led the FDA and EMA to consider mechanical heart valves as a contraindication for dabigatran therapy.

Heparin-induced Thrombocytopenia

Krauel et al.[82] demonstrated that neither dabigatran nor rivaroxaban had any effect on the interaction of PF4 or anti-PF4/heparin antibodies with platelets, thus making them potential options for anticoagulation in patients with HIT and possibly even for the treatment of HIT-induced thrombosis. However, there are neither randomized controlled trials nor anecdotal case reports describing the off-label use of NOAs in the treatment of HIT-induced thrombosis; hence, its use cannot be recommended until more evidence is available.

Cancer-associated VTE

The LMWH is superior to VKAs in treating cancer-associated VTE,[83] but studies evaluating NOAs for acute VTE were compared only with VKAs. Nevertheless, the RE-COVER study[47] found that dabigatran use was noninferior to VKA use (3.1% vs. 5.3%) in preventing recurrent symptomatic VTE/death in patients with cancer (9.5% of the study population). In the EINSTEIN DVT and PE studies,[59,60] patients with cancer (12% and <5%, respectively, of the study population) were included in the analysis. Neither study showed a difference between rivaroxaban use and VKA use in preventing recurrent VTE (acute DVT: 3.4% vs. 5.6% and PE study: 1.8% vs. 2.8%). Furthermore, the incidence of clinical bleeding between the treatment groups was comparable. Given the small number of patients with cancer in these studies, future trials testing the efficacy and safety of NOAs in patients with cancer are needed before they can be recommended.

MANAGEMENT OF BLEEDING COMPLICATIONS/OVERDOSE

Lack of specific agents that reverse the anticoagulant effect complicates the management of NOA associated bleeding events or the periprocedural reversal of anticoagulation. Management of minor bleeding, e.g. epistaxis, consists of addressing the potential anatomical defects, e.g. cauterization or nasal packing. The decision to hold the next dose of drug will hinge on the comorbidities and assessment of risks of drug discontinuation. Given the relatively short half-lives of the NOAs in patients with normal renal function, most of the anticoagulant effect should dissipate within 48 hours.[84] Administration of oral activated charcoal retards absorption of recently ingested drug, e.g. within a couple hours of presentation.[85] Given that only 35% of dabigatran is bound to plasma proteins, hemodialysis typically removes 60% of dabigatran and should be considered, especially in patients with impaired renal function.[86] However, given the extensive volume of distribution (50–70 L) of dabigatran, a "rebound" increase in dabigatran plasma levels may occur after hemodialysis. Although there are no data, dialysis is unlikely to be effective for rivaroxaban and apixaban as they are >85–90% protein bound.

Recombinant Factor VIIa

This agent has been used in clinical practice to help reverse life-threatening bleeds caused by NOAs. It decreases the bleeding time in animal models but does not reverse the anticoagulation effect on most other laboratory coagulation tests.[87] Other than anecdotal case reports, there are no randomized controlled studies confirming its benefit in these situations. One must keep in mind the potential serious adverse effects of recombinant factor VIIa, including disseminated intravascular coagulation and systemic thrombosis.

Prothrombin Complex Concentrates

In the United States, 3-factor prothrombin complex concentrates (PCCs) [Bebulin (Baxter), and Profilnine SD (Grifols)] are available with relatively similar concentrations of nonactivated factors II, IX, and X but low concentrations of nonactivated factor VII. In addition, there is an adverse effects of recombinant factor VIIa, inclut contains relatively similar concentrations of nonactivated factors II, IX, and X and activated factor VII. The use of either PCC may increase the risk of thrombosis, with the 3-factor PCC being less likely to do so.[88] A randomized controlled study using a nonactivated 4-factor PCC showed normalization of the PT alone in patients taking rivaroxaban but not dabigatran.[89] No studies have evaluated PCCs in patients receiving the NOAs with clinical bleeding; however, its use seems reasonable in the setting of serious bleeding.

CHOOSING AN ORAL ANTICOAGULANT

When identifying a long-term oral anticoagulant for a patient, it is important to adopt a personalized approach.[90] The NOAs are not all superior in terms of efficacy compared with warfarin; hence, patients who are stable with warfarin therapy with acceptable/minimal complications will not benefit from switching to an NOA. Warfarin remains the standard of care for the management of patients with valvular AF or mechanical heart valves until further safety and efficacy data regarding the use of NOAs in these situations is available.

Patients with hepatic dysfunction or associated coagulopathies or impaired renal function (CrCl < 30 mL/min per 1.73 m^2) are not good candidates for NOAs owing to their hepatic metabolism and renal excretion. If compliance is an issue, rivaroxaban, with its once-daily administration, might be a better choice than dabigatran or apixaban. Dabigatran is best avoided in patients with ulcer/nonulcer dyspepsia given its tartaric acid core and described associations with GI adverse effects. In patients with a recent history of GI bleeding, apixaban may be a better choice as it has a lower incidence of GI bleeding than dabigatran and rivaroxaban. Given the recent association of dabigatran with a trend toward an increase in the incidence of MI, rivaroxaban or apixaban should possibly be considered when selecting an NOA in this subset of patients. However, in patients with a history of ischemic strokes while taking warfarin, dabigatran and apixaban may be suitable alternatives as they are the only NOAs with a lower rate of ischemic stroke than warfarin.

SUMMARY

Antiplatelets and anticoagulants have extensively been studied and utilized for prevention and management of thrombosis. Novel anticoagulants have recently been developed from intense clinical research. These oral agents, due to their ease of administration as well as favorable pharmacodynamics, have the potential to replace the earlier drugs. Hemorrhage, however, remains the major adverse effect as with earlier agents. It is therefore imperative for the clinicians to have an in-depth knowledge of the applicability of these drugs so as to enable them to use these agents judiciously.

REFERENCES

1. Hirsh J, Guyatt G, Albers GW, et al. Executive summary: American College of Chest Physicians Evidence-Based Clinical Practice Guidelines, 8th edn. Chest. 2008;133:71S-109S.
2. Burch JW, Stanford N, Majerus PW. Inhibition of platelet prostaglandin synthetase by oral aspirin. J Clin Invest. 1978;61:314-9.
3. Becker RC, Meade TW, Berger PB, et al. The primary and secondary prevention of coronary artery disease: American College of Chest Physicians Evidence-Based Clinical Practice Guidelines, 8th edn. Chest. 2008;133:776S-814S.
4. Sobel M, Verhaeghe R. Antithrombotic therapy for peripheral artery occlusive disease: American College of Chest Physicians Evidence-Based Clinical Practice Guidelines, 8th edn. Chest. 2008;133:815S-43S.
5. Adams RJ, Albers G, Alberts MJ, et al. Update to the AHA/ASA recommendations for the prevention of stroke in patients with stroke and transient ischemic attack. Stroke. 2008;39:1647-52.
6. Cattaneo M. Resistance to antiplatelet drugs: molecular mechanisms and laboratory detection. J Thromb Haemost. 2007;5:230-7.
7. Schwartz KA, Schwartz DE, Ghosheh K, et al. Compliance as a critical consideration in patients who appear to be resistant to aspirin after healing of myocardial infarction. Am J Cardiol. 2005;95:973-5.
8. Eikelboom JW, Hankey GJ, Thom J, et al. Incomplete inhibition of thromboxane biosynthesis by acetylsalicylic acid: determinants and effect on cardiovascular risk. Circulation. 2008;118:1705-12.
9. Gurbel PA, Bliden KP, Hiatt BL, et al. Clopidogrel for coronary stenting: response variability, drug resistance, and the effect of pretreatment platelet reactivity. Circulation. 2003;107:2908-13.
10. Gori AM, Marcucci R, Migliorini A, et al. Incidence and clinical impact of dual nonresponsiveness to aspirin and clopidogrel in patients with drug-eluting stents. J Am Coll Cardiol. 2008;52: 734-9.
11. Erlinge D, Varenhorst C, Braun OO, et al. Patients with poor responsiveness to thienopyridine treatment or with diabetes have lower levels of circulating active metabolite, but their platelets respond normally to active metabolite added ex vivo. J Am Coll Cardiol. 2008;52:1968-77.
12. Gladding P, Webster M, Ormiston J, et al. Antiplatelet drug nonresponsiveness. Am Heart J. 2008;155:591-9.
13. Wiviott SD, Trenk D, Frelinger AL, et al. Prasugrel compared with high loading- and maintenance-dose clopidogrel in patients with planned percutaneous coronary intervention: the Prasugrel in Comparison to Clopidogrel for Inhibition of Platelet Activation and Aggregation-Thrombolysis in Myocardial Infarction 44 trial. Circulation. 2007;116:2923-32.
14. Wiviott SD, Braunwald E, McCabe CH, et al. Prasugrel versus clopidogrel in patients with acute coronary syndromes. N Engl J Med. 2007;357:2001-15.
15. Niitsu Y, Jakubowski JA, Sugidachi A, et al. Pharmacology of CS-747 (prasugrel, LY640315), a novel, potent antiplatelet agent with in vivo P2Y12 receptor antagonist activity. Semin Thromb Hemost. 2005;31:184-94
16. Weerakkody GJ, Jakubowski JA, Brandt JT, et al. Greater inhibition of platelet aggregation and reduced response variability with prasugrel versus clopidogrel: an integrated analysis. J Cardiovasc Pharmacol Ther. 2007;12:205-12.
17. Antman EM, Wiviott SD, Murphy SA, et al. Early and late benefits of prasugrel in patients with acute coronary syndromes undergoing percutaneous coronary intervention: a TRITON-TIMI 38 (TRial to Assess Improvement in Therapeutic Outcomes by Optimizing Platelet Inhibition with Prasugrel-Thrombolysis in Myocardial Infarction) analysis. J Am Coll Cardiol. 2008;51: 2028-33.
18. Eli Lilly and Co. Prasugrel Label. 2009. Available at: *http://www.fda.gov/NewsEvents/Newsroom/PressAnnouncements/ucm171497.html*
19. Angiolillo DJ, Bhatt DL, Gurbel PA, et al. Advances in antiplatelet therapy: agents in clinical development. Am J Cardiol. 2009;103:40A-51A.
20. Cannon CP, Husted S, Harrington RA, et al. Safety, tolerability, and initial efficacy of AZD6140, the first reversible oral adenosine diphosphate receptor antagonist, compared with clopidogrel, in patients with non-ST-segment elevation acute coronary syndrome: primary results of the DISPERSE-2 trial. J Am Coll Cardiol. 2007;50:1844-51.
21. Wallentin L, Becker RC, Budaj A, et al. Ticagrelor versus clopidogrel in patients with acute coronary syndromes. N Engl J Med. 2009;361:1045-57.
22. Schomig A. Ticagrelor: is there need for a new player in the antiplatelet-therapy field? N Engl J Med. 2009;361:1108-11.

23. Gurbel PA, Bliden KP, Butler K, et al. Response to ticagrelor in clopidogrel nonresponders and responders and effect of switching therapies: the RESPOND study. Circulation. 2010; 121:1188-99.
24. Husted S, Emanuelsson H, Heptinstall S, et al. Pharmacodynamics, pharmacokinetics, and safety of the oral reversible P2Y12 antagonist AZD6140 with aspirin in patients with atherosclerosis: a double-blind comparison to clopidogrel with aspirin. Eur Heart J. 2006;27:1038-47.
25. Gurbel PA, Bliden KP, Butler K, et al. Randomized double-blind assessment of the ONSET and OFFSET of the antiplatelet effects of ticagrelor versus clopidogrel in patients with stable coronary artery disease: the ONSET/OFFSET study. Circulation. 2009;120:2577-85.
26. AstraZeneca. Brilinta REMS Document. NDA 22-433. 2011. Available at: *http://www.fda.gov/NewsEvents/Newsroom/PressAnnouncements/ucm263964.html.*
27. Greenbaum AB, Ohman EM, Gibson CM, et al. Preliminary experience with intravenous P2Y12 platelet receptor inhibition as an adjunct to reduced-dose alteplase during acute myocardial infarction: results of the Safety, Tolerability and Effect on Patency in Acute Myocardial Infarction (STEP-AMI) angiographic trial. Am Heart J. 2007;154:702-9.
28. Bhatt DL, Lincoff AM, Gibson CM, et al. Intravenous platelet blockade with cangrelor during PCI. N Engl J Med. 2009;361: 2330-41.
29. Fugate SE, Cudd LA. Cangrelor for treatment of coronary thrombosis. Ann Pharmacother. 2006;40:925-30.
30. Schulman S, Beth RJ, Kearon C, et al. Hemorrhagic complications of anticoagulant and thrombolytic treatment: American College of Chest Physicians Evidence-Based Clinical Practice Guidelines, 8th edn. Chest. 2008;133:257S-98S.
31. Buller HR, Davidson BL, Decousus H, et al. Fondaparinux or enoxaparin for the initial treatment of symptomatic deep venous thrombosis: a randomized trial. Ann Intern Med. 2004;140: 867-73.
32. The Matisse Investigators. Subcutaneous fondaparinux versus intravenous unfractionated heparin in the initial treatment of pulmonary embolism. N Engl J Med. 2003;349:1695-702.
33. Cohen AT, Davidson BL, Gallus AS, et al., for the ARTEMIS Investigators. Efficacy and safety of fondaparinux for the prevention of venous thromboembolism in older acute medical patients: randomized placebo controlled trial. BMJ. 2006;332: 325-9.
34. Turpie AGG, Bauer KA, Eriksson BI, et al. Fondaparinux vs enoxaparin for the prevention of venous thromboembolism in major orthopedic surgery. A meta-analysis of 4 randomized double-blind studies. Arch Intern Med. 2001;162:1833-40.
35. Dager WE, Dougherty JA, Nguyen PH, et al. Heparin-induced thrombocytopenia: treatment options and special considerations. Pharmacotherapy. 2007;27:564-87.
36. Bijsterveld NR, Moons AH, Boekholdt M, et al. Ability of recombinant factor VIIa to reverse the anticoagulant effect of the pentasaccharide fondaparinux in healthy volunteers. Circulation. 2002;106:2550-4.
37. Di Nisio M, Middeldorp A, Buller HR. Direct thrombin inhibitors. N Engl J Med. 2005;353:1028-40.
38. Love JE, Ferrell C, Chandler W. Monitoring direct thrombin inhibitors with a plasma diluted thrombin time. Thromb Haemost. 2007;98:234-42.
39. Warkentin TE. Current agents for the treatment of patients with heparin-induced thrombocytopenia. Curr Opin Pulm Med. 2002;8:405-12.
40. Adams CD, Anger KA, Greenwood BC, et al. Antithrombotic pharmacotherapy. In: Irwin and Rippe (Eds). Intensive Care Medicine, 7th edn. Philadelphia, PA: Lippincott, Williams, and Wilkins; 2012. pp. 1224-42.
41. Elg M, Carlsson S, Gustafsson D. Effect of activated prothrombin complex concentrate or recombinant factor VIIa on the bleeding time and thrombus formation during anticoagulation with a direct thrombin inhibitor. Thromb Res. 2001;101:145-57.
42. Ageno W, Gallus AS, Wittkowsky A, et al. Oral anticoagulant therapy: Antithrombotic Therapy and Prevention of Thrombosis, 9th edn. American College of Chest Physicians Evidence-Based Clinical Practice Guidelines. Chest. 2012;141:44S-88S.
43. Holbrook A, Schulman, Witt DM, et al. Evidence-based management of anticoagulant therapy: Antithrombotic Therapy and Prevention of Thrombosis, 9th edn. American College of Chest Physicians Evidence-Based Clinical Practice Guidelines. Chest. 2012;141;152S-84S.
44. Oake N, Fergusson DA, Forster AJ, et al. Frequency of adverse events in patients with poor anticoagulation: a metaanalysis. CMAJ. 2007;176(11):1589-94.
45. Connolly SJ, Ezekowitz MD, Yusuf S, et al. Dabigatran versus warfarin in patients with atrial fibrillation. N Engl J Med. 2009; 361(12):1139-51.
46. Wallentin L, Yusuf S, Ezekowitz MD, et al. Efficacy and safety of dabigatran compared with warfarin at different levels of international normalised ratio control for stroke prevention in atrial fibrillation: an analysis of the RE-LY trial. Lancet. 2010; 376(9745):975-83.
47. Schulman S, Kearon C, Kakkar AK, et al. Dabigatran versus warfarin in the treatment of acute venous thromboembolism. N Engl J Med. 2009;361(24):2342-52.
48. Eriksson BI, Dahl OE, Rosencher N, et al. Oral dabigatran etexilate vs. subcutaneous enoxaparin for the prevention of venous thromboembolism after total knee replacement: the REMODEL randomized trial. J Thromb Haemost. 2007;5(11): 2178-85.
49. Ginsberg JS, Davidson BL, Comp PC, et al. Oral thrombin inhibitor dabigatran etexilate vs North American enoxaparin regimen for prevention of venous thromboembolism after knee arthroplasty surgery. J Arthroplast. 2009;24(1):1-9.
50. Eriksson BI, Dahl OE, Rosencher N, et al. Dabigatran etexilate versus enoxaparin for prevention of venous thromboembolism after total hip replacement: a randomised, double-blind, noninferiority trial. Lancet. 2007;370(9591):949-56.
51. Eriksson BI, Dahl OE, Huo MH, et al. Oral dabigatran versus enoxaparin for thromboprophylaxis after primary total hip arthroplasty (RE-NOVATE II*): a randomised, double-blind, non-inferiority trial. Thromb Haemost. 2011;105(4):721-9.
52. Sarah AS, Vincent JW. A patient's guide to taking Dabigatran etexilate. Circulation 2011;124:e209-e211.
53. Uchino K, Hernandez AV. Dabigatran association with higher risk of acute coronary events: meta-analysis of noninferiority randomized controlled trials. Arch Intern Med. 2012;172(5): 397-402.
54. Uchino K, Hernandez AV. Dabigatran association with higher risk of acute coronary events: meta-analysis of noninferiority randomized controlled trials. Arch Intern Med. 2012;172(5): 397-402.
55. Eriksson BI, Borris LC, Friedman RJ, et al. Rivaroxaban versus enoxaparin for thromboprophylaxis after hip arthroplasty. N Engl J Med. 2008;358(26):2765-75.
56. Kakkar AK, Brenner B, Dahl OE, et al. Extended duration rivaroxaban versus short-term enoxaparin for the prevention of

venous thromboembolism after total hip arthroplasty: a double-blind, randomised controlled trial. Lancet. 2008;372(9632):31-9.

57. Lassen MR, Ageno W, Borris LC, et al. Rivaroxaban versus enoxaparin for thromboprophylaxis after total knee arthroplasty. N Engl J Med. 2008;358(26):2776-86.
58. Turpie AGG, Lassen MR, Davidson BL, et al. Rivaroxaban versus enoxaparin for thromboprophylaxis after total knee arthroplasty (RECORD4): a randomised trial. Lancet. 2009;373(9676):1673-80.
59. Bauersachs R, Berkowitz SD, Brenner B, et al. Oral rivaroxaban for symptomatic venous thromboembolism. N Engl J Med. 2010;363(26):2499-510.
60. Buller HR, Prins MH, Lensin AW, et al. Oral rivaroxaban for the treatment of symptomatic pulmonary embolism. N Engl J Med. 2012;366(14):1287-97.
61. Patel MR, Mahaffey KW, Garg J, et al. Rivaroxaban versus warfarin in nonvalvular atrial fibrillation. N Engl J Med. 2011; 365(10):883-91.
62. Cohen AT. Rivaroxaban compared with enoxaparin for the prevention of venous thromboembolism in acutely ill medical patients. *http://my.americanheart.org/idc/groups/ahamah-public/@wcm/@sop/@scon/documents/downloadable/ucm_425442.pdf.*
63. Deborah C, John F. Rivaroxaban to prevent pulmonary embolism after hip or knee replacement. Circulation 2012;125:e542-e544.
64. Lassen MR, Raskob GE, Gallus A, et al. Apixaban or enoxaparin for thromboprophylaxis after knee replacement. N Engl J Med. 2009;361(6):594-604.
65. Lassen MR, Raskob GE, Gallus A, et al. Apixaban versus enoxaparin for thromboprophylaxis after knee replacement (ADVANCE-2): a randomised double-blind trial. Lancet. 2010; 375(9717):807-15.
66. Lassen MR, Gallus A, Raskob GE, et al. Apixaban versus enoxaparin for thromboprophylaxis after hip replacement. N Engl J Med. 2010;363(26):2487-98.
67. Connolly SJ, Eikelboom J, Joyner C, et al. Apixaban in patients with atrial fibrillation. N Engl J Med. 2011;364(9):806-17.
68. Granger CB, Alexander JH, McMurray JJ, et al. Apixaban versus warfarin in patients with atrial fibrillation. N Engl J Med. 2011; 365(11):981-92.
69. Agnelli G, Buller HR, Cohen A, et al. Apixaban for extended treatment of venous thromboembolism. N Engl J Med. 2013; 368(8):699-708.
70. Scaglione F. New oral anticoagulants: comparative pharmacology with vitamin K antagonists. Clin Pharmacokinet. 2013;52(2):69-82.
71. Hartter S, Koenen-Bergmann M, Sharma A, et al. Decrease in the oral bioavailability of dabigatran etexilate after co-medication with rifampicin. Br J Clin Pharmacol. 2012;74(3):490-500.
72. Huisman MV, Lip GY, Diener HC, et al. Dabigatran etexilate for stroke prevention in patients with atrial fibrillation: resolving uncertainties in routine practice. Thromb Haemost. 2012;107(5):838-47.
73. Hillarp A, Baghaei F, Fagerberg Blixter I, et al. Effects of the oral, direct factor Xa inhibitor rivaroxaban on commonly used coagulation assays. J Thromb Haemost. 2011;9(1):133-9.
74. Stangier J, Feuring M. Using the HEMOCLOT direct thrombin inhibitor assay to determine plasma concentrations of dabigatran. Blood Coagul Fibrinolysis. 2012;23(2):138-43.
75. van Ryn J, Stangier J, Haertter S, et al. Dabigatran etexilate: a novel, reversible, oral direct thrombin inhibitor: interpretation of coagulation assays and reversal of anticoagulant activity. Thromb Haemost. 2010;103(6):1116-27.
76. Schulman S, Crowther MA. How I treat with anticoagulants in 2012: new and old anticoagulants, and when and how to switch. Blood. 2012;119(13):3016-23.
77. De Smedt A, De Raedt S, Nieboer K, et al. Intravenous thrombolysis with recombinant tissue plasminogen activator in a stroke patient treated with dabigatran. Cerebrovasc Dis. 2010;30(5): 533-4.
78. Matute MC, Guillan M, Garcia-Caldentey J, et al. Thrombolysis treatment for acute ischaemic stroke in a patient on treatment with dabigatran. Thromb Haemost. 2011;106(1):178-9.
79. Fuster V, Ryden LE, Cannom DS, et al. 2011 ACCF/AHA/HRS focused updates incorporated into the ACC/AHA/ESC 2006 Guidelines for the management of patients with atrial fibrillation: a report of the American College of Cardiology Foundation/American Heart Association Task Force on Practice Guidelines developed in partnership with the European Society of Cardiology and in collaboration with the European Heart Rhythm Association and the Heart Rhythm Society. J Am Coll Cardiol. 2011;57(11):e101-e198.
80. Nagarakanti R, Ezekowitz MD, Oldgren J, et al. Dabigatran versus warfarin in patients with atrial fibrillation: an analysis of patients undergoing cardioversion. Circulation. 2011;123(2):131-6.
81. Dabigatran etexilate in patients with mechanical heart valves. *http://www.clinicaltrials.gov/ct2/show/NCT01452347?term¼NCT01452347&rank¼1.*
82. Krauel K, Hackbarth C, Furll B, et al. Heparin-induced thrombocytopenia: in vitro studies on the interaction of dabigatran, rivaroxaban, and low-sulfated heparin, with platelet factor 4 and anti-PF4/heparin antibodies. Blood. 2012; 119(5):1248-55.
83. Kearon C, Akl EA, Comerota AJ, et al. Antithrombotic therapy for VTE disease: Antithrombotic Therapy and Prevention of Thrombosis, 9th edn. American College of Chest Physicians Evidence-Based Clinical Practice Guidelines. Chest. 2012;141 (Suppl 2):e419S-e94S.
84. Kaatz S, Kouides PA, Garcia DA, et al. Guidance on the emergent reversal of oral thrombin and factor Xa inhibitors. Am J Hematol. 2012;87 (Suppl 1):S141-S5.
85. Van Ryn J, Sieger P, Kink-Eiband M. Adsorption of dabigatran etexilate in water or dabigatran in pooled human plasma by activated charcoal in vitro. Paper presented at: 51st American Society of Hematology Annual Meeting and Exposition; December 5-8, 2009; New Orleans, LA.
86. Chang DN, Dager WE, Chin AI. Removal of dabigatran by hemodialysis. Am J Kidney Dis. 2013;61(3):487-9.
87. Tinel H, Huetter J, Perzborn E. Recombinant factor VIIA partially reverses the anticoagulant effect of high-dose rivaroxaban a novel, oral, direct factor XA inhibitor in rats. J Thromb Haemost. 2007;5 (Suppl 2):Abstract P-W-652.
88. Dentali F, Marchesi C, Pierfranceschi MG, et al. Safety of prothrombin complex concentrates for rapid anticoagulation reversal of vitamin K antagonists: a meta-analysis. Thromb Haemost. 2011;106(3):429-38.
89. Eerenberg ES, Kamphuisen PW, Sijpkens MK, et al. Reversal of rivaroxaban and dabigatran by prothrombin complex concentrate: a randomized, placebocontrolled, crossover study in healthy subjects. Circulation. 2011;124(14):1573-9.
90. Weitz JI, Gross PL. New oral anticoagulants: which one should my patient use? Hematology Am Soc Hematol Educ Program. 2012;2012:536-40.

11

Drug Management of Arrhythmias: Newer Insights

Aseem Dhall, Satyendra Kumar Tiwari

INTRODUCTION

Tachyarrhythmias are broadly characterized as supraventricular tachycardia (SVT), defined as a tachycardia in which the driving circuit or focus originates, at least in part, in tissue above the level of the ventricle [i.e. sinus node, atria, atrioventricular (AV) node, or His bundle], and ventricular tachycardia (VT), defined as a tachycardia in which the driving circuit solely originates in ventricular tissue or Purkinje fibers. Because of differences in prognosis and management, the distinction between SVT and VT is critical early in the acute management of a tachyarrhythmia. In general (with the exception of idiopathic VT), VT often carries a much graver prognosis, usually implies the presence of significant heart disease, and therefore requires immediate attention to revert to sinus rhythm. However, SVT is usually not lethal and often does not result in hemodynamic collapse; therefore, more conservative measures can be applied initially to convert to sinus rhythm.

There have been several breakthroughs in the management of arrhythmias in the recent past.

- Persistent imperfections of currently available antiarrhythmic drugs and rapidly expanding technologies have led to continued explosion in the use of devices and ablative techniques for both supraventricular and ventricular arrhythmias.
- Atrial fibrillation (AF) has become active focus of research with the recognition that with our aging population it is now a major health hazard.
- Stroke is recognized as complication of AF, and with the introduction of new antithrombotic agents, stroke prevention has become important consideration in AF management.
- There has been increasing interest in the use of so-called upstream therapy in arrhythmia management. Upstream therapy targets the process leading to arrhythmia development (primary prevention) or reducing the arrhythmia recurrence after initial presentation (secondary prevention).

Antiarrhythmic drugs are important components of any therapeutic strategy even after the advances seen in ablation techniques and device based therapies. Antiarrhythmic drugs could be used for prevention of sudden cardiac death, ventricular tachycardia, or supraventricular tachyarrhythmia. Currently, the implantable cardioverter-defibrillator therapy is being used as the mainstay of treatment for most lethal ventricular tachyarrhythmias, and antiarrhythmic drugs for these arrhythmias are presently used as acutely to terminate or as adjuncts to device therapy. It has been seen that drugs used for atrial tachyarrhythmias are often limited by the effect of drug on the ventricles that led to development of drugs acting on ion channels located in the atria. The outward K current, the acetylcholine-activated outward K current, and both peak and late atrial Na currents have become principal targets for antiarrhythmic drugs.[1-4] Another strategy is to use such agents that affect multiple channels at the same time, while minimizing the toxicity. In this review, the properties and evidence-based future uses of these drugs will be discussed.

NEWER INSIGHTS IN ANTIARRHYTHMIC TREATMENT OF ATRIAL FIBRILLATION

Goals of therapy with the use of these drugs include a reduction in the frequency and duration of episodes of arrhythmia as well an emerging goal of reducing mortality and hospitalizations associated with AF. The use of these drugs has been limited by both proarrhythmic and noncardiovascular toxicities as well as often modest antiarrhythmic efficacy. Despite these limitations, antiarrhythmic drugs remain widely prescribed for the management of symptomatic AF, and a host of new antiarrhythmic drugs are in various stages of clinical development.

Goals of therapy in AF are as follows:

- Rate and rhythm control
- Prevention of thromboembolism

The outline of management of patients with newly diagnosed AF is outlined in Flow chart 11.1.

Flow chart 11.1 Pharmacological management of patients with newly discovered atrial fibrillation

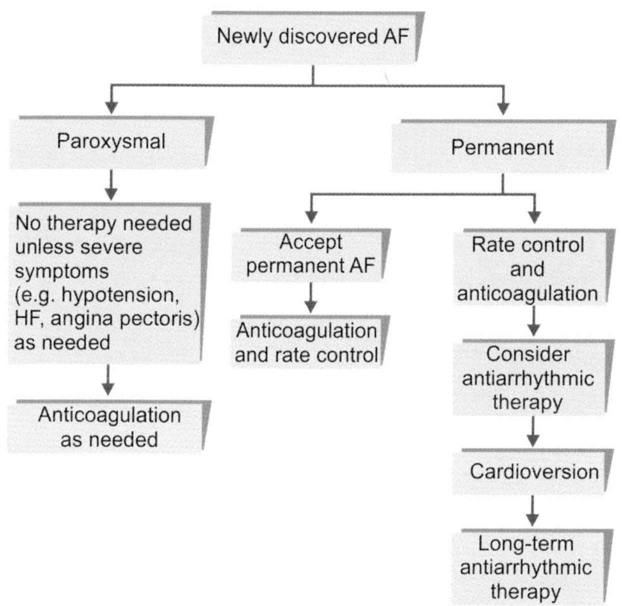

Abbreviations: AF, atrial fibrillation; HF, heart failure.

Rate Versus Rhythm Control

A multitude of studies have evaluated the health-related outcomes associated with a strategy of rate compared with rhythm control in patients with AF.[5-7] These studies, which included primarily patients aged >60 years with at least one risk factor for stroke, failed to demonstrate a mortality benefit associated with a rhythm control strategy. This equivalence in outcome was in part related to toxicities associated with antiarrhythmic drug therapy as well as excess stroke risk in patients in whom anticoagulation was discontinued.[8] At present, practice guidelines recommend antiarrhythmic therapy for patients with significant symptoms despite adequate rate control.[9]

How strict should the rate control be? Optimal criteria for rate control are presently unknown. Excess bradycardia may lead to syncope or fatigue; whereas consistently faster rate may result in tachycardia-induced cardiomyopathy. Strict rate control is a resting heart rate of <80 bpm and <110 bpm with exercise. RACE 2 (rate control versus electrical cardioversion for persistent atrial fibrillation) trial[10] showed that strict rate control is not essential, and that in selected patients a target heart rate <100 bpm may suffice.

Drugs for Cardioversion of AF (Rhythm Control)

It has been seen that rhythm conversion of AF while using antiarrhythmic drug therapy is much more for acute AF (<7 days) as compared to long-standing AF.

- *Ibutilide* is intravenous IKr channel blocking agent that is also known to enhance the late inward sodium current.[11] The drug is 50% effective to restore sinus rhythm and is more effective for atrial flutter than for AF.[11] Ibutilide causes QT prolongation and Torsdes de Points (TDP), so patients should be monitored for at least approximately 2 hours after drug infusion has been given.
- *Amiodarone* can be used intravenously as rhythm converting agent; but it is weak agent for rhythm control.[12] Intravenous amiodarone is also having rate-controlling effects and amiodarone while used orally can convert AF to sinus rhythm with conversion rate of 27% over time course of 3 weeks.
- *Propafenone and Flecainide* can be used as oral and intravenous agents. Flecainide (200–300 mg) or propafenone (450–600 mg) orally has been given for patients who present within 30 minutes approximately of arrhythmia onset and this approach is popularized as "pill in the pocket" approach. The conversion rate for AF was found to be approximately 85%.[13] The drugs should be used in patients with structurally normal heart.
- *Vernakalant* is a novel agent that has been tested in various trials for the rhythm control of AF.[14,15] In one of the study where intravenous amiodarone was compared with vernakalant, it was shown that there was 50% conversion rate of AF at 90 minutes with vernakalant while only 5% with amiodarone.[16]
- *Dronedarone* is an amiodarone analog. As compared to amiodarone, it is less lipophilic and without iodine moieties that cause thyroid dysfunction. Like amiodarone, dronedarone has multichannel blocker and antiadrenergic properties. It prolongs action potential duration and decreases heart rate, while lower potential of polymorphic ventricular tachycardia. Plasma level of dronedarone are reached to maximum within 1–4 hours and its plasma protein binding is around 98%, but oral bioavailability is about 15%. Mean concentrations of dronedarone are reached within 1 week of 400 mg twice daily. Dronedarone is metabolized by cytochrome P450 (CYP3A4) enzymes, with excretion of small amount of unchanged drug in bile and urine. The elimination half-life (about 24 hours) is shorter than that for the amiodarone. It is contraindicated in symptomatic heart failure.

A study was designed to see the effect of dronedarone on mortality in patients with congestive heart failure (CHF) and results showed a greater mortality in the dronedarone-treated group.[17] It was concluded that drug should not be used in patients with decompensated heart failure. A Placebo-Controlled, Double-Blind, Trial to Assess the Efficacy of Dronedarone 400 mg bid for the Prevention of Cardiovascular Hospitalization or Death From Any Cause in Patients With Atrial Fibrillation/Atrial Flutter (ATHENA) showed reduction in cardiovascular accidents while using dronedarone.[18] Dronedarone is the only antiarrhythmic drug that has shown a decrease risk of stroke in AF patients.

In the Permanent Atrial Fibrillation Outcome Study Using Dronedarone on Top of Standard Therapy (PALLAS), effect of dronedarone was evaluated in patients having permanent AF and it was concluded that there was more risk of stroke, cardiovascular death, and hospitalizations.[19]

Antiarrhythmic Efficacy of Dronedarone

A meta-analysis from various randomized controlled trials (DAFNE, EURIDIS, ADONIS, ATHENA, DIONYSOS trials). In all trials, dronedarone delayed the time to first recurrence of arrhythmia and decreased recurrence of these events and had modest antiarrhythmic efficacy. Also, dronedarone was found to have reduced efficacy in maintaining sinus rhythm, but only being modestly better tolerated than amiodarone.

Rate Control

Efficacy and Safety of Dronedarone for the Control of Ventricular Rate During Atrial Fibrillation (ERATO) trial was designed to see the efficacy of dronedarone 400 mg bid given for 6 months to control ventricular rate in permanent AF and dronedarone was found to reduce the ventricular rate of permanent AF and other types of AF patients as well. So, it can be concluded that dronedarone is having potential to control both rhythm and rate in patients with AF/AFL. But the antiarrythmic efficacy is half as compared with amiodarone.

Dronedarone safety has been evaluated in ANDROMEDA trial in which patients with symptomatic decompensated heart failure were enrolled with or without AF.[17] Due to increased mortality among dronedarone-treated patients, the trial was terminated prematurely. Excess mortality was probably due to decompensated heart failure, arrhythmia, and sudden cardiac death (SCD). Long-term effect of dronedarone was evaluated in ATHENA study, where dronedarone 400 mg bid was used against placebo for all-cause mortality in patients with a recent or current history of nonpermanent AF/AFL and additional risk factors.[20] The trial excluded the patients who were clinically decompensated. After the results of ATHENA trial, the FDA approved dronedarone in the treatment of AF/AFL so as to reduce the risk of cardiovascular hospitalization. Dronedarone use is contraindicated in decompensated heart failure, as a boxed warning issued by the FDA.[21]

Adverse Event Profile

- Nausea, vomiting, diarrhea, and rash can be seen with dronedarone.
- Sometimes transient elevation in serum creatinine can be seen with dronedarone that returns to baseline within a week after discontinuation of drug.[22]
- Dronedarone has no proarrhythmic effect and there is no data with oral anticoagulation therapy.

Recently, guidelines from American College of Cardiology/Heart Rhythm Society and European Society of Cardiology for selection of drugs in AF focused on the use of flecainide, propafenone, sotalol, dronedarone, or amiodarone in patients without underlying heart disease (i.e. coronary artery disease, heart failure, or left ventricular hypertrophy). Guidelines also agree on the use of amiodarone, sotalol, and dronedarone for patients with coronary artery disease and amiodarone for patients with symptomatic CHF. As per guidelines, for patients having left ventricular hypertrophy, same drugs should be used as in those with structurally normal heart (Flow chart 11.2).

Anticoagulation for AF

Atrial fibrillation is associated with an increased risk for stroke in significant proportion of patients. Loss of atrial systolic function results in sluggish blood flow in the atrium. Atrial distention disturbs the atrial endothelium and activates hemostatic factors leading to a hypercoagulable state. Several factors increase the risk for stroke in patients with AF. The primary risk factors are increased age, history of stroke or transient ischemic attack, hypertension, left atrial enlargement, diabetes, and CHF. The CHADS2 scoring system is now widely used and forms the basis for current guidelines. In CHADS2, one point is given for the following risk factors: recent CHF, hypertension, age older than 75 years, and diabetes: two points are given for a prior stroke. Patients with a CHADS2 score of 0 should not require antithrombotic therapy. Considering conventional treatment by warfarin, patients with a CHADS2 score of 1 may be treated with either aspirin or warfarin. Patients with a CHADS2 score of 2 or more should be treated with warfarin with a target international normalized ratio (INR) of 2–3. Regarding patients >75 years old, the Birmingham Atrial Fibrillation treatment of the Aged Study supported the use of warfarin, unless there are contraindications or the patient decides that the benefits are not worth the inconvenience.

Newer Antithrombotics

In general, antithrombotics have either been approved or are likely to be approved by the FDA and European authorities for stroke prevention in nonvalvular AF. The current recommendations are that when oral anticoagulant therapy is indicated, the new anticoagulants are preferable to warfarin for most patients. The major problem with all three drugs is the risk of rare but potentially fatal uncontrollable bleeding. No studies in patients have yet assessed the ability of prohemostatic drugs to antagonize excess anticoagulant effects. Regardless of the relatively short half-life of these agents, immediate reversal of the anticoagulant effect may be needed in case of major bleeding or emergency surgery. The major positive aspects of these agents include the following: (1) no need for monitoring of INR, as required for warfarin: (2) reduced risk of adverse interactions following a change in diet or concomitant drugs: and (3) an enhanced ability to prevent strokes.

Flow chart 11.2 Potential role for dronedarone in atrial fibrillation for the maintenance of sinus rhythm

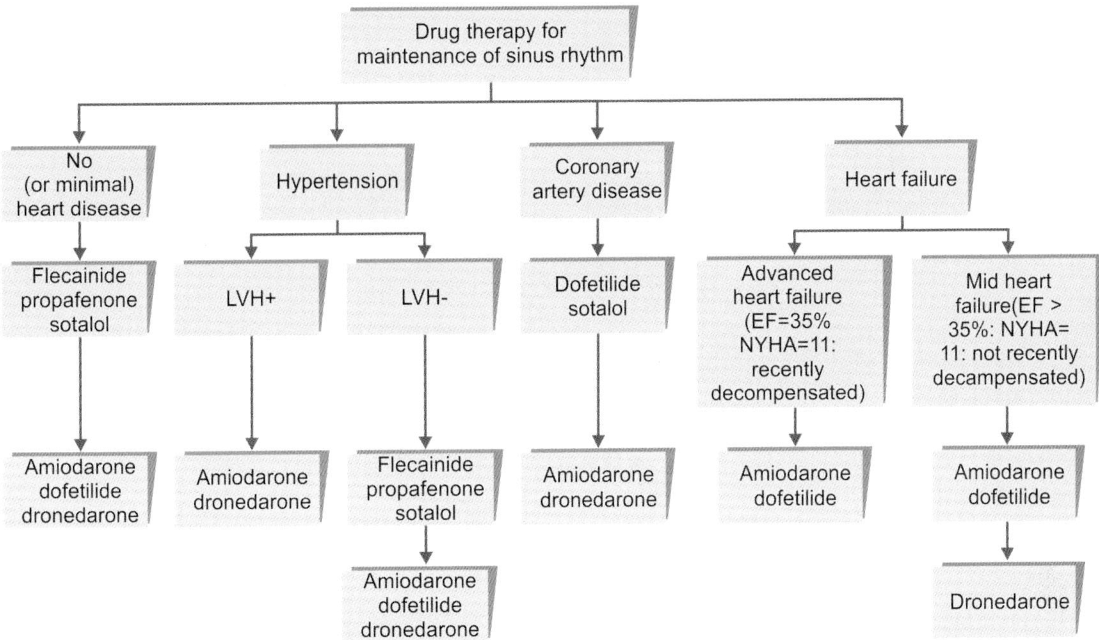

Abbreviations: EF, ejection fraction; LVH, left ventricular hypertrophy; NYHA, New York Heart Association.

Apixaban

Apixaban, a factor Xa inhibitor was superior to aspirin in patients with AF. The AVERROES trial study, which compared apixaban with aspirin, was terminated early because of a clear difference in favor of apixaban. Primary outcomes events (stroke) were reduced without any increase in major bleeding [hazard ratio (HR) 0.45: $P < 0.001$]. The decisive ARISTOTLE trial evaluated apixaban against warfarin in > 18,000 patients with AF. Apixaban was clearly superior to warfarin in preventing stroke or systemic embolism (HR, 0.79: $P = 0.01$ for superiority), caused less bleeding, and resulted in lower mortality ($P = 0.047$).

Dabigatran Etexilate (Pradaxa) and Rivaroxaban

Dabigatran etexilate is a prodrug that is converted to the active moiety dabigatran[23] (direct thrombin inhibitor). The Randomized Evaluation of Long-Term Anticoagulation Therapy (RE-LY) trial was a large, open-label, randomized trial in which dabigatran was compared with warfarin (goal INR 2.0–3.0) in 18,113 patients with nonvalvular AF. Primary outcome rate of all stroke or systemic embolism was found to be 1.71% per year in the warfarin group.[24,25] FDA, on October 19, 2010, approved dabigatran 150 mg orally twice daily for stroke prevention and prevention of peripheral embolism in patients with nonvalvular AF.[23] A dose of 75 mg twice daily was approved if creatinine clearance was 15–30 mL/min.

FDA approved rivaroxaban (Xarelto) 20 mg orally once daily for prevention of stroke in AF patients in 2011, after the results of the Rivaroxaban Once Daily Oral Direct Factor Xa Inhibition Compared with Vitamin K Antagonism for Prevention of Stroke and Embolism Trial[26] (ROCKET AF). Rivaroxaban is contraindicated in patients with creatinine clearance < 15 mL/min, and dose reduction to 15 mg once daily has been recommended. Dabigatran and rivaroxaban should not be used in patients with acute kidney injury. The 2011 American Heart Association/Heart Rhythm Society (ACCF/AHA/HRSA) Guidelines recommended dabigatran as an alternative to warfarin therapy for the prevention of stroke and systemic thromboembolism in patients with paroxysmal and permanent AF and with risk factors for stroke or systemic embolization.[27] As per guidelines, dabigatran should not be given to patients with prosthetic heart valve or significant valve disease, significant renal dysfunction (creatinine clearance < 15 mL/min), or chronic liver disease. Recently, the 2012 American College of Chest Physicians (ACCP) guidelines stated that anticoagulation or antiplatelet therapy should be offered to patients with a CHADS2 score of ≥1.[28]

Newer Antiarrhythmic Therapy for Supraventricular Arrhythmias and Ventricular Arrhythmias

Celivarone

Celivarone is benzofuran-derivative devoid of iodine with similar electrophysiological properties to amiodarone.[29] Efficacy of celivarone was tested at 300 mg or 600 mg daily doses for conversion of AF and atrial flutter (CORYFEE) and a dose-related study compared celivarone at 50, 100, 200, or 300 mg once daily with amiodarone for the maintenance of sinus rhythm (MAIA) have already been completed. Results showed the lowest rate of AF recurrence at the 50 mg dose without increased efficacy at the higher doses.[30]

Vernakalant

Vernakalant is an atrial depolarizing agent, acting on multiple ion channels, which has its major target IKur. It also blocks Ito and INa, but there is little effect on IKr or IKs.[31] The drug has been used in a multicenter, randomized trial, the CRAFT trial (conversion of rapid atrial fibrillation trial) that was performed in patients with AF to establish the safety and efficacy of intravenous vernakalant.[32] A 2-mg/kg vernakalant infusion over 10 minutes was given in AF patients and second dose was repeated at a dose of 3-mg/kg infusion if normal sinus rhythm was not restored within a period of 15 minutes and there was found a statistically significant difference in conversion to sinus rhythm when compared with placebo group (61% vs. 5%; $P = 0.0005$).

Vernakalant has its modest effect for rhythm conversion of recently detected AF with maintenance of sinus rhythm approximately 24 hours. Oral vernakalant can be useful alternative for maintenance of sinus rhythm, but phase 3 trials are still underway. If drug is found efficacious in these trials, then probably it would have more potential for clinical application while conversion attempts could be undertaken so as to restoration of long-term sinus rhythm. Adverse effects seen with vernakalant might be cough and dysgeusia.

Ivabradine

Ivabradine is selective 1f channel blocker (f denotes funny channel, so called because it had unusual properties compared with other current systems known at the time of its discovery) and inhibits the spontaneous pacemaker activity of the sinus node.[33] As a result, there is reduction in the heart rate without affecting myocardial contractility.[34] The blockage of 1f channel is dependent on heart rate and dose. Electrophysiological studies of ivabradine have already shown very little effect on conduction system or atrial and ventricular refractoriness. The drug is metabolized 80% in liver by CYP3A4 enzyme, so cannot be used if drugs inhibiting the same enzyme, such as macrolide and ketoconazole are being used simultaneously. Data analysis has shown that most of the side effects of ivabradine are dose related. Ivabradine also affects the ion channels in the retina that could be the mechanism for ivabradine's side effect, a visual luminous phenomenon, which is also known as phosphenes (14.5%). Visual luminous phenomenon generally abates over time while treatment is not interrupted. Significant sinus bradycardia is seen in approximately 3.3% of patients. Sometimes palpitations, nausea, headaches, vertigo, muscle cramps, hyperuricemia can be noted. There is not much trial data on the treatment of atrial tachyarrhythmias with ivabradine. Ivabradine is used off-label in Europe for the treatment of inappropriate sinus tachycardia.

Adenosine A1 Receptor Agonists

As we know, intravenous adenosine terminates AV nodal re-entry tachycardia or AV re-entry after stimulating the A1 adenosine receptor by creating transient AV block. Sometimes adenosine can give rise to serious adverse effect profile[35] like flushing (18%), dyspnea (12%), and chest pain (7%), and it has been correlated with activity of adenosine on the receptors A2A, A2B, and A3 adenosine receptor subtypes. Studies have been done to identify A1 receptor-selective agonists for SVT termination and control of rate in AF. Some of these agents are under trials presently, including tecadenoson and selodenoson. Tecadenoson is currently being tested in TEMPEST trial[36] that is a multicenter, double-blinded, placebo-controlled trial that randomly assigned 181 patients to receive placebo versus tecadenoson for SVT termination. Conversion rates were found to be 73.5% in the tecadenoson-treated patients and 6.7% in the placebo group. Side effects were mild and found to be dose-related, like 12 patients had second-degree heart block and two patients developed complete heart block. In few patients, flushing, dyspnea, and chest pain were reported.

Ranolazine

Ranolazine is piperazine-derivative having chemical structure similar to lidocaine while blocking multiple ion channels. It is new agent having the antianginal and antiarrhythmic activity. Its most potent ion channel blocking effect is seen on late sodium current.[37-40] Ranolazine belongs to Vaughan Williams Class IB agent and prolongs action potential duration, with QT interval prolongation. Experiments done on animals have shown antiarrhythmic effects in the ventricle also.[39,40] Ranolazine has shown clinically to reduce arrhythmic episodes, in patients presenting with acute coronary syndrome[38] in the Metabolic Efficiency with Ranolazine for Less Ischemia in Non-ST-Elevation Acute Coronary Syndrome–Thrombolysis in Myocardial Infarction 36 trial (MERLIN-TIMI 36) and despite causing QT prolongation, ranolazine was not found to be associated with increased risk of SCD compared with placebo.[41] Based on limited experience but often good clinical results, it appears that ranolazine can be used as add-on therapy to Class III antiarrhythmic agent in patients with recurrent VT.

Upstream Therapies for AF

The concept of preventing the development of atrial electric and mechanical remodeling and thereby reducing the likelihood of AF is referred to as "upstream" therapy. It is now recognized that AF originates from atrial tissue that has altered structure or function. Fibrosis within the atrium is one of the major mechanisms of atrial remodeling, which provide the substrate for AF generation and maintenance.[42] Potential agents in this category include blockers of the renin-angiotensin axis, aldosterone inhibitors, polyunsaturated fatty acids, and statins.[43] It is likely that agents in this category of upstream therapy will be most effective when administered before the development of significant atrial fibrosis.

Targets of Future Antiarrhythmic Agents

The commonly used antiarrhythmic for treatment of ventricular tachycardia/ventricular fibrillation acts on sodium channels (Class I agents) or potassium channels (Class III agents), but efficacy has not been constant and there is always risk for drug-related ventricular proarrhythmia. Newer targets for the treatment of ventricular arrhythmia are being explored and newer pharmacologic agents will be tested in future clinical trials in upcoming years. Newer targets have focused on the roles of sodium-calcium exchange, intracellular calcium, gap junctions, and adenosine triphosphate (ATP)-sensitive potassium channel blockade.[44] Altered intracellular calcium homeostasis has been implicated in development of ventricular arrhythmias.[45] Pharmacotherapies to normalize intracellular calcium handling by either stabilizing RyR2 activity or modulating associated proteins involved in diastolic SR calcium leakage so as to prevent ventricular arrhythmia may be a future insight in development of antiarrhythmic agents in this regard.

Gap Junctions

When cell-cell coupling is disrupted in the heart, it results in arrhythmogenesis since synchronization of depolarization and repolarization is lost. It has been suggested that restoration of coupling via gap junctions could be an effective antiarrhythmic target approach.[44] Connexin 43 has been implicated as the principal gap junction protein that maintains cell to cell coupling in ventricles, and its function is impaired during episodes of ischemia.[46]

Sodium-calcium Exchange

The sodium-calcium exchanger (NCX) is a cell membrane protein that removes a single calcium ion in exchange for the import of three sodium ions in the cardiomyocyte. It has been seen that increased expression of NCX is associated with cardiac contractile dysfunction, so an increased risk of arrhythmias in congestive cardiac failure.[47] Findings are promising but it has to be tested in clinical trials and larger studies.

Blockade of ATP-Sensitive Potassium Channel

During ischemia, there is increase in extracellular potassium, most probably that causes development of ventricular arrhythmias. In fact, ATP-sensitive potassium channels during ischemia cause potassium efflux and action potential duration is reduced along with impaired function of the sodium/potassium ATPase have also been postulated.[48] Ischemia causes potassium distribution heterogeneously that leads to dispersion of repolarization and thus creating availability of a substrate for re-entrant arrhythmias. Glibenclamide is an ATP-sensitive potassium channel inhibitor that reduces action potential duration in models of ischemia, and suppresses episodes of extrasystoles and ventricular fibrillation.[48]

REFERENCES

1. Page RL, Roden DM. Drug therapy for atrial fibrillation: where do we go from here? Nat Rev Drug Discov. 2005;4:899 -910.
2. Musco S, Conway EL, Kowey PR. Drug therapy for atrial fibrillation. Med Clin North Am. 2008;92:121-41.
3. Savelieva I, Camm AJ. Anti-arrhythmic drug therapy for atrial fibrillation: current anti-arrhythmic drugs, investigational agents, and innovative approaches. Europace. 2008;10:647-65.
4. Ehrlich JR, Biliczki P, Hohnloser SH, et al. Atrial-selective approaches for the treatment of atrial fibrillation. J Am Coll Cardiol. 2008;51:787-92.
5. Wyse DG, Waldo AL, DiMarco JP, et al. A comparison of rate control and rhythm control in patients with atrial fibrillation. N Engl J Med. 2002;347:1825-33.
6. Carlsson J, Miketic S, Windeler J, et al. Randomized trial of rate-control versus rhythm-control in persistent atrial fibrillation: the Strategies of Treatment of Atrial Fibrillation (STAF) study. J Am Coll Cardiol. 2003;41:1690-6.
7. Opolski G, Torbicki A, Kosior DA, et al. Rate control vs rhythm control in patients with nonvalvular persistent atrial fibrillation: the results of the Polish How to Treat Chronic Atrial Fibrillation (HOT CAFE) study. Chest. 2004;126:476-86.
8. Zimetbaum P. Is rate control or rhythm control preferable in patients with atrial fibrillation? An argument for maintenance of sinus rhythm in patients with atrial fibrillation. Circulation. 2005;111:3150-6.
9. Camm AJ, Kirchhof P, Lip GY, et al. Guidelines for the management of atrial fibrillation: the Task Force for the Management of Atrial Fibrillation of the European Society of Cardiology (ESC). Eur Heart J. 2010;31:2369-429.
10. Groenveld HF, Crijns HJ, Rienstra M, et al. Does intensity of rate control influence outcome in persistent atrial fibrillation? Data of the RACE study. Am Heart J. 2009;158:785-91.
11. Stambler BWM, Ellenbogen K. Ibutilide Repeat Dose Study Investigators. Efficacy and safety of repeated intravenous doses of ibutilide for rapid conversion of atrial flutter or fibrillation. Circulation. 1996;7:1613-21.
12. Galve E, Rius T, Ballester R, et al. Intravenous amiodarone in treatment of recent-onset atrial fibrillation: results of a randomized, controlled study. J Am Coll Cardiol. 1996;27:1079-82.

13. Alboni P, Botto GL, Baldi N, et al. Outpatient treatment of recent-onset atrial fibrillation with the "pill-in-the-pocket" approach. N Engl J Med. 2004;351:2384 -91.
14. Roy D, Pratt CM, Torp-Pedersen C, et al. Vernakalant hydrochloride for rapid conversion of atrial fibrillation:a phase 3, randomized, placebo-controlled trial. Circulation. 2008;117: 1518-25.
15. Kowey PR, Dorian P, Mitchell LB, et al. Vernakalant hydrochloride for the rapid conversion of atrial fibrillation after cardiac surgery: a randomized, double-blind, placebo-controlled trial. Circ Arrhythm Electrophysiol. 2009;2:652-9.
16. Camm AJ, Capucci A, Hohnloser SH, et al. A randomized active-controlled study comparing the efficacy and safety of vernakalant to amiodarone in recent-onset atrial fibrillation. J Am Coll Cardiol. 2011;57:313-21.
17. Kober L, Torp-Pedersen C, McMurray JJ, et al. Increased mortality after dronedarone therapy for severe heart failure. N Engl J Med. 2008;358:2678-87.
18. Connolly SJ, Crijns HJ, Torp-Pedersen C, et al. Analysis of stroke in ATHENA: a placebo-controlled, double-blind, parallel-arm trial to assess the efficacy of dronedarone 400 mg bid for the prevention of cardiovascular hospitalization or death from any cause in patients with atrial fibrillation/atrial flutter. Circulation. 2009;120:1174-80.
19. Connolly SJ, Camm AJ, Halperin JL, et al. Dronedarone in high risk permanent atrial fibrillation. N Engl J Med. 2011;365:2268-76.
20. Hohnloser SH, Crijns HJ, van Eickels M, et al. Effect of dronedarone on cardiovascular events in atrial fibrillation. N Engl J Med. 2009;360:668-78.
21. Dronedarone Label. Rockville, MD: Food and Drug Administration, 2009.
22. Singh BN, Connolly SJ, Crijns HJ, et al. Dronedarone for maintenance of sinus rhythm in atrial fibrillation or flutter. N Engl J Med. 2007;357:987-99.
23. Pradaxa (dabigatran etexilate capsules) prescribing information. Boehringer Ingelheim Pharmaceuticals Inc; Ridgefield, CT: January 2012.
24. Connolly SJ, Ezekowitz MD, Yusef S, et al. Dabigatran versus warfarin in patients with atrial fibrillation. N Engl J Med. 2009;361:1139 -51.
25. Connolly SJ, Ezekowitz MD, Yusuf S, et al. Newly identified events in the RE-LY trial. N Engl J Med. 2010;363:1875-6.
26. Rivaroxaban (Xarelto rivaroxaban tablets) prescribing information. Janssen Pharmaceuticals Inc; Titusville, NJ: December 2011.
27. Wann LS, Curtis AB, Ellenbogen KA, et al. 2011 ACCF/AHA/HRS focused update on the management of patients with atrial fibrillation (update on dabigatran). A report of the American College of Cardiology Foundation/American Heart Association Task Force on Practice Guidelines. Circulation. 2011;123:1144-50.
28. You JJ, Singer DE, Howard PA, et al. Antithrombotic therapy for atrial fibrillation: Antithrombotic therapy and prevention of thrombosis, 9th edn: American College of Chest physicians evidence-based clinical practice guidelines. Chest. 2012; 141(Suppl):e531S-e575S.
29. Wallentin L, Yusef S, Ezekowitz, et al. Efficacy and safety of dabigatran compared with warfarin at different levels of international normalised ratio control for stroke prevention in atrial fibrillation: an analysis of the RE-LY trial. Lancet. 2010;376:975-83.
30. Gautier P, Gillemare E, Djandjighian L, et al. In vivo and in vitro characterization of the novel antiarrhythmic agent SSR149744C: electrophysiological, antiadrenergic and anti-angiotensin II effects. J Cardiovasc Pharmacol. 2004;44:244-57.
31. Kowey PR, Aliot EM, Cappucci A, et al. Placebo-controlled, double-blind dose-ranging study of the efficacy and safety of SSR149744C in patients with recent atrial fibrillation/flutter [abstract]. Heart Rhythm. 2007;5(Suppl):S72.
32. Fedida D, Orth PM, Chen JY, et al. The mechanism of atrial antiarrhythmic action of RSD1235. J Cardiovasc Electrophysiol. 2005;16:1227-38.
33. Roy D, Rowe BH, Stiell IG, et al.; CRAFT Investigators. A randomized controlled trial of RSD 1235, a novel antiarrhythmic agent, in the treatment of recent onset atrial fibrillation. J Am Coll Cardiol. 2004;2355-61.
34. Savelieva I, Camm AJ. If Inhibition with ivabradine: electrophysiological effects and safety. Drug Safety. 2008;31:95-107.
35. Manz M, Reuter M, Lauck G, et al. A single intravenous dose of ivabradine, a novel If inhibitor, lowers heart rate but does not depress left ventricular function in patients with left ventricular dysfunction. Cardiology. 2003;100:149-55.
36. Elzein E, Zablocki J. A1 adenosine receptor agonists and their potential therapeutic applications. Exp Opin Investig Drugs. 2008;17:1901-10.
37. Ellenbogen KA, O'Neill G, Prystowsky EN, et al.; TEMPEST Study Group. Trial to evaluate the management of paroxysmal supraventricular tachycardia during an electrophysiology study with tecadenoson. Circulation. 2005;111:3202-8.
38. Vizzardi E, D'Aloia A, Quinzani F, et al. A focus on antiarrhythmic properties of ranolazine. J Cardiovasc Pharmacol Ther. 2012;17:353-6.
39. Scirica BM, Morrow DA, Hod H, et al. Effect of ranolazine, an antianginal agent with novel electrophysiological properties, on the incidence of arrhythmias in patients with non ST-segment elevation acute coronary syndrome: results from the Metabolic Efficiency With Ranolazine for Less Ischemia in Non ST-Elevation Acute Coronary Syndrome Thrombolysis in Myocardial Infarction 36 (MERLIN-TIMI 36) randomized controlled trial. Circulation. 2007;116:1647-52.
40. Frommeyer G, Kaiser D, Uphaus T, et al. Effect of ranolazine on ventricular repolarization in class III antiarrhythmic drug-treated rabbits. Heart Rhythm. 2012;9:2051-8.
41. Verrier RL, Pagotto VP, Kanas AF, et al. Low doses of ranolazine and dronedarone in combination exert potent protection against atrial fibrillation and vulnerability to ventricular arrhythmias during acute myocardial ischemia. Heart Rhythm. 2012;1:121-7.
42. Spach MS. Mounting evidence that fibrosis generates a major mechanism for atrial fibrillation. Circ Res. 2007;101:743-5.
43. Burstein B, Nattel S. Atrial fibrosis: mechanisms and clinical relevance for atrial fibrillation. J Am Coll Cardiol. 2008;51:802-9.
44. Savelieva I, Kakouros N, Kourliouros A, et al. Upstream therapies for management of atrial fibrillation: review of clinical evidence and implications for the European Society of Cardiology guidelines. Europace. 2011;13:308-28.
45. Mason PK, DiMarco JP. New pharmacological agents for arrhythmias. Circ Arrhythm Electrophysiol. 2009;2:588-97.
46. Thireau J, Pasquie JL, Martel E, et al. New drugs vs. old concepts: a fresh look at antiarrhythmics. Pharmacol Ther. 2011;132: 125-45.
47. Wit AL, Duffy HS. Drug development for treatment of cardiac arrhythmias: targeting the gap junctions. Am J Physiol Heart Circ Physiol. 2008;294:H16-8.
48. Antoons G, Sipido KR. Targeting calcium handling in arrhythmias. Europace. 2008;10:1364-9.

12

Chest Radiography and Cardiovascular Disease: Is It Still Relevant in the Era of Other Imaging Modalities?

Poonam Khurana, Rishabh Khurana

INTRODUCTION

Chest radiography is a frequently performed radiological study, which is reflected by the fact that majority of the medical centers worldwide still perform chest radiograph routinely for all hospital admissions. It remains one of the prime methods for investigations of the diseases of the lungs, heart, mediastinal structures, and pulmonary circulation, despite the remarkable advances in other noninvasive and invasive imaging modalities. It is admitted that only few fields in clinical medicine have shown more innovative and even sensational advances in recent years than has diagnostic imaging and its therapeutic applications. In the last three decades, new modalities and related technologies (ultrasound, computed tomography (CT), magnetic resonance imaging (MRI), and radionuclide studies) have been introduced and developed. These modalities have thrived far beyond our most optimistic expectations.

However, chest radiography still lies at the core of cardiac diagnosis in one way or the other. It is readily available, safe, inexpensive, and reproducible. A simple snapshot of the chest provides information on the pulmonary tree, heart, great arteries (vessels) and lungs, assessing cardiac chamber size and mass, thus providing a rapid means of evaluating the patient's status. The chest radiograph accurately depicts support device positioning, related complications, and is a useful guide for the assessment of daily interval change in thoracic disease. Chest radiography is responsible for approximately 30–40% of all X-ray examinations performed in a reputed hospital.[1] Studies are on record,[2-5] which reveal that the outcome of daily radiographs in intensive care units (ICUs), may lead to a change in patient's management to the extent of 65%. Besides, important advances have also taken place in chest radiography too, which will be discussed in this chapter in detail.

STATUS OF CHEST RADIOGRAPHY: PAST AND PRESENT

Applicability of Chest Radiograph in Cardiovascular-related Diseases and Ailments

The chest radiograph is an excellent method for evaluating pulmonary hemodynamics, including the signs of pulmonary edema and heart failure, both of which may appear before physical signs can be detected. In addition to that, it can diagnose increased pulmonary blood flow caused by intra- and extracardiac shunts, venous anomalies that also include arteriovenous fistulas, and any existing evidence of pulmonary hypertension.

The technique is still relevant as depicted in Table 12.1, whether it is the presentation of the patient with symptoms pointing to cardiac diseases, follow-up, monitoring, ruling out cardiac/extracardiac diseases, or deciding the need for further examination with other modalities. In most instances, a definite diagnosis cannot be made; however, the differential can be narrowed to a few likely diagnoses that can further guide and lead to several more studies and thus facilitates the institution of timely therapy in right direction.

These indications are in addition to routine radiographs for periodic health examinations, pre-employment health assessment, and preadmission and preoperative chest radiographs, which are also carried out to exclude certain cardiac-related pathological lesions.

Advancement

Chest radiography and clinicians

As stated earlier, patient with known or suspected heart disease undergoes routine conventional chest radiograph

Table 12.1 Indication of chest radiographs in various clinical scenarios

Clinical scenarios	Utility of chest radiograph
Presentation of patient signs and symptoms pointing to cardiac/ respiratory disease like chest pain, breathlessness, cough, pulmonary edema, and heart failure	• To diagnose/rule out cardiac disease • Even signs of pulmonary edema and heart failure may appear before physical signs can be detected by the physician. Refer to text for more information.
Follow-up of the patient with diagnosed cardiac disease	For the evaluation of improvement and progression
Monitoring of cardiac patient	• Patient with intra- and extracardiac shunts • Intensive care unit patients with supporting devices
Rule out the extracardiac diseases that resemble cardiac disease	Differential can be narrowed to a few likely diagnosis
For further examination with other modalities for the evaluation of cardiac chamber, great vessels, pulmonary hemodynamics, and calcification	For choosing the need for other modalities viz nuclear medicine, echocardiography, computed tomography (CT), magnetic resonance imaging (MRI)
Screening tests	Refer to text

at various healthcare centers to evaluate their clinical status. In addition, various indices of cardiac chamber and great vessels with respect to their size, shape, and position provide a wealth of information that facilitates the diagnosis of congenital and acquired heart disease, before and after treatment; calcification at various locations of heart helps to confirm and elucidate the nature and severity of heart disease. Indeed, information obtained from chest radiographic images is often provided in a convenient format with which all clinicians feel comfortable.

Inherent technical problems

Inherent technical problems of chest radiography are listed in Table 12.2.

Advancements in chest radiography

Over the past two decades, there has been a remarkable advancement in the technology pertaining to conventional chest radiography. New approaches to image acquisition and display have been introduced to circumvent the limitations of conventional film screen study. Computed radiography system has become the standard for bedside chest imaging in many developed countries and has made an encroachment at various sophisticated centers in India and other developing countries.[6] Digital radiography has also followed a similar pattern and is rapidly replacing fixed film-based chest units. The impetus for these changes can mainly be attributed to digital imaging technique.

Most important advances taken place in chest radiography are enlisted in Table 12.3, which has been bifurcated into Tables 12.3a and 12.3b.

In conventional chest radiography, the screen film detector happens to be the most commonly used image recorder that has limitations in its ability to provide contrast as well as overall image latitude.[7-9] New screen film systems in chest radiography have evolved the highly sensitive image receptors to radiation, which are capable to respond

Table 12.2 Inherent technical problems of chest radiography

- Large difference in tissue density present in the chest
- Wide latitude of X-ray transmission through the thorax
- Scattered radiation due to high X-ray photon energy and thick chest with large field of view
- Projection of a three-dimensional structure onto a two-dimensional image leading to overlay
- Perceptual limitations due to inexperienced radiologist

Table 12.3 Advances in chest radiography

Table 12.3a Road to user-friendly techniques: detector developments

Detector developments
a. Screen film detector
b. Digital chest radiography
c. Computed radiography system
d. Flat panel direct system
e. Charge-coupled devices (CCD) and complementary metal-oxide semiconductor (CMOS)-based detectors
f. Slot-scan technology

to a wide range of exposures. In past two decades, several innovations have been developed combined with gathering more information that can be recorded and displayed. It has minimized the need for repeat X-rays and omitted the fear of losing films. The image degradation caused by scatter radiation warrants the use of a grid.

Digital radiography with its wide exposure latitude, low scatter images, and flexible display capabilities has

Table 12.3b Road to user-friendly techniques: Advances made in image processing developments

Advances made in chest radiography	*Remarks*
Image processing developments:	
a. Image preprocessing	a. In preprocessing image, correction for detector defects or nonuniformities can be carried out along with scaling for optimal display of image after identification of the anatomically relevant range exposures and anatomic area of interest[8,12,13]
b. Image post-processing	b. After overcoming the inherent "flaws," digital radiography uses various algorithms to further enhance the finer details of image[14,15]
Display development	It is a soft copy display with monochrome monitor or color monitor that improves the brightness, reduces glare and reflection, and thus markedly improves the resolution for the review by radiologists/physicians[16-23]
Application developments a. Dual energy subtraction imaging b. Temporal subtraction c. Digital tomosynthesis	The concept of equalization radiography is used and developed to improve the visibility of lesions in the dense regions of chest that include retrocardiac area besides mediastinum and retrodiaphragmatic areas
Computer-aided detection (CAD) and computer-aided diagnosis (CADx) systems advancements	System aids the radiologist in detecting abnormalities

compensated for the limited spatial resolution in this radiographic system, which combined with modern computer technology made it feasible to replace film screen systems with superior and improved image acquisition through digital methodology. And this new technology offers transmission and storage capabilities also.[10,11]

STATUS OF CHEST RADIOGRAPHY IN INTENSIVE CARE UNIT: A UNIQUE AND INDISPENSABLE ROLE

Intensive Care Unit Patients and Chest Radiography

In ICU patients, portable radiograph still forms the basis of our diagnostic approach even in sophisticated centers and it is routinely performed. The drawback is that the bedside radiograph is never of the quality of standard radiograph. In spite of being readily available and inexpensive, it has technical and diagnostic limitations due to difference in film exposure and scattered radiation. The degree of inspiration on portable examinations is usually suboptimal, geometric unsharpness is always present, and the evaluation of cardiac size and posterior basal disease remains difficult.

The clinical assessment of the intensive care patient is reliant on imaging and the portable chest radiography continues to remain the most commonly requested radiographic examination. Here too, remarkable advancements have taken place to overcome the defects owing to differences in film exposure and scattered radiation, which improved the technique in obtaining diagnostic quality radiographs consistently. Thus, the intensive care radiography can be revolutionized in several ways mentioned below:

1. The implementation of a wide latitude screen film system, together with adequate scatter control utilizing a grid whenever possible.[24]
2. The introduction of a digital radiography with the features of exposure compensation and image processing.
3. Picture archiving and communication system (PACS) networks consist of image acquisition devices, image servers, or image archives and storage devices. The introduction of PACS has improved the efficiency of the radiology department and increased the utilization of radiological services.

Detection of Support Devices: Role of Chest Radiography for Their Correct Placement

Patients in ICU consist of either postoperative patients or the critically ill patients. In fact, both type of above-mentioned patients share many disorders in common. They suffer similar pulmonary insult and experience the benefits and mishaps of various monitoring and support procedures.[25-34] The clinical problems in them are often complex and rapidly changing. The respiratory and cardiac diseases are the most common causes of morbidity and the leading causes of mortality. Even when the disease process or surgery is initially extrathoracic, the heart and lungs are frequently involved secondarily.

Chest radiography is highly accurate in demonstrating support device positioning and complications. The role of portable radiographs are reliable and indispensable guide to correct device placement (Fig. 12.1), therefore always required for confirmation. Support devices are associated with a wide variety of complications ranging from suboptimal placement to life-threatening events.[35-43] Physical examination even by experienced operators is an unreliable guide to correct device placement, therefore solely dependent on portable radiography. The portable radiograph is highly accurate in demonstrating support device positioning and complication. The role of portable radiographs and other modalities for assessing correct placement has been shown in Table 12.4.

ROLE OF CHEST RADIOGRAPHY IN DETECTION AND DIAGNOSIS OF CONGENITAL HEART DISEASE

Chest radiograph can provide lot of information depending on the severity of the congenital heart disease, which is described briefly in Tables 12.5a and 12.5b. However, with

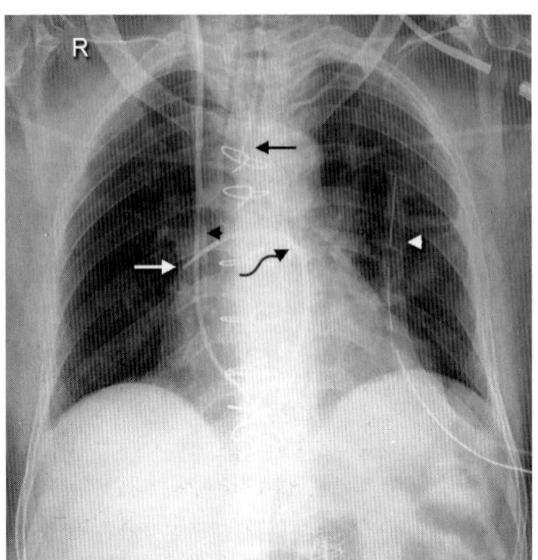

Fig. 12.1 Postoperative cardiac surgery chest radiograph shows that tip of endotracheal tube is above the carina (black arrow), central venous catheter in superior vena cava (black arrowhead), right jugular Swan–Ganz catheter with its tip in the right main pulmonary artery (white arrow), tip of intra-aortic balloon pump (IABP) in the descending thoracic aorta (curved arrow); also note chest tube left side (white arrowhead). Sternal wires are also present

the advent of echocardiography, cardiac CT, and MRI, the traditional and conventional film-screen photographic radiography is increasingly being replaced in imaging applications by these newer modalities.[44,45]

But once it comes to chest imaging of pediatric patients with congenital heart diseases admitted in ICU, the so-called unsophisticated portable radiograph continues to remain the cornerstone of diagnostic approach even in sophisticated centers. This issue has already been dealt in detail earlier in this chapter.

DEPENDENCY OF OTHER MODALITIES ON CHEST RADIOGRAPHY: DIAGNOSIS OF CARDIOVASCULAR DISEASE

Remarkable advances have been made during the past three decades in understanding diagnosis and treatment of heart diseases. The rise in the use of other cardiac imaging modalities including CT scan, MRI, nuclear medicine imaging, echocardiography, cardiac angiography and left ventriculography has not only resulted in facilitating morphologic diagnosis, but allowed quantification of morphologic changes, which include the following:

1. To differentiate functioning and dysfunctional myocardium
2. The instant physiologic aberration reflected in those changes
3. The resulting regional and global changes in cardiac function.

Such quantitative information had significant value providing the basis for risk stratification and objective assessment of the effects of medical or surgical treatment. But here too, chest radiography can play a role of a diagnostic tool, which helps clinicians in assessing the need and choosing the sequence of other modalities, to be undertaken for cardiovascular patients. Therefore, chest radiography still remains the mainstay of chest imaging despite the known diagnostic superiority and increasing availability of other imaging modalities.

NEED AND IMPORTANCE OF REPEAT IMAGING: CHEST RADIOGRAPHY AND OTHER MODALITIES

Many of the disease processes have a similar image appearance and are difficult to differentiate on the basis of a single imaging as picture keeps on changing with time particularly in ICU patients in whom repeat imaging is invariably required. In spite of the fact that several new imaging modalities have been introduced and developed, chest radiography remains a useful investigation being simple, quick, and cost-effective test that yields useful

Table 12.4 Status of portable radiographs/other modalities for correct placement of support devices: dominating role of portable radiographs (Fig. 12.1)

Serial No	Support device	Remarks
1.	Endotracheal tube	• Repositioned on the basis of chest radiograph finding • Correct and optimal positioning is of paramount importance • Low position result in right main bronchus intubation whereas too high placement is associated with a theoretical risk of inadvertent extubation and vocal cord injury • Following intubation, physical examination identified tube malposition in 2–5% of patients whereas the radiograph revealed suboptimal positioning in 10% to 25%[25,26]
2.	Enteric tube	• Chest radiograph is mandatory to confirm the tip of nasogastric tube in the stomach • It is important to ensure that distal side holes are in the stomach to prevent aspiration • Wrong placement may occur in major bronchi or pleural space
3.	Pulmonary artery catheter	• Ideal location for the pulmonary artery catheter tip is central lying within 2 cm of the hilar point • It should not extend beyond proximal interlobar arteries • Distal placement will lead to increase in risk of life-threatening vascular trauma and thromboembolic events[27-31]
4.	Intra-aortic balloon pump (IABP)	• The correct position of IABP tip in the descending aorta beneath the subclavian artery is identified on chest radiograph • Portable radiograph prevents the incorrect positioning that in turn may cause limb ischemia and vascular complications of various magnitude[32-34]
5.	Central venous catheter	• Exact location of central venous catheter tip within the superior vena cava is mandatory prior to commencement of total parental nutrition, chemotherapy, and vasopressors. • Complication ranges from hemothorax, pneumothorax, sepsis, and pneumonia
6.	Tracheostomy tube	• Radiograph is done to exclude postsurgical complications of hemorrhage or abnormal air collection secondary to placement of tracheostomy tube • Over distension is identified as bulging of the tracheal walls by the cuff. Thus, cuff-induced stenosis can be prevented
7.	Thoracostomy tube	• Normally positioned chest tube lies on the surface of the expanded lung, between the visceral and parietal pleura[35,36] • Both frontal and lateral chest radiographs are needed to accurately assess the position of tube
8.	Cardiac devices	• Radiograph is done to assess the correct placement of device, leads and associated complications

diagnostic information on thoracic diseases as well as providing a readily available documentation of related facts for serial comparison. Therefore, the main advantage of chest radiography is the speed at which they can be performed, acquired, repeated, and interpreted, at low cost and low radiation exposure and it will play an important role as a fast tool to rule out various cardiovascular diseases or to monitor response to therapy.

RADIOLOGIST, CLINICIANS, AND CHEST RADIOGRAPHY

In fact, the most significant limitation of chest radiography as a diagnostic tool is the experience and expertise of the individual interpreting the chest radiograph. An experienced and competent radiologist appreciates the significance of an observation that varies from normal findings. The skill and experience of the radiologist in performing and interpreting these radiographs remain crucial in maintaining the relevance and importance of chest radiography. Studies differ in how much a radiologist's perception and abilities are involved and how well they represent the clinical situation.

Many of the disease processes in ICU patients have a similar radiographic appearance and are difficult to differentiate on the basis of a single radiograph. Clues to their etiology can often be gained by careful attention to the time of onset relative to surgery or other insults, the speed of progression or resolution and the response to various therapeutic maneuvers. Therefore, a constant dialogue between the radiologist and the referring clinician is highly recommended to arrive at a correct diagnosis.

Table 12.5a Appearance of chest radiograph in various congenital heart diseases: conditions with respect to pulmonary vascularity

Serial No.	Congenital heart diseases	Chest radiograph findings
a	*Conditions with increased pulmonary vascularity (Fig. 12.2)* Atrial septal defect (ASD), ventricular septal defect (VSD), atrioventricular septal defect, patent ductus arteriosus (PDA), total anomalous pulmonary venous connection (TAPVC), transposition of the great arteries (TGA), truncus arteriosus	• *ASD/VSD:* Normal sizes heart/cardiomegaly, convex main pulmonary artery, and increase in pulmonary arterial markings • *PDA:* Mild cardiomegaly, convex main pulmonary artery, prominent aortic arch with increased pulmonary vascular markings • *TAPVC:* Cardiomegaly with increased pulmonary arterial markings, widening of superior mediastinum with classical "snowmen or figure of 8"appearance • *TGA:* Cardiomegaly with increased pulmonary blood flow and prominent hila
b	*Conditions with decreased pulmonary vascularity:* Tetralogy of Fallot (TOF) (Fig. 12.3), tetralogy/absent pulmonary valve syndrome, pulmonary atresia/VSD (pseudotruncus), tricuspid atresia, Ebstein's anomaly, TGA with pulmonary stenosis (TGA with PS) (Fig. 12.4), pulmonary hypertension/Eisenmenger's syndrome (Fig. 12.5)	• *TOF:* "Boot-shaped" heart with diminished pulmonary vascular markings • *Tricuspid atresia:* Enlarged right atrium with reduced pulmonary flow • *Ebstein's anomaly:* Marked cardiomegaly with right atrial dilatation and diminished pulmonary arterial markings • *TGA with PS:* Cardiomegaly with diminished pulmonary arterial markings • *Eisenmenger's syndrome:* Dilatation of main pulmonary artery with decreased peripheral vascular markings
c	*Conditions with normal pulmonary vascularity:* Aortic stenosis (AS) (Fig. 12.6), coarctation of the aorta (COA), interrupted aortic arch, cardiomyopathy, pulmonary stenosis (PS), mitral stenosis (MS) (Fig. 12.7), hypoplastic left heart syndrome, cor triatriatum, idiopathic pulmonary artery dilatation	• *AS:* Cardiomegaly with normal vasculature • *COA:* Rib notching, figure-three sign in left upper mediastinum secondary to poststenotic dilatation of aorta infracoarctation • *PS:* Normal cardiac size, convex main pulmonary artery with normal branch pulmonary arteries • *MS:* Cardiac enlargement with pulmonary venous congestion leading to Kerley B lines in lung bases

Table 12.5b Appearance of chest radiograph in various congenital heart diseases: conditions associated with other anomalies and therapeutic devices

Serial No.	Congenital heart diseases	Chest radiograph findings
a	*Aortic arch anomalies/vascular ring:* Double aortic arch, right aortic arch with aberrant left subclavian artery, right aortic arch with left ductus remnant	• *Double aortic arch:* Right-sided aortic arch is common with tracheal deviation. Descending aorta is usually contralateral to dominant arch • *Right aortic arch:* Chest radiograph demonstrates right sided aortic arch
b	*Malposition cardiac lesions:* Dextrocardia, situs inversus totalis (Fig. 12.8).	• *Dextrocardia:* Cardiac apex is on right side • *Situs inversus:* Chest radiograph demonstrates dextrocardia with gastric bubble on the right
c	*Postinterventional implant:* Pulmonary artery stent, coarctation stent, atrial septal defect (ASD) occlusion device (Figs 12.9A and B), patent ductus arteriosus (PDA) coil occlusion, aortopulmonary collateral coil embolization	• Devices and implants are visible on chest radiograph • Both PA and lateral radiograph is to be done for proper localization

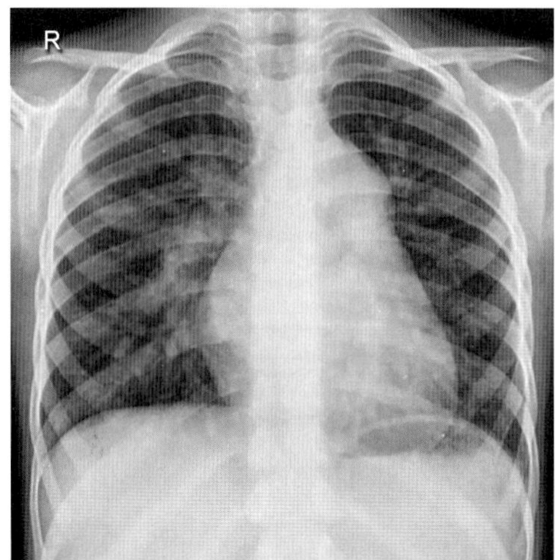

Fig. 12.2 Posteroanterior (PA) chest radiograph demonstrates cardiomegaly, convex main pulmonary artery segment and increased pulmonary arterial markings—case of large ventricular septal defect (VSD)

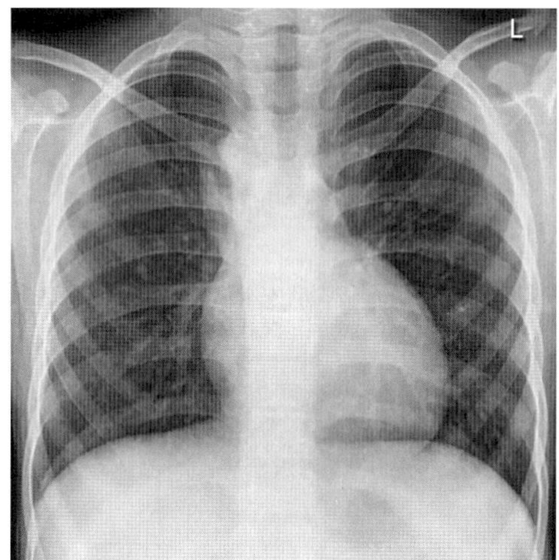

Fig. 12.3 Posteroanterior (PA) chest radiograph shows normal heart size with right ventricular contour and decrease pulmonary vascularity—case of tetralogy of Fallot (TOF), perimembranous ventricular septal defect (VSD) and severe pulmonary stenosis

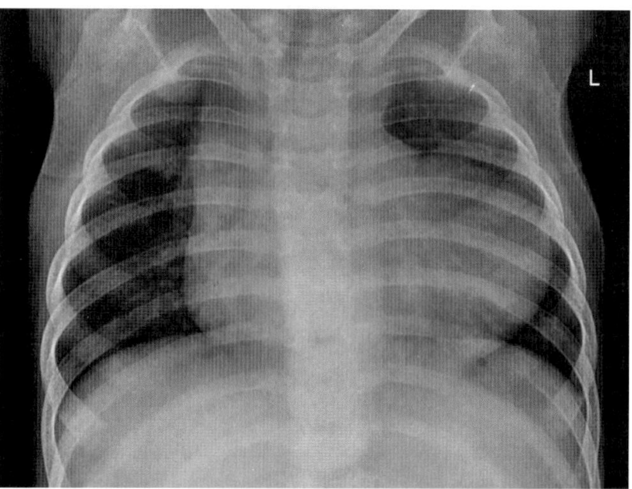

Fig. 12.4 Chest radiograph showing cardiomegaly with upturned right ventricle apex and reduced pulmonary arterial markings—case of dextro-transposition of the great arteries (d-TGA), hypoplastic left ventricle, pulmonary stenosis, and multiple ventricular septal defect (VSD)

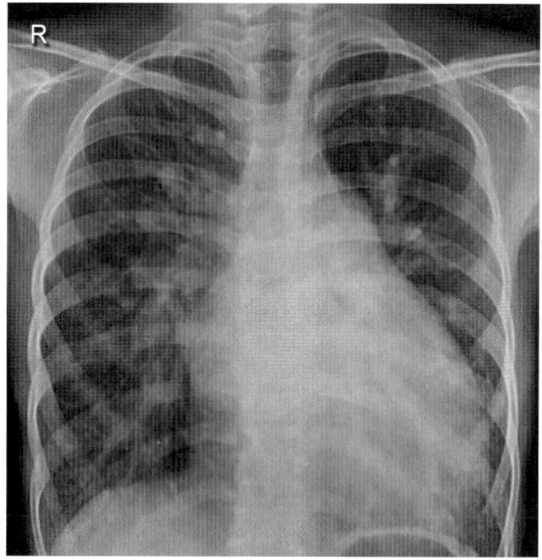

Fig. 12.5 Chest posteroanterior (PA) radiograph demonstrating cardiomegaly, prominent main pulmonary artery and hilar arterial markings with decreased peripheral vascular markings—case of ventricular septal defect (VSD), hypoplastic right ventricle and pulmonary arterial hypertension

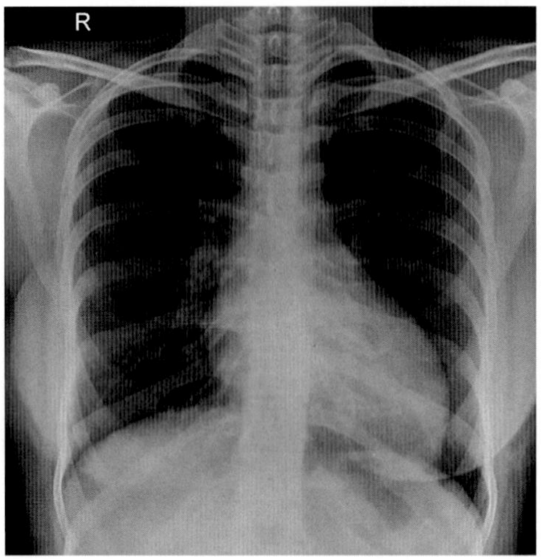

Fig. 12.6 Posteroanterior (PA) chest radiograph demonstrates cardiomegaly and displaced left ventricle apex—case of severe valvular aortic stenosis

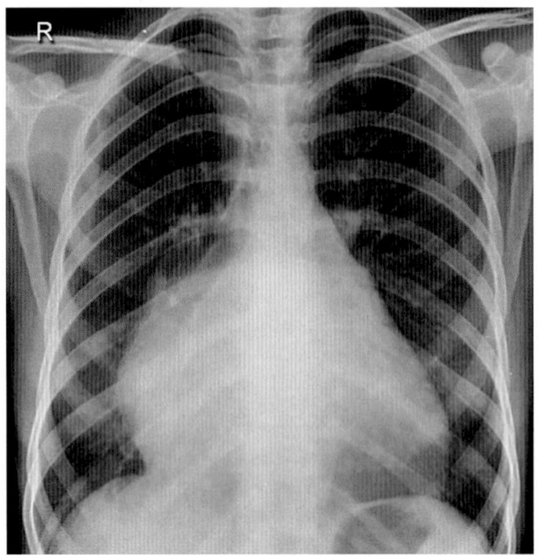

Fig. 12.7 Posteroanterior (PA) chest radiograph demonstrates cardiac enlargement with dilated left atrium, straightening of left cardiac border, and mild enlargement of left atrial appendage—case of rheumatic heart disease with severe mitral stenosis

The introduction of digital radiography and PACS has improved the efficiency of the radiology department and increased the utilization of radiological services. However, PACS has modified the relationship between the clinician and the radiologist, with a decrease in radiologic consultations due to improved viewing access at remote locations. As the effect of PACS on patient care is being evaluated, it is important to remember that dialogue between the clinicians is an important facet of patient management and an essential adjunct to the meaningful interpretation of imaging.

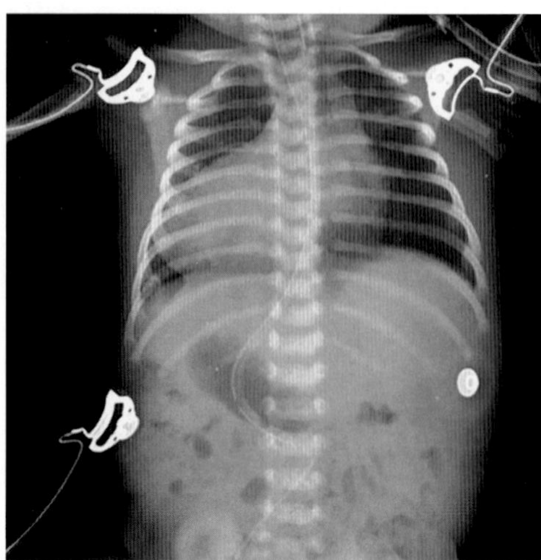

Fig. 12.8 Chest radiograph demonstrating dextrocardia with situs inversus, gastric bubble with ryles tube seen on right

CHEST RADIOGRAPHY AND CARDIOVASCULAR DISEASE: SUMMARY AND CONCLUSION

1. Chest radiography represents a significant percentage of the workload of a radiology department in a cardiac clinical setup, regardless of the level of healthcare delivery. If later has an active cardiothoracic surgery service, it generates large numbers of daily chest radiographs, many of which display support devices used to treat and monitor patients of all age groups. This is consequent to the advances in the treatment of the ICU patients that has increased the numbers of examination performed at patient's bedside. Obtaining a daily chest radiograph is standard practice and any change in patient's condition or an intervention can lead to several more studies in a given day based on the finding of chest radiograph.
2. The chest radiograph provides perhaps the most rapid, safe, and cost-effective screening for patient with cardiovascular disease. One of the most valuable contributions of chest radiography is its ability to facilitate the exclusion of noncardiac diseases, which may cause similar symptoms or may coexist with cardiovascular disease.
3. The portable chest radiography is an indispensable diagnostic tool and still plays a dominating role in the management of patients in ICU.
4. The introduction of digital radiography and PACS has further improved the efficiency and utility of radiological services; this has revolutionized the communication between radiologist and clinician that creates the best situation for making the correct diagnosis.

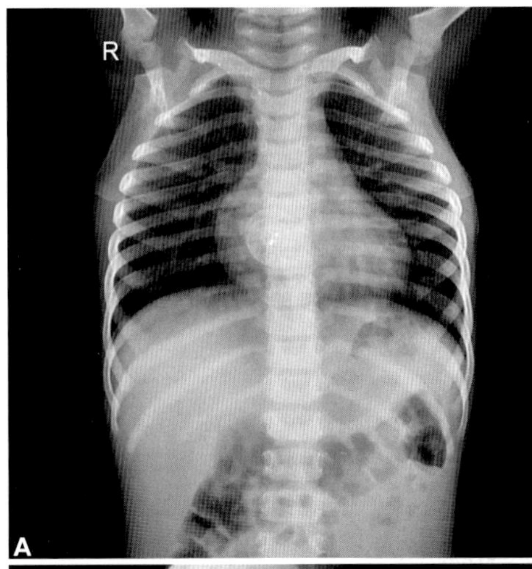

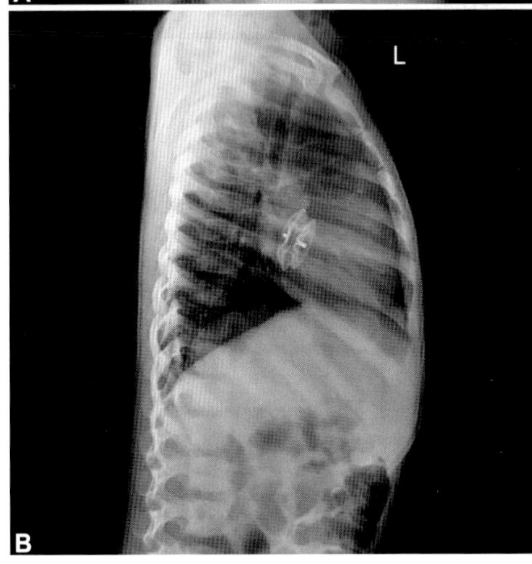

Figs 12.9A and B Case of fossa ovalis atrial septal defect (ASD)—posteroanterior (PA) and lateral chest radiographs demonstrate an ASD occlusion device located in the atrial septal defect

5. The chest radiography guides clinicians in assessing the need and choosing or omitting the sequence of other costly modalities for better management of cardiovascular patients. Therefore, the existing imaging system can be approached and utilized in cost effective manner.
6. Chest radiography is still relevant across the globe in the era of other imaging modalities and it is bound to stay.

REFERENCES

1. International Commission on Radiological Protection. Managing patient dose in digital radiology. Ann ICRP. 2004;34(1):1-73.
2. Henschke CI, Pasternack GS, Schroeder S, et al. Bedside chest radiography: diagnostic efficacy. Radiology. 1983;149:23-6.
3. Bekemeyer WB, Crapo RD, Calhoon S, et al. Efficacy of chest radiography in a respiratory intensive care unit. Chest. 1985;88: 691-6.
4. Strain DS, Kinasewitz GT, Vereen LE, et al. Value of routine daily chest X-rays in the medical intensive care unit. Crit Care Med. 1985;13:534-6.
5. Hall JB, White SR, Karrison T. Efficacy of daily routine chest radiographs in intubated, mechanically ventilated patients. Crit Care Med. 1991;19(5):689-93.
6. Sonoda M, Takano M, Miyahara J, et al. Computed radiography utilizing scanning laser stimulated luminescence. Radiology. 1983;148:833-8.
7. Van Metter R. Describing the signal-transfer characteristics of asymmetrical radiographic screen-film systems. Med Phys. 1992;19:53-8.
8. Haus AG, Jaskulski S. Basics of film processing in medical imaging. Madison, WI: Medical Physics; 1997.
9. Van Metter R, Dickerson R. Objective performance characteristics of a new asymmetric screen-film system. Med Phys. 1994;21: 1483-90.
10. Samei E, Flynn MJ. An experimental comparison of detector performance for computed radiography systems. Med Phys. 2002;29:447-59.
11. Korner M, Weber CH, Wirth S, et al. Advances in digital radiography: physical principles and system overview. Radio Graphics. 2007;27:675-86.
12. Haus AG. Advances in film processing systems technology and quality control in medical imaging. Madison, WI: Medical Physics; 2001.
13. Seibert JA. Digital radiographic image presentation: preprocessing methods. In: Samei E, Flynn MJ (Eds), 2003 Syllabus: Categorical Course in Diagnostic Radiology Physics—Advances in Digital Radiography. Oak Brook, IL: Radiological Society of North America; 2003. pp. 53-70.
14. Prokop M, Neitzel U, Schaefer-Prokop C. Principles of image processing in digital chest radiography. J Thorac Imaging. 2003;18:148-64.
15. Flynn MJ. Processing digital radiographs of specific body parts. In: Samei E, Flynn MJ (Eds). 2003 Syllabus: Categorical Course in Diagnostic Radiology Physics—Advances in Digital Radiography. Oak Brook, IL: Radiological Society of North America. 2003;71-8.
16. Uffmann M, Prokop M, Kupper W, et al. Soft-copy reading of digital chest radiographs: effect of ambient light and automatic optimization of monitor luminance. Invest Radiol. 2005;40: 180-5.
17. Oschatz E, Prokop M, Scharitzer M, et al. Comparison of liquid crystal versus cathode ray tube display for the detection of simulated chest lesions. Eur Radiol. 2005;15:1472-6.
18. Scharitzer M, Prokop M, Weber M, et al. Detectability of catheters on bedside chest radiographs: comparison between liquid crystal display and high-resolution cathode-ray tube monitors. Radiology. 2005;234(2):611-6.
19. Balassy C, Prokop M, Weber M, et al. Flat-panel display (LCD) versus high-resolution gray-scale display (CRT) for chest radiography: an observer preference study. AJR Am J Roentgenol. 2005;184:752-6.
20. Samei E, Badano A, Chakraborty D, et al. Assessment of display performance for medical imaging systems. Madison, WI: Medical Physics; 2005.
21. Badano A, Gagne RM, Jennings RJ, et al. Noise in flat-panel displays with subpixel structure. Med Phys. 2004;31:715-23.
22. Samei E, Wright SL. Effect of viewing angle response on DICOM compliance of liquid crystal displays. In: Ratib OM, Huang HK (Eds). Proceedings of SPIE: Medical Imaging 2004—PACS and

Imaging Informatics: Bellingham, Wash: International Society for Optical Engineering, 2004;5371:170-7.

23. Averbukh AN, Channin DS, Flynn MJ. Assessment of a novel, high-resolution, color, AMLCD for diagnostic medical image display: luminance performance and DICOM calibration. J Digit Imaging. 2003;16:270-9.
24. Wandtke J. Bedside chest radiography. Radiology. 1994;190:1-10.
25. Lotano R, Gerber D, Aseron C, et al. Utility of postintubation chest radiographs in the intensive care unit. Crit Care. 2000;4(1): 50-3.
26. Gray P, Sullivan G, Ostryzniuk P, et al. Value of postprocedural chest radiographs in the adult intensive care unit. Crit Care Med. 1992;20:1513-8.
27. Kaiser CW, Koornick AR, Smith N, et al. Choice of route for central venous cannulation: Subclavian or internal jugular vein? A prospective randomized study. J Surg Oncol. 1981;17:345-4.
28. Eckhardt WF, Iaconnetti J, Kwon JS, et al. Inadvertent carotid artery cannulation during pulmonary artery catheter insertion. J Cardiothorac Vasc Anesth. 1996;10:283-90.
29. Herbst CA Jr. Indications, management, and complications of percutaneous subclavian catheters. An audit. Arch Surg. 1978; 113:1421-5.
30. Boyd KD, Thomas SJ, Gold J, et al. A prospective study of complications of pulmonary artery catheterizations in 500 consecutive patients. Chest. 1983;84:245-9.
31. Kearney TJ, Shabot MM. Pulmonary artery rupture associated with the Swan-Ganz catheter. Chest. 1995;108:1349-52.
32. Baskett RJF, Ghali WA, Maitland A, Hirsch GM. The intra-aortic balloon pump in cardiac surgery. Ann Thorac Surg. 2002;74: 1276-87.
33. Kantrowitz A, Wasfie T, Freed P, et al. Intra-aortic balloon pumping 1967 through 1982: analysis of complications in 733 patients. Am J Cardiol. 1986;57:976-83.
34. Gottlieb S, Brinker J, Borkon A, et al. Identification of patients at high risk for complications of intra-aortic balloon counter-pulsation: a multivariate risk factor analysis. Am J Cardiol. 1984; 53:1135-9.
35. Swensen SJ, Peters SG, LeRoy AJ, et al. Radiology in the intensive-care unit. Mayo Clin Proc. 1991;66:396-410.
36. Maffessanti M, Berlot G, Bortolotto P. Chest roentgenology in the intensive care unit: an overview. Eur Radiol. 1998;8:69-78.
37. Landay MJ, Mootz AR, Estrera AS. Apparatus seen on chest radiographs after cardiac surgery in adults. Radiology. 1990;174: 477-82.
38. Wiener MD, Garay SM, Leitman BS, et al. Imaging of the intensive care unit patient. Clin Chest Med. 1991;12:169-98.
39. Henry DA, Jolles H, Berberich JJ, et al. The post-cardiac surgery chest radiograph: a clinically integrated approach. J Thorac Imaging. 1989;4:20-41.
40. Zarshenas Z, Sparschu RA. Catheter placement and misplacement. Crit Care Clin. 1994;10:417-36.
41. Trotman-Dickenson B. Radiology in the intensive care unit (part I). J Intensive Care Med. 2003;18:198-210.
42. Trotman-Dickenson B. Radiology in the intensive care unit (part 2). J Intensive Care Med. 2003;18:239-52.
43. Henschke CI, Yankelevitz DF, Wand A, et al. Chest radiography in the ICU. Clin Imaging. 1997;21:90-103.
44. Brant WE, Helms CA. Fundamentals of diagnostic radiology. Lippincott Williams & Wilkins; 2007.
45. Smevik B. Radiological Imaging of the Neonatal Chest. Springer; 2008.

13

Ambulatory Arrhythmia Monitoring Devices

Niti Chadha

IMPLANTABLE LOOP RECORDERS

Ambulatory arrhythmia monitoring is cardiac rhythm monitoring in an individual with no restriction of activities for the period for which monitoring is done. With the availability of newer monitoring devices, gone are the days when arrhythmia monitoring in an ambulatory individual was restricted to a 24-hour Holter monitor attached to the patient by a not so convenient belt/strap. Inconvenience aside, these Holter monitors had an ability of diagnostic catch only for very frequent rhythm disturbances. Infrequently occurring arrhythmias easily evaded such monitors keeping the diagnostic dilemma ongoing for the treating doctor concerned. With the current accessibility of a multitude of arrhythmia monitors, the field of arrhythmia monitoring is now facing a new era where the electrophysiologists can track each beat of their patient in real time and filter the wealth of information for the best interests of patients.

To better appreciate the differences in various newer modalities of ambulatory arrhythmia monitoring devices, we start our discussion with the good old Holter monitor.

HOLTER MONITOR

Named after physicist Norman J. Holter, telemetric cardiac monitoring marked its debut in 1949. However, clinical use of Holter began only in 1960 and since then has served the purpose of rhythm monitoring. A Holter monitor is a portable device for cardiac rhythm monitoring for a period of 24–72 hours, less often for 2 weeks. The monitor records electrical signals from the heart via a series of electrodes attached to the chest. The number and position of the electrodes vary by the model, but most Holter monitors use 3–8 electrodes. These electrodes are attached to a recording cassette that records the electrical data. After collecting the data, the digitized ECG signal is downloaded onto a computer and automatically processed using advanced data processing software. Holter monitors automatically recognize PQRST complex morphology and the system generates a single page report with details of normal and abnormal beats. These data are reviewed by trained personnel's before a final report is given to the patient. Most of the Holter monitors use the ECGs in two or three channels; however, 12-channel Holter monitors have been introduced that help in morphological analysis of arrhythmias (Fig. 13.1).

Advantages

Holter monitors have already made a place in the hearts of the cardiologists and electrophysiologists. This noninvasive and a relatively inexpensive rhythm monitoring technique has an easy availability. Fifty years of its use in clinical diagnostics has made the specialists well aware of its use and nuances. It gives fair information of a rhythm disturbance that is likely to recur in less than a week frequency.

Limitations

The attachment of sticky electrodes to the chest may act as irritant and cutaneous allergies to a few patients, though hypoallergenic electrodes are now available. The monitor itself is strapped to the body by a belt or hung around the neck that may be uncomfortable to the wearer. The recorded data may be affected by body motion and muscle activity and artifactual disturbances may occur.

EVENT MONITORS

Event monitors are of two main types: Continuous looping monitors and postevent recorders. The advantages and limitations of the event monitors are discussed here.

Advantages

The biggest advantage of these recorders is that they are comfortable for use to the patient. These devices provide

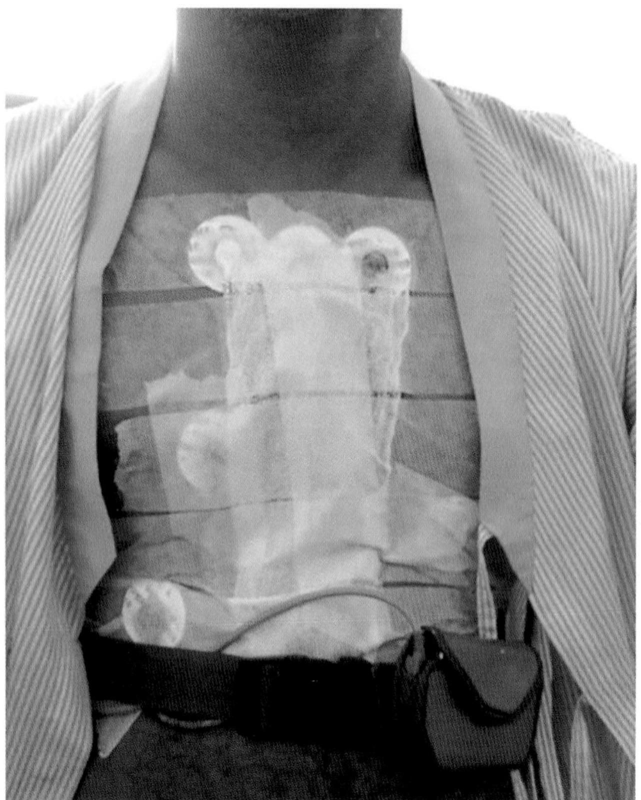

Fig. 13.1 Image showing a Holter monitor attached to the chest wall via electrodes

for monitoring up to 30 days and can be used for extended period of time also.

Limitations

The event monitors are not meant to capture the pre-event data, which is hence missed, leading to loss of valuable information. Another limitation is the inability to capture asymptomatic events as most event monitors require patients to activate the device to be able to store data. Patient compliance is also an issue. Patients need to carry the device with them at all times and need to be able to activate it. Some level of technical skill is required by the patient to be able to transmit the recordings through a telephone landline. It records only a single lead ECG strip and there is no trending data available like heart especially in patients with atrial fibrillation (AF).

Continuous Looping Monitors

Noninvasive continuous looping monitors, also referred to as external loop recorders (ELRs) are recorders that are attached to the chest wall and continuously monitor the cardiac rhythm. However, the total memory storage capacity of these devices is short, and hence, the entire data that is being recorded is not saved. A continuous process of recording and deleting the rhythm data goes on in these recorders. These need to be continuously worn, i.e. attached to the body by means of electrodes or patches and have a limited memory capacity of up to 6 minutes of recording. The device stops the process of erasing the rhythm data once it is activated.

Both patient-activated and auto-triggered recorders are available. The patient-activated device needs to be activated by the patient when he/she feels the symptoms. Auto-triggered monitors can be programmed to detect rhythm disturbances, bradyarrhythmias and tachyarrhythmias, and get activated on their own. Following the device activation, the data is stored that can then be transmitted to a central monitoring station where it is analyzed.

Advantages

Longer term monitoring is possible with these recorders. Up to 14–30-day recorders are now available. Initial loop recorders had to be attached through electrodes that were slightly cumbersome. Recent introduction of patch-type recorders is easier to use and provide good-quality recordings. Patients can carry about all their daily routine activities while wearing these recorders (Figs 13.2A to C).

Limitations

Recorders that need to be attached through electrodes reduce patient compliance that in turn leads to missing of useful information. This limitation is overcome by availability of patch-type monitors. A second limitation is the need for patient involvement in patient-activated type recorders limiting their role in evaluation of syncopal episodes for obvious reasons. A third limitation is a requirement of some technical sophistication to be able to transmit the data to the receiving station.

Post-event Recorders

These devices are not required to be worn continuously by the patient and are applied to the chest wall only when patient feels symptoms. Hence, such a recorder does not record data continuously (nonlooping) unlike loop recorders where continuous data recording goes on. No pre-event data is recorded in these monitors (Figs 13.3A to C).

Advantages

A significant advantage is that patients are not required to wear these recorders continuously. They need to be applied

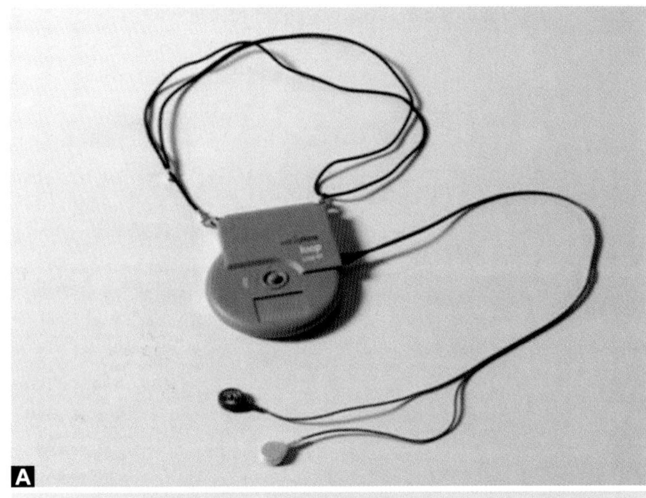

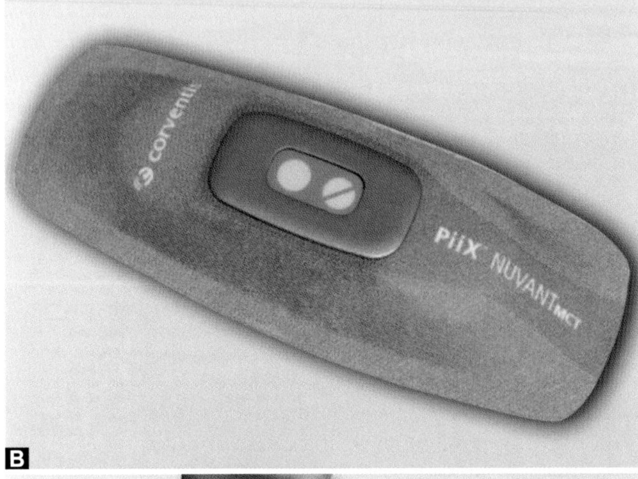

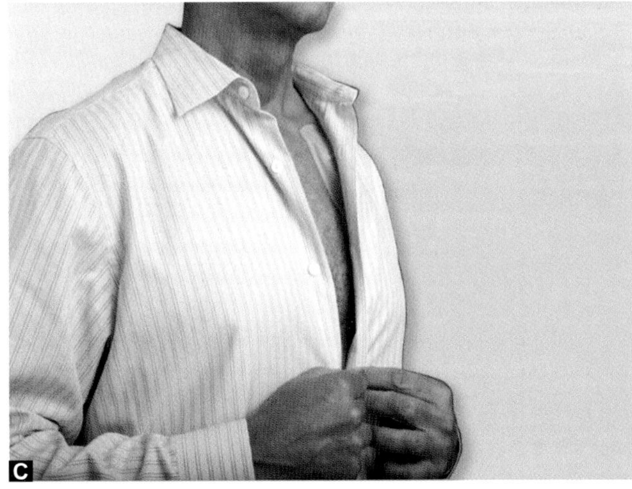

Figs 13.2A to C (A) External loop recorder; (B) Patch-type external loop recorder; (C) Loop recorder in functional state

to the chest wall only when symptoms develop. These are handy devices available with patients that can help detect symptomatic arrhythmias.

Limitations

The memory space for these recorders is short. Normally, the nonlooping memory systems have up to 6 minutes of memory storage space. Hence, after one to three episodes, the data needs to be transmitted to the central station to make space for further storage. Asymptomatic arrhythmias cannot be monitored with these devices. Moreover, significant data is missed following an event before the patient applies the device to the chest wall. Some amount of technical sophistication is required for the patient/family members to transmit a recording to the central monitoring station.

Implantable Loop Recorders

Implantable loop recorders (ILRs) are a relatively recent introduction to the armamentarium of cardiac rhythm specialists. These devices need to be implanted subcutaneously in the parasternal pocket and provide monitoring duration of up to 3 years. They have a loop memory space of recording up to 45 minutes of ECG storage. These ILRs have found place in rhythm monitoring especially in cases of infrequent syncopal episodes diagnosis of AF, pre- and postablation.

Advantages

The implantable loop memory recorders have overcome the limitations of the event recorders. They allow pre-event data to be captured and store it from the internal looping memory. The availability of pre-event, event, and post-event data helps guide the therapy decisions in a better way than the simple event monitors for obvious reasons. Long-term monitoring duration also helps in improving the diagnostic yield for detection of arrhythmias.

Limitations

ILRs need to be implanted in the body and this requires some surgical expertise for the implanter and some inconvenience to the patience at the time of implant. However, the diagnostic yield of these devices is high, and hence, the initial inconvenience may easily be overlooked.

Continuous Real-time Monitors

They are worn continuously and are similar in size to the standard ELR. Three electrodes are attached to battery-powered sensor that is held by the patient. They automatically record and transmit arrhythmic event data to an attended monitoring station (Fig. 13.4). Stored data are either directly transmitted to central station via cell phone network coverage or wirelessly to a portable monitor that has a built-in cell

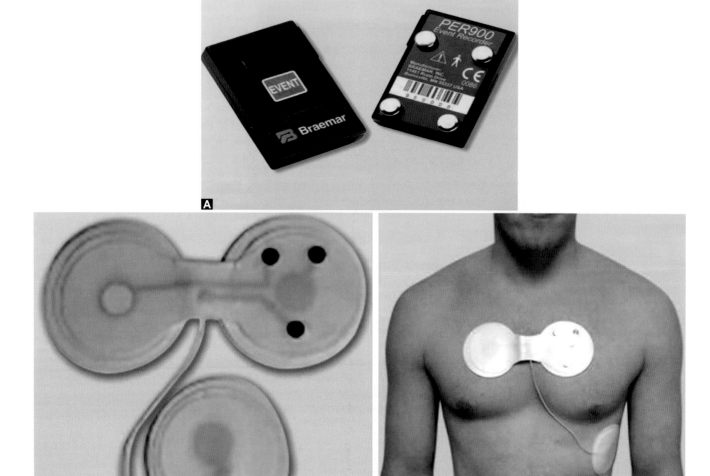

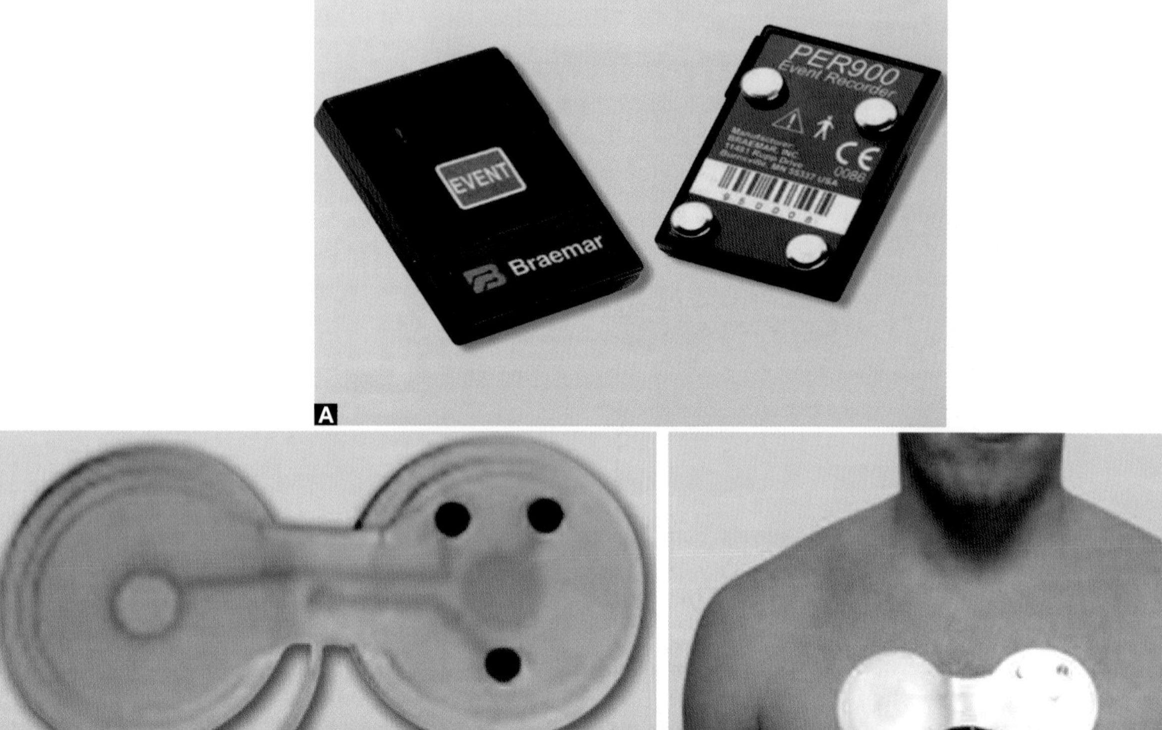

Figs 13.3A to C (A) Post-event recorder; (B) Patch-type event monitor; (C) Device is in functional state

phone; data is immediately analyzed by trained technicians who can contact the patient and/or the physician if an urgent intervention is needed. Hence, with these monitors 24*7 vigilance can be obtained on the cardiac rhythm of the patients (Fig. 13.3D).

Advantages

With these devices, continuous real-time ECG monitoring is available. Extended period of monitoring (up to 30 days) can be done. There is no need for patient activation or transmission of data. Real-time monitoring of data is done by technical experts at the monitoring station and alerts can be issued to the patient/family.

Remote Monitoring through Pacemakers and ICDs

Pacemakers and implantable cardioverter defibrillators (ICDs) can also be used for rhythm analysis. Newer technology allows Internet-based remote monitoring of arrhythmias and device therapies that are programmable in the devices. The physician can set parameters and alerts wherein he receives data and alerts if a certain parameter is violated.

Event Interpretation Summary of V Patch Device

Name of the Patient: Ramesh kumar
Name of the Ref Physician: Rajnish Jain
Hospital: Gangaram Hospital

AGE: 68
Sex: M

Monitoring Start date: 18/02/2013 Time
Monitoring end date: 25/02/2013 Time
Total Usage days: 8

Event Summary

Total event detected: 98
No. of automatic triggered event: 82
No. of patient triggered event: 16
No. of reportable significant event: 28

Report Impression by Technician

1. The patient has 1st degree AV block with pause (1.40 sec), PABs and PVCs
2. The patient heart rate ranges between 40 to 110 bpm during the monitoring periord
3. The reportable events as follows:
   a. Ist degree AV block with pasuse (1.40 sec) and PVCs
   b. Ist degree AV block with PABs

RAMESH KUMAR

Start Date: 18/02/2013
End Date: 25/02/2013

File ID	Device	Machine Interpretation	Date	Time	Analyst Interpretation	HR Min 8 pm	HR Max 8 pm	Reportable
254390	103188	Possible atrial fibrillation	2/18/2013	3:40	Ist degree AV block	80	90	NO
254424	103188	Possible atrial fibrillation	2/18/2013	6:14	Ist degree AV block with PVCs	80	90	NO
254432	103188	Possible atrial fibrillation	2/18/2013	9:05	Ist degree AV block with PVCs	90	100	NO
254440	103188	Possible atrial fibrillation	2/18/2013	9:48	Ist degree AV block	90	100	NO
254449	103188	Possible atrial fibrillation	2/18/2013	10:24	Ist degree AV block	90	100	NO
254489	103188	Possible atrial fibrillation	2/18/2013	11:13	Ist degree AV block with PVCs	90	100	NO
254490	103188	Possible atrial fibrillation	2/18/2013	12:07	Ist degree AV block with PVCs	80	90	NO
254507	103188	Possible atrial fibrillation	2/18/2013	14:37	Ist degree AV block with PVCs	70	80	NO
254513	103188	Possible atrial fibrillation	2/18/2013	15:44	Ist degree AV block	90	110	NO
254515	103188	Possible atrial fibrillation	2/18/2013	15:46	Ist degree AV block with pause (1,40 sec) and PVCs	80	100	NO
254566	103188	Possible atrial fibrillation	2/18/2013	17:59	Ist degree AV block with PABs	90	100	NO
254592	103188	Possible atrial fibrillation	2/18/2013	19:11	Ist degree AV block with PVCs	100	110	NO
254603	103188	Possible atrial fibrillation	2/18/2013	19:26	Ist degree AV block	100	110	NO
254506	103188	Possible atrial fibrillation	2/18/2013	19:31	Ist degree AV block	100	110	NO
254529	103188	Possible atrial fibrillation	2/18/2013	20:20	Ist degree AV block with PVCs	100	110	NO
254666	103188	Possible atrial fibrillation	2/18/2013	21:58	Ist degree AV block with PVCs	100	110	NO
254671	103188	Possible atrial fibrillation	2/18/2013	22:09	Ist degree AV block with PVCs	100	110	NO
254672	103188	Possible atrial fibrillation	2/18/2013	22:11	Ist degree AV block	100	110	NO
254673	103188	Possible atrial fibrillation	2/18/2013	22:14	Ist degree AV block	100	110	NO

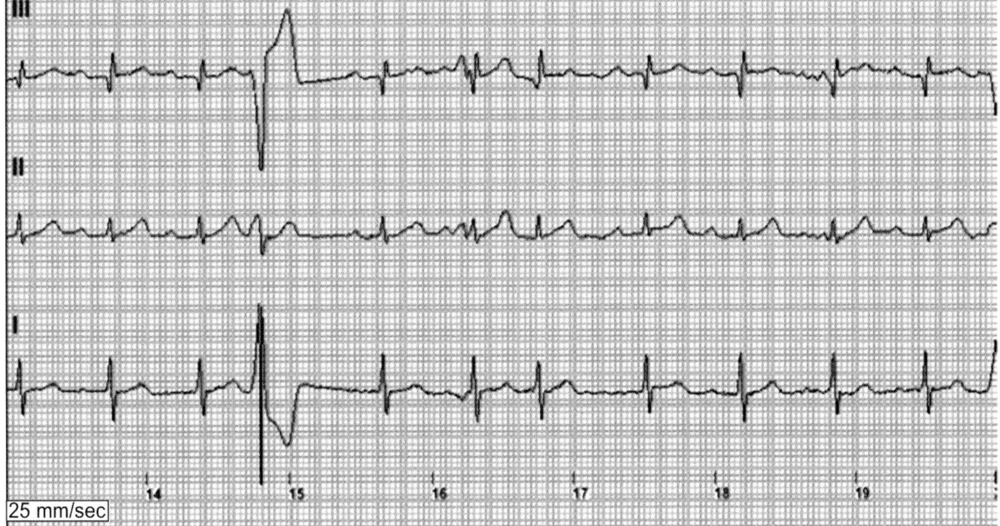

Fig. 13.3D Event interpretation summary for an event monitor

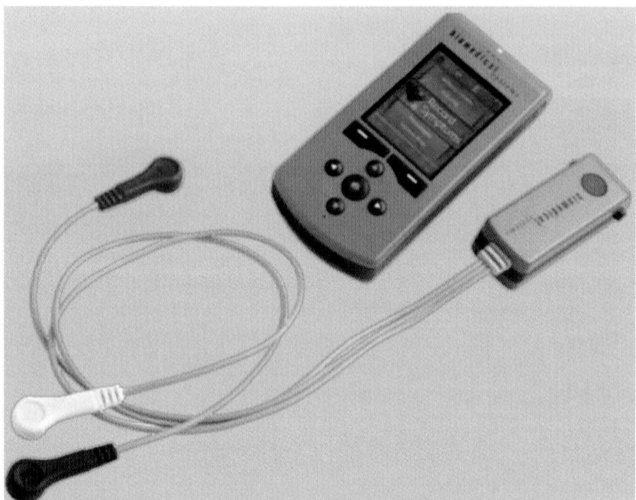

Fig. 13.4 Continuous real-time telemetry monitor

WHO ARE THE CANDIDATES FOR WHICH DEVICE?

With the availability of a multitude of these devices, the decision lies with the physicians to select an appropriate device for their patient. Not all the available devices are useful in all patients. Hence, choosing the right device is mandatory to increase the diagnostic yield of the symptom being evaluated. The main purposes for which these devices are utilized are evaluation of palpitation and syncope.

Three important criteria for selecting a device to evaluate symptoms of palpitations are as follows:

1. Technical ability of the patient/family to transmit the data
2. Length of an episode
3. Frequency of an episode.

Evaluation of Palpitations

- Patient able to activate a monitor and transmit the data
  - Episodes long enough to activate the monitor reliably
    - Post-event recorder
    - ELRs
  - Episodes not long enough to activate the monitor
    - ELRs
    - Real-time continuous telemetry device
- Patient not able to activate the monitor/transmit the data
  - Episodes occur daily
    - Holter monitor
  - Episodes do not occur daily
    - Real-time continuous telemetry device.

Evaluation of Syncope

- Symptom occurs at least once a month
  - Real-time continuous telemetry device
- Symptom recurrence in more than a month
  - ILR.

The decision regarding implant of one of these devices is taken based on symptom frequency. Frequently occurring symptoms can be monitored by Holter or an event monitor. Symptom recurrence in more than a week but less than month may be monitored by an event monitor or ELR. For infrequent symptoms, ILRs may be used (Flow charts 13.1 to 13.3).

STUDIES COMPARING THE DIAGNOSTIC YIELDS OF VARIOUS MONITORING DEVICES

In the evaluation of palpitations, studies directly comparing Holter monitor with 48-hour recording with a loop recorder with longer duration monitoring, the diagnostic yield of a loop recorder was up to 83% compared to 39% for Holter.[1,2] In another study of patients with infrequent palpitations (<1 episode per month lasting >1 minute), in the absence of severe heart disease, ILRs provided a diagnostic yield of 73% compared to 21% in the group evaluated with standard conventional therapy (24-hour Holter, EP study, ELRs).[3]

For patients with syncope, the diagnostic yield of external ambulatory monitors, especially those requiring patient initiated activation, is extremely limited. ELRs have been directly compared to Holter monitors in several small trials. The diagnostic yield has been between 56% for loop recorders worn for 1 month versus 22% for 48-hour Holters[4]. ILRs allow a prolonged period of monitoring and have been shown to increase the diagnostic yield for syncope to up to 85% in some studies.[5,6]

Monitoring devices for asymptomatic recurrences of AF have become a common indication for rhythm monitoring devices. These include event recorders with AF triggers, continuous telemetry devices, 2-week Holters, or ILRs with automatic triggers. A study comparing mobile telemetry devices with ELRs showed asymptomatic AF was detected in 17.3% of mobile telemetry devices versus 8.7% with ELRs when monitored up to 30 days.[7] Implanted devices (pacemakers, ICDs, ILRs) are useful for monitoring AF recurrences. A device detected AF duration of >24 hours is associated with a threefold increase in stroke risk and an AF duration of <5 hours may not carry an excess stroke risk (Fig. 13.5).[8]

Flow chart 13.1 Selection criteria for monitoring devices for evaluation of symptoms of palpitations

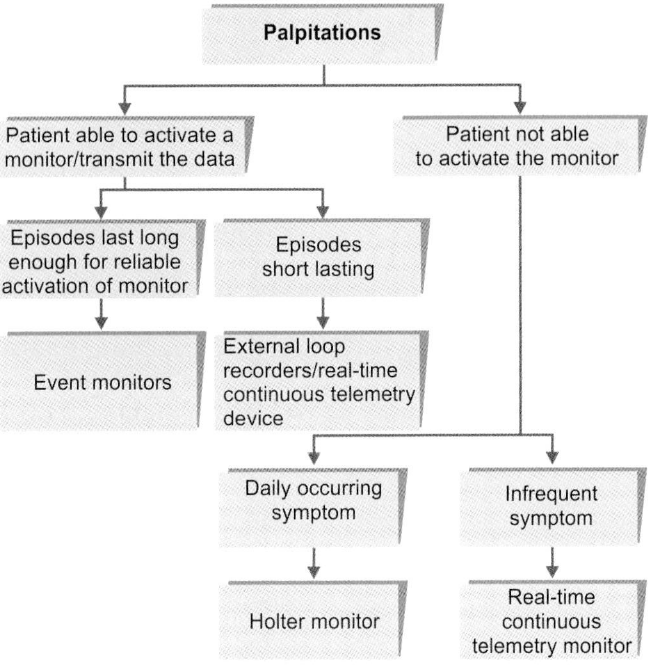

Flow chart 13.2 Selection criteria for recommending monitoring devices for the evaluation of symptoms of syncope

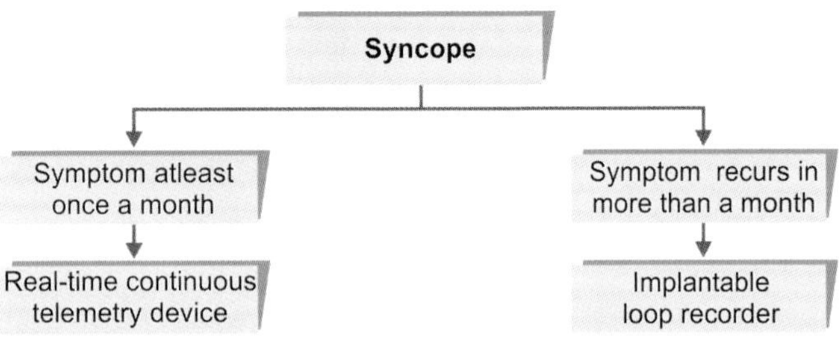

Flow chart 13.3 Selection criteria for the evaluation of asymptomatic arrhythmias

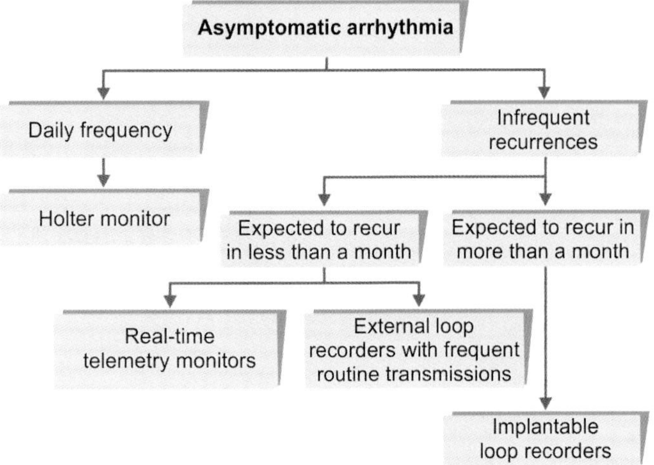

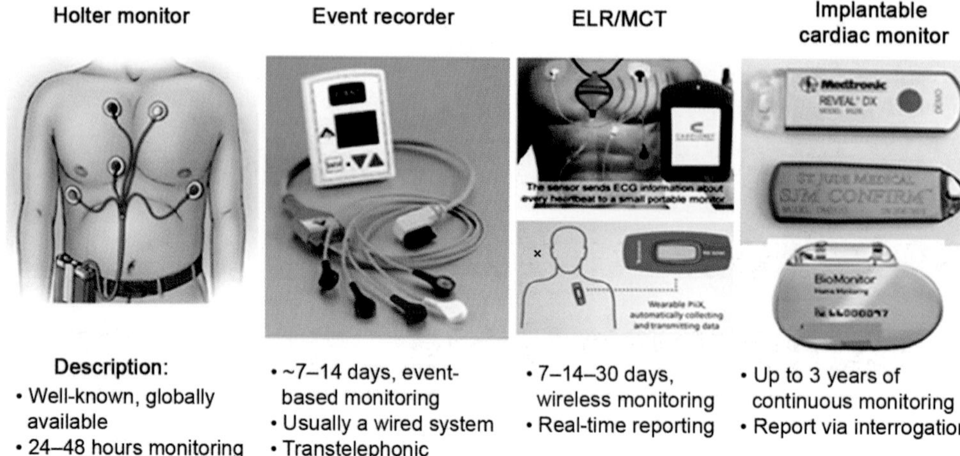

Fig. 13.5 Image showing a comparison of available cardiac rhythm monitoring devices

CONCLUSION

Ambulatory arrhythmia monitoring is a field that is rapidly crossing the traditional boundaries. The availability of a variety of newer monitoring devices is helping in diagnosing arrhythmias that would have evaded detection with the previous conventional monitors resulting in significant clinical benefits to our patients.

REFERENCES

1. Zimetbaum PJ, Kim KY, Josephson ME, et al. Diagnostic yield and optimal duration of continuous-loop event monitoring for the diagnosis of palpitations. Ann Intern Med. 1998;128:890-5.
2. Kinlay S, Leitch JW, Neil A, et al. Cardiac event recorders yield more diagnoses and are more cost-effective than 48-hour Holter monitoring in patients with palpitations. Ann Intern Med. 1996;124:16-20.
3. Giada F, Gulizia M, Francese M, et al. Recurrent unexplained palpitations (RUP) study: comparison of implantable loop recorder versus conventional diagnostic strategy. J Am Coll Cardiol. 2007;49:1951-6.
4. Sivakumaran S, Krahn AD, Klein GJ, et al. A prospective randomized comparison of loop recorders versus Holter monitors in patients with syncope or presyncope. Am J Med. 2003;115:1-5.
5. Krahn AD, Klein GJ, Skanes AC, Yee R. Use of implantable loop recorder in evaluation of patients with unexplained syncope. J Cardiovasc Electrophysiol. 2003;14(Suppl):S70-S3.
6. Krahn AD, Klein GJ, Norris C, et al. The etiology of syncope in patients with negative tile table and electrophysiological testing. Circulation. 1995;92:1819-24.
7. Rothman SA, Laughlin JC, Seltzer J, et al. The diagnosis of cardiac arrhythmias: a prospective multi-center randomized study comparing mobile cardiac outpatient telemetry versus standard loop event monitoring. J Cardiovasc Electrophysiol. 2007;18: 241-7.
8. Glotzer T, Daoud E, Wyse G, et al. The relationship between daily atrial tachyarrhythmia burden from implantable device diagnostics and stroke risk. Circ Arrhythmia Electrophysiol. 2009;2:474-80.

14

Exercise Stress Testing (Stress Echocardiography): Where does it Stand with Other Modalities?

Neel Bhatia, Sameer Shrivastava

OVERVIEW

The goal of cardiac testing is to help stratify patients thought to be at risk of symptomatic coronary artery disease (CAD), specifically for short-term complications such as myocardial infarction or sudden cardiac death. The tests reviewed include exercise stress testing, pharmacologic stress testing, myocardial perfusion imaging, stress echocardiography, and cardiac computed tomography (CCT), magnetic resonance imaging (MRI), and positron emission tomography (PET) scanning. These noninvasive tests can be performed in an outpatient setting, in a physician's office, in a hospital, or in an observation unit, as well as for admitted patients. An understanding of these tests is important.

Exercise stress echocardiography is the combination of echocardiography with physical exercise (i.e. is in form of treadmill or supine bicycle test). The diagnostic end point for the detection of myocardial ischemia is the induction of a transient worsening in regional function during stress.

Stress echocardiography requires a comparison of echocardiographic data obtained at the time of or after stress with baseline resting data, and it is essential to review resting and stress images side by side using digital acquisition and display.[1,2] Stress echocardiography also requires a great deal of patient cooperation as wall motion is transient, and imaging must be completed within 60–90 seconds before it begins to resolve. A positive stress echocardiogram is defined by stress-induced decrease in regional wall motion, decreased wall thickening, or regional compensatory hyperkinesias. In experienced hands, this can have a diagnostic accuracy similar to that of nuclear stress testing. However, results are operator dependent.

Bicycle and treadmill stress echocardiography are the two most common forms of exercise echocardiography. Supine and upright bicycle protocols have been used with similar results. However, bicycle stress may lead to submaximal stress. Most labs now use treadmill exercise because of the familiarity with treadmill protocols and the degree of stress that it produces. It should be remembered, however, that with treadmill stress echocardiography, unlike bicycle stress echocardiography, the images first acquired are immediate "post" exercise, rather than "peak" exercise.

INDICATIONS OF STRESS ECHOCARDIOGRAPHY

- Diagnosis of CAD
- Prognosis in patients with established diagnosis of CAD
- For preoperative assessment of CAD
- Follow-up after revascularization
- To locate site of ischemia
- Evaluation of severity of valvular stenosis
- Patients in whom the exercise treadmill test was nondiagnostic or yielded ambiguous results
- Left bundle branch block or significant resting electrocardiography (ECG) changes that makes any ECG interpretation during stress difficult
- Submaximal treadmill ECG
- Cardiac treadmill testing in women—They are more likely to have nonobstructive or single-vessel disease when compared to men. Treadmill testing in one study was shown to have a sensitivity and specificity of 61% and 70%, respectively, for women compared with higher sensitivity of 72% and 77%, respectively, for men. Exercise tolerance test is recommended by American Heart Association as still the initial test of choice for a low-risk or intermediate-risk symptomatic woman in whom there are no contraindications.[3]

ADVANTAGES

- It has shorter imaging time, immediate availability of the results, and lower cost.
- It has no associated radiation exposure.
- The test can be more readily performed in an office setting.
- No biohazards for the patient and the physician.
- It provides comparison in pulmonary pressure, valvular regurgitation, or filling pressures before and after a stress to identify pathological condition not evident at rest. It also provides information about chamber sizes and function, valves, pericardial effusion, aortic root disease, and wall thicknesses.
- In a meta-analysis that included data from 24 studies, Fleischmann et al. found that exercise echocardiography had a sensitivity of 85% and a specificity of 77% when compared with coronary angiography. The results were felt to be similar to those for SPECT imaging.[4]

DRAWBACKS OF EXERCISE STRESS ECHOCARDIOGRAPHY

Factors such as hyperventilation, obesity, lung disease, tachycardia, hypercontraction of normal walls, and excessive chest wall movement render the ultrasonic examination difficult during exercise. All these factors degrade image quality and in stress echo worse image quality dramatically leads to higher interobserver variability and lower diagnostic accuracy. The test is dependent on the experience of the operator. Up to 10% of cases have inadequate image quality.

PHARMACOLOGIC STRESS TESTING

Pharmacological stress echocardiography is for those patients who cannot do exercise. It differs from exercise stress testing as the patient is not supposed to do exercise but medication is used to increase persons' heart rate and cardiac oxygen demand. The drugs used for pharmacologic stress testing are dipyridamole, adenosine, regadenoson, and dobutamine.

Pharmacologic agents are used to stress the myocardium and produce the characteristic ECG or nuclear imaging findings. Test interpretation—The test interpretation is similar to exercise echocardiography. Pharmacologic stress testing along with nuclear imaging has a value equivalent to an exercise stress test with nuclear imaging at detecting CAD. Patients who undergo pharmacologic stress testing have more comorbidities; so, they have higher post-test probability of disease. A person with a normal pharmacologic stress test result has a 1-2% per year cardiac event rate and a person with normal exercise test result with nuclear imaging has a cardiac event rate <1% per year.[5]

Theophylline and caffeine have been found to reduce ischemic changes on the ECG with vasodilator stress testing. Calcium channel blockers, beta-blockers, and nitrates ideally should be withheld for 24 hours prior to pharmacologic stress testing as they can alter perfusion defects on pharmacologic stress tests. In patients with severe airway reactive disease or who have wheeze, drugs such as dipyridamole and adenosine are generally avoided as they can lead to bronchospasm. Dobutamine has been found to be safe in these patients.

Patients who have been found to have positive stress echocardiography that is occurring at low workload, with slow recovery and those showing akinesis or dyskinesis of more than five segments of the left ventricle, should be subjected to coronary intervention in form of coronary angiography. The findings of exercise echocardiography should be used as "a gatekeeper" to subsequent coronary intervention. With documented ischemia on exercise echocardiography, the benefit of coronary recanalization is much more compared to those who do not have documented ischemia.

Contraindications to stress echocardiography include active asthma, high-grade heart block, hemodynamically significant left ventricular (LV) outflow tract obstruction, tachyarrhythmias (including prior history of ventricular tachycardia), uncontrolled hypertension (blood pressure >200/110 mm Hg), aortic dissection or large aortic aneurysm, and hypotension. Regadenoson is relatively safe in asthma.[6] Beta-blockers should be discontinued so that response to dobutamine will not be attenuated.

APPROPRIATE USE CRITERIA 2011

"An appropriate imaging study is one in which the expected incremental information, combined with clinical judgment, exceeds the expected negative consequences by a sufficiently wide margin for a specific indication that the procedure is generally considered acceptable care and a reasonable approach for the indication."[7] In 2011, the technical panel had scored each indication as follows for stress echocardiography (i.e. through exercise and pharmacological stress):

Score (7–9), i.e. "A" Appropriate

The test is appropriate for specific condition (i.e. test is acceptable).

Score (4–6), i.e. "U" Uncertain

The test is uncertain for specific condition. It means that more research and/or patient information is required to classify the indication definitive.

Score (1–3), i.e. "I" Inappropriate

The test is inappropriate for specific condition (i.e. test is not acceptable).

EXERCISE ECHOCARDIOGRAPHY IN VALVULAR HEART DISEASE

It has been used to quantify severity of mitral regurgitation in patient who has rheumatic mitral valve disease with mild mitral stenosis and mitral regurgitation at rest.[8] Exercise echocardiography also helps in knowing significant mitral regurgitation (dynamic) in patients with LV systolic dysfunction. It has been found in some of the patients that dynamic mitral regurgitation can account for acute pulmonary edema, which predicts poor outcome. Patients who had an increase in the effective regurgitant orifice or increase in the pulmonary artery systolic pressure at peak exercise had higher morbidity and mortality incidence.[9]

DIAGNOSTIC ACCURACY

In a large comparison study (112 patients), the overall sensitivity and specificity of exercise echocardiography were 85% and 88%, respectively, and that of exercise thallium was 81% and 85%, respectively (Tables 14.1 to 14.10).

Table 14.1 Stress echocardiography in symptomatic or who had an Ischemic event for detection of coronary artery disease[7]

Pretest probability of coronary artery disease	*Score*
To evaluate people who had an ischemic event (nonacute) with stress echocardiography	
• *Low:*	
– ECG—interpretable and able to exercise	I
—uninterpretable or unable to exercise	A
• *Intermediate:*	
– ECG—interpretable and able to exercise	A
—uninterpretable or unable to exercise	A
• *High:*	
– Regardless of ECG interpretability and ability to exercise	A
Acute chest pain with stress echocardiography	
Possible ACS	
ECG: No ischemic changes or with LBBB or electronically paced ventricular rhythm	
Negative troponin levels. Peak troponin: borderline, equivocal, minimally elevated	
• TIMI score—low risk	
—high risk	A
Definite ACS	I

Abbreviations: ECG, electrocardiogram; ACS, acute coronary syndrome. A, appropriate; I, inappropriate; U, uncertain.

Table 14.2 Stress echocardiography in patients with comorbidities for detection of coronary artery disease (CAD) and for assessment of risk[7]

Indication	*Score*
In persons with left ventricular systolic dysfunction that is recent onset and those who have not been evaluated for CAD and are not being planned for coronary angiography	A
In persons with history of arrhythmias:	
• Sustained ventricular tachycardia	A
• Frequent premature ventricular complexes, exercise-induced ventricular tachycardia, or nonsustained ventricular tachycardia	A
• Infrequent premature ventricular complexes	I
• New-onset atrial fibrillation	U
In people who had syncope with global CAD risk: Low	I
: Intermediate or high	A
• In asymptomatic and those who do not have evidence of acute coronary syndrome (ACS) leaving elevated levels of troponin	A

Abbreviations: A, appropriate; I, inappropriate; U, uncertain.

The likelihood of a cardiac event (cardiac death, nonfatal infarct, or coronary revascularization) after normal stress echocardiography is extremely low. Among 1325 with normal findings on exercise echocardiography at Mayo Clinic, the event rate during 3 years of follow-up was <3%. The cardiac event rate per person-years of follow-up was 0.9%.[10]

CONCLUSION

Thus, exercise stress echocardiography is not only useful for diagnosis of ischemic heart disease but also useful in other forms of heart disease. Since there is no exposure to radiation in this test, it becomes easier to perform repeated studies if required. Also the results of the tests are immediately available. One also comes to know the hemodynamics, i.e. if there is worsening of diastolic dysfunction, or if there is significant increase in regurgitation, these details are not available from any other noninvasive tests. And future belongs to real-time three-dimensional (3D) echocardiography as it has the advantage of acquiring even small areas of wall motion abnormalities in a relatively shorter duration of image acquisition time. Few studies have recently used 3D echocardiography to assess wall motion abnormalities with dobutamine stress with and without contrast.[11]

3D echocardiography is the future of stress echocardiography. Further technical advances will lead in its

Table 14.3 Stress echocardiography in investigated patients[7]

Indication	Score
In people who have evidence of subclinical disease and are asymptomatic	
• Level of calcium in coronaries	
Agatston score <100	I
Agatston score between 100 and 400	U
—Low to intermediate global coronary artery disease (CAD) risk	
—High global CAD risk	A
Agatston score >400	
• Increase in carotid intimal medial thickness (i.e. >0.9 mm and/or presence of plaque)	U
• In patients who have undergone angiography, but a decision could not be taken on the basis of angiography.	A
For the evaluation of individuals who are asymptomatic or who have stable symptoms or who have a history of normal stress imaging and who have been found to have low global CAD risk.	I
Individuals with positive stress echocardiography or abnormal coronary angiography in past with no coronary revascularization and who have been asymptomatic.	
• Stress echocardiography study done <2 years ago	I
Stress echocardiography study done ≥2 years ago	U
Stress echocardiography in new or worsening symptoms	
• Individuals with abnormal stress echocardiography or angiography in the past	A
• Individuals with normal stress echocardiography or angiography in the past	U

Abbreviations: A, appropriate; I, inappropriate; U, uncertain.

Table 14.4 Perioperative risk assessment with stress echocardiography for noncardiac surgery without active cardiac conditions[7]

Indication	
Evaluation with stress echocardiography in low-risk surgery	
• Perioperative assessment of cardiac risk	I
Evaluation with stress echocardiography in intermediate-risk surgery	
• Asymptomatic individuals who had a normal coronary angiography in the past year or who have been found to have moderate to good functional capacity (≥4 METs)	I
• No risk factors	
• Individuals with more than one clinical risk factor Or who have poor or unknown functional capacity (<4 METs)	U
Evaluation with stress echocardiography in prior to vascular surgery	
• Asymptomatic individuals who had a normal coronary angiography in the past year or who have been found to have moderate to good functional capacity (≥4 METs)	I
• No risk factors	
• Individuals with poor or unknown functional capacity (i.e. <4 METs)	A

Abbreviations: A, appropriate; I, inappropriate; U, uncertain.

Table 14.5 Stress echocardiography for risk assessment in <3 months of an acute coronary syndrome (ACS)[7]

In individuals who are hemodynamically stable and who do not have recurrent chest pain symptoms, or signs of heart failure and in whom coronary status has not been evaluated post the event to evaluate for inducible ischemia	
• STEMI with stress echocardiography	A
• UA/NSTEMI with stress echocardiography	A
Post revascularization (PCI or CABG) assessment of asymptomatic patients who had an ACS prior to revascularization with stress echocardiography	
Just before initiation of cardiac rehabilitation (as a stand-alone indication)	I

Abbreviations: A, appropriate; I, inappropriate; U, uncertain.

ultimate widespread use in routine clinical practice. Stress echocardiography also helps in knowing diastolic dysfunction and defining its severity that is pretest and at peak stress, i.e. normal diastolic function at rest and during peak stress; initial damage will have normal diastolic function at rest and abnormal diastolic function (diastolic dysfunction) during stress; advanced damage will have diastolic dysfunction at rest, and fixed abnormality at peak stress. In patients with most advanced stages of apparent diastolic dysfunction, stress echocardiography helps in unmasking fixed versus reversible patterns, patients who show reversible pattern have comparatively better prognosis. Similarly a fixed restrictive pattern of diastolic dysfunction is more dangerous than a reversible restrictive pattern that can be partially normalized by nitroprusside infusion.[12]

Exercise stress echocardiography has become a test of choice in the diagnosis and prognostication of CAD. The low cost of equipment and immediate availability of result and no exposure to radiation have made it investigation of choice. Newer techniques in stress echocardiography, i.e. myocardial contrast echocardiography for the assessment of myocardial perfusion, evaluation of myocardial mechanics using strain rate imaging, and 3D imaging great are being

Table 14.6 Risk assessment in post-revascularization (i.e. after angioplasty or bypass surgery)[7]

Indications	*Score*
• In symptomatic individuals (i.e. who have ischemia equivalent symptoms)	A
In asymptomatic individuals	
• When complete revascularization was not done	A
• If additional revascularization is required	
CABG that is <5 years old	I
CABG that is ≥5 years old	U
Angioplasty that is <2 years old	I
Angioplasty that is ≥2 years old	U
• In individuals before initiation of cardiac rehabilitation	I

Abbreviations: A, appropriate; I, inappropriate; U, uncertain.

Table 14.7 Stress echocardiography for the evaluation of hemodynamics in valvular heart disease[7]

Long-standing valvular heart disease patients who have been asymptomatic	*Score*
• Mitral stenosis—Moderate	U
—Severe	A
• Aortic stenosis—Moderate	U
—Severe	U
• Mitral regurgitation—Moderate	
—Severe	U
Left ventricular (LV) size and function not meeting surgical criteria	A
• Aortic regurgitation—Moderate	U
—Severe	
LV size and function not meeting surgical criteria	A
Chronic valvular disease—symptomatic with stress echocardiography	
• Moderate mitral stenosis	A
• Severe mitral stenosis	I
• Severe aortic stenosis	I
• Evaluation of equivocal aortic stenosis	
Evidence of low cardiac output or left ventricular (LV) systolic dysfunction	
("low gradient aortic stenosis") Use of dobutamine only	A
• Mild mitral regurgitation	U
• Moderate mitral regurgitation	A
• Severe mitral regurgitation	
Severe LV enlargement or LV systolic dysfunction	I

Abbreviations: A, appropriate; I, inappropriate; U, uncertain.

Table 14.8 Stress echocardiography in patients with pulmonary artery hypertension[7]

Indications	*Appropriate use score*
• Suspected pulmonary artery hypertension Normal or borderline elevated estimated right ventricular systolic pressure on resting echocardiographic study	U
• Routine evaluation of patients with known resting pulmonary hypertension	I
• Re-evaluation of patient with exercise-induced pulmonary hypertension to evaluate response to therapy	U

Abbreviations: A, appropriate; I, inappropriate; U, uncertain.

Table 14.9 Sensitivity of exercise echocardiography for single, double and triple vessel disease[10]

Vessel involvement	*Sensitivity*	
	Exercise thallium	*Exercise echocardiography*
Single	61%	58%
Double	86%	86%
Triple	94%	94%

evaluated and appear to show promise in the field of stress echocardiography. Stress echocardiography is indicated in patients who are admitted with chest pain in the emergency ward especially when ECG stress test is submaximal, not feasible, or nondiagnostic for risk stratification purpose.[13,14]

FUTURE

Real-Time Three-Dimensional Imaging

Matrix probes used for real-time 3D echocardiography offer the unique feature of recording all LV segments simultaneously, which may be advantageous for stress studies. Initial studies with 3D echocardiography during stress echocardiography have been encouraging.[15,16]

Comparison with Competing Techniques

Myocardial Perfusion Imaging

As per the American College of Radiology guidelines for imaging, rest SPECT has been stated to be "test of choice" in patients with active chest pain, troponin negative, and

Table 14.10 Accuracy of exercise echocardiography for the detection of coronary artery disease

	Year	n	Type of exercise	Sensitivity (%)	Specificity (%)	Accuracy (%)
Marwick et al.[17]	1992	150	TME	84	86	85
Hecht et al.[18]	1993	180	SBE	93	86	91
Beleslin et al.[19]	1994	136	TME	88	82	88
Luotolahti et al.[20]	1996	118	UBE	94	70	92
Roger et al.[21]	1997	340	TME	78	41	69

Abbreviations: n, number of patients; SBE, supine bicycle exercise; TME, treadmill exercise; UBE, upright bicycle exercise.

an ECG with no ischemic changes; the absence of perfusion defect in such cases is associated with a very high negative predictive value for acute coronary syndrome. However, rest SPECT sensitivity compared to stress SPECT if the imaging is performed after the chest pain has subsided. If there is increase in size of perfusion defect or appearance of perfusion defect during stress, than it helps in diagnosing stress-induced ischemia.[22]

Stress echocardiography has been found to have higher specificity, convenience, and lower cost in comparison to nuclear imaging.[23] While stress perfusion imaging has been found to have a higher sensitivity (especially for single-vessel disease involving the left circumflex coronary artery), better accuracy when there is multiple resting LV wall motion abnormalities are present, and a more larger database for the evaluation of prognosis in comparison to stress echocardiography.[23,24] The effective dose of a single nuclear cardiology stress imaging scan ranges from 10 mSv to 27 mSv. When compared to chest X-rays, the radiation exposure dose equivalent to 500 chest X-rays (sestamibi), 1200 chest X-rays (Thallium), and 1300 chest X-rays (dual isotope protocol). According to BEIR VII estimates risk of cancer for a middle-aged patient ranges from 1 in 1000 (for a sestamibi) to 1 in 400 (for a dual isotope scan). But there is no radiation exposure in stress echocardiography, so, considering the risk-benefit ratio, stress echo was found to have more advantages when compared with nuclear imaging as far as radiation exposure is concerned.[25]

Soman et al. had studied on 473 patients with chest pain, of which two thirds had positive ST segment response to exercise. It was found that patients with normal technetium-99 sestamibi SPECT study results were associated with an annual mortality rate of 0.2%.[26] In 18 studies involving 1304 patients who were subjected to exercise or pharmacologic stress echocardiography along with thallium or technetium-labeled radioisotope imaging and results showed that stress echocardiography had 80% sensitivity and 86% specificity and corresponding values were 84% sensitivity and 77% specificity for myocardial perfusion imaging, respectively (Table 14.11).[10] The sensitivity and specificity of tests are reduced in present due to availability of coronary angiography as today the patients with negative result or normal response in noninvasive examinations are being subjected to coronary angiography.[27]

As per the findings, exercise stress echocardiography has an advantage in terms of sensitivity and specificity in comparison to treadmill test and exercise thallium scan.

CARDIAC COMPUTED TOMOGRAPHY

It can measure the density and extent of calcifications in coronary artery walls. No contrast is used. The coronary lumen itself is not visualized. A low and regular heart rate (typically sinus rhythm) is necessary for optimal imaging. Studies have shown that if a patient's heart rate can be brought below 60 beats/min, only about 3% of coronary segments will be unevaluable by the cardiac computed tomography (CCT), while at 61–65 beats/min, over 21% are unevaluable. Obtaining optimal images with the least radiation exposure depends on control of the heart rate.[28]

Interpretation

Test result is interpreted as positive or negative within the coronary arteries. Positive test is 100% specific for atheromatous coronary plaque but not help in quantifying the disease.[29] People with a negative test result has a 96–100% negative predictive value for obstructive lesions. Agatston scores have been used to categorize individuals, i.e. one with a score of <10 has minimal amount of calcification, one with score of 11–99 has moderate amount of calcification, one with score of 100–400 increased amount of calcification, and those who have score above 400 have extensive amounts of calcification.

Table 14.11 Comparison of stress echocardiography with treadmill and thallium scan

Type of test	Sensitivity	Specificity
Treadmill test	77%	56%
Exercise stress echo	85%	88%
Exercise thallium scan	81%	85%

There was increased occurrence of coronary revascularization procedures, i.e. bypass, stenting, angioplasty, and acute coronary events, i.e. myocardial infarction, cardiac death in individuals with Agatston scores >400 in a duration of 2–5 years after the test. Individuals had been found to have 20% chance of myocardial infarction or cardiac death within a year if their Agatston scores were very high (>1000). Overall risk can be assessed with calcium scores, but diagnosis of obstructing lesion cannot be assessed with calcium scores.[30]

Test utility: Thus, use in low-risk patients is the most important application of CCT. A negative predictive value of 98% has been reported for coronary chest pain or myocardial infarction in patients with acute symptoms and nonspecific ECG results.[31] CCT does not help in knowing about unstable plaque, but it will tell about presence of calcification and calcification is present more often than significant stenosis. And patients those who have coronary calcification and who undergo coronary angiography based on those findings have been found to have non-significant CAD.

CARDIAC CT ANGIOGRAPHY

Cardiac CT Angiography (CCTA) has been found to have good negative predictive value in comparison to conventional angiography and a normal study rules out significant coronary stenosis was considered negative if stenosis was found to be <50% in the coronaries and the calcium score was <100. Individuals with a negative result were discharged. On follow-up of the 407 individuals who were discharged, 402 had 30-day follow-up. Those with a negative result when they were reviewed after 30 days, none of them had died from a cardiovascular cause or had required a revascularization, or had an acute coronary event. The conclusion was that low-risk chest pain patients with a negative CCTA result can be discharge safely.[32]

However, it appears that enough evidence exists to allow safe discharge of patients without acute ECG changes, elevated markers, and benign CCTA examinations. Of course, this assumes other serious causes of chest pain have been considered and excluded as needed. Most of the studies can be interpreted as negative or positive, but sometimes it becomes difficult to read the test as in cases of suboptimal visualization; in these situations the experience of cardiologist is required for correct interpretation of the test. There is interobserver variability that is commonly encountered in medicine, and in cardiology it can be substantial with almost all diagnostic methods that include electrocardiography (rest and exercise), perfusion scintigraphy, and even conventional coronary angiography.

FUTURE DIRECTIONS IN NONINVASIVE TESTING

Magnetic Resonance Angiography and Cardiac Magnetic Resonance

Cardiac magnetic resonance (CMR) is one of the newest technique in the field of cardiac imaging.[33] The biggest advantage of this technique is that there is no radiation, but the test is costly and there is lower availability when compared to stress echocardiography. It has been found to have great value in spite of the costs, acquisition time, and low availability when stress echocardiography is not feasible or inconclusive.[34]

Cardiac magnetic resonance angiography (MRA) helps to assess coronary arteries by visualization of coronaries, without radiation or contrast dye. It can be used to assess myocardial viability by using contrast and with addition of vasodilators or dobutamine. By using new protocols, the patient is not required to hold his breathe during the test. Cardiac MRI/MRA continues to evolve; it has a great future as it can combine angiography with perfusion and wall motion assessments.

Combined Computed Tomography (CT) Studies for Chest Pain Evaluation: The "Triple Rule Out"

Computed tomography scan with contrast can do combine imaging of the coronary arteries, ascending aorta, and pulmonary arteries, that help to assess CAD, pulmonary embolism, and disease of the thoracic aorta (dissection) with a single study. But this technique is not cost-effective and involves radiation exposure. Since it is a single test that evaluates the coronaries, ascending aorta, and pulmonary arteries, it has been called the "triple rule out (TRO)." A review of the topic suggests that this approach may have utility under relatively limited circumstances.[35] In current practice, this type of imaging exposes patients to significant radiation but shows promise in appropriately selected patients.

Cardiac PET Scanning

There are two specific clinical applications of PET that have been proposed for the evaluation of patients with known or suspected CAD. Detection of CAD and estimation of severity are performed using a PET perfusion agent at rest and during pharmacologic vasodilation. The second clinical application of PET is the assessment of myocardial viability in patients with CAD and LV dysfunction.

The combined technique of PET/CT of the coronary arteries was shown in one study to compare favorably with the criterion standard of catheter coronary angiography. All patients underwent PET/CT, and the results were compared with that of invasive coronary angiography. It was found that CT angiography alone was not sufficient in assessing the severity of stenosis, and perfusion imaging alone could not always separate microvascular disease from epicardial stenosis, but diagnostic accuracy improved to 98% with hybrid PET/CT.[36]

SUMMARY

Risk stratification of patients with possible acute coronary syndrome can be done with noninvasive cardiac testing. There are advantages and disadvantages of the tests that exist. Selection of test is dependent on patient characteristics and resources available. There is variability in how noninvasive cardiac tests correlate with angiography, but still short-term risk of myocardial infarction and death can be determined. New diagnostic methods and technologies are being developed in field of noninvasive cardiology, so that treating physicians can assess patients risk of CAD in a better way and recommend further testing and interventions.

Stress echocardiography is cost-effective and has absence of environmental impact and biological effects for the patient and operator both[25] when compared to other imaging modalities.[37] The amount of radiation in cardiac CT angiography was found to be equivalent to 600 X-rays.[38] That is why even though that exercise stress echocardiography is dependent on operator's skills and training like any other tests, it still is the most cost-effective and risk-effective possible imaging choice for noninvasive diagnosis and prognostication of CAD. At present no single test has been found ideal; each test has been found to have advantages and disadvantages, and if a single test is used for detection of CAD, than one can miss some serious cases of CAD. The requirement of a test has to be decided on individual basis.

REFERENCES

1. Pellikka PA. Stress echocardiography for the diagnosis of coronary artery disease: progress towards quantification. Curr Opin Cardiol. 2005;20:395.
2. Armstrong WF, Zoghbi WA. Stress echocardiography: current methodology and clinical applications. J Am Coll Cardiol. 2005; 45:1739.
3. Mieres JH, Shaw LJ, Arai A, et al. Role of noninvasive testing in the clinical evaluation of women with suspected coronary artery disease: Consensus statement from the Cardiac Imaging Committee, Council on Clinical Cardiology, and the Cardiovascular Imaging and Intervention Committee, Council on Cardiovascular Radiology and Intervention, American Heart Association. Circulation. 2005;111(5):682-96.
4. Fleischmann KE, Hunink MG, Kuntz KM, et al. Exercise echocardiography or exercise SPECT imaging? A meta-analysis of diagnostic test performance. JAMA. 1998;280(10):913-20.
5. Navare SM, Mather JF, Shaw LJ, et al. Comparison of risk stratification with pharmacologic and exercise stress myocardial perfusion imaging: a meta-analysis. J Nucl Cardiol. 2004;11(5): 551-61.
6. Leaker BR, O'Connor B, Hansel TT, et al. Safety of regadenoson, an adenosine A2A receptor agonist for myocardial perfusion imaging, in mild asthma and moderate asthma patients: a randomized, double-blind, placebo-controlled trial. J Nucl Cardiol. 2008;15(3):329-36.
7. Douglas MJ, Garcia DEH, Wyman WL, et al. Appropriate use criteria for echocardiography. JACC. 2011;57(9):1126-66.
8. Tischler MD, Battle RW, Saha M, et al. Observations suggesting a high incidence of exercise induced severe mitral regurgitation in patients with mild rheumatic mitral valve disease at rest. J Am Coll Cardiol. 1995;25:128-33.
9. Lancellotti P, Gerard PL, Pierard LA. Long-term outcome of patients with heart failure and dynamic functional mitral regurgitation. Eur Heart J. 2005;26:1528-32.
10. Mann DL, Zipes DP, Libby P, Bonow RO (Eds), Braunwalds Heart Disease: A Textbook of Cardiovascular Medicine, 9th edn:229.
11. Takeuchi M, Otani S, Weinert L, et al. Comparison of contrast enhanced real-time live 3D dobutamine stress echocardiography with contrast 2D echocardiography for detecting stress-induced wall-motion abnormalities. J Am Soc Echocardiogr. 2006;19:294-9.
12. Maurizio Galderisi, Eugenio Picano. Diastolic Stress Echocardiography. 2009.pp.361-73.
13. Buchsbaum M, Marshall E, Levine B, et al. Emergency department evaluation of chest pain using exercise stress echocardiography. Acad Emerg Med. 2001;8:196-9.
14. Conti A, Sammicheli L, Gallini C, et al. Assessment of patients with low-risk chest pain in the emergency department: head-to-head comparison of exercise stress echocardiography and exercise myocardial SPECT. Am Heart J. 2005;149:894-901.
15. Ahmad M, Xie T, McCulloch M, et al. Real-time three dimensional dobutamine stress echocardiography in assessment stress echocardiography in assessment of ischaemia: comparison with two dimensional dobutamine stress echocardiography. J Am Coll Cardiol. 2001;37:1303-9.
16. Hung J, Lang R, Flachskampf F, et al. ASE. 3D echocardiography: a review of the current status future directions. J Am Soc Echocardiogr. 2007;20:213-33.
17. Marwick TH, Nemec JJ, Pashkow FJ, et al. Accuracy and limitations of exercise echocardiography in a routine clinical setting. J Am Coll Cardiol. 1992;19:74-81.
18. Hecht HS, DeBord L, Shaw R, et al. Digital supine bicycle stress echocardiography: a new technique for evaluating coronary artery disease. J Am Coll Cardiol. 1993;21:950-6.
19. Beleslin BD, Ostojic M, Stepanovic J, et al. Stress echocardiography in the detection of myocardial ischemia. Head-to-head comparison of exercise, dobutamine and dipyridamole tests. Circulation. 1994;90:1168-76.
20. Luotolahti M, Saraste M, Hartiala J. Exercise echocardiography in the diagnosis of coronary artery disease. Ann Med. 1996;28:73-7.
21. Roger VL, Pellikka PA, Bell MR, et al. Sex and test verification bias: impact on the diagnostic value of exercise echocardiography. Circulation. 1997;95:405-10.

22. American College of Radiology. ACR Appropriateness Criteria, 2010. ACR.org. Available at http://www.acr.org/Quality-Safety/Appropriateness-Criteria.
23. Gibbons RJ, Abrams J, Chatterjee K, et al. American College of Cardiology; American Heart Association Task Force on Practice Guidelines. Committee on the Management of Patients With Chronic Stable Angina. ACC/AHA 2002 guideline update for the management of patients with chronic stable angina: a report of the American College of Cardiology/American Heart Association Task Force on Practice Guidelines (Committee to Update the 1999 Guidelines for the management of Patients With Chronic Stable Angina). Circulation. 2003;107:149-58.
24. Geleijnse ML, Elhendy A. Can stress echocardiography compete with perfusion scintigraphy in the detection of coronary artery disease and cardiac risk assessment? Eur J Echocardiogr. 2000; 1:12-21.
25. Picano E. Informed consent in radiological and nuclear medicine examinations. How to escape from a communication Inferno. Education and debate. BMJ. 2004;329:578-80.
26. Soman P, Parsons A, Lahiri N, et al. The prognostic value of a normal Tc-99m sestamibi SPECT study in suspected coronary artery disease. J Nucl Cardiol. 1999;6(3):252-6.
27. Schinkel A, Bax J, Geleijnse M, et al. Non-invasive evaluation of ischemic heart disease: myocardial perfusion imaging or stress echocardiography? Eur Heart J. 2003;24:789-800.
28. Branch K, Hamilton-Craig C, Hansen M, et al. Safety of heart rate control and the relationship to radiation exposure from coronary CT angiography. *Society of Cardiovascular Computed Tomography 2012 Annual Scientific Meeting*. July 20, 2012; Baltimore, MD.
29. Budoff MJ, Achenbach S, Blumenthal RS, et al. Assessment of coronary artery disease by cardiac computed tomography: a scientific statement from the American Heart Association Committee on Cardiovascular Imaging and Intervention, Council on Cardiovascular Radiology and Intervention, and Committee on Cardiac Imaging, Council on Clinical Cardiology. Circulation. 2006; 114(16):1761-91.
30. Silber S, Richartz BM. Impact of both cardiac-CT and cardiac-MR on the assessment of coronary risk. Z Kardiol. 2005;94 Suppl 4:IV/70-80.
31. Bielak LF, Rumberger JA, Sheedy PF 2nd, et al. Probabilistic model for prediction of angiographically defined obstructive coronary artery disease using electron beam computed tomography calcium score strata. Circulation. 2000;102(4):380-5.
32. Chang AM, Litt HI, Baxt WG, et al. Efficacy of CT coronary angiography for disposition of low risk chest pain patients in the emergency department. Ann Emerg Med. 2008;51:482.
33. Paetsch I, Jahnke C, Fleck E, et al. Current clinical applications of stress wall motion analysis with cardiac magnetic resonance imaging. Eur J Echocardiogr. 2005;6:317-26.
34. Sicari R, Pingitore A, Aquaro G, et al. Cardiac functional stress imaging: a sequential approach with stress echo and cardiovascular magnetic resonance. Cardiovasc Ultrasound. 2007;5:47.
35. Gallagher MJ, Raff GL. Use of multislice CT for the evaluation of emergency room patients with chest pain: the so-called "triple rule-out". Catheter Cardiovasc Interv. 2008;71(1):92-9.
36. Kajander S, Joutsiniemi E, Saraste M, et al. Cardiac positron emission tomography/computed tomography imaging accurately detects anatomically and functionally significant coronary artery disease. Circulation. 2010;122(6):603-13.
37. Picano E. Stress echocardiography: a historical perspective. Special article. Am J Med. 2003;114:126-30.
38. Hausleiter J, Meyer T, Hermann F, et al. Estimated radiation dose associated with cardiac CT angiography. JAMA. 2009;301:5.

15

Three-dimensional Echocardiography: Utility in Clinical Practice

Vinay Kumar Sharma

Three-dimensional echocardiography (3DE) offers the most complete and comprehensive assessment of cardiac pathologies. Unlike cross-sectional imaging modalities [i.e. two-dimensional (2D) echocardiography], 3DE images provide en-face and anatomically oriented "real-life view" of intracardiac structures that is very similar to the view to be seen by the surgeon in the operation theater. The development of matrix array transducers, which imparted the capability of real-time 3D imaging of the beating heart, has brought 3DE in the realm of day-to-day clinical practice. The usefulness of 3DE has been demonstrated in (a) the evaluation of the cardiac chamber volumes and mass, (b) the assessment of regional left ventricular (LV) wall motion and 3DE stress imaging, (c) evaluation of the valvular heart disease, and (d) volumetric evaluation of the regurgitant lesions with 3 DE color Doppler imaging.[1]

DATA ACQUISITION MODES AND DISPLAY OF IMAGES

Three-dimensional dataset acquisitions involve sequential acquisitions of multiple narrow volumes of datasets over several heartbeats. These dataset can be viewed either separately as "real-time 3DE" or after stitching them together as "full-volume dataset" (Figs 15.1A and B):

- *Real-time 3D mode*: Real-time and focused wide sector mode offer higher temporal and spatial resolution and thus superior image details. Real-time datasets do not require cropping to visualize the structure of interest and thus as the name suggests can be seen in real time, making them invaluable during interventional procedures and intraoperative setting. Further, unlike full-volume datasets they do not suffer from problem of stitch artifacts.

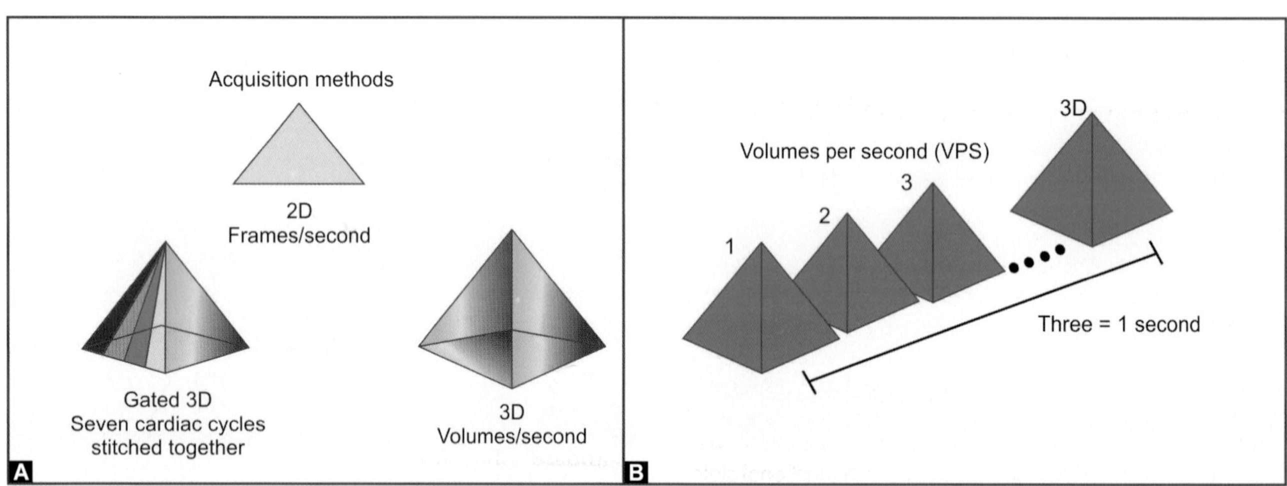

Figs 15.1A and B Multiple-beat three-dimensional echocardiography (3DE) acquisition acquires narrow volumes of information over several heartbeats (ranging from 2 to 7 cardiac cycles) that are then stitched together to create a larger volumetric dataset (A). This method of data acquisition compensates for the poor temporal resolution of single-beat full volumetric real-time 3DE acquisition, (B) but has the disadvantage of having stitch artifacts. From EAE/ASE recommendations for image acquisition and display using 3DE. Eur Heart J Cardiovasc Imaging. 2012;13(1):1-46

- *Focused wide sector—"ZOOM"*: This mode permits a focused, wide sector view of cardiac structures. However, it comes at cost of decrease in the spatial and temporal resolution relative to real-time 3DE.
- *Full-volume dataset*: Full-volume datasets, however, provide convenience of acquiring a single dataset encompassing entire heart that can later be cropped to any cardiac structure. Theoretically any cardiac structure can be visualized from this dataset by cropping away tissue planes other than the structure of interest. Surrounding structures can also be included in the same image to identify the spatial relation of the structure of interest to its surrounding structures. However, as one need to crop this dataset, i.e. crop away the tissue planes other than the structure of interest, this image cannot be seen in real time. Multiple-beat full-volume dataset also suffers from problem of stitching artifacts and has lower temporal and spatial resolution as compared to real-time imaging.
- Matrix array probe can also be used to image any cardiac structure in two orthogonal planes. The first image is typically a reference view of a particular structure, while the second image or "lateral plane" represents a plane rotated 30–1500 from the reference plane.

3D images are initially displayed as volume rendered images. Volume rendering is a technique that projects 3D images onto a two-dimensional (2D) plane for viewing. Volume-rendered 3DE datasets can be manipulated, cropped, and rotated to understand. Volume rendering brings out complex spatial relationships in a 3D display that is particularly useful for evaluating valves and adjacent anatomic structures.

ACQUISITION OF THE THREE-DIMENSIONAL DATASET

Theoretically, any intracardiac structure can be visualized from a single, full-volume 3D dataset. However, the choice of the dataset varies according to the pathology suspected and the operator must be aware of the optimal views to obtain datasets according to the suspected pathology. Detail discussion of these views is beyond the scope of this chapter and can be seen elsewhere.[1]

The quality of 3D images is critically dependent on gain settings before acquisition of the dataset. Low gain settings lead to echo dropouts in the image, while high gain settings lead to blurring of anatomical boundaries obscuring the fine structural details. There is no universally applicable method to predict optimal gain setting in every patient and it has to be found out for every patient. What we follow in our laboratory is to keep gain setting in mid range and acquire a dataset. This dataset is immediately cropped to see the quality of images. If there are echo dropouts, then the gain is increased before acquiring subsequent images. Similarly if the anatomical boundaries are getting blurred, then gain is decreased before acquiring next dataset.

Another common problem arises due to stitch artifacts. Since the wide-angle dataset is compiled by "stitching together" four narrower pyramidal scans obtained over four consecutive heartbeats, artifact can occur if the position of heart changes in between these four cycles. The most common cause of this problem is suboptimal ECG as the datasets are acquired by ECG gating. The second common cause is the translational movement of the heart due to respiration. So data should be acquired during suspended respiration to avoid translational movement and thus stitch artifact in the final 3D dataset.

CLINICAL APPLICATIONS OF THREE-DIMENSIONAL ECHOCARDIOGRAPHY

Assessment of Cardiac Chambers

Assessment of the LV Function

Quantification of LV ejection fraction (LVEF) is the most important contribution of 3DE in day-to-day clinical practice. The advent of matrix transducers, together with improved volumetric analysis software, has made 3DE a simple and fast imaging modality ready for everyday clinical use. 3DE can be used to quantify LV volumes and global LVEF, assessment of regional wall motion abnormalities (RWMAs) and LV structural changes including ventricular septal defects and masses such as LV thrombi or tumors.

Data acquisition and analysis: Apical views are the preferred approach for the acquisition of a full-volume LV dataset for the assessment of LV function. Acquisition of 3D dataset should be guided by the 2D image—it should be from the probe position where 2D image is least foreshortened and includes the entire LV. One can take help of volume rendered live 3D images or split screen orthogonal plane imaging to ensure that the entire LV is included in the full-volume dataset. Full-volume dataset is volume rendered and inspected for structural abnormalities such as thrombi and masses. Thereafter, quantification of LV is started. Most vendors offer software packages for online quantification of global and regional functional measurements. This process involves identification of anatomic landmarks, such as the tricuspid annulus and apex followed by blood endocardial interface detection to construct a surface-rendered cavity cast of the left ventricle (Figs 15.2A to D). The process is semiautomated so that manual corrections to the endocardial borders can be performed if necessary.[2] LV volume and LVEF can be computed from this casts without making any geometric assumptions.

Calculation of LVEF: 3D measurements are much more accurate as compared to 2D echocardiographic measurements of LV volumes. 2D echocardiographic methods have to assume a certain shape of the LV to compensate for the missing dimension to calculate LV volumes, and

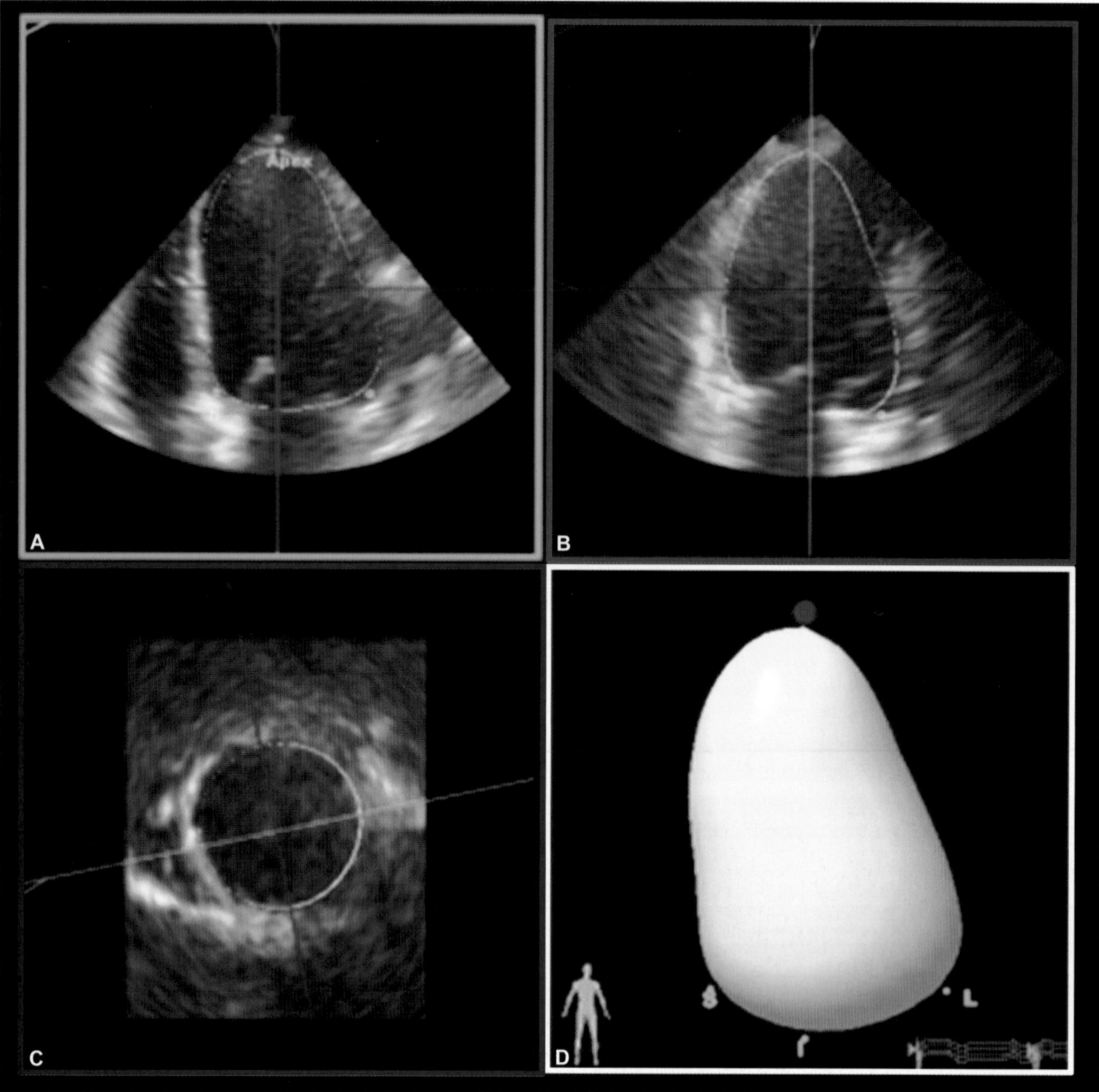

Figs 15.2A to D The raw three-dimensional (3D) dataset (A to C) is used to construct a cast corresponding to left ventricular (LV) cavity (D), which than can be used to assess the regional or global LV function

these assumptions can go terribly wrong in heart disease with grossly distorted chamber geometry. During 3D echocardiographic calculation of the volume of the LV, nothing is assumed regarding the shape of the LV and LV is displayed as it actually is in the form of an LV cast. The ability to assess LV volumes without making any geometrical assumption regarding shape of LV is the biggest advantage of 3DE over 2DE. 3D measurement of LV volume and function is rapid, more accurate and reproducible than with 2DE, and has an accuracy that is similar to magnetic resonance imaging (MRI).[3] Currently, 3D transthoracic echocardiographic (TTE) and transesophageal echocardiography (TEE) assessment of LVEF is recommended over the use of 2DE, as it has been clearly demonstrated to provide more accurate and reproducible measurements.[1]

Assessment of RWMA: It is a common day-to-day experience that endocardial definitions may not be optimal in all the patients and the operator often move and/or tilt the probe to improve image quality. However, the improved endocardial visualization often comes at cost of foreshortening of the views. These foreshortened images can make areas of RWMA appear normal and vice versa. A full-volume dataset can be easily and rapidly cropped to create nonforeshortened views similar to conventional 2C, 3C, and 4C views. Regional function can also be displayed as bulls' eye map to illustrate the spatial distribution of contraction and relaxation of different segments for easy comprehension.

***Utility of 3DE during stress echocardiography*:** During stress echocardiography (STEC), we are running against time to acquire images before heart rate settles down because RWMA can be transient and disappear as the heart rate comes down from peak values. The principal advantage of 3DE during STEC is that this avoids necessity of acquiring multiple datasets as a single full-volume dataset is enough to evaluate multiple segments. This cuts down acquisition time allowing image acquisition to be completed before the heart rate starts declining in recovery. A single, full-volume dataset of the left ventricle can be cropped to create all conventional 2D images including apical four-chamber, two-chamber, long-axis, and short-axis views (Figs 15.3A and B). Most vendors had made this process semiautomatic with option of manual correction if needed. 3DE also allows creation of nonforeshortened images, which is a major limitation of 2DE. Feasibility and accuracy of 3DE during STEC have been proven with both exercise[4,5] and dobutamine.[6,7]

Assessment of the Right Ventricular Function

Assessment of the right ventricular (RV) function is an important issue prior to valvular and congenital and coronary artery bypass surgery, because right-sided heart failure is one of the most frequent causes of morbidity and mortality in postoperative period after cardiovascular surgery.

Conventional 2D echocardiographic methods measure the chamber in two dimensions and then convert it into volumes by assuming the RV to be of certain shape to compensate for the missing dimension. The problem is that RV, because of its asymmetrical and pyramidal shape, does not conform to simple geometric assumptions. So direct visualization of the entire chamber with 3DE should overcome these limitations, and there is good amount of data to demonstrate accuracy of RV function assessment by 3DE and its superiority over 2DE assessment of RV function. Several clinical studies have documented a good correlation between cardiac magnetic resonance and 3DE volumes and ejection fraction of the right ventricle.[8,9] The use of 3D TTE for assessing RV function has been validated in patients with pulmonary regurgitation, secundum atrial septal defects (ASDs), tetralogy of Fallot repair, Ebstein's anomaly, and RV cardiomyopathy.[10-12]

***Data acquisition and analysis*:** 3D dataset is acquired in a full-volume mode from the four-chamber apical view taking care to include the entire right ventricle in the dataset. The dataset is volume rendered and inspected for structural abnormalities such as thrombi and masses. Most recently volumetric border detection software has become available.

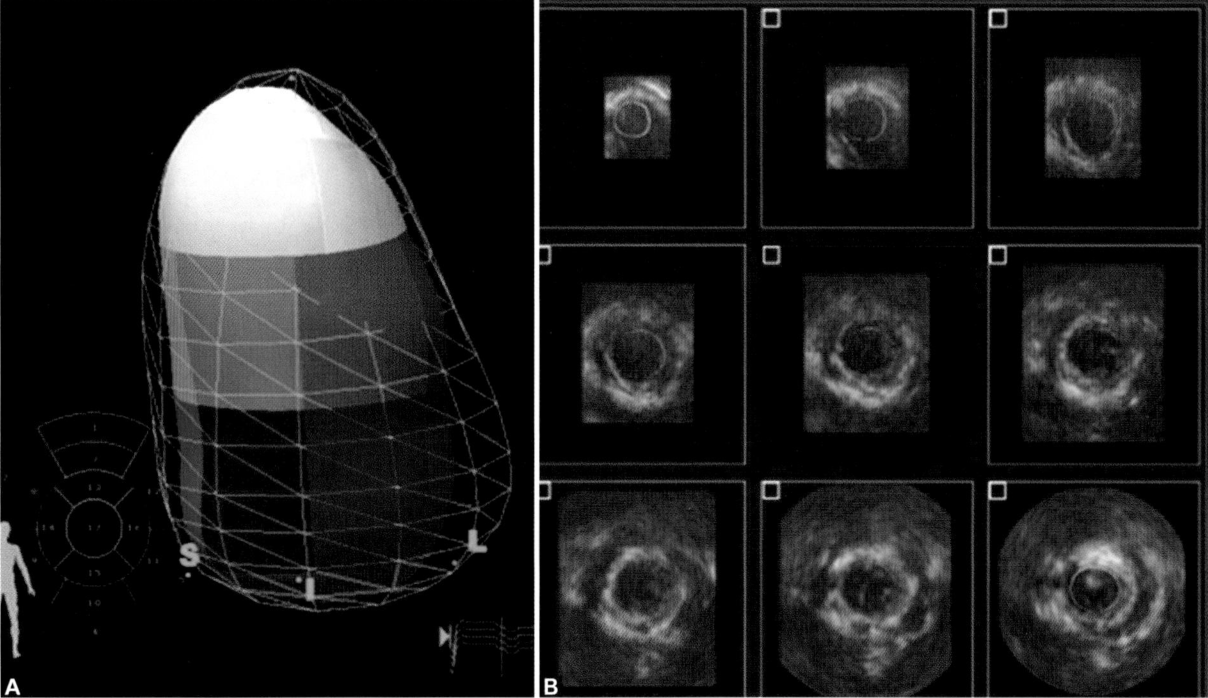

Figs 15.3A and B The left ventricular (LV) cast is used to derive global ejection fraction from LV diastolic and systolic volumes. (A) Regional function can be assessed in relation to a reference mesh corresponding to the end diastolic dimensions of LV. (B) It can also be used to construct multiple short-axis views of LV

This process involves identification of anatomic landmarks, such as the tricuspid annulus and apex followed by blood endocardial interface detection to construct a surface-rendered cavity cast of the left ventricle. The process is semiautomated so that manual corrections to the endocardial borders can be performed if necessary. RV volume can be computed from this casts without making any geometric assumptions. Segmental analysis of the three main sections of the right ventricle (inlet, apex, and outflow segments) may be performed. Curves of global and regional RV function may be generated and analyzed.

Evaluation of the Left Atrial Function

Left atrial (LA) volume has been shown to be accurately quantified by 3DE and correlate well with MRI and appears to have accuracy compared to 2D left atrial volume methods. 3DE provides anatomically oriented en-face view of atrial masses and clot. In addition, the 3DE can accurately define spatial location of the thrombus or mass in LA that can be so important in planning appropriate surgical procedure.

Assessment of Cardiac Valves

Assessment of Mitral Valve

TTE dataset acquisitions to visualize mitral valve can be made either from the parasternal or the apical approach. A zoomed acquisition provides best details of mitral valve leaflet anatomy and motion as it gives highest temporal and spatial resolution. Alternatively valve can be visualized by cropping a full-volume dataset. Irrespective of modality of acquisition valve is always displayed with aorta in 12 o'clock position because it resembles the intraoperative image of the mitral valve after the surgeon, standing on the patient's right side, opens the left atrium (i.e. why it is known as the "Surgeon's View").

- *Assessment of severity of mitral stenosis*: 3DE superior to 2DE in quantifying mitral stenosis severity. Mitral valve opening is funnel shaped with narrowest diameter at the tip of the funnel. Correct calculation of mitral valve area requires precise positioning of the cursor at the tip of the valve that is often not possible. 3DE provides en-face view of the valve, allowing en-face visualization of the narrowest appoint of the funnel that corresponds to the true anatomical area of the valve (Figs 15.4A and B). 3DE area measurements have been shown to correlate strongly with area measurements derived invasively using the Gorlin formula.[13,14]
- *Assessment of severity of mitral regurgitation*: 3DE has been shown to be much more accurate than 2D techniques to define effective regurgitant orifice area and the vena contracta (VC). Accuracy of 2D VC measurement is limited by the fact that it is noncircular in most patients, especially those with functional mitral regurgitation. 3DE provides en-face view of the VC, allowing direct planimetry of VC. En-face 3D images of the mitral valve allow direct visualization and measurement of anatomic regurgitant orifice area.

3DE is an excellent method to evaluate details of morphological abnormalities of the mitral valve apparatus that is very important in formulating the appropriate plans for surgical repairs. Each component of mitral valve apparatus can be visualized as follows:

- 3DE provides exquisite details of morphological abnormalities of the mitral valve leaflets in cases of mitral valve prolapse (MVP) and flail valves. The anterior mitral valve leaflet (AML) is attached to about one-third of the annular circumference. The posterior mitral leaflet (PML) is attached to remaining two-thirds of the annulus. Both leaflets are reciprocally shaped to ensure proper cooptation. Both leaflets are segmented into three scallops: A_1, A_2, and A_3 scallops of AML and P_1, P_2 and P_3 segments of PML (from left to right, respectively). Prolapsing segments of the leaflets can be precisely localized in terms of scallops. The cooptation line can be checked for visible leaks while in the closed position.
- En-face views of the mitral valve from the LV perspective provide excellent visualization of mitral valve apparatus and allow reliable diagnosis of chordal rupture with flail or prolapsed leaflets. Subvalvular apparatus involves papillary muscles and chordate tendinae insertions on the tips (primary chordae), body (secondary chordae), and base (tertiary chordae) of the mitral valve leaflets.
- 3DE can visualize the shape of mitral annulus, which has important implication in ring repair of the mitral valve. Mitral annulus is saddle shaped with high points that are anterior and posterior and low points that are lateral and medial and this complex shape can only be appreciated by 3DE. However, a dedicated separate software is required for construction of the image.

Assessment of Aortic Valve

3D TTE dataset acquisitions for aortic valve visualization can be made either from the parasternal or the apical approach. Alternatively valve can be visualized by cropping a full-volume dataset. Irrespective of modality of acquisition valve is best examined from aortic perspective for valve cusp morphology.

- *Assessment of aortic stenosis*: 3DE is superior to 2DE in quantifying aortic valve area (AVA) for assessment of severity of aortic stenosis. Exact en-face alignment of aortic valve opening is often very difficult during 2DE due to poor window and/or aortic root dilatation. 3DE provides en-face view of the valve allowing easy identification of the narrowest area (Figs 15.4C and D). Improved

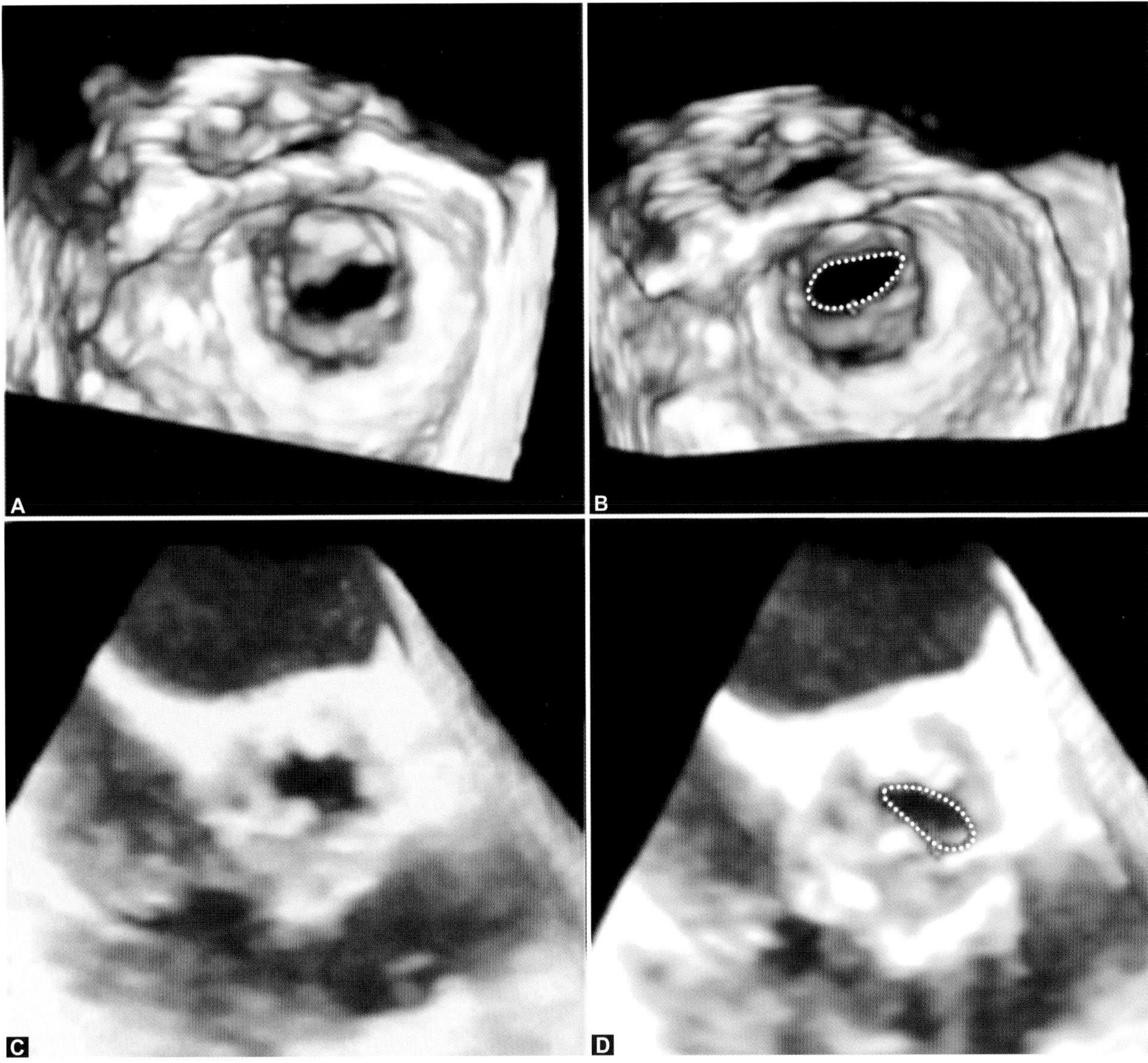

Figs 15.4A to D (A and B) En-face images of mitral valve: (B and C) En-face images of the aortic valve. The valve area calculated from these en-face images is very accurate and correlate very closely with cardiac catheterization derived valve areas. Images of mitral valve have been oriented anatomically with aorta in 11 o'clock position

identification of cuspal opening on 3DE also decreases interobserver variability. 3DE area measurements have been shown to be better than with either 2D planimetry[15,16] or the continuity equation.[17,18] 3DE calculation of AVA correlates better to invasively measured AVA compared with 2D TEE values.[17]

- *Quantification of aortic regurgitation*: 3DE has been shown to be much more accurate than 2D techniques to define effective regurgitant orifice area and the VC. Accuracy of 2D VC measurement is limited by the fact that it assumes the VC to be circular while it is noncircular in many patients, especially those with functional mitral regurgitation. 3DE profiles the VC en-face allowing direct planimetry of VC. 3DE measurement of VC has been shown to have a good correlation with aortographic grading of aortic regurgitation.

Assessment of Pulmonary Valve

Three-dimensional echocardiography provides en-face short-axis view of the pulmonary valve (PV) that is nearly impossible to get by 2DE allowing assessment of all three leaflets simultaneously.

3DE has been shown to be useful for defining cusp number, thickness, and mobility and for assessment of pulmonary regurgitation.[19] However, 3D TTE images remain less than satisfactory. Transesophageal approach provides better images, but there is no current evidence supporting the routine use of 3D TEE for the evaluation of the pulmonic valve disease.[1]

Assessment of Tricuspid Valve

Three-dimensional transthoracic echocardiographic dataset acquisitions for tricuspid valve (TV) visualization can be made either from the parasternal or the apical approach. A zoomed acquisition provides best details of TV leaflet anatomy and motion as it gives highest temporal and spatial resolution. Alternatively valve can be visualized by cropping a full-volume dataset. Irrespective of modality of acquisition en-face view of TV is always displayed with the septal leaflet located in the 6 o'clock position.

As in the case of mitral valve, 3DE has been shown to be superior to 2DE for assessment of tricuspid regurgitation and tricuspid stenosis. A recent article by Velayudhan et al. demonstrated efficacy in measuring the VC of the tricuspid regurgitant jet using 3D color Doppler data.[20] En-face view of TV is helpful in localizing leaflet pathologies such as prolapse, perforation, or vegetation, as well as localizing the origin of regurgitation jets, or planimetering the tricuspid orifice area to assess severity of tricuspid stenosis.[21,22] En-face views of the TV from the RV perspective allow diagnosis of chordal rupture with flail or prolapsed leaflets. Tricuspid annulus is also saddle shaped with higher points (toward the right atrium) along the anterior and posterior aspects of the annulus and the low or inferior points (toward the right ventricle) along the medial and lateral aspects of the annulus.

Assessment of Congenital Heart Disease

The complex nature of these defects can make a thorough anatomic evaluation difficult and require multiple 2D views. The perspective provided by 3DE provide a more complete preoperative assessment of the extent and severity of the defect and its relation to its surrounding structures. Clinical investigations have emphasized the unique perspective provided by 3D imaging in both simple and complex congenital heart disease (CHD).[16] The ability to analyze the entire cardiac structure and to display complex spatial relationships is potential advantages of 3D imaging over 2DE. In addition, the decreased examination time afforded by RT 3DE may reduce the need for sedation in some children.

Evaluation of the ASDs

Atrial septal defects (ASDs) are commonest CHD in adult and adolescents, with ostium secundum variety alone accounting for 30–40% of all CHDs seen in this age group.[23] There is intense interest in a certain subgroup of patients with ostium secundum ASDs where percutaneous devise closure can be offered in place of surgical closure.[24-26] The primary requirement for selecting patients for device closure is to demonstrate adequacy of the surrounding margins to hold the device. Echocardiography plays a very important role in identifying these patients. TEE is by far very superior to TTE, as TEE is not hindered by problem of poor echocardiographic window. In fact, an ASD is never taken up for devise closure without first doing a TEE study to assess adequacy of its margins to hold the device.

3D TEE has opened an exciting new vista to evaluate patient with ASD. All the margins and size of the ASD can be assessed in a single 3D TEE image (Figs 15.5A to C), which otherwise would have taken a series of 2D TEE views. 3DE can record the size and shape, precise location, and, most important, the adequacy of the margins to hold the devise. 3DE has been used for both selecting the candidates for devise closure and to evaluate the success of the procedure. In our laboratory, we routinely do 3D reconstruction of the interatrial septum before taking up the patient for devise closure.[27]

Evaluation of the Ventricular Septal Defects

Three-dimensional imaging can interrogate the entire septum and can also measure the shape and size of the color flow jet, which allows for accurate measurement of the magnitude of shunting in patients with isolated ventricular septal defects.[28]

Evaluation of the Ventricular Function in CHD

The advantages of 3D over 2D echocardiographic techniques are obvious as no geometrical assumptions are needed to calculate the volume and ejection fraction. This becomes very important to assess the RV function as the RV's asymmetrical shape invalidates the simple geometric assumptions used for volume calculations. In patients with CHDs that involve RV pathology, 3DE correlates well with MRI for the measurement of RV volume.[29]

Miscellaneous Uses

Three-dimensional echocardiography has been successfully applied to the detection and assessment of several anatomic defects such as circumferential extent and severity of discrete subaortic membranes and congenital malformations of the mitral valve. With the apical view, a unique en-face image of the subaortic membrane can be recorded, which permits analysis of the effective orifice area and the dynamic nature of the defect.

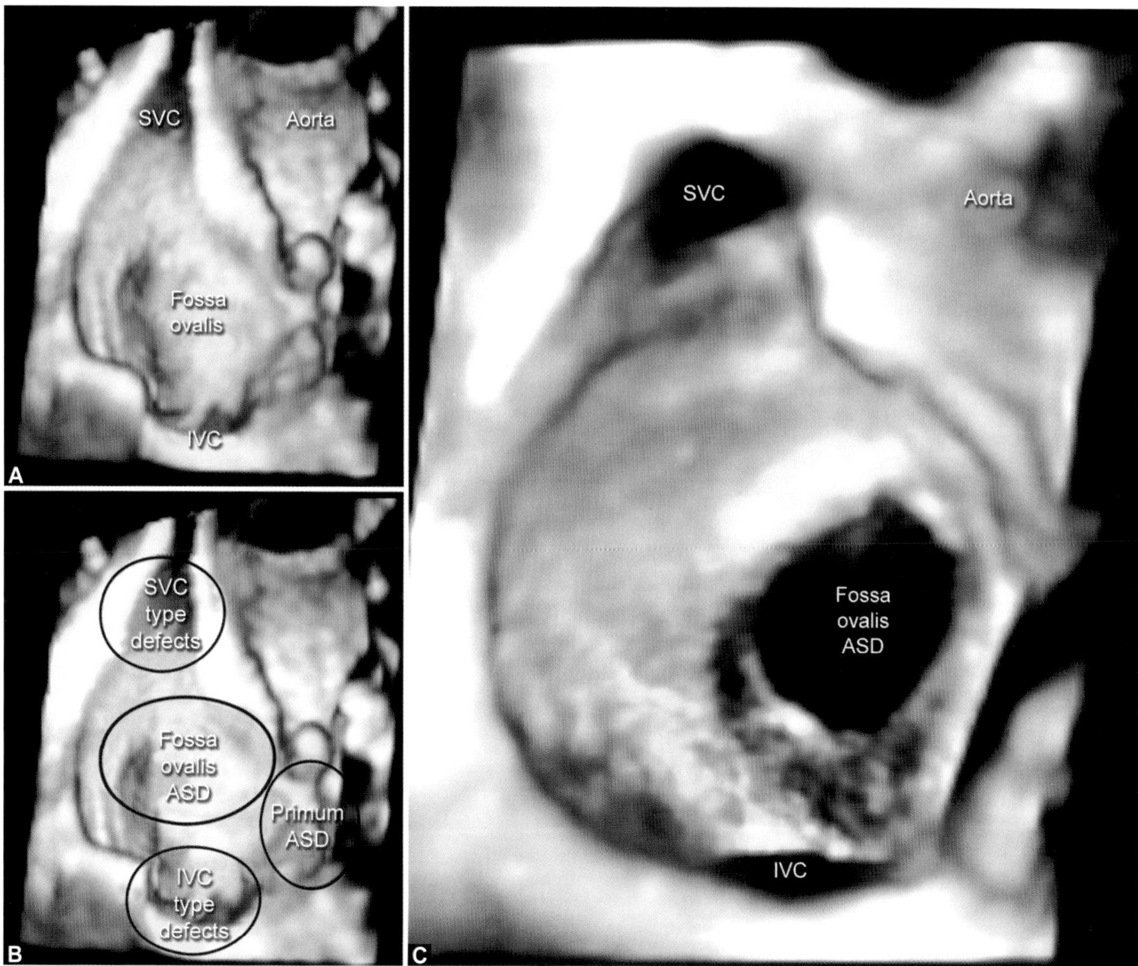

Figs 15.5A to C (A) Appearance of normal interatrial septum as seen from the right atrial perspective. Note the position of the aorta, superior vena cava (SVC), and tricuspid valve (TV) and inferior vena cava (IVC) in relation to the interatrial septum because they are used as anatomical landmarks to define the margins of the atrial septal defects; (B) Illustrates the typical position of various types of atrial septal defects; (C) From a patient with large fossa ovalis type atrial septal defect and one can see all good around margins. This patient underwent successful device closure

Three-dimensional Transesophageal Echocardiography

2D TEE as such is very superior to 2D TTE as TEE is not hindered by problem of poor echocardiographic window. 3D TEE is further superior to 2D TEE as it provides unique anatomically oriented en-face view of cardiac structure and often provides all the needed information in a single view, which otherwise would take a series of 2D TEE views. 3D TEE is also superior to 3D TTE due to better temporal and spatial resolution leading to better image resolution. Development of 3D TEE has thrown up several exciting possibilities. However, 3D TEE probes are costly and need special operating skills. Most of the images used in this chapter have been taken from transesophageal approach.

Utility of 3D TEE during Interventional Procedures

The real-time images provided by 3D TEE are invaluable in several interventional procedures. Unique en-face view provided by 3DE results in accurate diagnoses and improved clinical decision making.

Device Closure of ASD

An ASD is never taken up for devise closure without first doing a TEE study to assess adequacy of its margins to hold the device. 3D TEE also potentially very useful during the procedure of device closure. It confirms the proper positioning of the device across all the margins in a single view that otherwise would require a series of 2D views. A single postprocedure 3D TEE image can tell whether the device is excessively mobile or whether it is encroaching onto AV valves or pulmonary veins or SVC or IVC orifices.

Device Closure of Paravalvular Leaks

High mortality associated with reoperation has led to development of percutaneous transcatheter closure procedures. However, transcatheter PVL closure is not successful in the entire patient (success rate is only 60–90% patients in patients with mitral PVL). In most cases, technical failure results from inability to adequately visualize the 3D anatomy of the defect with 2D imaging modalities, e.g. fluoroscopy and 2D TEE. 3D TEE provides en-face view of entire valve and entire extant of the dehiscence allowing proper planning of the procedure. 3DE can be used immediately before deployment of device to ensure that the device is not encroaching over PHV struts.

Visualization of Atrial Architecture

Real-time imaging of atrial structure is very useful in electrophysiologic procedures and several left-sided interventional procedures require septal puncture. These procedures are usually done under fluoroscopic guidance. However, many structures that are target of catheter-based procedures and septal puncture like crista terminalis, coronary sinus ostium, and fossa ovale are difficult to visualize by fluoroscopy. 3D TEE provides exquisite images of these structures as they are posteriorly situated and thus are very close to the TTE probe.

Percutaneous Closure of the Left Atrial Appendage

Accurate assessment of left atrial appendage (LAA) orifice area is mandatory requirement to determine appropriate device size. 3D TEE measurements from the en-face view of LAA orifice area have been shown to be more accurate than 2D TEE and correlate well with computed tomographic values.

CONCLUSION

Three-dimensional echocardiography is not a substitute for 2DE. Rather it should act as a supplement to 2DE. Thus, the current clinical practice is to use a focused examination, where we start with 2D imaging to localize the structure of interest, then switch to live 3DE imaging to check if the structure of interest is encompassed within the volume of interest, and then obtain a 3D acquisition in the full volume or zoom mode. Thereafter, the 3D dataset is cropped to reveal structure of interest and oriented anatomically. Development of matrix array probes has made it possible to do 3DE in real time. The drastic decrease in acquisition time and more user friendly software has brought 3DE in day-to-day clinical care. Development of single-heartbeat full-volume dataset and live 3DE color Doppler imaging with a larger angle has tremendously enhanced utility of 3DE in day-to-day clinical practice.

REFERENCES

1. Roberto M Lang, Luigi P Badano, Wendy Tsang, David H Adams, Eustachio Agricola, et al. EAE/ASE recommendations for image acquisition and display using three-dimensional echocardiography. Eur Heart J Cardiovasc Imaging. 2012;13(1):1-46.
2. Muraru D, Badano LP, Piccoli G, et al. Validation of a novel automated border-detection algorithm for rapid and accurate quantitation of left ventricular volumes based on three-dimensional echocardiography. Eur J Echocardiogr. 2010;11:359-68.
3. Mor-Avi V, Jenkins C, Kuhl HP, et al. Real-time 3-dimensional echocardiographic quantification of left ventricular volumes: multicenter study for validation with magnetic resonance imaging and investigation of sources of error. JACC Cardiovasc Imaging. 2008;1:413-23.
4. Walimbe V, Garcia M, Lalude O, et al. Quantitative real-time 3-dimensional stress echocardiography: a preliminary investigation of feasibility and effectiveness. J Am Soc Echocardiogr. 2007;20:13-22.
5. Peteiro J, Pinon P, Perez R, et al. Comparison of 2- and 3-dimensional exercise echocardiography for the detection of coronary artery disease. J Am Soc Echocardiogr. 2007;20:959-67.
6. Aggeli C, Giannopoulos G, Misovoulos P, et al. Real-time three-dimensional dobutamine stress echocardiography for coronary artery disease diagnosis: validation with coronary angiography. Heart. 2007;93:672-5.
7. Matsumura Y, Hozumi T, Arai K, et al. Noninvasive assessment of myocardial ischaemia using new real-time three-dimensional dobutamine stress echocardiography: comparison with conventional two-dimensional methods. Eur Heart J. 2005;26:1625-32.
8. Niemann PS, Pinho L, Balbach T, et al. Anatomically oriented right ventricular volume measurements with dynamic three-dimensional echocardiography validated by 3-Tesla magnetic resonance imaging. J Am Coll Cardiol. 2007;50:1668-76.
9. Kjaergaard J, Petersen CL, Kjaer A, et al. Evaluation of right ventricular volume and function by 2D and 3D echocardiography compared to MRI. Eur J Echocardiogr. 2006;7:430-8.
10. Kjaergaard J, Hastrup SJ, Sogaard P, et al. Advanced quantitative echocardiography in arrhythmogenic right ventricular cardiomyopathy. J Am Soc Echocardiogr. 2007;20:27-35.
11. Acar P, Abadir S, Roux D, et al. Ebstein's anomaly assessed by real-time 3-D echocardiography. Ann Thorac Surg. 2006;82:731-3.
12. Grewal J, Majdalany D, Syed I, et al. Three-dimensional echocardiographic assessment of right ventricular volume and function in adult patients with congenital heart disease: comparison with magnetic resonance imaging. J Am Soc Echocardiogr. 2010;23:127-33.
13. Zamorano J, Cordeiro P, Sugeng L, et al. Real-time three-dimensional echocardiography for rheumatic mitral valve stenosis evaluation: an accurate and novel approach. J Am Coll Cardiol. 2004;43:2091-6.
14. Perez de Isla L, Casanova C, Almeria C, et al. Which method should be the reference method to evaluate the severity of

rheumatic mitral stenosis? Gorlin's method versus 3D-echo. Eur J Echocardiogr. 2007;8:470-73.
15. de la Morena G, Saura D, Oliva MJ, et al. Real-time three-dimensional transoesophageal echocardiography in the assessment of aortic valve stenosis. Eur J Echocardiogr. 2010;11: 9-13.
16. Nakai H, Takeuchi M, Yoshitani H, et al. Pitfalls of anatomical aortic valve area measurements using two-dimensional transoesophageal echocardiography and the potential of three-dimensional transoesophageal echocardiography. Eur J Echocardiogr. 2010;11:369-76.
17. Gutierrez-Chico JL, Zamorano JL, Prieto-Moriche E, et al. Real-time three-dimensional echocardiography in aortic stenosis: a novel, simple, and reliable method to improve accuracy in area calculation. Eur Heart J. 2008;29:1296-306.
18. Poh KK, Levine RA, Solis J, et al. Assessing aortic valve area in aortic stenosis by continuity equation: a novel approach using real-time three-dimensional echocardiography. Eur Heart J. 2008;29:2526-35.
19. Pothineni KR, Wells BJ, Hsiung MC, et al. Live/real time three-dimensional transthoracic echocardiographic assessment of pulmonary regurgitation. Echocardiography. 2008;25:911-7.
20. Velayudhan DE, Brown TM, Nanda NC, et al. Quantification of tricuspid regurgitation by live three-dimensional transthoracic echocardiographic measurements of vena contracta area. Echocardiography. 2006;23:793-800.
21. Muraru D, Badano LP, Sarais C, et al. Evaluation of tricuspid valve morphology and function by transthoracic three-dimensional echocardiography. Curr Cardiol Rep. 2011;13:242-9.
22. Badano LP, Agricola E, Perez de Isla L, et al. Evaluation of the tricuspid valve morphology and function by transthoracic real-time three-dimensional echocardiography. Eur J Echocardiogr. 2009;10:477-84.
23. Dickinson DF, Arnold R, Wilkinson JL. Congenital heart disease among 160480 live born children in Liverpool 1960 to 1969-Implications for surgical treatment. Br Heart J. 1981;46:55-62.
24. Das GS, Voss G, Jarvis G, et al. Experimental atrial septal defect closure with a new, transcatheter, self-centering device. Circulation. 1993;88:1754-64.
25. Chan KC, Godman MJ. Morphological variations of fossa ovalis atrial septal defects (secundum): feasibility for transcutaneous closure with the clam-shell device. Br Heart J. 1993;69:52-5.
26. Hellenbrand WE, Fahey JT, McGowan FX, et al. Transoesophageal echocardiographic guidance of transcatheter closure of atrial septal defect. Am J Cardiol. 1990;66:207-13.
27. Sharma VK, Radhakrishnan S, Shrivastava S. Three-dimensional trans-esophageal echocardiographic evaluation of atrial septal defects: a pictorial essay. Images Paediatr Cardiol. 2011;13(3): 1-18.
28. Ishii M, Hashino K, Eto G, et al. Quantitative assessment of severity of ventricular septal defect by three-dimensional reconstruction of color Doppler-imaged vena contracta and flow convergence region. Circulation. 2001;103:664-9.
29. Heusch A, Rubo J, Krogmann ON, et al. Volumetric analysis of the right ventricle in children with congenital heart defects: comparison of biplane angiography and transthoracic 3-dimensional echocardiography. Cardiol Young. 1999;9:577-84.

16

Coronary CT Angiography Current Perspective: Redefining the Gold Standard for Coronary Angiography

Mona Bhatia

BACKGROUND

Imaging of the coronary arteries requires high temporal and spatial resolution. Even if spatial and temporal resolution have been the prime differentiators favoring invasive coronary angiography (ICA), over the past few decades, coronary CT Angiography (CCTA) has almost bridged the gap owing to recent technological advances in hardware and software. The resultant high diagnostic performance of CCTA as a noninvasive alternative to ICA in the detection and exclusion of obstructive CAD has been demonstrated with a per-patient sensitivity and specificity of 100% and 93.6%, respectively, and an average negative predictive value of 98%[1-5] (Figs 16.1A to D). The newer CT scanners having wider scan range, faster acquisitions, and the ability to image the entire heart in a single heartbeat,[6] with dual source imaging and spectral capabilities, combined with advanced image postprocessing. Thus, CCTA contributes, in a single study, to much more than a "lumenography".

The unique strength of CCTA is in imaging the coronary tree anatomically in three dimensions. Importantly, CCTA enables in addition to lumen assessment, coronary artery wall evaluation for positive and negative remodeling, plaque assessment, calcium scoring, fractional flow rate, and myocardial perfusion assessment.[7]

All these provide new insights in the evaluation, risk stratification, and prognostication of future cardiac events in patients suspected of CAD with incremental value in therapy guidance. Coronary CT angiography is thus playing an increasingly important role as a viable, effective, and noninvasive alternative in patient evaluation and planning for cardiovascular interventions in CAD.

LUMENOGRAPHY

Invasive coronary angiography, the current gold standard, is a lumenography with several shortcomings which today questions its very position.[7] These shortcomings include insufficient sampling, quantitation of minimum luminal area and diameter, overlap and foreshortening, and plaque severity and characterization; all of which impact technical and clinical decision making.

INSUFFICIENT SAMPLING

A typical selective coronary angiography comprises approximately five left coronary and two or three right coronary artery acquisitions. Given that most lesions are eccentric, it is extremely unlikely that this insufficient sampling of the 3D coronary tree displayed in limited two dimensional standard angiographic view,[7] chosen subjectively, with intra- and interobserver variability could capture the true minimum luminal diameter. As a result, lesions may be missed or underestimated, with subsequent incorrect stent selection (diameter and length) and inaccurate placements. Some of these shortcomings are addressed by rotational angiography.[8] The tomographic nature of CCTA, however, permits evaluation of the artery from every possible angle with measurement of the true minimum luminal diameter measurement (Figs 16.2A and B).

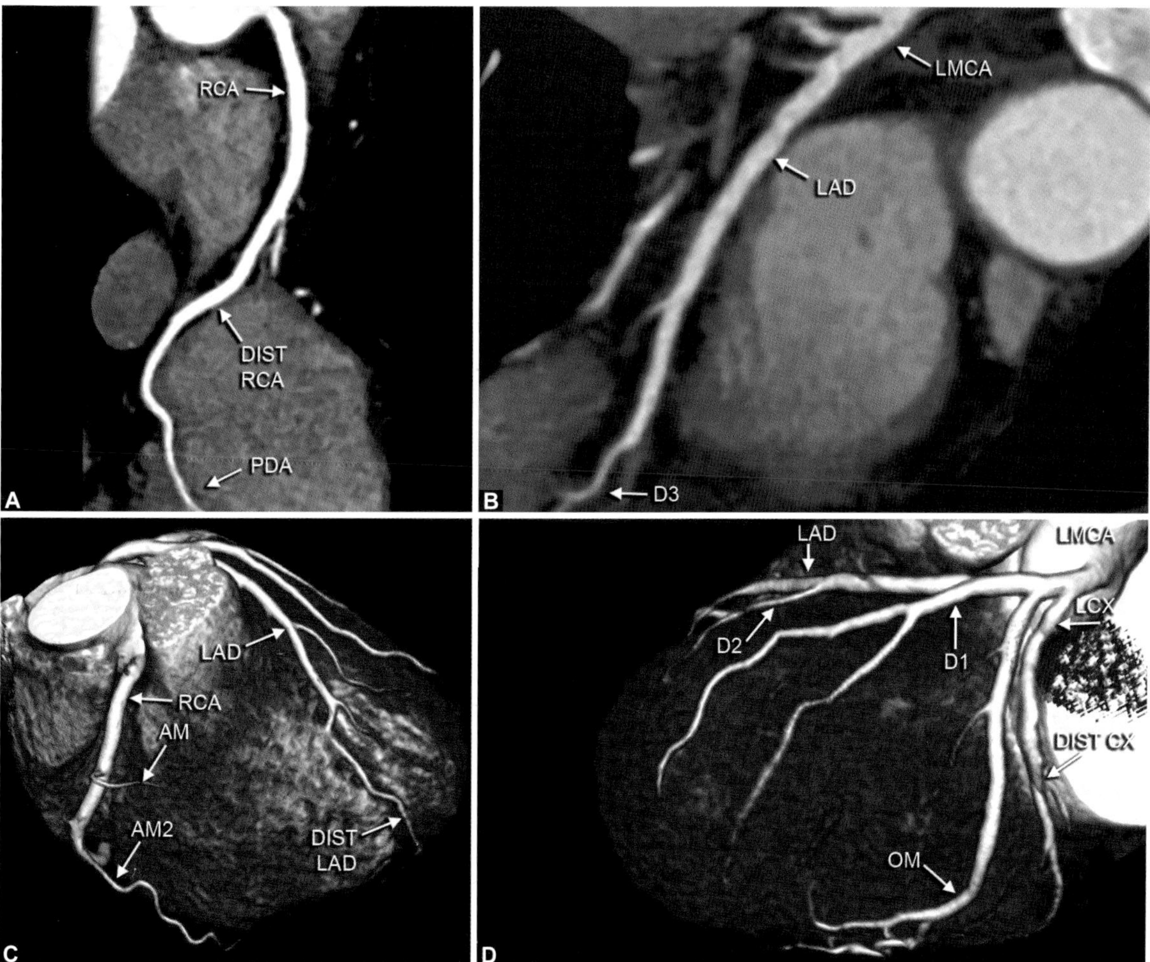

Figs 16.1A to D Coronary CT angiography demonstrating exclusion of coronary artery disease. Curved multiplanar reconstructed images demonstrate the right coronary artery (RCA) and posterior descending artery (PDA) (A), the left main coronary artery (LMCA), left anterior descending coronary artery (LAD), and third diagonal branch (D3) (B), volume-rendered CCTA images demonstrate the anatomy and branching pattern of the RCA with visualization of the acute marginal branches (AM, AM2) (C), and LMCA, LAD, diagonal (D1, D2, D3), and obtuse marginal (OM) branches (D)

Abbreviations: DIST, distal; DISTCX, distal circumflex; LCX, left circumflex; LAD, left anterior descending

QUANTITATION OF MINIMUM LUMINAL AREA AND MINIMUM LUMINAL DIAMETER

From the physiological perspective, measurement of the minimum luminal cross-sectional area is more relevant as it integrates all possible vessel diameters than minimum luminal diameter,[7,9-11] which has no relation to flow limitation, with the exception of perfectly concentric lesions. Minimum luminal area measurement is obtainable from tomographic intravascular analysis. Further, the frequent positive remodeling adjacent to areas of stenosis results in inaccurate quantitative measurements and overestimation of minimum luminal diameter, as they use adjacent "normal" proximal and distal segments.[7]

Coronary CT angiography, however, due to its cross-sectional capability has the advantage of measuring minimum luminal area along with the minimum luminal diameter, with identification of vessel wall remodeling and even plaque quantification and characterization.[7]

OVERLAP AND FORESHORTENING

Coronary stenosis evaluation by selective coronary angiography is complicated by foreshortening and vessel overlap on account of the projection angle. Specific clinical scenarios

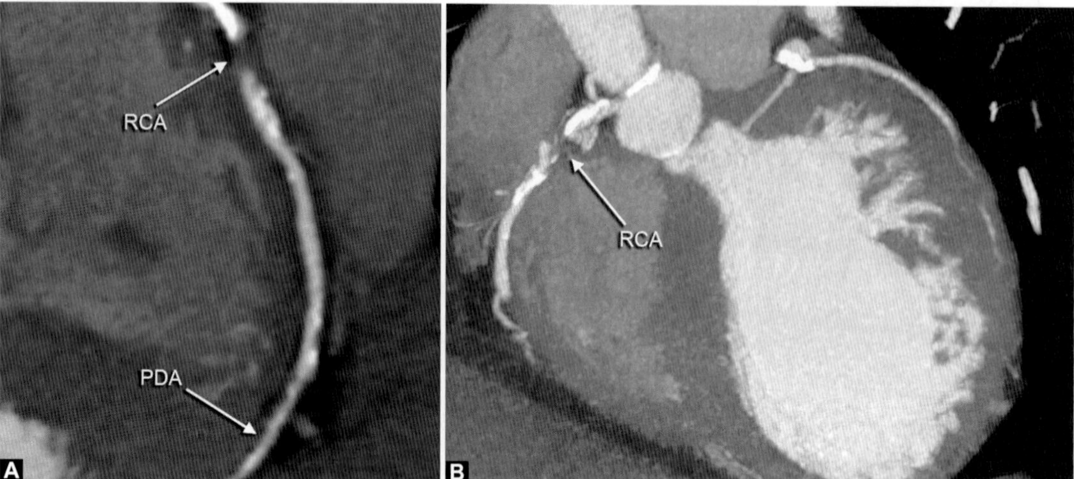

Figs 16.2A and B Curved multiplanar reconstruction (A) and maximum intensity projection (B) images demonstrate focal segment of soft noncalcified plaque with near total occlusion of the right coronary artery (RCA), 1 cm distal to the ostium with good distal reformation and runoff. In addition, multiple eccentric calcified plaques are seen

Abbreviation: PDA, posterior descending artery

where this is applicable are left main and ostial disease (Fig. 16.3), which may be difficult to assess using the standard limited projections of ICA.[12,13] Inadequate visualization and passage of percutaneous intervention hardware through regions of diseased left main artery en route to the lesion may demonstrate lesions in subsequent studies not initially present. Coronary CT angiography by permitting evaluation and tracking of individual vessels from all possible angles eliminates the chance of foreshortening and vessel overlap.[7] Further, CCTA can clearly delineate the path to the lesion, thereby guiding the treatment plan.

In diffuse coronary artery disease, in the absence of an adjacent "normal" reference segment, ICA may underestimate the degree of stenosis. Coronary CT angiography has the advantage of being immune to this problem, as both the vessel lumen and wall are viewed in cross section for measurement of maximum lumen area.

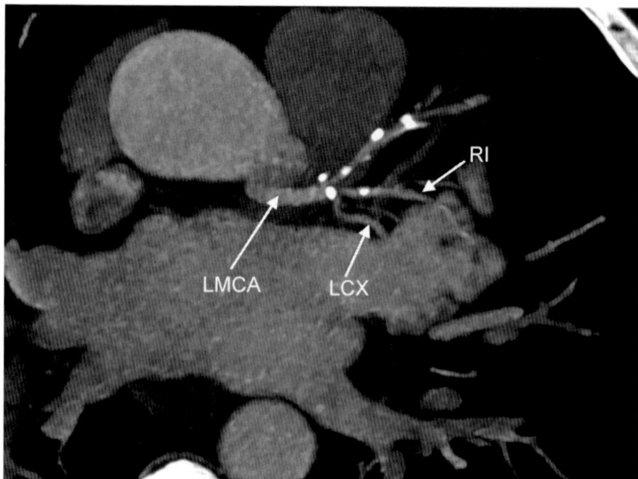

Fig. 16.3 Curved multiplanar reconstruction images demonstrate trifurcation of the left main coronary artery (LMCA) into the left anterior descending, ramus intermedius (RI) and left circumflex artery (LCX) with calcific plaques causing ostial disease

PLAQUE COMPOSITION, DISTRIBUTION, AND SEVERITY

Of immense clinical relevance is evaluation of coronary plaques. Noncalcified plaques have been found to be more prevalent in the culprit lesions when compared with stable lesions in patients with acute coronary syndrome and stable angina.[9,10,14] Odds ratios have shown that patients with mixed plaque are nearly four times as likely to have significant coronary stenosis. A similar odds ratio is observed for diffuse plaque. Among patients with both mixed and diffuse plaque, nearly 92% had clinically significant CAD.[14]

Thus, plaque composition and delineation of obstructive and nonobstructive coronary plaques (Figs 16.4A and B) is an important factor in the evaluation of the true risk of the patient that guides diagnosis, treatment, and prognostication in a way that is meaningful to patients and physicians.

Coronary CT angiography can accurately delineate and characterize coronary plaques. Plaque composition is defined as soft (>75% soft), calcified (>75% calcified), or mixed (<75%

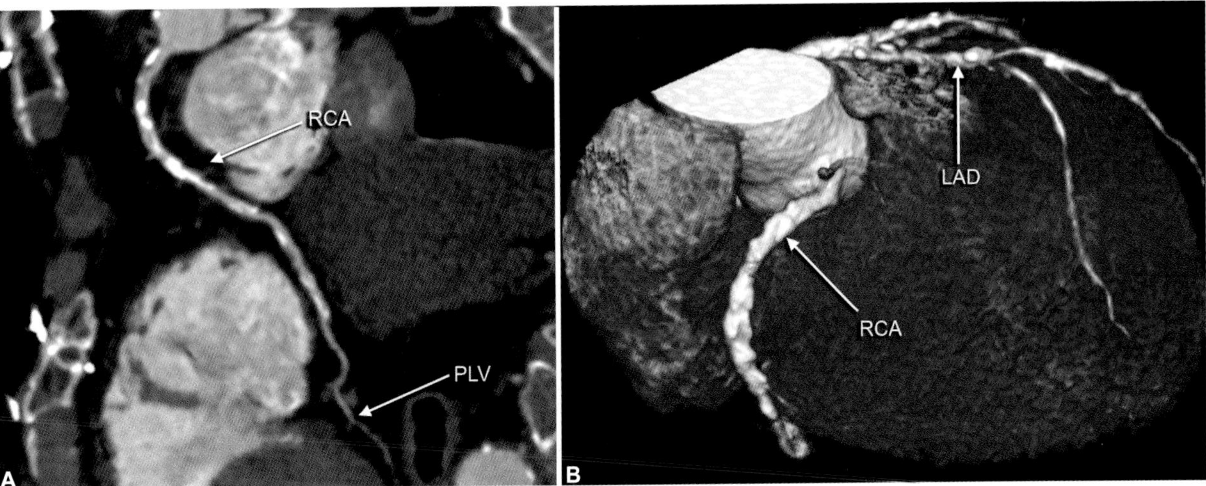

Figs 16.4A and B Curved multiplanar reconstruction (A) and volume-rendered images (B) demonstrate diffuse, mixed atheromatous plaques along the entire length of the right coronary artery (RCA), causing significant 70–80% stenosis in the mid-segment. The posterolateral ventricular (PLV) branch is seen

Abbreviation: LAD, left anterior descending

soft and <75% calcified).[14] A study by Leber et al. showed that soft plaque, intermediate or mixed, and calcified plaques have varying densities and Hounsfield units (HU) with an average density of 49 HU, 91 HU, and 391 HU, respectively. However, components of soft plaque—lipid, fibrous, and/or thrombotic tissues, and water—have HU densities that tend to overlap and hence CT is unable to differentiate these.[15]

Coronary CT angiography by individually tracking each vessel can accurately define plaque distribution, focal i.e. ≤3 discrete sites or diffuse i.e. >3 sites, or ≤3 sites with continuous plaque encompassing more than one third of the vessel. Further stenosis may be mild (<25% stenosis); moderate (25-50% stenosis); or severe (>50% stenosis).[14]

While cardiologists have traditionally evaluated >70% stenosis of the coronary arteries, 86% of people have a <70% stenosis prior to myocardial infarction (MI).[10] Myocardial infarctions can result from low-grade stenosis and majority of noncalcified plaques, often the culprit lesions, result in luminal narrowing of <50%.

Plaque burden, the number of diseased segments, segments with significant CAD, noncalcified (Fig. 16.5) and mixed plaque are significant predictors of events. While CCTA is extremely beneficial, invasive coronary angiography has an extremely limited contribution in this field.

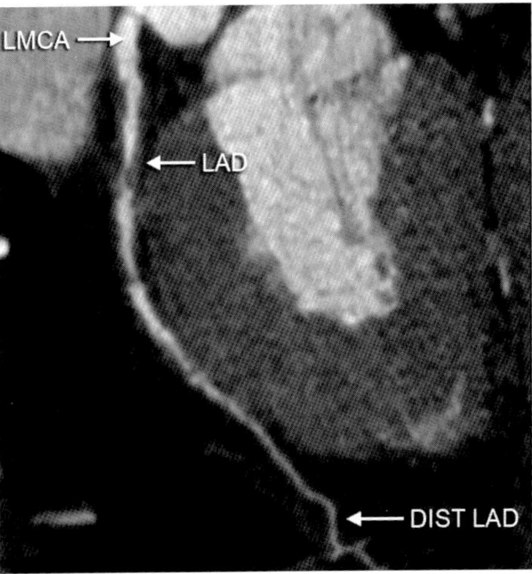

Fig. 16.5 Curved multiplanar reconstruction images demonstrate noncalcified soft plaque causing 70–80% stenosis in the proximal left anterior descending (LAD) artery. The normal left main coronary artery (LMCA) is seen free of atheromatous disease

TECHNICAL DECISION MAKING AND PROCEDURE PLANNING USING CORONARY COMPUTED TOMOGRAPHY ANGIOGRAPHY

Preprocedural knowledge of the complexity of the vascular system, e.g. its course, tortuosity, size, and the length of the vessels, is of enormous benefit to a diagnostic and therapeutic procedure. Recently 3D arterial models have been developed from 2D invasive coronary angiography. Prior CCTA provides identical and valuable information contributing to preprocedural planning of appropriate choice of guidewire, catheter, balloon, and stent[7] (Fig. 16.6). Prior stent sizing may avoid longitudinal misses and provide accurate assessment of the degree of positive and negative remodeling in the axial dimension, which may guide ideal stent diameter and allowable degree of poststent dilatation.

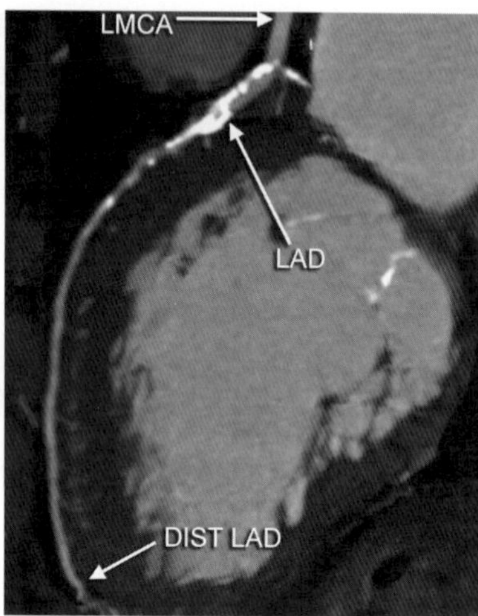

Fig. 16.6 Curved multiplanar reconstruction images demonstrate multiple calcific eccentric plaques causing diffuse long segment 40–60% stenosis with good distal runoff

Abbreviations: LMCA, left main coronary artery; LAD, left anterior descending; DIST LAD distal left anterior descending

Successful intervention to treat a chronic total occlusion is dependent on measure of its length and diameter, tortuosity of the vessel proximal to the lesion, ability to identify the route and course of the totally occluded arterial segment, with visualization of the distal vessel beyond the occlusion, and nature of plaque within the occlusion, which, if heavily calcified, may be a contraindication to the procedure. In general, shorter, less calcified chronic total occlusions are easier to open.[16] Coronary CT angiography is ideally suited to provide all the requisite data. Although angiographic parameters that facilitate or impede stent tracking or delivery are well known, CTA plaque severity and calcification assessment may be helpful in guiding equipment selection besides avoiding trauma to less well-appreciated areas of severe plaque formation.

Currently, CCTA data can be imported into the catheterization laboratory that provides the operator with optimum C-arm orientation from the CTA-determined optimal angiographic views with minimum foreshortening for the given lesion. Benefits of this hybrid approach include decreased fluoroscopy time and radiation exposure, decreased contrast, improved device selection, increased laboratory throughput, and, most importantly, better patient outcomes.[17]

Thus, prior CCTA has positive implications on preprocedural planning that guide technical decision making in complex, multivessel, multilesion interventional procedures in the presence of vessel overlap and bifurcations making them safe and more efficient.

CLINICAL DECISION MAKING

The ultimate goal of imaging is to guide the best therapeutic strategy for patients. Coronary CT angiography has the requisite capability to enable triage of patients to medical therapy or angiographic evaluation, and enable decisions regarding need for revascularization and appropriate choice of revascularization procedure.[2] Various studies confirm a high per-patient sensitivity (85–95%), specificity (96–98%), and negative predictive value (93–100%) of CCTA.[4] Sensitivity and specificity of 64-slice CT for significant coronary stenosis by segment was found to be 95% and 86%, respectively; by artery, 92% and 91%; and by patient, 90% and 95%.[18]

Studies have demonstrated that CCTA correctly excluded obstructive CAD in all patients with angiographically normal vessels at catheterization. Coronary CT angiography helped correctly predict the need for revascularization in 95% of patients with an angiographic diagnosis of CAD and the eventual revascularization procedure in 92% of cases. These statistics demonstrate the excellent performance and safety of CCTA for therapeutic decision making in patients suspected of CAD.[2] Thus, there is a strong potential for reducing unnecessary and inconsequential invasive diagnostic catheterization procedures if CCTA is integrated into the diagnostic algorithm of suspected CAD.[19]

Absence of stenosis in excess of 50% on CTA with maintained adequate minimum luminal area measurements do not warrant stress testing or selective coronary angiography routinely, while presence of stenosis in excess of 75% stenosis in the left main or proximal vessel are an indication for selective coronary angiography with subsequent PCI or CABG as required. Patients with intermediate stenosis in the 50–75% benefit from additional stress testing followed by selective coronary angiography if indicated. Intravascular ultrasound or fractional flow reserve (FFR) measurements may be useful in equivocal cases.[7]

ADDITIONAL ADVANTAGES OF CORONARY COMPUTED TOMOGRAPHY ANGIOGRAPHY

Calcium Scoring

Calcium scoring (CS) is an extremely useful tool for additional risk stratification of asymptomatic patients, given its added advantage to traditional risk assessment. Absence of calcium is linked to a low likelihood of severe future cardiac events; however, a negative CS may be seen in a small proportion of cases associated with noncalcified plaques.[20]

Calcium scoring has been shown to provide important prognostic information in symptomatic patients.[21] The annualized event rate in patients without any coronary calcium was 1.1%, 1.4% at CS 1–99, 3.7% at CS 100–399, and 4.8% at CS

400–999 with 8.5% at CS ≥ 1000.[20] Coronary CT angiography enables quantitation of calcium scoring, an important factor in risk stratification and prognostication of asymptomatic and symptomatic patients of coronary artery disease.

EVALUATION OF MYOCARDIAL PERFUSION

It is now established that mere anatomic assessment of the coronary artery luminal narrowing (lumenography) is not sufficient and that functional assessment for myocardial ischemia is critical for assessing future adverse outcome.[6] Revascularization therapies are most effective when the culprit lesion is identified both anatomically and functionally with demonstrable ischemia.[22] Hybrid imaging with CCTA is possible combining evaluation of coronary anatomy, first-pass and delayed perfusion together with functional imaging, thereby assessing myocardial ischemia and viability. Stress CT perfusion has further additional value for demonstrating stress-induced hemodynamically significant ischemia.[23] Thus, CT can provide the "one stop shop" for coronary evaluation, with stress-rest ischemia testing, function, and viability assessment. CT stress myocardial perfusion imaging has diagnostic accuracy comparable to SPECT.[24]

FRACTIONAL FLOW RESERVE

Fractional flow reserve at the time of invasive coronary angiography is the current gold standard for determination of ischemia. Recent technological innovations enable noninvasive calculation of FFR from CT. Fractional flow reserve CT is superior to anatomic assessment of stenosis in coronary CTA for the diagnosis of ischemia-causing lesions on both a per-patient and a per-vessel basis having a significantly higher diagnostic performance than anatomic assessment alone.[25]

LIMITATION OF CORONARY COMPUTED TOMOGRAPHY ANGIOGRAPHY

Variability in scanner specifications, analysis software, ability and experience of the technologist and interpreting physician are potential factors that impact the performance of CCTA. Further coronary artery calcification, obesity, high and irregular heart rates are known to be challenges that impact CT image acquisition and interpretations.[5]

The spatial resolution of CCTA still does not match invasive angiography, limiting analysis of smaller side branches and distal vessel segments. Also, there is a tendency to overestimate the degree of stenosis in CT as compared with the invasive angiogram. Finally, coronary CT angiography is limited to diagnosis. In patients with a high pretest likelihood of disease, performing an invasive, catheter-based coronary angiogram will often be much more appropriated because it offers the option of immediate treatment.

ADVANCES IN CORONARY COMPUTED TOMOGRAPHY ANGIOGRAPHY ACQUISITIONS

The latest generation of CT scanners provides increased coverage (8–16 cm per rotation) and shorter acquisition times. The newer 256, 320, and 640 slice scanners decrease the likelihood of patient motion, respiration, and heart rate variations that degrade image quality. Improved temporal resolution is seen with faster rotation speeds, while dual source imaging further minimizes motion artifacts. The new detector technology provides improved spatial resolution, and improved image quality. Recent dual energy imaging minimizes the effects of calcified plaque and may allow distinction between types of plaque. Apart from this continuous development in the hardware, smarter acquisition protocols, improved injection profiles and reconstruction softwares have demonstrated a CCTA sensitivity of 96.4%, specificity of 98.5%, and a diagnostic study rate of 96.6%.[17] Overall, these studies have consistently shown a negative predictive value in the 95–99% range.[26] By combining more intelligent acquisition protocols and improved hardware capabilities, some manufacturers predict a complete diagnostic study with <2 mSv.

CONCLUSION

While invasive angiography may have held the position of the clinical gold standard for coronary artery visualization, important quantitative information such as cross-sectional lumen area, size, distribution and composition of plaque, remodeling of the vessel wall, and calcium scoring remain unavailable.[1] It also has several shortcomings due to its projectional nature, besides being an invasive procedure with inherent morbidity and mortality, requiring elaborate equipment, trained staff and associated higher costs.

Coronary CT angiography with its tomographic nature allows for easier and detailed identification of the 3D anatomy of the coronary vessels. Furthermore, its cross-sectional nature permits visualization not only of the contrast-enhanced coronary artery lumen but also of the vessel wall for plaque burden, severity, composition, calcium scoring, and myocardial assessment. In the presence of significant CAD, the number of diseased segments, obstructive segments, segments with noncalcified plaque, and the number of segments with mixed plaque remain independent predictors with incremental prognostic value over clinical variables.

Thus, even if, invasive coronary angiography is to be considered superior to CCTA for the detection of luminal stenosis, today, CCTA offers far more than the mere lumenography, by identifying clinically relevant disease, the patient's true risk of myocardial infarction, and cardiac death. It addresses the critical questions of both patients and physicians by identifying both obstructive and high-risk nonobstructive lesions related to coronary stenosis, guides the management strategy (conservative treatment versus revascularization) and choice of revascularization procedure PCI versus CABG with additional insight into patient prognosis.

REFERENCES

1. Dewey M, Zimmermann E, Deissenrieder F, et al. Noninvasive coronary angiography by 320-row computed tomography with lower radiation exposure and maintained diagnostic accuracy: comparison of results with cardiac catheterization in a head-to-head pilot investigation. Circulation. 2009;120(10):867-75.
2. Moscariello A, Vliegenthart R, Schoepf UJ, et al. Coronary CT angiography versus conventional cardiac angiography for therapeutic decision making in patients with high likelihood of coronary artery disease. Radiology. 2012;265:385-92.
3. Abdulla J, Abildstrom SZ, Gotzsche O, et al. 64-multislice detector computed tomography coronary angiography as potential alternative to conventional coronary angiography: a systematic review and meta-analysis. Eur Heart J. 2007;28(24):3042-50.
4. Miller JM, Rochitte CE, Dewey M, et al. Diagnostic performance of coronary angiography by 64-row CT. N Engl J Med. 2008;359(22):2324-36.
5. Raff GL, Gallagher MJ, O'Neill WW, et al. Diagnostic accuracy of noninvasive coronary angiography using 64-slice spiral computed tomography. J Am Coll Cardiol. 2005;46:552-7.
6. Albert de Roos. Myocardial perfusion imaging with multidetector CT: beyond lumenography. Radiology. 2010;254:321-3.
7. Hecht HS, Roubin G. Usefulness of computed tomographic angiography guided percutaneous coronary intervention. Am J Cardiol. 2007;99(6):871-5.
8. Green NE, Chen SY, Messenger JC, et al. Three-dimensional vascular angiography. Curr Probl Cardiol. 2004;29:104-42.
9. Hausleiter J, Meyer T, Hadamitzky M, et al. Prevalence of noncalcified coronary plaques by 64-slice computed tomography in patients with an intermediate risk for significant coronary artery disease. J Am Coll Cardiol. 2006;48:312-8.
10. Hoffmann U, Moselewski F, Nieman K, et al. Noninvasive assessment of plaque morphology and composition in culprit and stable lesions in acute coronary syndrome and stable lesions in stable angina by multidetector computed tomography. J Am Coll Cardiol. 2006;47:1655-62.
11. Leber AW, Becker A, Knez A, et al. Accuracy of 64-slice computed tomography to classify and quantify plaque volumes in the proximal coronary system (A comparative study using intravascular ultrasound). J Am Coll Cardiol. 2006;47:672-7.
12. Isner JM, Kishel J, Dent KM. Accuracy of angiographic determination of left main coronary arterial narrowing. Circulation. 1981;63:1056-61.
13. Ge J, Liu F, Gorge G, et al. Angiographically "Silent" plaque in the left main coronary artery detected by intravascular ultrasound. Coron Artery Dis. 1995;6:805-10.
14. Min JK. Coronary CTA versus cardiac catheterization: where do we stand today? Suppl Appl Radiol. 2006:32-40.
15. Leber AW, Knez A, von Ziegler F, et al. Quantification of obstructive and nonobstructive coronary lesions by 64-slice computed tomography: a comparative study with quantitative coronary angiography and intravascular ultrasound. J Am Coll Cardiol. 2005;46:147-54.
16. Mollet NR, Hoye A, Lemos PA, et al. Value of pre-procedure multislice computed tomographic coronary angiography to predict outcome of percutaneous recanalization of chronic total occlusions. Am J Cardiol. 2005;95:240-3.
17. Wink O, Hecht HS, Ruijters D. Coronary computed tomographic angiography in the cardiac catheterization laboratory: current applications and future developments. Cardiol Clin. 2009;27(3):513-29.
18. Fine JJ, Hopkins CB, Ruff N, et al. Comparison of accuracy of 64-slice cardiovascular computed tomography with coronary angiography in patients with suspected coronary artery disease. Am J Cardiol. 2006;97:173-4.
19. Chow BJW, Abraham A, Wells GA, et al. Diagnostic accuracy and impact of computed tomographic coronary angiography on utilization of invasive coronary angiography. Circ Cardiovasc Imaging. 2009;2(1):16-23.
20. van Werkhoven JM, Schuijf JD, Gaemperli O, et al. Incremental prognostic value of multi-slice computed tomography coronary angiography over coronary artery calcium scoring in patients with suspected coronary artery disease. Eur Heart J. 2009;30(21):2622-9.
21. Detrano R, Hsiai T, Wang S, et al. Prognostic value of coronary calcification and angiographic stenoses in patients undergoing coronary angiography. J Am Coll Cardiol. 1996;27:285-90.
22. Wijns W, Kolh P. Appropriate myocardial revascularization: a joint viewpoint from an interventional cardiologist and a cardiac surgeon. Eur Heart J. 2009;30(18):2182-5.
23. Rocha-Filho JA, Blankstein R, Shturman LD, et al. Incremental value of adenosine-induced stress myocardial perfusion imaging with dual-source CT at cardiac CT angiography. Radiology. 2010;254(2):410-19.
24. Blankstein R, Shturman LD, Rogers IS, et al. Adenosine-induced stress myocardial perfusion imaging using dual-source cardiac computed tomography. J Am Coll Cardiol. 2009;54(12):1072-84.
25. Grunau GL, Min JK, Leipsic J. Modeling of fractional flow reserve based on coronary CT angiography. Curr Cardiol Rep. 2012;15:336-8.
26. Hecht HS. Applications of multislice coronary computed tomography angiography to percutaneous coronary intervention: how did we ever do without it? Catheter Cardiovasc Interv. 2008;71:490-503.

17

Role of Nuclear Imaging for Damaged Ventricles

Atul Verma, Sanjeev Pandey

Nuclear cardiology is a well-established, noninvasive method for evaluating patients with known or suspected heart disease with very high sensitivity. The clinical utility of myocardial perfusion scintigraphy (MPS) has been well known and globally accepted.[1-5] This chapter describes the role of nuclear imaging in the evaluation of damaged ventricles.

A discordant coronary blood flow and myocardial oxygen demand may lead to myocardial damage. The most important cause of myocardial damage is atherosclerotic heart disease. The other causes include myocarditis, cardiomyopathies, hypertension/afterload mismatch, postoperative stage, sepsis, and toxins.

MYOCARDIAL INFARCTION

Myocardial infarction (MI) is one of the leading causes of myocardial damage leading to heart failure. The most important conditions leading to development and progression of heart failure include myocardial blood flow and sympathetic innervations.

Nuclear cardiology procedures include gated single photon emission computed tomography (G-SPECT) and positron emission tomography (PET) represent one of the important imaging modality for the evaluation of myocardial blood flow. These help in the evaluation, risk stratification, and prognostication of patients with myocardial damage and heart failure especially after acute coronary syndrome (ACS).

123-iodine metaiodobenzyl-guanidine (123-I MIBG) has been used for sympathetic innervations of the failing heart. This helps in the prediction of cardiac arrhythmias and the need of device implants to reduce the sudden cardiac deaths due to ventricular tachycardias. In addition, a number of novel imaging techniques have been developed for the early detection and prediction of heart failure.

ROLE OF NUCLEAR IMAGING IN ACUTE CORONARY SYNDROME

The spectral distribution of acute coronary syndrome (ACS) ranges from ST-segment elevation MI (STEMI), non-ST-elevation MI (NSTEMI) as well as unstable angina. The rupture of atherosclerotic plaque constitutes one of the most important causes of ACS that can lead to either partial or complete thrombosis of the infract-related artery. In such cases, the decision of appropriate therapeutic strategy including the interventional therapy is an urgency for salvaging the myocardium at risk and reduces the mortality and morbidity.

Left ventricular (LV) dysfunction and jeopardized/reversible viable myocardium comprise the two important parameters in the assessment of prognosis of patients with ACS. Both of these parameters can be assessed by nuclear cardiology techniques that help to find out the extent of permanent damage as well as the myocardium at risk with high sensitivity and predictivity. In fact, both the myocardial perfusion and wall motion abnormalities can be seen in the same sitting and can differentiate very well scarred from hibernating and stunned myocardial segments.

Left Ventricular Function

In acute MI, proper assessment of LV dysfunction constitutes a major predictor of patient's outcome. Multicenter Post-infarction Research Group (MPRG) used predischarged radionuclide angiography[6] and found that the 1 year mortality was inversely proportional to left ventricular ejection fraction (LVEF).[7] This was confirmed by CAMI study in the thrombolytic era of the 1990s.[8] It has also been confirmed by many studies that no significant events were reported in patients with LVEF in more than 40% cases. Simoons et al. inferred that in cases with left ventricular ejection fraction less than 30%, the 5-year survival rate was approximately 40% as compared to about 75% when EF is more than 40%.[9]

Nuclear imaging plays an important role in the evaluation of LV dysfunction and EF. This can best be achieved by multigated blood pool acquisition or radionuclide ventriculography (MUGA) as well as the rest gated myocardial perfusion SPECT imaging. Determination of LV function using radionuclide angiography has been shown to be a powerful predictor of outcome in patients who present with an acute MI. With the advent of new solid-state detector gamma cameras, gated myocardial perfusion imaging (G-MPI) can also give adequate LVEFs and volumes. The advantage of G-MPI is that it can simultaneously see myocardial perfusion and myocardial contractility in the same sitting and can very well differentiate myocardial infarction, hibernation, and stunning in patients with ACS and thus provides a very important information to the cardiologists to plan the intervention or treat by medical management.

Jeopardized Viable Myocardium

Nuclear myocardial perfusion imaging provides an accurate identification and quantification of jeopardized viable myocardium that helps in the risk stratification after acute MI. The advantages of nuclear MPS for the evaluation after MI include:

1. High sensitivity for the detection of ischemia.
2. High prognostic value by accurate risk stratification.
3. Evaluation of myocardial viability.
4. Evaluation of myocardial perfusion and myocardial contractility in the same sitting, thus differentiating MI, myocardial hibernation, and myocardial stunning with the adequate LV function.
5. Early risk stratification by the use of vasodilator stress.

The presence of transient perfusion defect, its extent, as well as the severity of ischemia predicts the future cardiac events and helps in the decision making for the intervention.[10,11] Ladenheim et al. found that among clinical and scintigraphic indices, the number of reversible perfusion defects on stress thallium-201 images was the best predictor of future cardiac events.[12]

ACUTE ST-SEGMENT ELEVATION MYOCARDIAL INFARCTION

G-MPI plays a very important role in the diagnosis, risk assessment, and prognostication in patients with acute MI. Gibson et al.[13] were the first to report the prognostic value of stress MPI in the post-acute myocardial infarction period. The submaximal stress Tl-201 MPS after acute STEMI was conducted and compared with clinical evaluation, exercise, and coronary angiography for the prediction of future cardiac events.

The study inferred that reversible myocardial defects especially involving multiple coronary territories and presence of lung uptake were the most important prognostic markers on MPI and detect patients at risk with very high sensitivity. This helps in discrimination of low-risk patients who do not require intervention with high sensitivity. Subsequently, many studies confirmed the prognostic value of exercise MPI in patients presenting with an acute MI.[10,11] Wilson et al.[14] demonstrated that in patients with acute MI and single-vessel disease, future cardiac events were related to the presence and extent of transient defects on submaximal exercise MPI but not to clinical or exercise electrocardiographic data. A rest G-SPECT MPI using Tc99m MIBI was able to rule out ACS in emergency department with a high negative predictive value (>99%) and to rule out any evidence of MI.[14-22]

Kontos et al.[17,18] studied 361 patients who got admitted in the emergency department within 6 hours of symptoms. In their study only two patients (0.6%) with a negative MPS results had MI within 5 days of hospitalization. In a study involving six centers, Heller et al. found only 1% (2 out of 204) with normal myocardial perfusion had acute MI during the hospital stay.[15] A rest G-MPS SPECT is capable of depicting the future adverse cardiac events with utmost accuracy.

The negative predictive value of a rest G-MPS study has a very important role in discriminating myocardial scar from myocardial hibernation and stunning. This is because of simultaneous visualization of myocardial perfusion and myocardial contractility in the same sitting. A grossly hypocontractile/akinetic LV segment with maintained myocardial perfusion infers myocardial stunning, whereas concordant hypoperfusion and hypocontractility of myocardial segment refer to myocardial hibernation.

The INSPIRE study, a multinational clinical trial, was performed in 728 patients to find out the role of SPECT radionuclide myocardial perfusion scanning for the risk assessment of stable patients after MI within 10 days of the episode. It included same day nitrate enhanced rest MPI and stress imaging with adenosine. They inferred that coronary angiography can be safely avoided in cases with defect size ≤20% and ischemic burden ≤10% with preserved LV function.[23-25]

There is also the role of ischemic memory imaging in ACS. In many cases of ACS, metabolic stunning can be present. In fact in ACS, normalization of myocardial blood flow is preceded by restoration of coronary blood flow and this can take many hours. This process of metabolic alteration is described as ischemic memory or metabolic stunning. This metabolic phase can be used to evaluate patients in whom the chest pain has subsided upon arrival to the emergency department. Radioactive glucose (FDG) PET imaging demonstrates selective tracer uptake in stunned myocardium if the patient is injected at a fasting state.[26-28]

Ischemic memory imaging has been tested with I-123 BMIPP SPECT, a free fatty acid analogue.[29,30] It has confirmed the incremental prognostic value of residual jeopardized viable myocardium post-MI. It has got the incremental prognostic value of jeopardized viable myocardium post-MI. In addition to myocardial perfusion, I123-BMIPP is also sensitive to metabolic changes induced by ischemia.[26] I-123 BMIPP SPECT images are the mirror images of FDG: normal myocardium concentrates I-123 BMIPP, whereas stunned myocardium does not. When imaged in conjunction with resting 201Tl imaging, a mismatch in uptake (normal 201Tl uptake, reduced 123I-BMIPP uptake) indicates an area of myocardium with normal resting flow but with a recent history of ischemic insult. Kawai et al.[31,32] have shown the potential use of I-123 BMIPP ischemic memory imaging in the emergency department.

In a group of 111 patients with ACS who underwent I-123 BMIPP SPECT and coronary angiography within 1–4 days and found the sensitivity and specificity of 74% and 92%, respectively, for obstructive coronary disease or spasm, Nanasato et al.[33] found that in patients with acute STEMI, 123I-BMIPP–201Tl mismatch and total 123I-BMIPP defect score added significant prognostic value to LV function and extent of angiographic coronary artery disease (CAD) for predicting cardiac events. All the patients underwent primary coronary intervention.

It has also been shown by two randomized studies[19,21] that a rest SPECT myocardial perfusion scintigraphic studies reduced healthcare costs and length of hospital stay. First study by Stowers et al.[19] have shown a reduction in hospital costs by $1843 for patients in hospitals where SPECT imaging was present. The second study (Erase Chest Pain) that is randomized study and in which 2475 patients were enrolled from seven institutions showed that hospital stay was reduced by 10% where rest SPECT myocardial perfusion studies were performed (reduced from 52% to 42%). But the logistic constraints included that the nuclear cardiology services should be available round the clock because of the importance of timing of the injection that should be done at the time or within few hours of the episode.

Another approach is rubidium-82 (^{82}Rb) myocardial perfusion PET that provides good accuracy and reduced imaging times. It mimics thallium-201 in kinetics except that myocardial extraction fraction is less than Tl201. In a retrospective study, which included 1177 patients who presented with chest pain, underwent rest/stress ^{82}Rb myocardial perfusion PET.[34] Out of the total cases, 95.4% had normal images and 4.6% had abnormal images. Of the abnormal group, 52% had obstructive CAD at coronary angiography, while 41% were confirmed to have ACS by clinical assessment.

There are various indirect prognostic markers associated with radionuclide MPS, which include:

1. Increased 201Tl lung uptake on exercise MPI has been shown to reflect stress-induced rises in LV filling pressure[35,36] and has been associated with severe CAD and resting and exercise-induced LV dysfunction.
2. Transient LV dilation on stress compared with rest imaging also has been related to extensive CAD and LV dysfunction, and has been associated with increased risk of cardiac events.[37-39]
3. Prominence of right ventricular cavity on stress.

UNSTABLE ANGINA AND NON–ST-SEGMENT ELEVATION MYOCARDIAL INFARCTION

Patients with unstable angina or NSTEMI are another ACS cohort for whom traditional management has involved an aggressive invasive approach because of the presumption that the syndrome is an immediate precursor to MI (unstable angina) or is associated with an incomplete and unstable infarction (NSTEMI).

Nuclear cardiology plays an important role in the risk stratification and the need of aggressive interventional approach in patients with unstable angina as well as non-Q or non-ST elevation MI. The symptomatic patients were first stabilized by medicines and then subjected to stress MPI. It is valid to find out the role of stress MPI in the risk stratification once the patient stabilizes. Various studies have been done to validate the need of stress MPI. Risk stratification in patients with unstable angina first was evaluated by Hillert et al. who performed submaximal exercise 201Tl-MPI in patients with unstable angina and stabilized over a 12-week follow-up period. Amongst them, 15 of 19 patients with reversible defects developed MI or had class III or IV angina compared with only 2 of 18 patients without reversible defects ($P < 0.001$).[40] In a larger series of 158 patients admitted with an acute non-MI coronary syndrome, an acute MI or cardiac death occurred in 21% of patients with reversible exercise 201Tl defects compared with only 3% without reversible defects over a median 14-month follow-up period.[41] When compared with Holter, electrocardiography, stress electrocardiography, and cardiac catheterization data, the extent of reversible defects on MPI was the only significant multivariate predictor of cardiac events.[42]

Brown[43] has described a series of 52 patients presenting with unstable angina who responded to initial medical treatment and underwent exercise 201Tl-MPI before discharge. The only significant multivariate predictor of cardiac death or MI over a 39-month follow-up period was the presence of reversible defects. Cardiac death or MI occurred in 26% of patients with reversible defects compared with only 3% of patients without reversible defects (<1% annual rate).

NON–ST-SEGMENT ELEVATION MYOCARDIAL INFARCTION

The symptoms of NSTEMI are similar to unstable angina Not all such infarctions are subendocardial or incomplete. Pathologic studies have shown that although the infarcts tend to be smaller, the transmural distribution is not much different from Q-wave or STEMI.[44] The smaller size of the non–Q-wave infarction is associated with a higher frequency of residual jeopardized viable myocardium that makes it feasible for intervention. Gibson et al.[45] have evaluated clinical and stress MPI results in patients with acute non–Q-wave MI and found that infarct zone reversible defects were present in 60% of patients compared with 36% with Q-wave MI ($P < 0.01$). Only 1 of 35 (3%) non–Q-wave MI patients without infarct zone reversibility on MPI developed recurrent MI over a mean 27-month follow-up period compared with 15 of 52 patients (29%) with infarct zone reversibility. Stress MPI also has predictive value in patients with NSTEMI and atypical presentation. In a series of 156 patients with elevated troponin levels but without typical symptoms or ischemic electrocardiogram, changes, an abnormal stress MPI was associated with a sevenfold increase in the annual cardiac death or MI rate compared with patients with normal stress MPI (12.5% vs. 1.7%; $P = 0.02$).[46] The TIMI IIIB trial examined the effect of thrombolysis and the possible benefit of an early nonselective invasive strategy in 1473 patients with unstable angina or non–Q-wave MI.[47] Thrombolysis was harmful in this cohort, with a higher incidence of fatal and nonfatal MI (7.4%) compared with placebo (4.9%; $P < 0.05$).

Cardiomyopathy

The definition proposed by American Heart Association (AHA) consensus panel defines cardiomyopathies as a heterogeneous group of diseases of the myocardium associated with mechanical and/or electrical dysfunction that usually exhibit inappropriate ventricular hypertrophy or dilatation. They are confined to the heart or are part of generalized systemic disorders, often leading to cardiovascular death or progressive heart failure-related disability. The important question lies in the differentiation of ischemic from nonischemic cardiomyopathies. Nuclear cardiac imaging has got a role in takotsubo cardiomyopathy.

It includes ballooning of LV apical wall that can mimic acute MI and is associated with significant ST-T changes simulating myocardial ischemic changes. In all such cases, coronary angiography showed normal coronaries. Also it is associated with significantly increased plasma catecholamine levels.[69] Many studies tried to find out the role of nuclear MPI studies in takotsubo cardiomyopathy.

Ito et al.[70] performed the serial resting MPI imaging in 10 patients with takotsubo cardiomyopathy. All patients had normal angiographic coronaries but resting G-MPI showed apical perfusion defects acutely. This perfusion defect got resolved at 3–9 days and 1 month later as seen on the serial nuclear G-MPI that also showed improved wall motion abnormalities. The authors speculated that impaired microcirculation was a causative factor. At 5 days after presentation, radionuclide imaging with iodine-123-beta-methyl-iodophenyl-pentadecanoic (I123 BMIPP), a tracer for myocardial fatty acid, showed more extensive defects than resting 201Tl-MPI, consistent with metabolic changes caused by an ischemic insult. The 123I-BMIPP defects resolved with serial imaging over 30 days. Burgdorf et al.[71] also imaged rest G-MPI and 123-I MIBG imaging in 10 patients with takotsubo cardiomyopathy. They found decreased apical MIBG cardiac uptake and rapid washout consistent with alterations in cardiac presynaptic washout and elevated norepinephrine levels in patients with this syndrome who showed decreased 123I-BMIPP uptake consistent with an ischemic insult. Such neurohumeral abnormalities may play an important role in the pathophysiologic mechanism of this condition. Similar findings were reported by Uchida et al.[72]

NUCLEAR IMAGING IN HEART FAILURE

Heart failure represents a very important condition with markedly increased morbidity and mortality rates. The AHA statistics and stroke statistics committee showed that the estimated life-time risk for the development of heart failure is about 20% at the age of 40 years.[48] A number of underlying mechanisms have been identified in heart failure. One of the important factor is sympathetic denervation that can result in cardiac arrhythmias, which can be life threatening. In such cases, the decision to put an implantable cardioverter-defibrillator (ICD) device is an important aspect. MPS plays an important role in the diagnosis and prognostication in heart failure.[49] The sympathetic innervations imaging is coming up in a big way and can be used in heart failure for risk stratification. A considerable improvement in nuclear imaging technology has changed the paradigm from assessment of myocardial perfusion and sympathetic innervation to the characterization of molecular processes at the cardiac tissue level. Moreover, an increasing number of molecular-targeted radiotracers is now being introduced that may extend the current possibilities for molecular imaging of biologic processes. The improvement in technology like solid-state SPECT gamma cameras, hybrid imaging using SPECT-CT, and PET-CT as well as improvements in software like resolution recovery and 3D iterative reconstruction facilitate the high-resolution images and hence increased sensitivity, specificity as well as predictivity.[50] The myocardial blood flow and viability can be assessed by SPECT and PET. The various radiopharmaceuticals used include:

SPECT Tracers (Kinetic Properties)

1. *Thallium-201 (^{201}Tl as thallous chloride)*: Acts through $Na^{+}K^{+}$ ATPase system.
2. *^{99m}Technetium (^{99m}Tc)- Sesta MIBI (methoxyisobutyl)/ tetrofosmin (1,2-bis[di-(2-ethoxyethyl) phosphino] ethane)*: Binds at the mitochondrial level.

PET Tracers (Kinetic Properties)

1. *^{13}N NH_3*: Metabolic trapping
2. *^{82}Rb*: Na/K ATPase channel
3. *^{15}O H_2O*: Freely diffusible
4. *^{18}F BMS747158*: Binds to mitochondrial complex-1.

Although myocardial perfusion SPECT is still the clinical mainstay, PET imaging is being increasingly utilized in clinical cardiovascular imaging practice. It has been shown that PET imaging allows accurate detection of significant CAD, which may be superior to SPECT imaging in particular subsets of patients such as the differentiation of ischemic v/s nonischemic cardiomyopathy.[51] The high temporal resolution of PET has the upper hand over SPECT for the absolute quantification of myocardial blood flow and flow reserve thus helping in the identification of ischemic cardiomyopathy. However, the advent of solid-state detector SPECT technology and the image resolution has improved comparable to PET.

The PET tracers as approved by the US Food and Drug Administration (FDA) and commonly used include N-13 ammonia ($^{13}NH_3$) and ^{82}Rb for myocardial perfusion and ^{18}F-fluorodeoxyglucose (FDG) for metabolism. Both $^{13}NH_3$ and ^{82}Rb can be used for the absolute quantification of myocardial blood flow as well as relative regional perfusion analysis. O-15 because of its first pass myocardial extraction fraction of 100% is considered to be most ideal to evaluate myocardial blood flow as well as coronary flow reserve. Also F-18-labeled compound BMS747158 (^{18}F-BMS) is considered another high potent tracer for myocardial flow imaging as it shows a first-pass extraction percentage exceeding 90%.[52,53]

Early studies demonstrated that flow-metabolism studies by PET using ^{13}N-labeled ammonia ($^{13}NH_3$) and the glucose analog FDG acquired after an oral glucose load can distinguish scars and viable myocardial segments. Regions that showed a concordant reduction in both myocardial blood flow and FDG uptake ("flow-metabolism match") were indicative of scar with no reversible viability, whereas regions in which FDG uptake was relatively preserved or increased despite having a perfusion defect ("flow-metabolism mismatch") were considered ischemic but still viable. These studies were having a lot of limitations that include the dietary status, LVEF, sympathetic innervations, and ischemic burden. Many such patients are insulin resistant that can hinder the maximum stimulation of myocardial glucose/FDG uptake. To reduce these problems, the role of hyperinsulinemic euglycemic clamp came into existence although cumbersome but with good effects. In this there is a gross reduction in plasma-free fatty acids and thus the insulin-sensitive tissue switches to glucose use. This results in good uptake of FDG even in patients with insulin resistance. This has been proved by European multicenter study.

CARDIAC AUTONOMIC IMAGING WITH SPECT TRACERS

An important aspect in heart failure is the role of neurohormonal system. This includes sympathetic nervous system as well as the renin–angiotensin–aldosterone axis (RAS). In heart failure, the reduction in cardiac output results in the activation of sympathetic nervous system by baroreceptors of the left ventricle, aortic arch, and carotid sinus, thus leading to increased peripheral vasoconstriction, heart rate, as well as the improved myocardial contractility.[54,55] Also reduction in effective renal arterial perfusion activates RAS that helps in maintaining the cardiac output by providing positive inotropic and chronotropic support to the dysfunctional heart. RAS activation leads to the retention of sodium and water and its direct action on arterial smooth muscle leading to vasoconstriction. This leads to the preservation of systemic arterial pressure. Thus, we see that sympathetic stimulation is one of the main compensatory mechanisms in the failing heart. As the heart failure progresses, cardiac stores of norepinephrine are depleted, but circulating norepinephrine concentration is elevated. This has direct effect on degree of LV dysfunction and life-threatening risk. Cardiac sympathetic nerve imaging with 123-I MIBG has often presently been used for the assessment of cardiac innervation. A large number of studies have shown that an abnormal myocardial sympathetic innervation, as assessed with 123-I MIBG imaging, is associated with increased mortality and morbidity rates in patients with heart failure. It also helps in the risk stratification for ventricular arrhythmias or sudden cardiac death. In fact this imaging is the better predictor than myocardial perfusion as well as the EF in the assessment for the need of device implantation.

The production, uptake, and release of norepinephrine from the presynaptic cleft are the mediators for the function of sympathetic nervous system. The uptake-1 (neuronal) and uptake-2 (non-neuronal) mechanisms are the controlling mechanisms for the amount of norepinephrine within the presynaptic cleft once tyrosine gets converted to norepinephrine. This gets cleared from the synaptic clefts by either the norepinephrine transporter (NET) protein (uptake-1) or sodium-dependent non-neuronal transport mechanism (uptake-2). These can be used for nuclear cardiological imaging of sympathetic innervations and activation patterns in heart failure.[56,57] Both SPECT and PET can perform the above said imaging and can assess the probability of life-threatening cardiac arrhythmias. Viable myocardium with reduced or absent sympathetic innervations can result in triggering of cardiac arrhythmias.[58,59]

There are several studies to assess the role of cardiac 123-I MIBG imaging for prediction of ventricular arrhythmias, sudden cardiac death, or appropriate ICD before discharge.[60,61] Jacobson et al.[62] evaluated 961 patients with heart failure and inferred after the median follow-up of 17 months that patients with preserved myocardial sympathetic innervation (H/M ratio ≥1.60) had significantly less arrhythmic events when compared to patients depressed sympathetic innervation (H/M ratio <1.60) (HR 0.37, 95% CI 0.16–0.85, P = 0.02). In addition, regional abnormalities in sympathetic innervation are also likely to play a role in the development of ventricular tachyarrhythmias.

The role of cardiac sympathetic nerve imaging with 123-I MIBG was also evaluated in 116 patients with advanced heart failure who were clinically referred for ICD implantation.[64] Patients with ventricular arrhythmias causing appropriate ICD discharge (primary endpoint) showed significantly more regional sympathetic denervation (as expressed in summed 123-I MIBG SPECT defect score) when compared to patients without appropriate ICD discharge (P<0.05). Moreover, late 123-I MIBG SPECT defect score was independently associated with the occurrence of appropriate ICD discharges (HR 1.13, 95% CI 1.05–1.21, P<0.01).

Tamaki et al.[63] evaluated 106 patients with chronic heart failure and LVEF<40% with the aim to determine the value of 123-I MIBG imaging for the prediction of sudden arrhythmic death in 106 outpatients with chronic heart failure and LVEF<40%. Patients with sudden cardiac death showed significantly lower early (1.72 ± 0.29 vs. 1.87 ± 0.26, P = 0.036) and late (1.54 ± 0.25 vs. 1.76 ± 0.31, P<0.01) H/M ratio as well as significantly higher myocardial washout rate (39.9 ± 15.2% vs. 27.6 ± 14.2%, P<0.01) than patients who survived the mean follow-up of 65 ± 31 months. Importantly, only myocardial washout rate (HR = 1.052, 95% CI 1.020–1.085, P<0.01) and LVEF (HR = 0.930, 95% CI 0.870–0.995, P = 0.0341) were independent predictors for sudden arrhythmic death.

Abnormal MIBG uptake occurs in patients with ventricular tachycardia even in absence of CAD and its uptake is reduced in 85% of patients in arrhythmogenic right ventricular dysplasias. In addition to I123-MIBG SPECT, a number of PET radiotracers are used for neuronal imaging. These include radiolabeled catecholamines and radiolabeled catecholamine analogs.

1. *Radiolabeled catecholamines* mimic endogenous neurotransmitters and hence undergo similar uptake, release, and metabolic pathways within the myocardium and sympathetic neurons.
2. *Radiolabeled catecholamine analogs* (also referred to as false neurotransmitters) mimic uptake and release mechanisms but not metabolized.

Hydroxyephedrine labeled with carbon-11 (^{11}C-HED) constitutes one of the most frequently used PET tracers for cardiac sympathetic nerve imaging because of its high affinity for the uptake-1 transporter located on the presynaptic nerve terminal. Also it can be used to determine neuronal function. Hartmann et al.[65] in a group of 29 patients with severely dilated cardiomyopathy and heart failure with 8 normals as the control group. They assessed cardiac sympathetic innervation patterns. Gated blood-pool imaging was performed to obtain LV systolic function. In all patients, the PET imaging protocol consisted of a resting perfusion scan with $^{13}NH_3$ combined with a dynamic PET scan using ^{11}C-HED. It was reported that global retention of ^{11}C-HED was significantly lower in patients diagnosed with heart failure when compared to the healthy control patients [6.2 (1.6) %/min vs. 10.7 (1.0) %/min, P<0.01]. Also significant regional neuronal defects in apical (P<0.01) and inferoapical (P<0.05) myocardial segments of patients with heart failure were also demonstrated by PET imaging. In these segments, the ^{11}C-HED/perfusion ratio showed a progressive and significant (P<0.05) decline when compared to the basal cardiac segments.

Nuclear cardiac imaging has also tried to explore cardiac reinnervation in patients with cardiac transplants.[66] Cardiac reinnervation was observed in a study by Bengel et al.[66] in patients with previous orthotopic heart transplantation by PET imaging using ^{11}C-HED. In a group of 27 patients, about 50% showed cardiac innervations. Di Carli[68] also studied ^{11}C-HED PET imaging in 14 asymptomatic patients previous with previous cardiac transplants and showed that cardiac innervations was maximum in the myocardial areas supplied by left anterior descending coronary artery. Furthermore, novel nuclear imaging techniques are being used for the risk stratification and the need for device implantation that may provide more detailed information for the detection of heart failure in an early phase as well as for monitoring the effects of new therapeutic interventions in patients with heart failure.

FUTURE PROSPECTS OF NUCLEAR IMAGING IN HEART FAILURE

In addition, a number of molecular targeted tracers are being evaluated that targets on:

1. Prediction of early development of heart failure.
2. Novel therapeutic interventions.

It has been demonstrated that matrix metalloproteinases, which are proteolytic enzymes, play an important role in remodeling of the heart.[67] Also the role of novel therapeutic interventions such as gene and cell therapy has come into picture. This happened because of better understanding of the heart failure etiology and pathophysiology. Presently In-111 oxin and ^{18}F-fluorodeoxyglucose for nuclear imaging have been used to label therapeutic cells.

Some of the SPECT images (Figs 17.1 to 17.3) are attached herewith using different protocols.

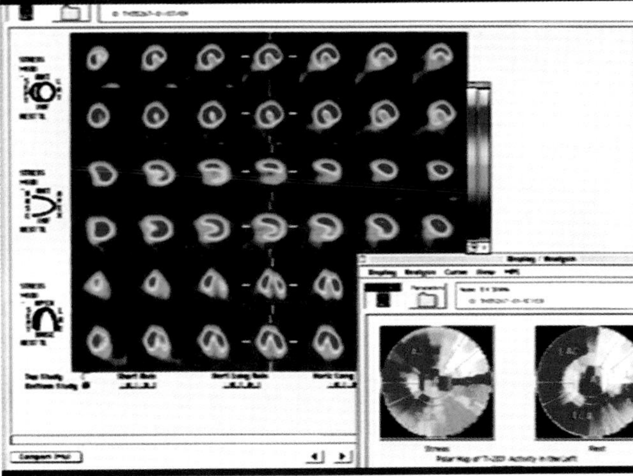

Fig. 17.1 Dual Isotope Protocol: Ischemia in apical, inferior, and inferolateral walls

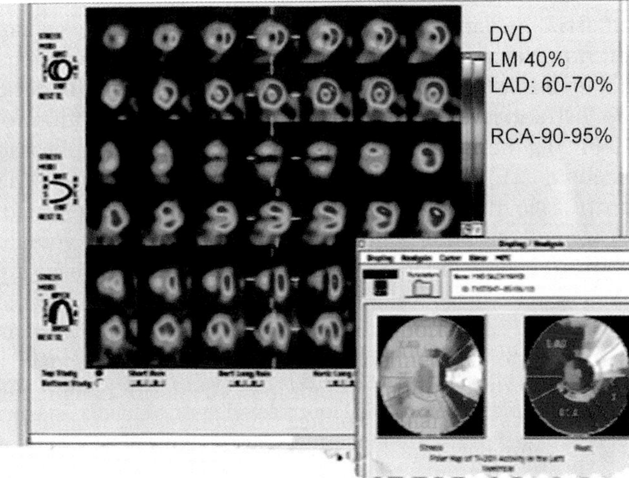

Fig. 17.2 Ischemia in anterior, apical, septal/anteroseptal and inferior walls

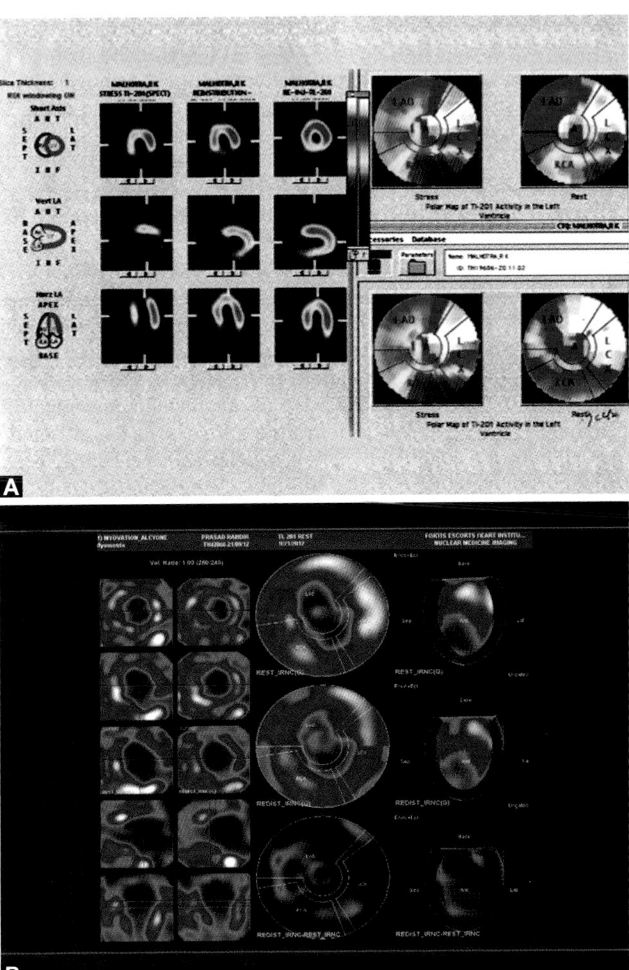

Figs 17.3A and B Rest-redistribution thallium-201 study: Ischemic cardiomyopathy

REFERENCES

1. Klocke FJ, Baird MG, Lorell BH, et al. ACC/AHA/ASNC guidelines for the clinical use of cardiac radionuclide imaging—executive summary: A report of the American College of Cardiology/American Heart Association Task Force on Practice Guidelines (ACC/AHA/ASNC Committee to Revise the 1995 Guidelines for the Clinical Use of Radionuclide Imaging). J Am Coll Cardiol. 2003;42:1318-33.
2. Shaw LJ, Iskandrian AE. Prognostic value of gated myocardial perfusion SPECT. J Nucl Cardiol. 2004;11:171-85.
3. Hamad EA, Travin MI. The complementary roles of radionuclide myocardial perfusion imaging and cardiac computed tomography. Semin Roentgenol. 2012;47:228-39.

4. Iskander S, Iskandrian AE. Risk assessment using single-photon emission computed tomographic technetium-99m sestamibi imaging. J Am Coll Cardiol. 1998;32:57-62.
5. Hachamovitch R, Berman DS, Shaw LJ. Incremental prognostic value of myocardial perfusion single photon emission computed tomography for the prediction of cardiac death: differential stratification for risk of cardiac death and myocardial infarction. See comment in PubMed Commons below Circulation. 1998; 97(6):535-43.
6. Risk stratification and survival after myocardial infarction. The Multicenter Post Infarction Research Group. N Engl J Med. 1983;309:331-6.
7. Zaret BL, Wackers FJ, Terrin ML, et al. Value of radionuclide rest and exercise left ventricular ejection fraction in assessing survival of patients after thrombolytic therapy for acute myocardial infarction: Results of Thrombolysis in Myocardial Infarction (TIMI) phase II study. The TIMI Study Group. J Am Coll Cardiol. 1995;26:73-9.
8. Rouleau JL, Talajik M, Sussex B, et al. Myocardial infarction patients in the 1990s their risk factors, stratification and survival in Canada: The Canadian Assessment of Myocardial Infarction (CAMI) Study. J Am Coll Cardiol. 1996;27:1119-27.
9. Simoons ML, Vos J, Tijssen JG, et al. Long-term benefit of early thrombolytic therapy in patients with acute myocardial infarction: 5-year follow-up of a trial conducted by the Interuniversity Cardiology Institute of the Netherlands. J Am Coll Cardiol. 1989;14:1609-15.
10. Brown KA. Prognostic value of thallium-201 myocardial perfusion imaging: A diagnostic tool comes to age. Circulation. 1991;83:363-81.
11. Brown KA. Prognostic value of myocardial perfusion imaging: state of the art and new developments. J Nucl Cardiol. 1996;3: 516-37.
12. Ladenheim ML, Pollack BH, Royanski A, et al. Extent and severity of myocardial reperfusion as predictors of prognosis in patients with suspected coronary artery disease. J Am Coll Cardiol. 1986;7:464-71.
13. Gibson RS, Watson DD, Craddock GB, et al. Prediction of cardiac events after uncomplicated myocardial infarction: A prospective study comparing predischarge exercise thallium-201 scintigraphy and coronary angiography. Circulation. 1983;68:321-36.
14. Wilson WW, Gibson RS, Nygaard TW, et al. Acute myocardial infarction associated with single vessel coronary artery disease: an analysis of clinical outcome and the prognostic importance of vessel patency and residual ischemic myocardium. J Am Coll Cardiol. 1988;11:223-34.
15. Heller GV, Stowers SA, Hendel RC, et al. Clinical value of acute rest technetium-99 m tetrofosmin tomographic myocardial perfusion imaging in patients with acute chest pain and nondiagnostic electrocardiograms. J Am Coll Cardiol. 1998;31:1011-7.
16. Hilton TC, Thompson RC, Williams HJ, et al. Technetium-99 m sestamibi myocardial perfusion imaging in the emergency room evaluation of chest pain. J Am Coll Cardiol. 1994;23:1016-22.
17. Kontos MC, Jesse RL, Anderson FP, et al. Comparison of myocardial perfusion imaging and cardiac troponin I in patients admitted to the emergency department with chest pain. Circulation. 1999;99:2073-8.
18. Kontos MC, Jesse RL, Schmidt KL, et al. Value of acute rest sestamibi perfusion imaging for evaluation of patients admitted to the emergency department with chest pain. J Am Coll Cardiol. 1997;30:976-82.
19. Stowers SA, Eisenstein EL, Th Wackers FJ, et al. An economic analysis of an aggressive diagnostic strategy with single photon emission computed tomography myocardial perfusion imaging and early exercise stress testing in emergency department patients who present with chest pain but nondiagnostic electrocardiograms: results from a randomized trial. Ann Emerg Med. 2000;35:17-25.
20. Tatum JL, Jesse RL, Kontos MC, et al. Comprehensive strategy for the evaluation and triage of the chest pain patient. Ann Emerg Med. 1997;29:116-25.
21. Udelson JE, Beshansky JR, Ballin DS, et al. Myocardial perfusion imaging for evaluation and triage of patients with suspected acute cardiac ischemia: a randomized controlled trial. JAMA. 2002;288:2693-2700.
22. Varetto T, Cantalupi D, Altieri A, et al. Emergency room technetium-99m sestamibi imaging to rule out acute myocardial ischemic events in patients with nondiagnostic electrocardiograms. J Am Coll Cardiol. 1993;22:1804-8.
23. Mahmarian JJ, Dakik HA, Filipchuk NG, et al. An initial strategy of intensive medical therapy is comparable to that of coronary revascularization for suppression of scintigraphic ischemia in high-risk but stable survivors of acute myocardial infarction. J Am Coll Cardiol. 2006;48:2458-67.
24. Mahmarian JJ, Shaw LJ, Filipchuk NG, et al. A multinational study to establish the value of early adenosine technetium-99m sestamibi myocardial perfusion imaging in identifying a low-risk group for early hospital discharge after acute myocardial infarction. J Am Coll Cardiol. 2006;48:2448-57.
25. Mahmarian JJ, Shaw LJ, Olszewski GH, et al. Adenosine sestamibi SPECT post-infarction evaluation (INSPIRE) trial: a randomized, prospective multicenter trial evaluating the role of adenosine Tc-99m sestamibi SPECT for assessing risk and therapeutic outcomes in survivors of acute myocardial infarction. J Nucl Cardiol. 2004;11:458-69.
26. Chikamori T, Yamashina A, Hida S, et al. Diagnostic and prognostic value of BMIPP imaging. J Nucl Cardiol. 2007;14:111-25.
27. Abbott BG, Liu YH, Arrighi JA. [18F]Fluorodeoxyglucose as a memory marker of transient myocardial ischaemia. Nucl Med Commun. 2007;28:89-94.
28. He ZX, Shi RF, Wu YJ, et al. Direct imaging of exercise-induced myocardial ischemia with fluorine-18-labeled deoxyglucose and Tc-99m-sestamibi in coronary artery disease. Circulation. 2003; 108:1208-13.
29. Jain D, He ZX. Direct imaging of myocardial ischemia: a potential new paradigm in nuclear cardiovascular imaging. J Nucl Cardiol. 2008;15:617-30.
30. Dilsizian V, Bateman TM, Bergmann SR, et al. Metabolic imaging with beta-methyl-p-[(123)I]-iodophenyl-pentadecanoic acid identifies ischemic memory after demand ischemia. Circulation. 2005;112:2169-74.
31. Kawai Y, Morita K, Nozaki Y, et al. Diagnostic value of 123I-beta-methyl-piodophenyl- pentadecanoic acid (BMIPP) single photon emission computed tomography (SPECT) in patients with chest pain. Comparison with rest-stress 99mTc-tetrofosmin SPECT and coronary angiography. Circ J. 2004;68:547-52.
32. Kawai Y, Tsukamoto E, Nozaki Y, et al. Significance of reduced uptake of iodinated fatty acid analogue for the evaluation of

patients with acute chest pain. J Am Coll Cardiol. 2001;38: 1888-94.
33. Nanasato M, Hirayama H, Ando A, et al. Incremental predictive value of myocardial scintigraphy with 123I-BMIPP in patients with acute myocardial infarction treated with primary percutaneous coronary intervention. Eur J Nucl Med Mol Imaging. 2004;31:1512-21.
34. Moore B, Pitts S, Sasson C, et al. Chest pain evaluation in the emergency department: A new application for positron emission tomographic [PET} Rb-82 myocardial perfusion imaging. J Nucl Med. 2007;48 (Suppl 2):213P.
35. Boucher CA, Zir LM, Beller GA, et al. Increased lung uptake of thallium-201 during exercise myocardial imaging: Clinical, hemodynamic and angiographic implications in patients with coronary artery disease. Am J Cardiol. 1980;46:189-96.
36. Brown KA, McKay R, Heller GV, et al. Hemodynamic determinants of lung thallium-201 uptake in patients during atrial pacing stress. Am Heart J. 1986;111:103-7.
37. Lette J, Lapointe J, Waters D, et al. Transient left ventricular cavity dilation during dipyridamole-thallium imaging as an indicator of severe coronary artery disease. Am J Cardiol. 1990;66:1163-70.
38. Stolzenberg J. Dilatation of left ventricular cavity on stress thallium scans as an indicator of ischemic disease. Clin Nucl Med. 1980;5:289-91.
39. Weiss AT, Berman DS, Lew AS, et al. Transient ischemic dilation of the left ventricle on stress thallium-201 scintigraphy: a marker of severe and extensive coronary artery disease. J Am Coll Cardiol. 1987;9:752-9.
40. Hillert MC, Narahara KA, Smitherman TC, et al. Thallium-201 perfusion imaging after the treatment of unstable angina pectoris: relationship to clinical outcome. West J Med. 1986;145:355-40.
41. Madsen JK, Stubgaard M, Utne HE, et al. Prognosis and thallium-201 scintigraphy in patients admitted with chest pain without confirmed acute myocardial infarction. Br Heart J. 1988;59: 184-9.
42. Marmur JD, Freeman MR, Langer A, et al. Prognosis in medically stabilized unstable angina: early Holter ST segment monitoring compared with predischarge exercise thallium tomography. Ann Intern Med. 1990;113:575-9.
43. Brown KA. Prognostic value of thallium-201 myocardial perfusion imaging in patients with unstable angina who respond to medical treatment. J Am Coll Cardiol. 1991;17:1053-7.
44. Phibbs B, Marcus F, Marriott HJ, et al. Q-wave versus non-Q wave myocardial infarction: A meaningless distinction. J Am Coll Cardiol. 1999;33:576-82.
45. Gibson RS, Beller GA, Gheorghiade M, et al. The prevalence and clinical significance of residual myocardial ischemia 2 weeks after uncomplicated non-Q-wave myocardial infarction: prospective natural history study. Circulation. 1986;73:1186-98.
46. Dorbaala S, Giugliano RP, Logsetty G, et al. Prognostic value of SPECT myocardial perfusion imaging in patients with elevated cardiac troponin I levels and atypical clinical presentation. J Nucl Cardiol. 2007;14:53-8.
47. TIMI Study Group. Effects of tissue plasminogen activator and a comparison of early invasive and conservative strategies in unstable angina and non-Q-wave myocardial infarction. Results of the TIMI IIIB trial. Circulation. 1994;89:1545-56.
48. Rosamond W, Flegal K, Furie K, et al. Heart disease and stroke statistics—2008 update: a report from the American Heart Association Statistics Committee and Stroke Statistics Subcommittee. Circulation. 2008;117:25-146.
49. Hendel RC, Berman DS, Di Carli MF, et al. ACCF/ASNC/ACR/AHA/ASE/SCCT/SCMR/SNM 2009 appropriate use criteria for cardiac radionuclide imaging: a report of the American College of Cardiology Foundation Appropriate Use Criteria Task Force, the American Society of Nuclear Cardiology, the American College of Radiology, the American Heart Association, the American Society of Echocardiography, the Society of Cardiovascular Computed Tomography, the Society for Cardiovascular Magnetic Resonance, and the Society of Nuclear Medicine. Circulation. 2009;119:561-87.
50. Bengel FM, Higuchi T, Javadi MS, et al. Cardiac positron emission tomography. J Am Coll Cardiol. 2009;54:1-15.
51. Di Carli MF, Dorbala S, Meserve J, et al. Clinical myocardial perfusion PET/CT. J Nucl Med. 2007;48(5):783-93.
52. Higuchi T, Nekolla SG, Huisman MM, et al. A new 18F-labeled myocardial PET tracer: myocardial uptake after permanent and transient coronary occlusion in rats. J Nucl Med. 2008;49: 1715-22.
53. Di Carli MF, Dorbala S, Meserve J, et al. Clinical myocardial perfusion PET/CT. J Nucl Med. 2007;48:783-93.
54. Bristow MR. The adrenergic nervous system in heart failure. N Engl J Med. 1984;311:850-51.
55. Braunwald E, Fauci AS, Kasper DL, et al. Principles of internal medicine. Harrison's. 2001;15:1316-23.
56. Mann DL, Bristow MR. Mechanisms and models in heart failure: the biomechanical model and beyond. Circulation. 2005;111: 2837-49.
57. Triposkiadis F, Karayannis G, Giamouzis G, et al. The sympathetic nervous system in heart failure physiology, pathophysiology, and clinical implications. J Am Coll Cardiol. 2009;54:1747-62.
58. Bengel FM, Higuchi T, Javadi MS, et al. Cardiac positron emission tomography. J Am Coll Cardiol. 2009;54:1-15.
59. Langer O, Halldin C. PET and SPECT tracers for mapping the cardiac nervous system. Eur J Nucl Med Mol Imaging. 2002;29: 416-34.
60. Schafers M, Wichter T, Lerch H, et al. Cardiac 123I-MIBG uptake in idiopathic ventricular tachycardia and fibrillation. J Nucl Med. 1999;40:1-5.
61. Paul M, Schafers M, Kies P, et al. Impact of sympathetic innervation on recurrent life-threatening arrhythmias in the follow-up of patients with idiopathic ventricular fibrillation. Eur J Nucl Med Mol Imaging. 2006;33:866-70.
62. Jacobson AF, Senior R, Cerqueira MD, et al. Myocardial iodine-123 meta-iodobenzylguanidine imaging and cardiac events in heart failure results of the prospective ADMIRE-HF (AdreView Myocardial Imaging for Risk Evaluation in Heart Failure) study. J Am Coll Cardiol. 2010;55:2212-21.
63. Tamaki S, Yamada T, Okuyama Y, et al. Cardiac iodine-123 metaiodobenzylguanidine imaging predicts sudden cardiac death independently of left ventricular ejection fraction in patients with chronic heart failure and left ventricular systolic dysfunction: results from a comparative study with signal-averaged electrocardiogram, heart rate variability, and QT dispersion. J Am Coll Cardiol. 2009;53:426-35.
64. Boogers MJ, Borleffs CJW, Henneman MM, et al. Cardiac sympathetic denervation assessed with 123-I MIBG imaging predicts ventricular arrhythmias in implantable cardioverter-defibrillator patients. J Am Coll Cardiol. 2010;55:2769-77.

65. Hartmann F, Ziegler S, Nekolla S, et al. Regional patterns of myocardial sympathetic denervation in dilated cardiomyopathy: an analysis using carbon-11 hydroxyephedrine and positron emission tomography. Heart. 1999;81:262-70.
66. Bengel FM, Ueberfuhr P, Schiepel N, et al. Myocardial efficiency and sympathetic reinnervation after orthotopic heart transplantation: a noninvasive study with positron emission tomography. Circulation. 2001;103:1881-6.
67. Mann DL, Spinale FG. Activation of matrix metalloproteinases in the failing human heart: breaking the tie that binds. Circulation. 1998;98:1699-1702.
68. Di Carli MF, Tobes MC, Mangner T, et al. Effects of cardiac sympathetic innervation on coronary blood flow. N Engl J Med. 1997;336:1208-15.
69. Gianni M, Dentali F, Grandi AM, et al. Apical ballooning syndrome or Takotsubo cardiomyopathy: a systematic review. Eur Heart J. 2006;27:1523-9.
70. Ito K, Sugihara H, Katoh S, et al. Assessment of Takotsubo (ampulla) cardiomyopathy using 99mTc-tetrofosmin myocardial SPECT—comparison with acute coronary syndrome. Ann Nucl Med. 2003;17:115-22.
71. Burgdorf C, von Hof K, Schunkert H, et al. Regional alterations in myocardial sympathetic innervation in patients with transient left-ventricular apical ballooning (Tako-Tsubo cardiomyopathy). J Nucl Cardiol. 2008;15:65-72.
72. Uchida Y, Nanjo S, Fujimoto S, et al. Scintigraphy studies on the etiology of ampulla cardiomyopathy. J Cardiol. 2008;51:121-30.

18

Blood Banking for Patient-care has Evolved

RC Khurana

Blood transfusion is an integral part of clinical management of patients. Historically, there has been a serious concern about transmitting infectious diseases from donor to the recipient of blood. With the rapid strides made in the science and technology of transfusion medicine and availability of NAT technology, the transmission of viral diseases has been mostly eliminated.

A strict hemovigilance, i.e. tracing transfusion-related adverse events, has been added to the blood safety. Attention has been paid to improve donor selection, preparation of donation site, processing of blood/blood products, testing techniques, delivery and monitoring of transfusion. This has helped to avoid, detect, and eliminate adverse transfusion events to a great extent.

Blood transfusion, however, has not become totally safe. The present attention of hematologists, blood transfusion specialists, and clinicians has been focused on noninfectious causes of transfusion-related adverse events.

These include:

1. Transfusion-related acute lung injury (TRALI)
2. Transfusion-associated cardiac overload (TACO)
3. Transfusion-related immunomodulation (TRIM)
4. Transfusion-associated graft versus host disease (TA-GVHD)
5. Post-transfusion iron overload.

Efforts are being made to make blood universally safe to avoid above melodies. The transfusion medicine is also currently focused on cellular therapy and cryopreservation of hemopoietic progenitor cells to treat conditions that were, hitherto, not amenable to treatment, and has helped prolong and preserve life.

TRANSFUSION-RELATED ACUTE LUNG INJURY

Transfusion-related acute lung injury (TRALI) is a serious blood transfusion complication characterized by acute onset of noncardiogenic pulmonary edema following blood transfusion. The symptoms come up within 4–6 hours of blood transfusion. It usually follows transfusion of fresh frozen plasma and platelet transfusions, though occasionally it has been noticed with red blood cell (RBC) transfusion. Acute lung injury is caused by the presence of granulocyte antibodies [human leukocyte antigen (HLA) class I and II] in the donor plasma. Patients with pre-existing infection of the lungs are more susceptible to acute lung injury.

Leukoagglutination with release of leukocyte granules occurs in the lungs with release of cytokines that affect the endothelial lining of the pulmonary microvasculature. This increases the vascular permeability and results in acute pulmonary edema and respiratory distress. The exact incidence of the disease is not known because it is virtually impossible to distinguish it from adult respiratory distress syndrome.

The plasma obtained from multiparous women and multitransfused men with HLA antibodies is more likely to cause this melady. The sudden onset of dyspnea, hypoxemia, hypotension, and pyrexia occurring within 6 hours of transfusion should attract the attention to TRALI. Supportive care with oxygen supplementation, vasopressors, and corticosteroids is the mainstay of therapy in TRALI. Diuretics should be avoided because they may aggravate hypotension and cause death due to shock. Leukocyte reduction of blood components has been effective in preventing TRALI and alloimmunization to white cell antigens.

TRANSFUSION-ASSOCIATED CARDIAC OVERLOAD

Cardiogenic pulmonary edema results from infusion of larger volume of blood/blood products. It usually occurs in young children and persons above 60 years of age. Symptoms include dyspnea, orthopnea, cyanosis, increased blood pressure, and tachycardia. Jugular venous distension and pedal edema may be present besides headache and dry cough. Chest radiographs reveal an enlarged cardiac silhouette and bilateral pulmonary edema. It is important to clinically identify the condition and differentiate it from TRALI.

Brain natriuretic peptide (BNP), a neurohormone, is a useful biochemical investigation to differentiate the two. BNP is always elevated in congestive cardiac failure. In a study by Zhou et al., a post-transfusion to pretransfusion BNP ratio of 1.5, as a cutoff point, yields a sensitivity of 81% for transfusion-associated cardiac overload (TACO). Once TACO is diagnosed, transfusion should be stopped. Oxygen should be administered immediately and patient should be put on diuretics to reduce plasma volume. If symptoms persist, therapeutic phlebotomy may be resorted to.

TRANSFUSION-RELATED IMMUNOMODULATION

Exposure to a foreign antigen can induce both immune activation and immune suppression in the recipient. Allogeneic blood transfusion exposes the recipient to numerous foreign antigens both cellular and soluble ones. TRIM encompasses effects attributable to immunomodulatory responses of the body to these antigens. This concept potentially explains many clinical observations and suggests proinflammatory and immunosuppression effects.

Transfusion-related immunomodulation (TRIM) effects may be mediated by allogeneic mononuclear cells (type II HLA antigen) and white blood cells-derived soluble mediators.

The effects of immunomodulation are as follows:

1. Impaired natural killer blood cell functions, thus increasing the chances of neoplasia
2. Alterations in T lymphocyte ratio
3. Suppression of lymphocytic blastogenesis (decreased CD4/CD8 ratio)
4. Decreased macrophage phagocytic functions
5. Decreased interleukin 2 (IL-2) secretion.

Clinically the results of these actions are as follows:

1. Prolonged graft survival in solid organ transplant, due to immunosuppression
2. Increased tumor recurrence
3. Increased postoperative infections/postoperative complications
4. Increased progression of human immunodeficiency virus.

Host defenses may thus be severely compromised after allogeneic transfusion. It has been observed that prestorage leukocyte depletion and use of autologous blood mitigate some of the ill effects of allogeneic transfusion. Studies comparing postoperative infection rate after transfusion of allogeneic blood with transfusion of autologous blood or nontransfused patients showed statistically significant increased rate of postoperative infection in allogeneic products transfused patients.

POST-TRANSFUSION IRON OVERLOAD

Post-transfusion iron overload is a problem in multitransfused patients like those suffering from thalassemia, aplastic anemia, refractory sideroblastic anemia, and myelodysplastic syndrome. These patients are transfusion dependents and receive excess of iron that body is unable to excrete. Each unit of transfused blood has approximately 250 mgm of iron that gradually accumulates in various organs/tissues.

Hepcidin, a peptide synthesized in liver, reduces iron export into the plasma by binding to iron protein ferroportin 1 (FPN-1) on the surface of enterocytes, macrophages, and other cells causing degradation of these cells. When the plasma iron binding protein, transferrin, is over saturated, as in transfused iron overload, the excess free iron is taken up by liver and other tissues. Transferrin-bound iron is also taken up by these cells through hepcidin mechanism. This excessive iron damages the tissues. Hemosiderin is an abnormal, insoluble form of iron storage. Unlike ferritin, it does not circulate in the blood but is deposited in the tissues. Major organs affected by this surplus iron are heart, lungs, liver, and endocrine glands.

Widespread subclinical organ dysfunction can result from transfusional iron overload. With the increasing use of transfusion support for patients, the incidence of hemochromatosis has increased. Left ventricular cardiac function gets impaired, especially in patients with coexisting coronary artery disease. Patients develop glucose in tolerance with significantly reduced insulin secretion. Pituitary ACTH and gonadotropin hormones get affected. Liver biopsy showed portal fibrosis. Iron chelating therapy improves the quality of life and extends the survival rate of the patient.

TRANSFUSION-ASSOCIATED GRAFT VERSUS HOST DISEASE

Transfusion-associated graft versus host disease (TA-GVHD) is a rare, possibly under reported and usually fatal complication of blood transfusion that is seen in immunocompromised individuals and occasionally in immunocompetent ones. When immunologically competent cells from allogeneic donor are transplanted to recipient, whose own immune response is impaired, the lymphoid cells from the donor colonize in the recipient. The transferred cells attack the tissues of the recipient, after perceiving the host tissue as antigenically foreign, and mount fulminant immune response against any cell of the recipient host.

Grafted immunoreaction cells infiltrate skin, intestines, spleen, and liver, which result in hepatosplenomegaly, dermatitis, and diarrhea. The disease occurs in acute and chronic form. The acute or fulminant form is normally observed within 100 days post-transplant and is associated with high morbidity and mortality. The chronic form of graft versus host disease (cGVHD) normally occurs after 100 days. It is a slowly progressive disease that adversely affects long survival. The disease is more severe in older people. The disease starts with maculopapular skin rash, especially on palms, abdominal cramps, and diarrhea. Hepatocellular necrosis occurs. Bacterial and viral infections follow.

A 72-year-old male patient received blood transfusion, postemergency coronary artery bypass grafting. He recovered well and was discharged on fifth postoperative day. He came back on 21st postoperative day with fever, skin rash, diarrhea, leukopenia, and hepatic dysfunction and died in 3 days. The diagnosis of GVHD was confirmed by skin and bone marrow biopsy. Surgeons, intensivists, transfusion medicine consultants, and hematologists should be aware of this rare but devastating complication of blood transfusion after cardiac surgery. It can be prevented/suppressed by administration of cyclosporin A, prednisolone, and anti-lymphocytic globulins. Response is rather poor. Mortality rate is 90%.

AVOIDING DELETERIOUS EFFECTS OF TRANSFUSION

There has been a serious concern regarding increased morbidity and mortality associated with liberal transfusion practices. There is no benefit of maintaining hemoglobin level of 10 g/dL as opposed to 7 g/dL.

It is advisable to practice restrictive transfusion policies, particularly in critical care and cardiac surgery cases. Minimal or "no use" of blood/blood products is being practiced in most of cardiac surgery centers. If the hemoglobin level of patient is good, it is advisable to use autologous donation and liberal use of cell salvage devices. Use of "off-pump" techniques reduces the use of blood, besides other proven advantages. The use of ecosprin and clopidogrel should be avoided, at least 1 week prior to planned surgery. The use of blood from first-degree relatives should be avoided and GVHD should be eliminated. Request of directed donation should be discouraged.

Recent researchers have found that modifying the donor blood prior to transfusion can reduce the incidence of adverse reactions. Using selective male plasma and platelets may eliminate transmission of certain antibodies that are found in previously pregnant women and multitransfused males. Removing white blood cells (leukodepletion) or gamma irradiation of blood products virtually eliminates the transmission of cytomegalovirus and reduces the risk of alloimmunization. Newer technologies permit collecting larger amount of red cells and platelets from the same donor to be transfused to the same recipient, thus reducing the exposure of multiple donors to one recipient.

Multiple top up transfusions in pediatric practice can be achieved by using Penta Bag. Apheresis process has revolutionized blood component delivery. It is now possible to collect desired blood components in good quantity and quality in clinical practice. Automated immunohematology systems are now available to do HLA typing and phenotyping of blood so that blood can be matched at molecular level to prevent future adverse reactions.

UNIVERSALLY SAFE BLOOD

Efforts have been made, recently, to eliminate the need to "type" blood and matching of donor's and recipients blood, before transfusion.

There are, basically, two methods to achieve this:

One is an enzymatic process to cleavage the immunodominant sugar (which expresses the blood group) from complex carbohydrate chain on the surface membrane of group A and B cells with the help of bacterial glycosidase. Due to complexity of group A RBCs (especially A1 RBC), this method has not been very successful.

Another method is pegylation, i.e. covering the blood group antigen with a layer of nonimmunogenic molecule such as polyethylene glycol. This hides the RBCs antigens from antibodies that trigger the immune reaction. The process acts as an "immunocamouflage" and provides "all purpose" red cells for transfusion. Oxygen can, however, still penetrate the polymer shell and RBCs can still continue to supply oxygen to all parts of the body. Life span of RBCs still remains intact (approximately 50 days). The technology has been used to produce universal RBCs from stem cells. This technology needs further evaluation before it can be used in clinical practice.

NOVEL CELLULAR THERAPIES

The last decade has seen phenomenal developments and innovative techniques in cellular therapy and bioengineering. It is now possible to collect specialized hematopoietic progenitor cells from circulating blood, bone marrow, and cord blood. Transplantation of these cells has now replaced bone marrow transplantation in aplastic anemia and leukemias. Umbilical cord stem cells, cryopreserved at the time of birth, are used as rich source of stem cells for transplantation therapy at anytime during the life span of an individual. These cells can also be modified with the help of growth factors and interleukins to convert into neurons, cardiac myocytes, beta cells of pancreas, skin, and cartilage. In future, this could become a preferred method of treatment of diabetes, myocardial infarction osteoarthritis, and burns. Bioengineering techniques have helped to convert stem cells into various functional tissues. The patients in future may obtain liver and kidney from stem cell labs.

BIBLIOGRAPHY

1. Clarke DA, Blajchman MA. Transfusion-related immunomodulation. Transfusion. 2008;48:814-21.
2. Gajic O, Moore SB. Transfusion-related acute lung injury. Mayo Clin Proc. 2005;80(6):766-70.
3. Mezrow CK, Bergstein I, Tartter PI. Post-operative infections following autologous and homologous blood transfusion. Transfusion. 1992;32:17-30.
4. Nielsen HJ. Br J Surg. 2005;82:582-7.
5. Noami LC Luban MD. Advances in Transfusion Medicine. American Society of Haematology Journal December 2008.
6. Patricia M, Kopko MD, Carol SJ. J Am Med Ass. (JAMA). 2002; 287:1968-71.
7. Roback JD, Cambs MR, Hillyer CD. American Association of Blood Banks - Technical Manual, 16th edition. Maryland, USA.
8. Rogalski J, Perry S. Centre for Blood Research Health Science Mall. Vancouver BC Canada.
9. Tobian AA, Sokall LJ, Ness PM. BNP as a useful diagnostic marker for transfusion associated circulatory overload. Transfusion. 2007;47:7A.
10. Zhou L, Gia Cherian D, Cooling L, et al. Use of BNP as a diagnostic marker in transfusion associated circulatory overload. Transfusion. 1995;45:1056-63.
11. Zimrin AB, Hess JR. Current issues relating to transfusion of stored RBCs. VOX Sang. 2009;96:93-103.

19

Risk Markers for Atherothrombosis

Dheeraj Gandotra, Subhash Chandra

Atherothrombosis, defined as atherosclerotic plaque disruption with superimposed thrombosis, is a leading cause of mortality worldwide. Atherosclerosis is a diffuse process that starts early in childhood and progresses asymptomatically through adult life. Later in life, it is clinically manifested as coronary artery disease (CAD), stroke, and peripheral arterial disease.[1] Atherothrombosis can no longer be considered a disease of the developed world, because myocardial infarction and stroke are increasingly prevalent worldwide, across all socioeconomic strata. By 2025, cardiovascular disease (CVD) mortality will surpass that of every disease including infection, cancer, and trauma.[2,3]

From our current perspective, it is perhaps surprising that the formal conceptual basis for considering specific cardiovascular risk factors and risk markers has emerged as recently as the 1960s, when the findings of the Framingham Heart Study began to appear. From an epidemiologic perspective, a risk marker is a characteristic or feature of an individual or population that presents early in life and associates with an increased risk of developing future disease.

Early detection and risk stratification continues to be some of the main focus of atherothrombotic research. In parallel with the quest for novel biomarkers, the substantial impact of the conventional risk factors was emphasized in several reports. We therefore present here a review of literature and update on risk markers for atherothrombotic disease. The review will include discussion on conventional risk factors, novel atherothrombotic risk factors including inflammatory markers, imaging risk markers including molecular imaging, and genetic determinants of atherothrombotic disease.

Risk markers for atherosclerosis can be broadly classified into conventional risk factors and others, which include novel atherosclerotic risk markers, imaging markers, genetic markers, and direct plaque imaging. Early identification and management of these is the basis for CVD prevention.

CONVENTIONAL RISK FACTORS

These have well-established association with atherothrombosis substantiated by multiple population-based studies and the treatment of these results in prevention of CAD.

Smoking

Other than advanced age, smoking is the single most important risk factor for coronary artery disease. Cigarette consumption is the leading preventable cause of death in the United States, where it accounts for >400,000 deaths annually.[4] Ischemic heart disease causes 35–40% of all smoking-related deaths, with an additional 8% attributable to second hand smoke exposure. Despite the relative stability in prevalence of current smokers in the United States, rates of tobacco use are increasing among adolescents, young adults, and women.[5] Smoking has a particularly large impact in the developing world. In China alone, more than 670,000 deaths annually are already attributable to smoking[6] and, by the end of 2010, 930,000 adult deaths may occur from smoking-related causes in India.[7]

Hypertension

High blood pressure often confers silent cardiovascular risk, and its prevalence is steadily increasing. Hypertension is a well-established cardiovascular risk factor evidenced by multiple trials. Blood pressure reduction as small as 4–5 mm Hg results in significant reduction in the risk for stroke, vascular mortality, congestive heart failure, and total coronary heart disease (CHD) in middle aged subjects, older adults, and high risk groups such as those with diabetes and peripheral arterial disease.[8]

Pulse pressure, generally reflecting vascular wall stiffness, also predicts first and recurrent myocardial infarction. Defined as the difference between systolic and diastolic blood pressures, pulse pressure appears to predict cardiovascular events independently, particularly heart failure.[9]

Dyslipidemia

Hyperlipidemia and Elevated Low-density Lipoprotein Cholesterol (LDL-C)

Cross-sectional population studies have consistently revealed relationship between serum cholesterol levels and CHD death. High levels of LDL-C increase CAD risk, evidenced by reduction in risk by statin use. The Heart Protection Study showed that statins can reduce stroke and coronary events in those with pre-existing vascular disease.[10] Several head-to-head trials comparing different statin regimens have shown that even more aggressive LDL reduction is associated with greater clinical improvements.

High-density Lipoprotein Cholesterol (HDL-C), Apolipoproteins, and Other Lipid Subclasses

As is the case with LDL-C, abundant prospective cohort studies have demonstrated a strong inverse relationship between HDL-C, and vascular risk. In general, each increase of HDL-C by 1 mg/dL is associated with a 2–3% decrease in risk of total CVD. In contrast to LDL, however, we currently lack evidence that increasing HDL-C levels reduce risk.[11,12]

Several investigators have suggested that the measurement of apolipoproteins A-I and B100 would predict cardiovascular risk better than HDL-C and LDL-C in clinical practice. Two recent prospective cohort studies have shown this to be the case for men[13] and women.[14] However, both of these studies also found that non–HDL-C (defined as total cholesterol minus HDL-C) provided clinical risk information at least as strong as that of apolipoprotein B100; this was an unsurprising observation, because non–HDL-C correlates very closely with apolipoprotein B100 levels. Thus, despite evidence favoring apolipoproteins A-I and B100 in univariate analyses as replacements for HDL-C and LDL-C, there remain little clinical data that use of these measures improves overall risk prediction compared with standard lipid testing.

Triglyceride-rich Lipoproteins and Cardiovascular Risk

In contrast to compelling evidence favoring a causal role for LDL-C in atherogenesis, the role of triglycerides remains controversial. Part of this controversy reflects the inverse correlation of triglyceride levels with HDL-C. Adjustment for HDL-C attenuates the relationship between triglycerides and CVD. A recent meta-analysis has suggested that the adjusted risk ratio for coronary disease among those in the top third of triglyceride levels, compared with the bottom third, decreases from approximately 2.0–1.5 after accounting for HDL-C.[15] Thus, current guidelines do not establish a target value of triglycerides.

Metabolic Syndrome, Insulin Resistance, and Diabetes

Insulin resistance and diabetes rank among the major cardiovascular risk factors; in one major survey, the presence of diabetes conferred an equivalent risk to aging 15 years, an impact higher than that of smoking.[16] Patients with diabetes have two- to eightfold higher rates of future cardiovascular events as compared with age- and ethnicity-matched nondiabetic individuals, and 75% of all deaths in diabetic patients result from CHD. Diabetes is considered as CAD equivalent.

Although hyperglycemia associates with microvascular disease, insulin resistance itself promotes atherosclerosis even before it produces frank diabetes, and available data corroborate the role of insulin resistance as an independent risk factor for atherothrombosis. This finding has prompted recommendations for increased surveillance for the metabolic syndrome, a cluster of glucose intolerance, and hyperinsulinemia accompanied by hypertriglyceridemia, low HDL levels, hypofibrinolysis, hypertension, microalbuminuria, a predominance of small, dense LDL particles, and central obesity. Several studies have documented that individuals with the metabolic syndrome have elevated vascular event rates. The most recent definition of metabolic syndrome from the National Heart, Lung, and Blood Institute includes a proinflammatory state.[17]

Thus, inflammatory biomarkers such as high-sensitivity C-reactive protein (hsCRP) may help further stratify clinical risk and improve the prognostic value of metabolic syndrome. The current controversy regarding the concept of the metabolic syndrome, its validity, and its clinical usefulness may present a false dichotomy. Given the growing epidemic of obesity and the foreseen burden of cardiovascular risk that it entails, professionals should reach beyond pedantic arguments regarding the nosology of the metabolic syndrome and combine forces to address the risk factors that comprise this cluster.

In particular, there is not enough evidence to reject the notion that the sum of the risk factors outweighs the parts in younger populations, in whom concern regarding obesity and cardiovascular risk has become urgent.

Exercise, Weight Loss, and Obesity

Most epidemiologic studies have demonstrated a strong graded association between levels of physical activity and reduced rates of cardiovascular morbidity and all-cause mortality. Observational studies have cast doubt on the long-held belief that exercise must be vigorous to be beneficial. In both men and women, exercise levels achieved with as little as 30 minutes of walking daily provide major cardiovascular benefits.[18]

Mental Stress, Depression, and Cardiovascular Risk

Both depression and mental stress predispose to increased vascular risk. The adrenergic stimulation of mental stress can augment myocardial oxygen requirements and aggravate myocardial ischemia. Mental stress can cause coronary vasoconstriction, particularly in atherosclerotic coronary arteries, and hence can influence myocardial oxygen supply as well.

In the INTERHEART study evaluating postinfarction patients from 52 countries, psychosocial stress was associated with vascular risk, with a magnitude of effect similar to that of the major coronary risk factors.[19]

NOVEL ATHEROSCLEROTIC RISK MARKERS

Current screening programs for risk detection and disease prevention, but clinical data continue to accrue that demonstrate the hazard of relying solely on classic risk factors. In one analysis of >120,000 patients with CHD, 15% of the women and 19% of the men had no evidence of hyperlipidemia, hypertension, diabetes, or smoking, and >50% had only one of these general risk factors.[20] In another large analysis, between 85% and 95% of participants with coronary disease had at least one conventional risk factor, but so did those participants without coronary disease, despite follow-up for as long as 30 years.[21] Thus, because of the considerable need to improve vascular risk detection, much research over the past 10 or 15 years has focused on the identification and evaluation of novel atherosclerotic risk factors.

Serum Biomarkers

Serum biomarkers can be classified as under:

Inflammatory Markers

Inflammation characterizes all phases of atherothrombosis and provides a critical pathophysiologic link between plaque formation and acute rupture, which lead to occlusion and infarction.[22]

Various inflammatory makers studied in CAD are as under:
1. High-sensitivity C-reactive protein (hsCRP)
2. Lipoprotein-associated phospholipase A2 (Lp-PLA2)
3. Soluble adhesion molecules (sICAM-1)
4. Serum amyloid A (SAA)
5. Interleukins (IL-6, IL-18)
6. Myeloperoxidase
7. Soluble CD40 ligand (s CD40 L)
8. Pregnancy-associated plasma protein A (PrPPA)

High-sensitivity C-reactive Protein

The acute phase reactant, CRP, has now emerged as a major cardiovascular risk marker.[23] Regardless of whether CRP is a marker or mediator, a large series of prospective epidemiologic studies has demonstrated that CRP, when measured with high-sensitivity assays (hsCRP), strongly and independently predicts risk of myocardial infarction, stroke, peripheral arterial disease, and sudden cardiac death in apparently healthy individuals, even when LDL-C plasminogen activator inhibitor-1 levels are low.[24] In recent comprehensive meta-analyses, the multivariable hazard associated with hsCRP was, if anything, larger than that associated with either blood pressure or cholesterol.[25] These data apply to women and men across all age levels and have been consistent in diverse populations. Most importantly, hsCRP adds prognostic information at all LDL-C levels and at all levels of risk, as determined by the Framingham Risk Score.[26] Current status of hsCRP evaluation in risk prediction—The American Heart Association and the Centers for Disease Control and Prevention issued a statement in 2003 regarding the use of hsCRP in clinical practice. Briefly, hsCRP levels <1, 1 to 3, and >3 mg/L should be interpreted as lower, moderate, and higher relative vascular risk, respectively, when considered along with traditional markers of risk, a finding recently corroborated within the Framingham Heart Study itself.[27] Screening for hsCRP should be done at the discretion of the physician as part of global risk evaluation, not as a replacement for LDL and HDL testing.

Although hsCRP predicts risk across the entire population spectrum, it likely has greatest usefulness for those at intermediate risk—i.e. those with anticipated 10-year event rates between 5% and 20%.[28]

The use of statin therapy to reduce vascular risk in individuals with elevated hsCRP, even when LDL-C levels are low, represents a fundamental change in treatment strategies for the prevention of CVD. Most importantly, in the recent JUPITER trial 102 of apparently healthy men and women with LDL-C levels lower than 130 mg/dL who were at increased risk because of hsCRP levels of 2 mg/L or higher, the use of rosuvastatin resulted in a 44% reduction in the trial primary endpoint of all vascular events ($P < 0.000001$), a 54% reduction in myocardial infarction ($P = 0.0002$), a 48% reduction in stroke ($P = 0.002$), a 46% reduction in the need for arterial revascularization ($P < 0.001$), and a 20% reduction in all-cause mortality ($P = 0.02$).[29]

Other Markers of Inflammation

These include cytokines such as IL-6, soluble forms of certain cell adhesion molecules such as soluble ICAM-1 (sICAM-1), P-selectin, or the mediator CD40 ligand, as well as the total white blood cell count and markers of leukocyte activation such as myeloperoxidase. Other inflammatory markers associated with lipid oxidation, such as Lp-PLA2 and PrPPA, have also shown promise.[30,31] Like hsCRP, Lp-PLA2 has shown efficacy in the prediction of stroke, demonstrating again the independence of inflammatory biomarkers from lipid parameters like LDL-C that are not closely related to stroke risk.[32]

Many of these alternative inflammatory biomarkers, however, have analytic issues that need careful evaluation before routine clinical use. Nonetheless, several of these inflammatory biomarkers can shed critical pathophysiologic light on the atherothrombotic process, particularly at the time of plaque rupture. Similarly, myeloperoxidase may provide prognostic information in cases of acute ischemia beyond that associated with troponin or CRP.[33]

Markers of Altered Thrombosis

These include:

- Tissue plasminogen activator
- Plasminogen activator inhibitor-1
- Fibrinogen
- Homocysteine
- D-dimer

Fibrinogen

Although also an acute-phase reactant and thus often considered an inflammatory biomarker, plasma fibrinogen additionally influences platelet aggregation and blood viscosity, interacts with plasminogen binding and, in combination with thrombin, mediates the final step in clot formation and the response to vascular injury.[34] In addition, fibrinogen associates positively with age, obesity, smoking, diabetes, and LDL-C level, and inversely with HDL-C level, alcohol use, and physical activity/exercise level.

Given these relationships, it is not surprising that fibrinogen was among the first novel risk factors evaluated. Early reports from the Gothenburg, Northwick Park, and Framingham heart studies all found significant positive associations between fibrinogen levels and future risk of cardiovascular events. Since then, a number of other prospective studies have confirmed these findings and, in a meta-analysis, there was an approximately linear logarithmic association between usual fibrinogen level and risk of CHD and stroke.[35] Three have evaluated the potential benefits of fibrinogen reduction, and all have found disappointing results.[35-37]

Given these results, continued evaluation of novel inflammatory biomarkers may provide targets for or monitors of therapy, particularly in the setting of acute coronary ischemia. However, in a comprehensive overview conducted by the National Academy of Clinical Biochemists that included multiple inflammatory biomarkers, only hsCRP met all the stated clinical criteria for acceptance as a biomarker for risk assessment in primary prevention.[38]

Homocysteine

Homocysteine is a sulfhydryl-containing amino acid derived from the demethylation of dietary methionine. Patients with rare inherited defects of methionine metabolism can develop severe hyperhomocysteinemia (plasma levels >100 mmol/L) and have a markedly elevated risk of premature atherothrombosis and venous thromboembolism. In contrast to severe hyperhomocysteinemia, mild-to-moderate elevations of homocysteine (plasma levels >15 mmol/L) are more common in the general population, primarily because of insufficient dietary intake of folic acid. Despite the availability of newer assays, measurement of homocysteine remains controversial, and recent guidelines have not advocated their use. This lack of enthusiasm reflects modest overall effects in prospective cohort studies and the results of several large trials of homocysteine reduction.

With regard to clinical trials of homocysteine reduction, several major studies have shown no substantive benefit (Vitamin Intervention for Stroke Prevention (VISP) trial,[39] Norwegian Vitamin Trial (NORVIT),[40] and Heart Outcomes Prevention Evaluation (HOPE-2).[41]

Despite reduced enthusiasm and lack of evidence that homocysteine reduction lowers risk, there remain specific patient populations for whom homocysteine evaluation may prove appropriate, including those lacking traditional risk factors, those with renal failure, or those with markedly premature atherosclerosis or a family history of myocardial infarction and stroke at a young age.[42] It is also crucial to continue folate supplementation in the general population to reduce the risk of neural tube defects, an inexpensive practice that has been in place in the United States for over a decade, yet remains a public health challenge for much of Europe and the developing world.[43]

Other Biomarkers

- Oxidative stress; oxidized LDL
- Altered lipids; lipoprotein (a) [Lp(a)]
- Heart fatty acid binding protein
- Asymmetric dimethylarginine

Lipoprotein (a) [Lp(a)] consists of an LDL particle with its apolipoprotein B-100 (apo B100) component linked by a disulfide bridge to apolipoprotein(a) [apo(a)], a variable-length protein that has sequence homology to plasminogen. Many prospective cohort studies have supported a role for Lp(a) as a determinant of vascular risk. In an updated meta-analysis of 36 prospective studies that included >12,000 cardiovascular endpoints, the adjusted risk ratios for each standard deviation increase in plasma Lp(a) level were 1.13 for CHD and 1.10 for ischemic stroke.[44] Adjustment for classic cardiovascular risk factors only modestly attenuated these effects, in part because there is little correlation between Lp(a) and other markers of risk.[45]

NONINVASIVE, IMAGING MARKERS/ MODALITIES TO EVALUATE ATHEROTHROMBOSIS

In addition to the use of inflammatory markers and family history, strategies to detect vascular disease will likely take several forms. One approach eschews risk factor measurement but identifies preclinical disease through the noninvasive detection of atherosclerotic plaque. Such an approach can never truly prevent disease; it can only lead to early detection. Various modalities for early evaluation of atherosclerosis are as follows:

- Ankle brachial pressure Index (ABI)
- Brachial artery flow-mediated dilatation (BAFMD)
- Pulse wave velocity (PWV)/pulse wave analysis (PWA)
- Carotid intima media thickness (CIMT)
- Coronary artery calcium scoring (CACS).

Ankle Brachial Index

The ABI is defined as ratio of systolic blood pressure in ankle to that in the arms. Normal ABI is >1. In 6647 participants enrolled in Multi-Ethnic Study of Atherosclerosis (MESA), the ABI was predictive of incident CHD, stroke, or other atherosclerotic cardiovascular death independent of traditional risk factors, serum biomarkers, electrocardiographic abnormalities, the CIMT, and the coronary calcium score.[46] Thus, ABI is an inexpensive, easily available, and reproducible test for early detection of atherosclerosis.

Brachial Artery Flow-mediated Dilatation

This is useful to assess endothelial function, which precedes the development of atherosclerosis. Flow-mediated dilatation <4.5% implies endothelial dysfunction. BAFMD is still not being used in day-to-day practice.[47-49]

***PWV/PWA*:** These are noninvasive markers of arterial stiffness. In the ARIC study, Liao et al. found a correlation between arterial stiffness and hypertension and atherosclerosis.[32] In 2232 participants of the Framingham Heart Study followed up for a median of 7.8 years, arterial stiffness as reflected by aortic PWV was also associated with incident major cardiovascular events after adjusting for standard risk factors, including systolic blood pressure or history of hypertension.[50]

Carotid Intima Media Thickness

Carotid intima media thickness has emerged as a quick, valid, reproducible, and inexpensive modality for evaluating atherosclerosis and has a good correlation with coronary artery stenosis. A cutoff point of 1.1 mm is taken to define atherosclerosis.[51,52]

Coronary Artery Calcium Scoring

Coronary artery calcium scoring was used for risk stratification of asymptomatic persons in many trials. In MESA study, 5878 nondiabetic participants were followed up for a mean of 5–8 years and it was found that addition of calcium score to conventional risk stratification scores improved the coronary risk classification in 25% of the subjects, particularly in those with intermediate risk.[53] In another study, coronary computed tomography (CT) was found to be an independent predictor of cardiac death and myocardial infarction in >2000 mostly symptomatic patients followed up for 16 ± 8 months. It was suggested that beyond disease severity and left ventricular ejection fraction, a score of plaque burden provided incremental prognostic information for the prediction of all course mortality and nonfatal myocardial infarction.[54]

DIRECT PLAQUE IMAGING

Plaque morphology and vulnerability can be studied by various modalities including intravascular ultrasound (IVUS), optical coherence tomography (OCT), and vascular magnetic resonance imaging (MRI).

INTRAVASCULAR ULTRASOUND

Data analyses from six clinical trials using serial IVUS studies revealed that baseline burden of coronary atherosclerosis progression was independently associated with major cardiovascular events, in particular revascularization during follow-up.[55] In another IVUS study, plaque regression occurred in >20% of the patients who achieved LDC-C <70 mg/dL.[56]

Another study involving serial IVUS demonstrated the highly dynamic nature of coronary atherosclerosis. In this study, symptomatic patients receiving conventional medical therapies, during 12 months period, it was found that as much as 75% of nonculprit thin-cap fibroatheroma at baseline transformed into a more stable lesion, whereas new fibroatheroma developed.[57] These findings could be of relevance regarding risk stratification based on plaque feature from a single point time or a lesion-targeted therapeutic strategies.

MOLECULAR IMAGING

Various molecular imaging techniques used for detection of atherosclerosis are as follows:

- Positron emission tomography (PET)
- MRI
- Spectral CT.

Positron Emission Tomography

The PET, using 18-fluorodeoxyglucose (FDG), can be used for the evaluation of vascular inflammation. In a study of carotid PET in patients with impaired fasting glucose and overt diabetes, it was found that vascular inflammation is present in both subsets of patients. However, inflammatory activity was higher in presence of overt diabetes.[58]

Vascular MRI

Vascular MRI, using contrast agent targeted to activated platelets, was studied in experimental model of disease for detection of intravascular thrombi.[59] This modality is being utilized for studying vascular inflammation in various device trials.

Spectral CT

Spectral CT is a novel technique based on X-ray differentiation properties, which enables differentiation of various contrast agents in a single scan. This imaging modality demonstrated potential for simultaneous depiction of arterial inflammation and calcification.[60] Genetic markers of atherothrombosis—deciphering the genetic underpinnings of atherothrombosis presents considerable challenges because of major gene-environment interactions. Also, atherothrombosis represents a prototypic complex disease in which multiple small effects accumulate and have a substantial population-attributable risk.[61] Some genetic determinants of atherothrombotic CVD were initially described on a candidate gene basis and have been replicated in multiple cohorts.

Perhaps the best known of these is the relationship between polymorphisms in the apolipoprotein E (apo E) gene that codes for three common isoforms (E2, E3, and E4), which in turn are associated with differential risks of coronary heart disease.[62]

Genome-wide association study (GWAS) has made it possible to discover gene loci that previously were not anticipated as determinants of vascular risk.[63] For example, a common polymorphism on chromosome 9p21 has repeatedly been found to be associated with CAD that is not strongly related to any known intermediate phenotype, such as cholesterol or blood pressure.[64,65] Yet, despite clear replication in more than a dozen cohorts to date, no study has shown that measurement of 9p21 alters global risk prediction.[66]

Although a considerable biologic insight into mechanisms and pathogenesis has already come from large-scale genomic studies of vascular disease, currently available data do not support the use of genetic biomarkers as clinical tools in the prediction or prevention of CVD.

These risk markers should be used for early detection and identification of individuals at risk of atherosclerosis and CAD. Based on these risk markers, various approaches and risk models have been proposed for identification at risk individuals.

Novel approaches to global risk detection—In the half century since the identification of the major coronary risk factors of age, hypertension, smoking, and hyperlipidemia, our understanding of atherothrombosis has expanded to include the biology of hemostasis, thrombosis, inflammation, and endothelial function. Despite this more ample view of pathophysiology, the variables in current risk assessment algorithms remain largely unchanged from those evaluated a half-century ago.

An expanded and updated approach—An expanded and updated approach to vascular risk detection is needed so that primary care physicians can be guided by the most modern biologic constructs. New risk prediction algorithms must involve rigorous evaluation, with particular care given not only to the concepts of discrimination but also to calibration and reclassification.[67] This change in focus for prevention must include an understanding that reliance on the C-statistic as a traditional method for selecting variables for inclusion in risk prediction models is outmoded and subject to considerable error.[68] Careful investigation has shown that inappropriate reliance on the C-statistic would actually eliminate LDL-C, HDL-C, and blood pressure from most global prediction models. Furthermore, continued reliance on 10-year risk estimates rather than estimates of lifetime risk may actually restrain more effective prevention efforts.[69]

Current status of novel risk markers in risk calculation and risk scores evaluation—data in the Women's Health Study, nine variables—age, current smoking, systolic blood pressure, HbA_{1c} among diabetics, hsCRP, apo B100, apo A-I, Lp(a), and a parental history of premature atherosclerosis—were found to improve risk prediction substantially when compared with traditional Framingham covariates.[3]

Both hsCRP and parental history of premature atherothrombosis, the two novel parameters included in the Reynolds Risk Score, have also been shown to improve risk reclassification within the Framingham Heart Study.[70] Other major epidemiologic investigations,[71-73] but not all,[74] have reported similar results, underscoring continued controversy in this arena. As a general rule, those studies that have not found novel biomarkers to add risk information have been conducted in very low-risk cohorts with only small numbers of individuals at intermediate risk for whom reclassification is possible.

CONCLUSION

Atherosclerosis is a multifactorial disease. Novel risk markers, newer imaging diagnostic modalities and genetic markers in addition to traditional risk, should be utilized for risk stratification of individuals at risk of CVD. This might enable the health care systems across the globe to become more proactive, moving the focus away from treatment of end staged CAD toward early detection and prevention of CAD.

REFERENCES

1. Corti R, Fuster V, Badimon JJ. Pathogenetic concepts of acute coronary syndromes. J Am Coll Cardiol. 2003;41:S7-S14.
2. Bhatt DL, Steg PG, Ohman EM, et al. International prevalence, recognition, and treatment of cardiovascular risk factors in outpatients with atherothrombosis. JAMA. 2006;95:180.
3. He J, Gu D, Wu X, et al. Major causes of death among men and women in China. N Engl J Med. 2005;353:1124.
4. Centers for Disease Control and Prevention (CDC). Smoking-attributable mortality, years of potential life lost, and productivity losses—United States. JAMA. 2009;301:593.
5. Centers for Disease Control and Prevention (CDC). Cigarette smoking among adults—United States. JAMA. 2009;301:373.
6. Gu D, Kelly TN, Wu X, et al. Mortality attributable to smoking in China. N Engl J Med. 2009;360:150.
7. Jha P, Jacob B, Gajalakshmi V, et al. A nationally representative case-control study of smoking and death in India. N Engl J Med. 2008;358:1137.
8. Nissen SE, Tuzcu EM, Libby P, et al. Effect of antihypertensive agents on cardiovascular events in patients with coronary disease and normal blood pressure: The CAMELOT study: A randomized controlled trial. JAMA. 2004;292:2217.
9. Haider AW, Larson MG, Franklin SS, et al. Systolic blood pressure, diastolic blood pressure, and pulse pressure as predictors of risk for congestive heart failure in the Framingham Heart Study. Ann Intern Med. 2003;38:10.
10. Collins R, Armitage J, Parish S, et al. Effects of cholesterol-lowering with simvastatin on stroke and other major vascular events in 20,536 people with cerebrovascular disease or other high-risk conditions. Lancet. 2004;363:757.
11. Barter PJ, Caulfield M, Eriksson M, et al. Effects of torcetrapib in patients at high risk for coronary events. N Engl J Med. 2007;357:2109.
12. Rader DJ. Illuminating HDL—is it still a viable therapeutic target? N Engl J Med. 2007;357:2180.
13. Pischon T, Girman CJ, Sacks FM, et al. Non-high-density lipoprotein cholesterol and apolipoprotein B in the prediction of coronary heart disease in men. Circulation. 2005;112:3375.
14. Ridker PM, Rifai N, Cook NR, et al. Non-HDL cholesterol, apolipoproteins A-I and B100, standard lipid measures, lipid ratios, and CRP as risk factors for cardiovascular disease in women. JAMA. 2005;294:326.
15. Sarwar N, Danesh J, Eiriksdottir G, et al. Triglycerides and the risk of coronary heart disease: 10,158 incident cases among 262,525 participants in 29 Western prospective studies. Circulation. 2007;115:450.
16. Booth GL, Kapral MK, Fung K, et al. Relation between age and cardiovascular disease in men and women with diabetes compared with non-diabetic people: a population-based retrospective cohort study. Lancet. 2006;368:29.
17. Grundy SM, Brewer HB Jr, Cleeman JI, et al. Definition of metabolic syndrome: Report of the National Heart, Lung, and Blood Institute/American Heart Association conference on scientific issues related to definition. Circulation. 2004;109:433.
18. Manson JE, Greenland P, LaCroix AZ, et al. Walking compared with vigorous exercise for the prevention of cardiovascular events in women. N Engl J Med. 2002;347:716.
19. Rosengren A, Hawken S, Ounpuu S, et al. Association of psychosocial risk factors with risk of acute myocardial infarction in 11119 cases and 13648 controls from 52 countries (the INTERHEART study): Case-control study. Lancet. 2004;364:953.
20. Khot UN, Khot MB, Bajzer CT, et al. Prevalence of conventional risk factors in patients with coronary heart disease. JAMA. 2003;290:898.
21. Greenland P, Knoll MD, Stamler J, et al. Major risk factors as antecedents of fatal and nonfatal coronary heart disease events. JAMA. 2003;290:89.
22. Libby P, Ridker PM, Hansson GK. Inflammation in atherosclerosis: From pathophysiology to practice. J Am Coll Cardiol. 2009;54:2129.
23. Ridker PM. C-reactive protein: eighty years from discovery to emergence as a major risk marker for cardiovascular disease. Clin Chem. 2009;55:209.
24. Ridker PM. C-reactive protein and the prediction of cardiovascular events among those at intermediate risk: moving an inflammatory hypothesis toward consensus. J Am Coll Cardiol. 2007;49:2129.
25. Kaptoge S, Di Angelantonio E, Lowe G, et al. C-reactive protein concentration and risk of coronary heart disease, stroke, and mortality: an individual participant meta-analysis. Lancet. 2010;375:132.
26. Ridker PM, Rifai N, Rose L, et al. Comparison of C-reactive protein and low-density lipoprotein cholesterol levels in the prediction of first cardiovascular events. N Engl J Med. 2002;347:1557.
27. Wilson PWF, Pencina M, Jacques P, et al. C-reactive protein and reclassification of cardiovascular risk in the Framingham Heart Study. Circ Cardiovasc Qual Outcomes. 2008;1:92.
28. Genest J, McPherson R, Frohlich J, et al. Canadian Cardiovascular Society/Canadian guidelines for the diagnosis and treatment of dyslipidemia and prevention of cardiovascular disease in the adult—2009 recommendations. Can J Cardiol. 2009;25:567.
29. Ridker PM, Danielson E, Fonseca FA, et al. Reduction in C-reactive protein and LDL cholesterol and cardiovascular event rates after initiation of rosuvastatin: a prospective study of the JUPITER trial. Lancet. 2009;373:1175.
30. Zalewski A, Macphee C. Role of lipoprotein-associated phospholipase A2 in atherosclerosis: Biology, epidemiology, and possible therapeutic target. Arterioscler Thromb Vasc Biol. 2005;25:923.
31. Cosin-Sales J, Christiansen M, Kaminski P, et al. Pregnancy-associated plasma protein A and its endogenous inhibitor, the proform of eosinophil major basic protein (proMBP), are related to complex stenosis morphology in patients with stable angina pectoris. Circulation. 2004;109:1724.

32. Nambi V, Hoogeveen RC, Chambless L, et al. Lipoprotein-associated phospholipase A2 and high-sensitivity C-reactive protein improve the stratification of ischemic stroke risk in the Atherosclerosis Risk in Communities (ARIC) study. Stroke. 2009;40:376.
33. Morrow DA, Sabatine MS, Brennan ML, et al. Concurrent evaluation of novel cardiac biomarkers in acute coronary syndrome: myeloperoxidase and soluble CD40 ligand and the risk of recurrent ischaemic events in TACTICS-TIMI 18. Eur Heart J. 2008;29:1096.
34. Kerlin B, Cooley BC, Isermann BH, et al. Cause-effect relation between hyperfibrinogenemia and vascular disease. Blood. 2004;103:1728.
35. Danesh J, Lewington S, Thompson SG, et al. Fibrinogen Studies Collaboration: Plasma fibrinogen level and the risk of major cardiovascular diseases and nonvascular mortality: An individual participant meta-analysis. JAMA. 2005;294:1799.
36. Tanne D, Benderly M, Goldbourt U, et al. A prospective study of plasma fibrinogen levels and the risk of stroke among participants in the bezafibrate infarction prevention study. Am J Med. 2001;111:457.
37. Meade T, Zuhrie R, Cook C, et al. Bezafibrate in men with lower extremity arterial disease: randomised controlled trial. BMJ. 2002;325:1139.
38. Myers GL, Christenson RH, Cushman M, et al. National Academy of Clinical Biochemistry Laboratory Medicine Practice guidelines: emerging biomarkers for primary prevention of cardiovascular disease. Clin Chem. 2009;55:378.
39. Toole JF, Malinow MR, Chambless LE, et al. Lowering homocysteine in patients with ischemic stroke to prevent recurrent stroke, myocardial infarction, and death: the Vitamin Intervention for Stroke Prevention (VISP) randomized controlled trial. JAMA. 2004;291:565.
40. Lange H, Suryapranata H, De Luca G, et al. Folate therapy and in-stent restenosis after coronary stenting. N Engl J Med. 2004;350:2673.
41. Bonaa KH, Njolstad I, Ueland PM, et al. Homocysteine lowering and cardiovascular events after acute myocardial infarction. N Engl J Med. 2006;354:1578.
42. Loscalzo J. Homocysteine trials—clear outcomes for complex reasons. N Engl J Med. 2006;354:1629.
43. Eichholzer M, Tonz O, Zimmermann R. Folic acid: a public-health challenge. Lancet. 2006;367:1352.
44. The Emerging Risk Factors Collaboration. Lipoprotein(a) concentration and the risk of coronary heart disease, stroke, and nonvascular mortality. JAMA. 2009;302:412.
45. Kamstrup PR, Benn M, Tybjaerg-Hansen A, et al. Extreme lipoprotein(a) levels and risk of myocardial infarction in the general population: The Copenhagen City Heart Study. Circulation. 2008;117:176.
46. Criqui MH, McClelland RL, McDermott MM, et al. The anklebrachial index and incident cardiovascular events in the MESA (Multi-Ethnic Study of Atherosclerosis). J Am Coll Cardiol. 2010;56:1506-12.
47. Raitakari OT, Celermajer DS. Flow-mediated dilatation. Br J Clin Pharmacol. 2000;50(5):397-404.
48. Bae JH. Non-invasive evaluation of endothelial function. Am J Cardiol. 2001;37(1):89-92.
49. Anderson TJ. Assessment and treatment of endothelial dysfunction. J Cardiovasc Pharmacol. 1998:32(3):29-32.
50. Course JR. Predictive value of carotid 2-dimensional ultrasound. Am J Cardiol. 2001;8:27E-30E.
51. Pignoli P, Tremoli E, Poli E, et al. Intimal plus medial thickness of the arterial wall: a direct measurement with ultrasound imaging. Atherosclerosis. 1986;74:1399-406.
52. Mitchell GF, Hwang SJ, Vasan RS, et al. Arterial stiffness and cardiovascular events: the Framingham Heart Study. Circulation. 2010;121:505-11.
53. Polonsky TS, McClelland RL, Jorgensen NW, et al. Coronary artery calcium score and risk classification for coronary heart disease prediction. JAMA. 2010;303:1610-6.
54. Chow BJ, Wells GA, Chen L, et al. Prognostic value of 64-slice cardiac computed tomography severity of coronary artery disease, coronary atherosclerosis, and left ventricular ejection fraction. J Am Coll Cardiol. 2010;55:1017-28.
55. Nicholls SJ, Hsu A, Wolski K, et al. Intravascular ultrasound-derived measures of coronary atherosclerotic plaque burden and clinical outcome. J Am Coll Cardiol. 2010;55:2399-407.
56. Bayturan O, Kapadia S, Nicholls SJ, et al. Clinical predictors of plaque progression despite very low levels of low-density lipoprotein cholesterol. J Am Coll Cardiol. 2010;55:2736-42.
57. Kubo T, Maehara A, Mintz GS, et al. The dynamic nature of coronary artery lesion morphology assessed by serial virtual histology intravascular ultrasound tissue characterization. J Am Coll Cardiol. 2010;55:1590-7.
58. Kim TN, Kim S, Yang SJ, et al. Vascular inflammation in patients with impaired glucose tolerance and type 2 diabetes: analysis with 18F-fluorodeoxyglucose positron emission tomography. Circ Cardiovasc Imaging. 2010;3:142-8.
59. Klink A, Lancelot E, Ballet S, et al. Magnetic resonance molecular imaging of thrombosis in an arachidonic acid mouse model using an activated platelet targeted probe. Arterioscler Thromb Vasc Biol. 2010;30:403-10.
60. Cormode DP, Roessl E, Thran A, et al. Atherosclerotic plaque composition: analysis with multicolor CT and targeted gold nanoparticles. Radiology. 2010;256:774-82.
61. Bayturan O, Kapadia S, Nicholls SJ, et al. Clinical predictors of plaque progression despite very low levels of low-density lipoprotein cholesterol. J Am Coll Cardiol. 2010;55:2736-42.
62. Kubo T, Maehara A, Mintz GS, et al. The dynamic nature of coronary artery lesion morphology assessed by serial virtual histology intravascular ultrasound tissue characterization. J Am Coll Cardiol. 2010;55:1590-7.
63. Nambi V, Chambless L, Folsom AR, et al. Carotid intima-media thickness and presence or absence of plaque improves prediction of coronary heart disease risk: the ARIC (Atherosclerosis Risk In Communities) study. J Am Coll Cardiol. 2010;55:1600-7.
64. Giannarelli C, Ibanez B, Cimmino G, et al. Contrast-enhanced ultrasound imaging detects intraplaque neovascularization in an experimental model of atherosclerosis. J Am Coll Cardiol Imaging. 2010;3:1256-64.
65. Parmar JP, Rogers WJ, Mugler JP III, et al. Magnetic resonance imaging of carotid atherosclerotic plaque in clinically suspected acute transient ischemic attack and acute ischemic stroke. Circulation. 2010;122:2031-8.
66. Polonsky TS, McClelland RL, Jorgensen NW, et al. Coronary artery calcium score and risk classification for coronary heart disease prediction. JAMA. 2010;303:1610-6.
67. Cook NR, Ridker PM. Advances in measuring the effect of individual predictors of cardiovascular risk: the role of reclassification measures. Ann Intern Med. 2009;150:795.
68. Cook N. Use and misuse of the ROC curve in the medical literature. Circulation. 2007;115:928.

69. Ridker PM, Cook N. Should age and time be eliminated from cardiovascular risk prediction models? Rationale for the creation of a new national risk detection program. Circulation. 2005;111:657.
70. Andersen LB, Harro M, Sardinha LB, et al. Physical activity and clustered cardiovascular risk in children: a cross-sectional study (The European Youth Heart Study). Lancet. 2006;368:299.
71. Zethelius B, Berglund L, Sundstrom J, et al. Use of multiple biomarkers to improve the prediction of death from cardiovascular causes. N Engl J Med. 2008;358:2107.
72. Shlipak MG, Ix JH, Bibbins-Domingo K, et al. Biomarkers to predict recurrent cardiovascular disease: the Heart and Soul Study. Am J Med. 2008;121:50.
73. McMurray JJ, Kjekshus J, Gullestad L, et al. Effects of statin therapy according to plasma high-sensitivity C-reactive protein concentration in the Controlled Rosuvastatin Multinational Trial in Heart Failure (CORONA): a retrospective analysis. Circulation. 2009;120:2188.
74. Melander O, Newton-Cheh C, Almgren P, et al. Novel and conventional biomarkers for prediction of incident cardiovascular events in the community. JAMA. 2009;302:49.

20

Cardiovascular Diseases in Women: Does the Gender Bias Exist?

Malay Shukla, Aparna Jaswal

INTRODUCTION

Cardiovascular Diseases in Women: The Problem

Cardiovascular diseases (CVDs) are the leading cause of mortality both in men and women.[1] Before menopause, women have a lower risk of cardiac events, but this protection fades after menopause thus leaving women vulnerable to develop myocardial infarction (MI), heart failure (HF), and sudden cardiac death. Furthermore, clinical as well as diagnostic manifestations of ischemic heart disease are different in women from men and this factor may account for under-recognition of the disease in women.

CVDs in Women: Perception and Its Impact on Overall Mortality and Morbidity

Studies have shown that awareness among women regarding heart diseases as the major cause of mortality has increased. However, it is still widely perceived to be a male-related illness among the female population. This unfortunately acts a deterrent in promoting health education among women (to reduce cardiovascular risk factors), and also delays accessing appropriate medical care.

Does Gender Play a Role?

It is widely propagated that CVDs present and behave differently in women. This is reflected in clinical manifestation as well as response to medical management. This difference seems to be multifactorial, and can be explained by different lifestyles in both sexes, difference in body weight and BMI (women tend to have lower BMI and higher fat proportion), and differences in drug metabolism. A meta-analysis reviewed data from "Women's Health Study" and trials involving men with no history of CVD.[2] It shows that giving daily aspirin to this group (women and men with no relevant cardiovascular history) has no effect on the incidence of MI in females. It, however, significantly reduces the risk of MI in general male population.

CVDs in Women: Are They Under-represented in the Clinical Trials?

The above-mentioned meta-analysis also reflects upon the under-representation of women in the clinical trials. Reflecting on the earlier paragraph, we lack clarity on the reasons behind these differences, and further clinical trials are needed. They could target these differences, with emphasis on appropriate representation of female population.

Hypertension in Women

Women have higher prevalence of hypertension than men, especially elderly women. In premenopausal females, oral contraceptives are associated with risk of hypertension. Hypertensive women are at increased risk for development of complication like congestive heart failure. Also, more women who suffer from stroke have history of hypertension. In spite of this, hypertension remains more under-recognized and under-treated in women than men.

Coronary Heart Diseases in Women

It is well documented that coronary heart disease (CHD) manifests differently in women, and this has been shown in various studies. This could be atypical chest pain or "vague symptoms" (e.g. abdominal pain, restlessness, and fatigue). Women also tend to have higher proportions of silent ischemia and MI.

Furthermore, there are issues in diagnosis of CHD in women. Exercise tolerance test (ETT) tends to be less accurate in women. It can give false-positive results in young women with an unlikely CHD, whereas it can give false-negative results in women with single vessel disease.

The "Euro Heart Survey of Stable Angina"[3] presents interesting facts (women comprised 42% of the patients presenting "de novo" to cardiologists with stable angina). It shows that women were less likely to be referred for functional testing, angiography, and revascularization, and were less likely to receive secondary prevention at initial assessment and at 1 year (in those with proven coronary disease). It is noteworthy that the risk of morbidity and mortality was higher in women with proven coronary disease, and that they seemed underinvestigated and undertreated.

There is a paradox of ischemic heart disease (IHD) in women. Although women have higher myocardial I schemes and mortality than men with IHD, they have lesser prevalence of obstructive coronary artery disease. This highlights the importance of recognizing and instituting appropriate therapy for microvascular dysfunction in females.

Difference in Revascularization Procedures

A higher proportion of women (as compared to men) suffer from secondary risk factors like hypertension, hypercholesterolemia, and diabetes mellitus.[4] In spite of these differences, women undergoing cardiac bypass surgery show similar outcomes than men.[5]

Women also have smaller coronary arteries,[6] and this influences the choice of device used for percutaneous revascularization, resulting in reduction in the use of endovascular stents in women.[7] The risks of adverse events (e.g. coronary artery dissection and bleeding) during and after the procedure remain higher in women.

We know that success rates of percutaneous coronary intervention (PCI) revascularization, new antithrombotic drugs, drug-eluting stents, and primary angioplasty during MI are similar in both sexes. However, women seem to have increased risk of reinfection, stroke, and 6-month mortality as per the "PAMI study."[8] The overall mortality in women undergoing primary stenting for acute MI also seems to be higher than men.

Heart Failure: Gender Differences

The prevalence of HF is similar in men and women and increases with age. HF is more common in women above 75 years of age. Hypertensive,[9] diabetic,[10] and post-MI women[11] are more likely to develop HF than men. They also seem to be more symptomatic of their HF symptoms, and can result in more frequent emergency hospital admissions.[12,13] Despite being more symptomatic of their disease, women with HF have a better life expectancy as compared to similar cohort of men as depicted in therapeutic intervention trials and large databases.[14,15]

Unfortunately women continue to be under-represented in trials and studies focusing on HF management—MADIT II, COMPANION, and SCD-HeFT trials advising use of ICD in patients with HF, and CARE-HF trial (advice on resynchronization therapy in patients with HF).

Stroke: Gender Differences

Stroke continues to be a major contributor to significant morbidity and mortality in patients. Stroke occurs in more men than women until advanced age when women have higher incidence.

Women also seem to have greater neurological impairment (NIH stroke scale) and disability (Barthel index) at hospital discharge. The pattern continued when 1 year outcomes of above parameters were evaluated for these patients. Although women have first stroke at higher age than men that may account for poorer functional outcomes, studies analyzed after age control show mixed results.[2,17] So, this makes women a population subset with more life expectancy and stoke severity, and hence a higher disability that highlights importance of aggressive stroke risk factor modification in females.

There seems to be difference in managing stroke in male and female patients. A multicenter study conducted in Europe[18] concluded that women were investigated to lesser extent (brain imaging, Doppler ultrasound examination, ECHO, and angiography) than male patients. It also revealed that carotid artery surgery was less frequently performed than on female patients.

Atrial Fibrillation and Risk of Stroke in Men and Women

Cardiogenic embolus due to atrial fibrillation (AF) is one of the major causes of stroke in women, as compared to men.[19] We are also aware that AF is more frequent in women who suffer from stroke. Women have higher CHADS-2 scores associated with AF as shown by the "EURO Heart Survey." The increased correlation between risk of stroke and AF is higher in women as shown by "ATRIA study" (including 15000 patients with AF, and showed that the risk of stroke was more in women). In spite of this, a lesser proportion of women with AF were treated with oral anticoagulation therapy prior to stroke as compared to their male counterparts.

WHAT NEXT?

Patient education and risk factor management remains the mainstay of patient management. This is important to improve the outcome including quality of life. It is indeed challenging for patients and clinicians alike because of many factors—lack of opportunities to promote health due to limited patient visits, lack of training in counseling patients about behavioral changes, lack of dedicated time and staff to help achieve this, presence of multiple comorbidities, and lack of perceived incentives (monetary and qualitative).

We will also have to be women centric in our approach and will have to find ways to convey the message to the target audience. This could be looking for opportunities to promote cardiovascular health when reviewing them for other illnesses and advise on weight management by using methods like wall posters/in house campaigns to help weight reduction. Particular emphasis should be given to postmenopausal women as the risk increases in this subset of patients. Until recently postmenopausal hormone replacement therapy (HRT) was considered beneficial for prevention of CVD; recent data, from HERS study, however, refutes these claims.

Emphasis should be laid on prevention and management of contributing risk factors like hypertension, hypercholesterolemia, and diabetes mellitus. Current NCEP guidelines recommend aggressive targets for managing triglycerides and high-density lipoprotein (HDL) cholesterol levels.

REFERENCES

1. World Health Organization Statistical Information System 2004. *www.who.int/whosis/*
2. Ridker PM, Cook NR, Lee IM, et al. A randomized trial of low-dose aspirin in the primary prevention of cardiovascular disease in women. N Engl J Med. 2005;352:1293-304.
3. Daly CA, Clemens F, Sendon JL, et al. Euro Heart Survey Investigators. The clinical characteristics and investigations planned in patients with stable angina presenting to cardiologists in Europe: from the Euro Heart Survey of Stable Angina. Eur Heart J. 2005;26:996-1010.
4. Jacobs AK. Coronary revascularization in women 2003. Sex revisited. Circulation. 2003;107:375-7.
5. Jacobs AK, Kelsey SF, Brooks MM, et al. Better outcome for women compared with men undergoing coronary revascularization: a report from the bypass angioplasty revascularization investigation (BARI). Circulation. 1998;98:1279-85.
6. Dodge JT Jr, Brown BG, Bolson EL, et al. Lumen diameter of normal human coronary arteries. Influence of age, sex, anatomic variation, and left ventricular hypertrophy or dilation. Circulation. 1992;86:232-46.
7. Schunkert H, Harrell L, Palacios IF. Implications of small reference vessel diameter in patients undergoing percutaneous coronary revascularization. J Am Coll Cardiol. 1999;34:40-8.
8. Stone GW, Grines CL, Browne KF, et al. Predictors of in-hospital and 6-month outcome after acute myocardial infarction in the reperfusion era: the Primary Angioplasty in Myocardial Infarction (PAMI) trial. J Am Coll Cardiol. 1995;25:370-7.
9. Levy D, Larson MG, Vasan RS, et al. The progression from hypertension to congestive heart failure. JAMA. 1996;275:1557-62.
10. Shindler DM, Kostis JB, Yusuf S, et al. Diabetes mellitus, a predictor of morbidity and mortality in the Studies of Left Ventricular Dysfunction (SOLVD) Trials and Registry. Am J Cardiol. 1996;77:1017-20.
11. McMurray J, McDonagh T, Morrison CE, et al. Trends in hospitalization for heart failure in Scotland 1980–1990. Eur Heart J. 1993;14:1158-62.
12. Petrie MC, Dawson NF, Murdoch DR, et al. Failure of women's hearts. Circulation. 1999;99:2334-41.
13. McMurray J, McDonagh T, Morrison CE, et al. Trends in hospitalization for heart failure in Scotland 1980–1990. Eur Heart J. 1993;14:1158-62.
14. Adams KF Jr, Sueta CA, Gheorghiade M, et al. Gender differences in survival in advanced heart failure. Insights from the FIRST study. Circulation. 1999;99:1816-21.
15. Simon T, Mary-Krause M, Funck-Brentano C, et al. Sex differences in the prognosis of congestive heart failure: results from the Cardiac Insufficiency Bisoprolol Study (CIBIS II). Circulation. 2001;103:375-80.
16. Rosamond W, Flegal K, Friday G, et al. Heart disease and stroke statistics – 2007 update: a report from the American Heart Association Statistics Committee and Stroke Statistics Subcommittee. Circulation. 2007;115:e69-e171.
17. Eriksson M, Norrving B, Terent A, et al. Functional outcome 3 months after stroke predicts long-term survival. Cerebrovasc Dis. 2008;25:423-9.
18. Di Carlo A, Lamassa M, Baldereschi M, et al. European BIOMED Study of Stroke Care Group. Sex differences in the clinical presentation, resource use, and 3-month outcome of acute stroke in Europe: data from a multicenter multinational hospital-based registry. Stroke. 2003;34:1114-9.
19. Goulené K, Santalucia P, Leonetti G, et al. Gender differences in the clinical presentation and outcome of acute stroke. Stroke. 2006;37:648.

21

What is Optimal Medical Therapy and What does it Achieve: Medical Management of Coronary Artery Disease—Is it a Full Circle Traveled?

Amitesh Chakravarty, Vijay Kumar

INTRODUCTION

Cardiology has seen new approaches both medical and surgical including guidelines for treatment of coronary artery disease (CAD). New sophisticated surgical techniques including robotics and percutaneous coronary intervention (PCI) technology to deal with difficult lesions, and of course, drug therapy for cardiovascular diseases (CVDs) have changed the scenario for good.[1] Medications that modify CV risk factors and improve survival include aspirin and P2Y12 antagonists, neuroendocrine axis modifiable agents (ACE-I, ARBs, β-blockers), and HMG CoA antagonist (atorvastatin, rosuvastatin) have revolutionized medical therapy. Optimal medical therapy (OMT) is the application of the above-mentioned agents in clinically applicable doses in CAD that provide both survival and symptomatic benefits without causing adverse effects and improves quality of life (QOL).[2-4] Optimal medical therapy is applicable to a large spectrum of stable CAD patients with invasive approaches kept for high risk or unstable acute coronary patients.

Indians have a tendency to develop early atherosclerosis that has led to a spurt in CAD and diabetes in the last few years, all thanks to lifestyle and eating habits with rise in obesity. Clinical features divide the patients of CAD into two groups, one with an acute presentation and the other with chronic but stable CAD. The treatment of stable CAD patients includes aggressive guideline based therapy of risk factors with patients although such patients require PCI/CABG (coronary artery bypass graft) when the symptoms are not controlled by medication to an extent hampering the QOL. Newer generation stents over and above balloon angioplasty and bare metal stents have improved revascularization in CAD patients who become symptomatic. Surgical advances in bypass surgery including off-pump, robotic, and hybrid surgery are useful approaches in diabetics, extensive CAD, and those with left ventricular (LV) dysfunction. Patients with acute presentation especially those at high risk are best managed at centers with available PCI and surgical backup. From presentation to the initiation of invasive procedure, it is mandatory to provide patients best medical care that too aggressively include aspirin, P2Y12 inhibitors, hypolipidemic agents and anticoagulants like heparin/LMWH, and usage of GP2B/3A inhibitors in high-risk cases. In India, thrombolysis still remains the most common approach to reperfusion, although cardiac centers with catheterization facilities are fast becoming the norm. This is especially important in acute presentations and complicated ST-elevation myocardial infarction (STEMI), where early aggressive invasive therapy is the most beneficial. The new guidelines help the clinician in formulating a proper protocol for each case. Rise in CAD has helped catheterization laboratories proliferate and improve treatment from predominantly medical management to medical and invasive approach.

Stable angina patients derive adequate benefit with OMT as compared to revascularization seen in the light of mortality, cardiac events such as myocardial infarction (MI), or even cerebrovascular events as the evidence suggests.

STICH: SURGICAL TREATMENT FOR ISCHEMIC HEART FAILURE

STICH trial gave evidence on similar lines on medical therapy versus and medical therapy plus CABG in death from any cause, although cardiac-cause-related deaths were lower in the surgery. Consensus has given CABG an edge over medical therapy and PCI in multivessel disease especially with LV dysfunction, but PCI scores more when it is the culprit artery in STEMI, although the recent PRAMI trial telling otherwise. To select the best possible strategy is the best approach even if it means discussion with the family when nothing is clearly justified.

POLYPILL FOR INCREASE IN TREATMENT COMPLIANCE

Invasive approach or invasive and medical management approach whatever be the case, secondary prevention becomes the common. Even in CAD patients aged >70–75 years, secondary prevention as per guidelines improves survival. Evidence from studies like clinical outcomes utilizing revascularization and aggressive drug evaluation (COURAGE), BARI-2D is that only one in two patients is getting to targets set for hypertension, lipid or sugar control, related to non-compliance to medical therapy. Polypill is supposedly the answer to this issue accounting for perhaps quite a few social as well as economic constraints. Wald and Law (2003) came up with this idea of multiple combination of well-known drugs in a single formulation ~~that will~~ be inexpensive as well. Most cardiac-oriented polypills address CVD risks in a single go such as blood pressure and cholesterol reduction with a platelet inhibitor. Compliance is increased and the costs per medication decreased. A total of 3.2 million CAD events and 1.7 million strokes over 10 years in general population may well be prevented as per a US-based consensus, and 0.9 million CAD events and 0.5 million strokes in those with CVDs. Several randomized studies are underway in proving this concept.

BACKGROUND

Assumed through evidence-based medicine is that by 40 years, the CAD risk in males is 50% and in females is around 30%.[5] Atherosclerosis affecting coronaries initiates early in life with continual progression through all ages gradually.[6]

Interheart showed that 90% of males and 94% of females have the following nine variables as the major risk factors contributing to the population attributable risk of CAD: dyslipidemia, hypertension, smoking, diabetes, abdominal obesity, diet poor in daily consumption of fruit and vegetables, lack of regular physical activity, alcohol intake, and psychological factors (mainly depression).[7]

Hypercholesterolemia begets atherosclerosis. Evidence indicates that a low density lipoprotein (LDL) cholesterol level decreases the risk of CAD by up to 80% compared with the general population. Intensive LDL reduction reduces the risk of CVD by 40–50%.[8]

GLOBAL SCENARIO

Most of the developed nations are seeing a decrease in CV-related deaths owing to aggressive evidence-based cholesterol management treatment of blood pressure and smoking cessation. Risk factor reduction through secondary prophylaxis especially after revascularization is the mainstay in such cases. Each death prevented by treating a CAD patient yields an additional 7.5 years of life. Risk factor reduction has been shown to account for up to 79% of the total life years gained in some registry data. Would not it be fruitful to start CV risk reduction much earlier in life to reduce the impact by early recognition and treatment to prevent new trends from spreading like hypertension, obesity, and diabetes mellitus when we know that CVD is increasing?[9]

USEFUL THERAPIES

Smoking is one of the most important risk factor where its cessation causes 36% relative mortality risk reduction.[10] Smoking cessation after suffering a MI causes 37% decrease in mortality risk.

Observational studies persistently reported a decreased number of CV events in patients who perform regular aerobic activity. Even 1 hour of walking/week is associated with a lower risk.

The decrease of about 1.5 mmol/L LDL cholesterol lessens the risk of cardiac events and stroke by 30%.[11]

Reducing dietary salt by 3 g/day can reduce blood pressure, new cases of CVD, stroke and mortality by a level similar to other risks.[12]

Aspirin reduces the relative risk of a nonfatal MI by 23%, but has no effect on mortality when used in primary prevention, although when used in secondary prevention aspirin reduces the same risk by a 31% and mortality by 9%.[13]

Clopidogrel is useful in patients having allergy to aspirin. CAPRIE: Clopidogrel versus Aspirin in Patients at Risk of Ischemic Events study found that clopidogrel treatment was associated with 8.7% decrease in vascular mortality rate including stroke and MI. CHARISMA: Clopidogrel for high atherothrombotic risk and ischemic stabilization, management and avoidance trial proved that usage of both aspirin and clopidogrel in place of aspirin alone is not more beneficial.

Niacin decreases major cardiac events especially coronary by one fourth according to a meta-analysis.[14]

In patients with stable CAD and a no LV dysfunction, angiotensin-converting enzyme (ACE) inhibitors (ACE-I) decrease mortality by 13% and nonfatal MI by 17% as shown in a meta-analysis.[15] In the same meta-analysis, ARBs decreased MI stroke and death by 12%.

Beta-blockers, used as a secondary prevention measure can reduce death and reinfarction by 23%.[16]

The use of N-3 PUFA after a MI decreases sudden cardiac death (SCD) by 45% CV-related mortality by 30%.[17]

Newer Agents

- *Ranolazine*: Late sodium current inhibitor that is a useful in angina reduction and helps in ischaemia management.
- *Fasudil*: ρ-kinase inhibitor that increases time to ECG changes, including ST depression and increase total exercise duration.
- *Trimetazidine*: Metabolic modulator and partial fatty acid oxidation (pFOX) inhibitor that is beneficial in stable-angina patients.
- *Ivabradine*: Noninferior to β-blockers in INITIATIVE: International trial on the treatment of angina with ivabradine versus atenolol study for reduction in angina. BEAUTIFUL: Ivabradine for patients with stable coronary artery disease and left ventricular systolic dysfunction study showed improvement in angina-related results.
- *Nicorandil*: In impact of nicorandil in angina (IONA) trial, beneficial effect in terms of CAD death and nonfatal MI was seen with nicorandil use.

EFFICACY OF OPTIMAL MEDICAL THERAPY

In a large trial, the use of five drugs [aspirin, clopidogrel, β-blocker, statin, renin-angiotensin system blocker (ACE-I/angiotensin II receptor blocker (ARB)] was tested versus the use of one of these drugs or none in survivors of a first MI, and it was found the use of the five drugs reduced death from any cardiac cause at 1 year by 74% versus one or none of the drugs used.[18]

In the chronic table angina patients, noncompliance to OMT was associated with a 10–40% increase in risk of hospital admissions from a cardiac cause and a 50–80% rise in death.[19]

ADDITIONAL THERAPIES

Use of folate and vitamin B supplementation to reduce homocysteine level which is widely considered a potential risk factor, failed to show any benefit. Homocysteine reduction in view of studies considering it as a potential risk factor, by using folate and vitamins especially the B group did not confirm the same assumption.[20]

DISCUSSION

Cardiovascular-related mortality especially due to coronary atherosclerosis is the leading cause of death all over the world. Secondary prevention is the important mainstay including risk factor reduction and medication for modifiable risks. Revascularization in addition to OMT has been shown to improve survival especially in acute coronary cases although studies have found it hard to prove the same in stable CAD. COURAGE trial included 2,287 patients having myocardial ischemia and significant CAD (≥70% in at least one proximal epicardial coronary artery) and found that PCI over and above medical management as an initial management strategy in stable CAD did not reduce hard endpoints proving that complication rate in chronic stable angina is less. Deduction that optimized medication therapy is as beneficial as PCI in chronic stable CAD. Interestingly what COURAGE trial implemented in terms of optimal intensity medical therapy is difficult to reproduce. Recent large registries suggested that stable CAD patients undergoing PCI <50% were receiving OMT before revascularization and only 60–65% were receiving OMT at discharge, even after COURAGE trial. Post COURAGE trial, PCI outcomes have improved with the availability of new generation drug eluting stents, calculation of FFR (fractional flow reserve) in intermediate lesions and extensive IVUS (intravascular ultrasound) usage.[21]

FAME II (Fractional Flow Reserve-Guided PCI vs. Medical Therapy in Stable Coronary Disease) enrolled 1,220 stable patients with CAD and implemented FFR measurement to detect hemodynamically important stenosis (FFR < 0.80) with randomization to either PCI or OMT in patients with one such lesion. FAME II found that PCI requiring patients with significant FFR had 66% fewer primary endpoint events; 4.3% versus 12.7% compared to medical therapy due to less rate of urgent revascularization in the PCI group (0.7%) compared to medical therapy group (9.5%), although there was no significant difference in mortality or MI in PCI plus medical therapy group and medical therapy alone group.

Patients with a >0.8 FFR had a cardiac event rate of 3.0% with medical therapy that was justified because of the concept of OMT. Also confirmed that angiography alone, as in COURAGE, is not enough in detecting patients with adverse outcomes. When deciding between revascularization and OMT, FFR be it invasive or noninvasive proclaims justification as seen by FAME II that channels this FFR strategy as standard of care for stable CAD patients. These studies proved that PCI did reduce symptoms and QOL it did not prevent mortality or acute coronary events in stable CAD. FAME II also reduced emergency revascularization procedures due to improvement in secondary endpoints because of FFR and newer drug eluding. Patients of stable CAD who demonstrate severe ischemia as in a hemodynamically significant FFR or a positive stress tests may be regarded as high risk and should be taken up for an early invasive approach. The ongoing ISCHEMIA (The International Study of Comparative Health Effectiveness with Medical and Invasive Approaches) trial is a randomized trial that is enrolling stable CAD patients with moderate-to-severe ischemia on stress test who will undergo a coronary CTA to exclude LM disease and to confirm the presence of stenotic coronaries due to atherosclerosis.

Patients will be divided into revascularization and OMT or OMT alone hoping to provide the initial best strategy possible.

CONCLUSION

Optimal medical therapy is not merely the absence of invasive therapy, instead it involves appropriate and aggressive medical management according to the latest guidelines for symptomatic benefit and maintenance of a stable physiological and clinical state of the patient.

REFERENCES

1. Lloyd-Jones D, Adams R, Carnethon M, et al. Heart disease and stroke statistics—2009 update: a report from the American Heart Association Statistics Committee and Stroke Statistics Subcommittee [published corrections appear in Circulation. 2009;119(3):e182, and Circulation. 2010;122(1):e11]. Circulation. 2009;119(3):e21-e181.
2. Third report of the National Cholesterol Education Program Expert Panel on detection, evaluation, and treatment of high blood cholesterol in adults (Adult Treatment Panel III). NIH Publication No. 02-5215. September 2002.
3. Fraker TD Jr, Fihn SD, Gibbons RJ, et al. 2007 chronic angina focused update of the ACC/AHA 2002 Guidelines for the management of patients with chronic stable angina: a report of the American College of Cardiology/American Heart Association Task Force on Practice Guidelines Writing Group to develop the focused update of the 2002 Guidelines for the management of patients with chronic stable angina. J Am Coll Cardiol. 2007;50(23):2264-74.
4. Fuster V, Badimon L, Badimon JJ, et al. The pathogenesis of coronary artery disease and the acute coronary syndromes (1). N Engl J Med. 1992;326(4):242-50.
5. Lloyd-Jones DM, Larson MG, et al. Life-time risk of developing coronary artery disease. Lancet. 1999;353:89-92.
6. Berenson GS, Pickoff AS. Preventive cardiology and its potential influence on the early natural history of adult heart disease: the Bogulusa Heart Study and the Heart SMART Program. Am J Med Sci. 1995;310(Suppl 1):S133-S138.
7. Yusuf S, Hawken S, Ounpuu S, et al. Effect of potentially modifiable risk factor associated with myocardial infarction in 52 countries (the INTERHEART study): case-control study. Lancet. 2004;364:937-52.
8. Grundy SM. Is lowering low-density lipoprotein (LDL) an effective strategy to reduce cardiac risk? Circulation. 2008;117: 569-73.
9. Brown JR, O'Connon GT. Coronary heart disease and prevention in the United States. N Engl J Med. 2010;362:2150-3.
10. Critchley JA, Capewell S. Mortality risk reduction associated with smoking cessation in patients with coronary heart disease: a systematic review. JAMA. 2003;290:86-97.
11. Baigent C, Keech A, Kearney PM, et al. Cholesterol Treatment Triallist (CTT) Collaboration. Efficacy and safety of cholesterol-lowering treatment: prospective metaanalysis of data from 90056 participations in 14 randomised trials of statins. Lancet. 2005;366:1267-78.
12. Bibbens-Domingo K, Chertow GM, Coxson PG, et al. Projected effect of dietary salt reductions on fatal cardiovascular disease. N Engl J Med. 2010.10.1056/NEJM oa 0907355.
13. Baigent C, Blackwell L, Collins R, et al. Aspirin in the primary and secondary prevention of vascular disease: collaborative meta-analysis of individual participant data from randomised trials. Lancet. 2009;373:1849-60.
14. Bruckert E, Labreuche J, Amarenco P. Meta-analysis of the effect of nicotinic acid alone or in combination on cardiovascular events and atherosclerosis. Atherosclerosis. 2010;210:353-61.
15. Baker WL, Coleman CI, Kluger J, et al. Systematic review: comparative effectiveness of angiotensin converting enzyme inhibitors or angiotension-II-receptor blockers for ischaemic heart disease. Ann Intern Med. 2009;151:861-71.
16. Chae CJ, Hennekens CH. Beta blockers. In: Hennekens CH (Ed). Clinical Trials in Cardiovascular Disease: a Companion to Braunwald's Heart Disease. Philadelphia, PA: WB Saunders; 1999. p. 84.
17. Khavandi A, Khavandi K, Greenstein A, et al. N-3 polyunsaturated fatty acids are still underappreciated and underused post myocardial infarction. Heart. 2009;85:540-41.
18. Bramlage P, Messer C, Bitterlich N, et al. The effect of optimal medical therapy on 1-year mortality after acute myocardial infarction. Heart. 2010;96:604-9.
19. Ho PM, Magid DJ, Shetterly SM, et al. Medication non-adherence is associated with a broad range of adverse outcomes in patients with coronary artery disease. Am Heart J. 2008;155:772-9.
20. Lewis SJ. Prevention and treatment of atherosclerosis: a Practitioner's guide for 2008. Am J Med. 2009;122:S38-S50.
21. Boden WE , O'Rourke RA, Teo KK, et al. Optimal Medical Therapy with or without PCI for Stable Coronary Disease COURAGE Trial Research Group N Engl J Med. 2007;356:1503-16.

22

Optimal Medical Therapy: What does it Mean and Deliver?

Mitu A Minocha, Sachin V Chaudhary

INTRODUCTION

Coronary artery disease (CAD) is the leading cause of death worldwide. Stable angina is the initial clinical manifestation in most of the patients. Angina can be disabling and can lead to increased morbidity and mortality.

The management of patients with stable angina is a major clinical challenge for health care providers. Large randomized trials suggest that people with stable angina have a good prognosis with an all-cause mortality of around 1.5% a year but population-based studies have reported substantially higher annual cardiovascular (CV) death rates.[1,2]

There have been marked advances in medical, percutaneous interventional and surgical treatments for the management of CAD during the past decade. There is enough data to suggest that for patients with stable angina, optimal medical therapy (OMT) is equally effective for lowering the risk of major CV events as are revascularization procedures, such as coronary artery bypass grafting (CABG) or percutaneous coronary intervention (PCI). Medical management comprises of various lifestyle changes, drug therapy to improve long-term outcome, and drug therapy to improve symptoms. Optimal selection of the procedure and/or medical management strategy that is most likely to benefit an individual CV patient is of prime importance.

Optimal medical therapy is defined as one or two antianginal drugs as required in addition to drugs for secondary prevention of cardiovascular disease (CVD).[3] It consists of antiplatelet agent, anti-ischemic drugs, and aggressive lipid and blood pressure management. Revascularization procedures need to be added to OMT if patients persist with significant symptoms or are intolerant to drugs or have high-risk coronary lesions.

MANAGEMENT OF STABLE CORONARY ARTERY DISEASE

The aim of management of stable CAD is to reduce symptoms and improve prognosis. The management of CAD patients encompasses lifestyle modification, management of CAD risk factors, and evidence-based drug therapy.

Lifestyle Modifications and Control of Risk Factors

Smoking

Smoking being an independent risk factor of CAD, smoking cessation should be encouraged for all patients with stable CAD. Cigarette smoking may be responsible for aggravating angina other than through the progression of atherosclerosis. It may increase myocardial oxygen demand and reduce coronary blood flow by an α-adrenergically mediated increase in coronary artery tone, thereby causing ischemia.

Quitting smoking is complex because it is both pharmacologically and psychologically addictive. Various measures for smoking cessation include counseling, regular follow-up, referral to cessation programs, and pharmacotherapy. Nicotine replacement therapy should be routinely offered as it is safe in patients with CAD.[4] Safety of Bupropion and varenicline have been reported in patients with stable CAD in some studies,[5] although the safety of varenicline has recently been questioned in a meta-analysis,[6] being associated with a small but significant increase in CVD.

Quitting smoking is probably the most effective of all measures of secondary prevention, being associated with a reduction in mortality of 36% after myocardial infarction (MI).[7]

Diet and Physical Activity

A healthy diet reduces CVD risk. Patients should be encouraged for weight maintenance/reduction through appropriate lifestyle measures including balanced calorie intake, physical exercise, and structured behavioral programs to maintain or achieve a body mass index between 18.5 and 24.9 kg/m^2 and a waist circumference <102 cm (40 in.) in men and <88 cm (35 in.) in women.[8]

The current recommendations are to reduce intake of saturated fats (<10% of total energy intake) and increase PUFA intake through fish consumption, as it is associated with beneficial effects, especially reduction in triglycerides.[8] Recently, the largest study ever conducted with a so-called Mediterranean diet, supplemented with extravirgin olive oil or nuts, reduced the incidence of major CV events in patients at high-risk of CV events but without prior CV disease.[9]

Both overweight and obesity can lead to increased risk of CAD. Weight reduction in overweight and obese people has favorable effects on blood pressure, dyslipidemia, and glucose metabolism.[8] The initial goal of weight loss therapy should be weight reduction by 5–10% from the baseline.

Regular physical activity leads to reduction in CV morbidity and mortality in patients with CAD and physical activity should therefore be incorporated into daily life. A structured cardiac rehabilitation program should be advised to patients with CAD to initiate them into aerobic exercise. Patients with stable CAD should undergo thrice weekly sessions of moderate-to-vigorous intensity aerobic exercise for 30 minutes per session. Sedentary patients should be initiated to light-intensity exercise programs after proper exercise-related risk stratification (Table 22.1).[8]

Blood Pressure Management

Hypertension is a major risk factor for CAD as well as heart failure, cerebrovascular disease and renal failure. It is recommended that systolic blood pressure (BP) be maintained <140 mm Hg and diastolic BP < 90 mm Hg in CAD patients with hypertension.[10] Based on current data, it may be prudent to recommend lowering SBP/DBP to values within the range 130–139/80–85 mm Hg. In diabetic patients, the goal is <140/85 mm Hg[8,11] and it is prudent to include angiotensin converting enzyme (ACE) inhibitor or angiotensin receptor blocker because of the renal protective effects.[8,10] The choice of antihypertensive agent should be based on patient characteristics and should include ACE inhibitors and/or β-blocker while other drugs such as thiazides or calcium channel blockers (CCBs) may be added as required.

Table 22.1 Recommended diet intakes

Saturated fatty acids to account for <10% of total energy intake, through replacement by polyunsaturated fatty acids
Transunsaturated fatty acids <1% of total energy intake
<5 g of salt per day
30–45 g fiber per day, from whole grain products, fruits, and vegetables
200 g fruit per day (2–3 servings)
200 g vegetables per day (2–3 servings)
Fish at least twice a week, one being oily fish
Consumption of alcoholic beverages should be limited to 2 glasses per day (20 g/day of alcohol) for men and 1 glasses per day (10 g/day of alcohol) for nonpregnant women

Diabetes Mellitus

The risk of atherosclerotic vascular disease is significantly higher in patients of diabetes mellitus. Diabetes is a strong risk factor that multiplies the risk of CV complications and enhances the risk of progression of coronary disease. Optimum management of diabetes is of prime importance in this subset of patients. A goal glycosylated hemoglobin (HbA_{1c}) of <7.0% (53 mmol/mol) generally and <6.5–6.9% on an individual basis is reasonable.[8,11] Glucose control should be based on individual considerations, including age, presence of complications, and diabetes duration.

Lipid Management

Patients with established CAD are at high-risk for CV events and statin treatment is indicated in them irrespective of low-density lipoprotein (LDL) cholesterol (LDL-C) levels.

Dyslipidemia management includes lifestyle and pharmacological interventions. Multiple large studies have shown that lipid lowering with statins reduces not only the risk of major acute cardiac events but also the need for revascularization and decreases the signs and symptoms of myocardial ischemia.

The goals of treatment are LDL-C <70 gm/dL or >50% LDL-C reduction when target level cannot be achieved. In the majority of patients, this is achievable through statin monotherapy. Fibrates, resins, nicotinic acid, and ezetimibe may lower LDL cholesterol but no benefit on clinical outcomes has been reported for these alternatives.

Although elevated levels of triglycerides and low-HDL cholesterol (HDL-C) are associated with increased CVD risk, clinical trial evidence is insufficient to specify treatment targets.

PHARMACOLOGICAL MANAGEMENT OF STABLE CAD PATIENTS

The aim of pharmacological management of stable CAD patients includes relief of symptoms and prevention of CV events.

ANTI-ISCHEMIC DRUGS

Nitrates

Nitrates are endothelium-independent vasodilators. They reduce the myocardial oxygen requirement and improve myocardial perfusion. Hence, they are effective in relieving both demand and supply ischemia.

Nitroglycerine administered sublingually can be used to treat the acute onset of angina symptoms, as well as a prophylaxis prior to an activity when angina is expected to occur. The recommended dose of sublingual nitroglycerine is 0.3–0.6 mg every 5 minutes until the pain goes or a maximum of 1.2 mg has been taken within 15 minutes.[12] Isosorbide dinitrate (5 mg sublingually) helps to abort anginal attacks for about 1 hour.

Long-term control of angina symptoms can be achieved with long-acting nitrates like isosorbide dinitrate and its active metabolite isosorbide mononitrate used as an oral preparation.[13] The dosing should provide a minimum of 10–12 hours nitrate-free interval to tackle the problem of nitrate tolerance during long-term therapy.[14] Once daily regimens of extended release preparations like transdermal nitrate patches and isosorbide mononitrate help to improve compliance.

In patients with chronic stable angina, nitrates improve exercise tolerance, time to onset of angina, and ST-segment depression during the treadmill exercise test. In combination with β-blockers or calcium antagonists, nitrates produce greater antianginal and anti-ischemic effects in patients with stable angina.[15]

The most common side effects include facial flushing and headache and the most serious is hypotension. Nitrates should be avoided within 24 hours of taking phosphodiesterase inhibitors (like sildenafil) as hypotension may ensue.

β-Blockers

β-Blockers are recommended as first-line therapy in CAD and patients with stable angina without contraindications. β-Blockers reduce heart rate and contractility, and myocardial oxygen demand. In post-MI patients, β-blockers achieved a 30% risk reduction for CV death and MI[16] and appear to be effective in controlling symptomatic and asymptomatic ischemic episodes. There is evidence for prognostic benefits from the use of β-blockers in post-MI patients, or in heart failure. Extrapolation from these data suggests that β-blockers may be the first-line antianginal therapy in stable CAD patients without contraindications.

All β-blockers are equally effective in alleviating angina pectoris, although optimal doses may vary. The most widely used β-blockers are those with predominant β1-blockade, such as metoprolol,[17] bisoprolol, atenolol, or nebivolol. Carvedilol, a nonselective β-α1 blocker, is also often used.

Nebivolol and bisoprolol are partly secreted by the kidney, whereas carvedilol and metoprolol are metabolized by the liver, hence being safer in patients with renal compromise. Important side effects are bradycardia, bronchoconstriction, fatigue, depression, impotence, and worsening of peripheral vascular diseases.

Calcium Channel Blockers

Calcium channel blockers promote coronary and peripheral vasodilation by blocking the entry of calcium into the myocardial and vascular smooth muscle cells. Calcium channel blockers, a heterogenous group, are classified into dihydropyridines (DHPs) and nondihydropyridines. Dihydropyridine CCBs (amlodipine, nicardipine, nifedipine, felodipine) have a greater effect on vascular smooth muscle cells and are particularly effective in reducing systemic arterial blood pressure. Nondihydropyridine CCBs (verapamil, diltiazem) affect conduction through the atrioventricular node and tend to reduce heart rate, thus explaining the antianginal properties. All CCBs have been shown to be effective in chronic stable angina.[18]

Dihydropyridines

Dihydropyridines reduce the frequency of angina episodes, improve exercise duration, and reduce the need for nitroglycerin.

***Amlodipine*:** The very long half-life and good tolerability of amlodipine make it an effective once-a-day antianginal and antihypertensive agent. Exercise-induced ischemia is more effectively reduced by amlodipine than by the β-blocker atenolol and the combination is even better.[19] Side effects are mainly ankle edema.

***Others*:** Felodipine and cilnidipine share the standard properties of other long-acting DHPs.

Short-acting nifedipine has an increased incidence of CV events and is not recommended for patients with acute coronary syndrome (ACS) or unstable angina.[20]

Nondihydropyridines

***Verapamil*:** Among CCBs, verapamil is useful in all varieties of angina (effort, vasospastic, unstable) and hypertension. Indirect evidence suggests good safety but with risks of heart block, bradycardia, and heart failure. Compared with metoprolol, the antianginal activity was similar.[17] Compared with atenonol in hypertension with CAD, verapamil gave less new diabetes, fewer anginal attacks,[21] and less psychological depression. β-Blockers combined with verapamil is not advised (due to risk of heart block), instead, use DHP-β-blockade.

***Diltiazem*:** It, because of its low side-effect profile, has advantages, compared with verapamil, in the treatment of effort angina.[22] Like verapamil, it acts by peripheral vasodilation, relief of exercise-induced coronary constriction, a modest negative inotropic effect and sinus node inhibition. There are no outcome studies comparing diltiazem and verapamil. The combination of diltiazem with β-blockers, as well as the use in patients with CAD and left ventricular dysfunction is best avoided.

Calcium channel blockers are generally as efficacious as β-blockers in reducing angina and improving exercise time to onset of angina or ischemia.

NEWER AGENTS

Nicorandil

Nicorandil a nicotinamide nitrate acts mainly by dilation of the large coronary arteries, as well as by reduction of pre and after load. It is approved for the treatment and prevention of angina.[23] It has a dual mechanism of action, both activation of potassium channels and a nitrate-like effect. In the IONA study, 5,126 patients with stable angina were followed for a mean of 1.6 years; major coronary events including ACS were reduced. Occasional side effects include oral, intestinal, and perianal ulceration.

Ivabradine

Ivabradine is a new drug that lowers the heart rate by acting on SA node by inhibiting the I(*f*) current, and thereby decreasing the myocardial oxygen demand without effect on inotropism or BP.[24] In the INITIATIVE study, ivabradine was found to be noninferior to β-blockers for reliving angina. In the BEAUTIFUL trial, which included CAD patients with LV dysfunction, it was proven that though there was no long-term reduction in MACE with ivabradine, there was significant reduction in angina compared with placebo.[25] The reduction of heart rate with ivabradine leads to anti-ischemic and antianginal effect equivalent to that of atenolol without any other known CV effects. It is therefore an important therapeutic alternative or addition to the current antianginal drugs.

European Society of Cardiology recommends ivabradine for the treatment of stable angina in patients who do not tolerate β-blockers or as an addition to β-blockade in patients with persistent angina and whose heart rate exceeds 60 bpm.[24] Ivabradine is well tolerated with occasional side effects of transient visual disturbances and bradycardia.

Ranolazine

Ranolazine is a newer antianginal drug that acts by selective inhibition of late sodium current. It inhibits the exaggerated late inward sodium current that occurs during ischemia, thereby preventing rise in intracellular sodium and intracellular calcium overload. The rise in intracellular calcium leads to an increase in diastolic LV stiffness compressing the intramyocardial vessels, thus reducing coronary blood flow. Ranolazine prevents this abnormal increase in late inward sodium and the downstream effects of increased LV stiffness and thereby reducing ischemia.

Trials of ranolazine in patients with stable angina (MARISA, CARISA, and ERICA) and with non-ST elevation acute coronary syndromes (MERLIN-TIMI 36) have shown that it improves exercise tolerance, reduces angina and nitrate intake, compared to placebo.

Doses of 500–2,000 mg daily reduce angina and increase exercise capacity without affecting heart rate or blood pressure.[26] Ranolazine plasma levels increase with cytochrome P3A (CYP3A) inhibitors (diltiazem, verapamil, macrolide antibiotics). Ranolazine clearance is reduced in renal and liver dysfunction. Ranolazine is recommended as a second-line adjunctive antianginal in patients of chronic stable angina with persistent symptoms in spite of treatment with first-line agents such as β-blockers and rate-limiting CCBs.[26] Ranolazine should be used cautiously in patients with QT prolongation or on QT-prolonging drugs, as it can also prolong QT.[27]

Trimetazidine

Trimetazidine is an antianginal with no hemodynamic effects. It acts by metabolic modulation and inhibition of partial fatty acid oxidation. Short-term clinical studies have demonstrated significant reduction in frequency of angina episodes and improved exercise tolerance, but large long-term trials are needed.[28] In diabetic patients with CAD, it decreased blood glucose, increased forearm glucose uptake, and improved endothelial function.[29]

Allopurinol

Allopurinol, an inhibitor of xanthine oxidase, is also antianginal. There is limited clinical evidence but, in a study of 65 patients with stable CAD, allopurinol 600 mg/day increased time to ST-segment depression and to chest pain.[30] High doses may have toxic side effects in patients with renal impairment.

Molsidomine

Molsidomine is a direct nitric oxide (NO) donor with anti-ischemic effects similar to those of isosorbide dinitrate.[32] The long-acting, once-daily 16 mg formulation is as effective as 8 mg twice daily.[31]

DRUGS FOR EVENT PREVENTION

Antiplatelet Agents

Aspirin is the backbone of secondary prevention of arterial thrombosis. In secondary prevention trials, the use of aspirin was associated with a significant reduction of nonfatal MI, stroke, and vascular death.[32] Lifelong aspirin is recommended in all patients with stable angina who do not have either aspirin resistance or allergy.

Clopidogrel is a thienopyridine derivative and P2Y12 inhibitor, which also inhibits platelet aggregation. In the CAPRIE trial, clopidogrel was slightly more effective than aspirin in reducing the combined risk of MI, ischemic stroke, or vascular death. Clopidogrel alone led to 8.7% relative decrease in MI, vascular death, or ischemic stroke.[33] However, the clopidogrel benefit was driven by the peripheral vascular disease subgroup and the dose of aspirin with which it was compared (325 mg/day) may not be the safest dose. Clopidogrel is proposed as a second-line treatment, especially for aspirin-intolerant CAD patients.

CHARISMA trial did not demonstrate any benefit of the use of dual antiplatelet therapy with aspirin (75–162 mg daily) and clopidogrel (75 mg daily) over aspirin alone.[34] The composite endpoint of death from CV causes MI or stroke in patients with stable CAD, or multiple CV risk factors were not significantly different between the two groups.

Prasugrel and ticagrelor are new P2Y12 antagonists that achieve greater platelet inhibition, compared with clopidogrel. Prasugrel and ticagrelor are both associated with a significant reduction of CV outcomes as compared with clopidogrel in ACS patients,[35,36] but no clinical studies have evaluated the benefit of these drugs in stable CAD patients.

Lipid-Lowering Agents

Data from numerous clinical trials support the use of statins for both primary and secondary prevention in stable CAD. The benefit of statins in reducing death, MI, and stroke has been amply demonstrated. The aggressive efforts to lower LDL levels to <70 mg/dL has been driven by a consistent and positive relationship between LDL cholesterol and the risk of CAD.[37] Statins are pleiotropic agents that reduce LDL to 30–60% of baseline, stabilize atherosclerotic plaque,[38] improve endothelial dysfunction, and promote plaque regression.[39] Statins also have anti-inflammatory effects which have been proved by reduction seen in C-reactive protein (CRP) levels.[40] The reduction in the progression of atherosclerosis in native as well as graft vessels after CABG can be achieved with intensive (LDL <70 mg/dL) compared with moderate (<100 mg/dL) lipid lowering.[41]

Cholestyramine and/or niacin can be used in patients with statin intolerance, or for statin failure. Fibrate therapy can be considered for elevated non-HDL-C despite statin therapy. Ezetimibe is to be considered if the above fail.

Renin–Angiotensin–Aldosterone System Blockers

Angiotensin converting enzyme inhibitors are beneficial in all patients with stable angina, especially those who have coexisting diabetes mellitus, previous MI, or left ventricular systolic dysfunction.[12]

Angiotensin converting enzyme inhibitors reduce ventricular and vascular remodeling, progression of atherosclerosis, and destabilization of coronary plaque.

The HOPE trial demonstrated that ACE inhibition with ramipril led to significant reduction in MI, CV death, and stroke in patients with vascular disease in the absence of heart failure.[42] Enalapril (CONSENSUS study) and captopril (SAVE study) produced similar results arguing in favor of the benefit being a class effect. The best ACE inhibitor for patients with CAD continues to be a controversy.

Angiotensin-receptor blockers are recommended in patients with stable CAD in whom ACE inhibition is recommended but not tolerated. The indications for the use of aldosterone antagonists like spironolactone or eplerenone include post-MI patients with LVEF ≤ 40% and either diabetes or heart failure[43] and are receiving therapeutic doses of an ACE inhibitor and a β-blocker in absence of hyperkalemia of renal dysfunction.

Nonpharmacological Antianginal Approaches (Tables 22.2 and 22.3)

The various nonpharmacological options to treat angina include enhanced external counterpulsation (EECP) and spinal cord stimulation (SCS). Randomized studies with EECP have demonstrated reduction in the frequency and severity of angina. It has been approved by FDA for treatment of stable angina. The potential mechanisms of benefit of EECP include coronary collateral formation and improvement in endothelial function.[44] Spinal cord stimulation is another antianginal strategy. Spinal cord stimulation may help by reducing neurotransmission of pain, release of endogenous opioids, and redistribution of myocardial blood flow.[45] The symptom relief provided by SCS in angina may be equivalent to CABG. These strategies are not widely available and not used routinely. These approaches may be beneficial in patients with refractory angina especially in those with coronary disease not amenable to any revascularization (Table 22.1).

OPTIMAL MEDICAL THERAPY OR MYOCARDIAL REVASCULARIZATION THERAPY FOR STABLE ANGINA-RECENT EVIDENCE

Percutaneous Coronary Intervention versus Medical Therapy

Last few decades have seen remarkable progress in the revascularization strategies, including PCI and CABG. Revascularization reduces symptoms and improves survival

Table 22.2 Major side effects, contraindications, drug–drug interactions (DDI), and precautions of anti-ischemic drugs

Drug class	*Side effects**	*Contraindications*	*DDI*	*Precautions*
Short-acting and long-acting nitrates	• Headache • Flushing • Hypotension • Syncope and postural hypotension • Reflex tachycardia • Methemoglobinemia	• Hypertrophic obstructive cardiomyopathy	• PDES inhibitors (sildenafil or similar agents) • α-Adrenergic blockers • CCBs	–
β-Blockers[†]	• Fatigue, depression • Bradycardia • Heart block • Bronchospasm • Peripheral vasoconstriction • Postural hypotension • Impotence • Hypoglycemia/ mask hypoglycemia signs	• Low heart rate or heart conduction disorder • COPD caution; may use cardioselective β-blockers if fully treated by inhaled steroids and long-acting β-agonists • Severe peripheral vascular disease • Decompensated heart failure • Vasospastic angina	• Heart-rate lowering CCB • Sinus-node or AV conduction depressors	• Diabetics • COPD
CCBs: Heart-rate lowering	• Bradycardia • Heart conduction defect • Low ejection fraction • Constipation • Gingival hyperplasia	• Low heart rate or heart rhythm disorder • Sick sinus syndrome • Congestive heart failure • Low BP	• Cardiodepressant (β-blockers, flecainide) • CYP3A4 substrates	–
CCBs: Dihydropyridines	• Headache • Ankle swelling • Fatigue • Flushing • Reflex tachycardia	• Cardiogenic shock • Severe aortic stenosis • Obstructive cardiomyopathy	• CYP3A4 substrates	–
Ivabradine	• Visual disturbances • Headache, dizziness • Bradycardia • Atrial fibrillation • Heart block	• Low heart rate or heart rhythm disorder • Allergy • Severe hepatic disease	• QTc prolonging drugs • Macrolide antibiotics • Anti-HIV • Anti-fungal	• Age >75 years • Severe renal failure
Nicorandil	• Headache • Flushing • Dizziness, weakness • Nausea • Hypotension • Oral, anal, gastro-intestinal ulceration	• Cardiogenic shock • Heart failure • Low blood pressure	• PDES inhibitors (sildenafil or similar agents)	–
Trimetazidine	• Gastric discomfort • Nausea • Headache • Movement disorders	• Allergy • Parkinson disease • Tremors and movement disorders • Severe renal impairment	• None reported	• Moderate renal impairment • Elderly
Ranolazine	• Dizziness • Constipation • Nausea • QT prolongation	• Liver cirrhosis	• CYP450 substrates (digoxin, simvastatin, cyclosporine) • QTc prolonging drugs	–
Allopurinol	• Rash • Gastric discomfort	• Hypersensitivity	• Mercaptopurine/ azathioprine	• Severe renal failure

Abbreviations: AV, atrioventricular; CCBs, calcium channel blockers; CHF, congestive heart failure; COPD, chronic obstructive pulmonary disease; DDI, drug–drug interactions; HIV, human immunodeficiency virus; PDES, phosphodiesterase type 5; BP, blood pressure.

*Very frequent: may vary according to specific drugs within the therapeutic class.

[†]Atenolol, metoprolol CR, bisoprolol, carvedilol.

Table 22.3 Pharmacological treatments in stable coronary artery disease patients

Indication	Class*	Level†
General considerations		
Optimal medical therapy indicates at least one drug for angina/ischemia relief plus drugs for event prevention.	I	C
It is recommended to educate patients about the disease, risk factors, and treatment strategy.	I	C
It is indicated to review the patient's response soon after starting therapy.	I	C
Angina/ischemia‡ relief		
Short-acting nitrates are recommended.	I	B
First-line treatment is indicated with β-blockers and/or calcium channel blockers to control heart rate and symptoms.	I	A
For second-line treatment it is recommended to add long-acting nitrates or ivabradine or nicorandil or ranolazine, according to heart rate, blood pressure and tolerance.	IIa	B
For second-line treatment, trimetazidine may be considered.	IIb	B
According to comorbidities/tolerance it is indicated to use second-line therapies in selected patients.	I	C
In asymptomatic patients with large areas of ischemia (>10%) ß-blockers should be considered.	IIa	C
In patients with vasospastic angina, calcium channel blockers and nitrates should be considered and β-blockers avoided.	IIa	B
Event prevention		
Low-dose aspirin daily is recommended in all stable CAD patients.	I	A
Clopidogrel is indicated as an alternative in case of aspirin intolerance.	I	B
Statins are recommended in all stable CAD patients.	I	A
It is recommended to use ACE inhibitors (or ARBs) if presence of other conditions (e.g. heart failure, hypertension, or diabetes).	I	A

*Class of recommendation.

†Level of evidence.

‡No demonstration of benefit on prognosis.

in selected subset of patients. Nowadays treatment strategy has shifted largely away from an initial pharmacological approach to one that focuses on revascularization.

There are now multiple contemporary RCTs that address the large group of stable CAD patients. COURAGE trial tested the hypothesis that PCI coupled with OMT would reduce the risk of death or MI in patients with stable CAD, as compared with OMT alone.[46] A total of 2,287 patients with objective evidence of MI and significant CAD were enrolled in this study. A total of 1,149 patients underwent PCI with OMT and 1,138 received OMT alone. The primary outcome was all-cause death or nonfatal MI during a median follow-up of 4.6 years. The study found no significant difference in the composite primary outcome between the two treatment strategies. Percutaneous coronary intervention in addition to OMT did not produce significant differences in other outcomes as well such as stroke or hospitalization for ACS. The study did not support addition of PCI to OMT as an initial management strategy.

The evidence from COURAGE and other previous randomized trials of PCl versus medical therapy highlight the importance of optimum medical therapy for secondary prevention of CV events in patients with stable CAD.

Coronary Artery Bypass Grafting versus Medical Therapy

While individual studies have not shown a significant reduction in death or MI for CABG compared with medical therapy, CABG has been proven to be beneficial in certain subsets of patients with left main stem coronary disease or three-vessel CAD and LV systolic dysfunction. Long-term follow-up of these trials have indicated that as an initial strategy of routine CABG compared to initial medical therapy significantly reduced the risk of death by about 25%, with the largest benefits being observed in those with left main disease and those with three-vessel CAD.

Flow chart 22.1 Medical management of patients with stable coronary artery disease

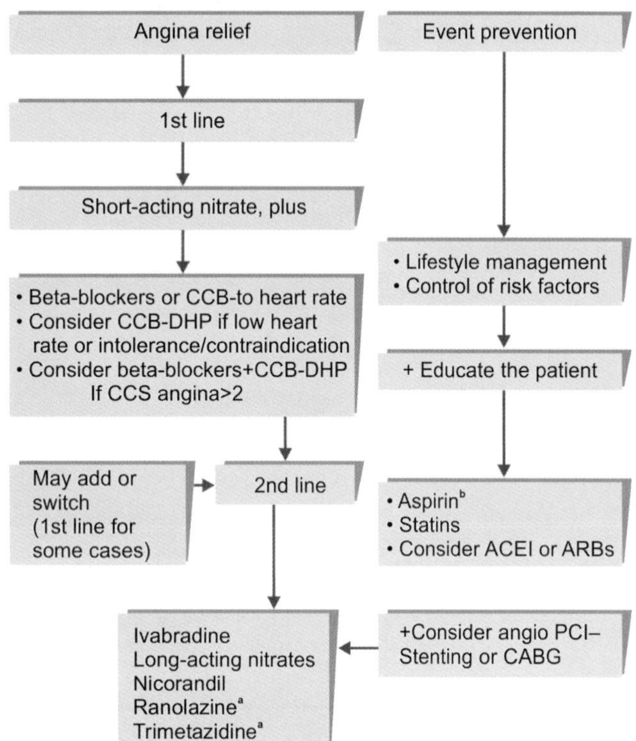

Abbreviations: ACEI, angiotensin converting enzyme inhibitor; CABG, coronary artery bypass graft; CCB, calcium channel blockers; CCS, Canadian Cardiovascular Society; DHP, dihydropyridine; PCI, percutaneous coronary intervention; ARBs, angiotensin II receptor blockers. [a]Data for diabetics. [b]If intolerance, consider clopidogrel

The indicators of survival benefit from CABG over medical therapy seen in randomized trials include greater severity of ischemia, a greater extent of disease, presence of LV systolic dysfunction, significant left main CAD, and three-vessel CAD that includes the proximal left anterior descending (LAD) coronary artery.

BARI-2D trial randomized 2,368 diabetic patients with CAD to prompt revascularization versus delayed/ no revascularization and OMT. There was no significant difference between prompt revascularization (PCl or CABG) versus OMT for the trial primary endpoint of all-cause death.[47] Patients with severe CAD were allotted to CABG. BARI-2D results reinforce the results of the COURAGE trial; that is, there is no additional benefit of an initial strategy of PCI over optimum medical therapy, and an "OMT-first" instead of a "PCI-first" strategy is reasonable in many diabetic patients with CAD.

In summary, based on the COURAGE and BARI-2D trials, in angiographically selected patients with chronic stable angina and preserved LV function, there is no benefit from coronary revascularization on death and MI. These results are consistent with almost three decades of trials and emphasize that current mortality rates in patients with chronic stable angina on intensive medical therapy receiving aggressive secondary prevention are low and unlikely to be improved by revascularization. In general, the concept of "the greater the risk, the greater the benefit from revascularization over medical therapy" applies to patients with left main CAD, multi-vessel disease, and in particular in conjunction with LV dysfunction, severe angina, and proximal LAD coronary disease (Flow chart 22.1).

Finally, as the controversy over management strategies in stable CAD patients continues, the key take-home message is that OMT is a safe and effective initial management strategy in these patients.

Advances in OMT have kept pace with those in interventional and surgical revascularization. Aggressive risk factor reduction and OMT need to be the backbone of patient management to prevent progression of disease and occurrence of adverse CV events in patients with stable CAD, regardless of the decision to revascularize.

REFERENCES

1. Sekhri N, Feder GS, et al. How effective are rapid access chest pain clinics? Prognosis of incident angina and non-cardiac chest pain in 8762 consecutive patients. Heart. 2007;93:458-63.
2. Jones M, Rait G, Falconer J, et al. Systematic review: prognosis of angina in primary care. Fam Pract. 2006;23:520-8.
3. Henderson RA, O'Flynn N. Management of stable angina summary of NICE guidelines. Heart. 2012;98(6):500-7.
4. Ludvig J, Miner B, Eisenberg MJ. Smoking cessation in patients with coronary artery disease. Am Heart J. 2005;149:565-72.
5. Rigotti NA, Thorndike AN, Regan S, et al. Bupropion for smokers hospitalized with acute cardiovascular disease. Am J Med. 2006;119:1080-7.
6. Singh S, Loke YK, Spangler JG, et al. Risk of serious adverse cardiovascular events associated with varenicline: a systematic review and meta-analysis. CMAJ. 2011;183:1359-66.
7. Critchley J, Capewell S. Smoking cessation for the secondary prevention of coronary heart disease. Cochrane Database Syst Rev. 2004(1):CD003041.
8. Perk J, De Backer G, Gohlke H, et al. European Guidelines on cardiovascular disease prevention in clinical practice (version 2012): The Fifth Joint Task Force of the ESC. Eur Heart J. 2012;33: 1635-1701.
9. Estruch R, Ros E, Salas-Salvado J, et al. The PSI. Primary prevention of cardiovascular disease with a Mediterranean diet. N Eng J Med. 2013;368(14):1279–90.
10. Mancia GF, Narkiewicz K, Redon J, et al. 2013 ESH/ESC Guidelines for the management of arterial hypertension: the Task Force for the management of arterial hypertension of the ESH and of the ESC. Eur Heart J. 2013.
11. Umpierrez GE, Hellman R, Korytkowski MT, et al. Endocrine S. Management of hyperglycemia in hospitalized patients in non-critical care setting: an endocrine society clinical practice guideline. J Clin Endocrinol Metab. 2012;97:16-38.
12. Zamorano JL, Achenbach S, Baumgartner H, et al. ESC guidelines on the management of stable coronary artery disease. The Task

Force on the management of stable coronary artery disease of the European Society of Cardiology; 2013:240-1.
13. Abrams J. Nitroglycerin and long-acting nitrates in clinical practice. Am J Med. 1983;74:85-94.
14. Parker JO. Eccentric dosing with isosorbide-5-mononitrate in angina pectoris. Am J Cardiol. 1993;72:871-6.
15. Waysbort J, Meshulamb N, Brunner D. Isosorbide-5-mononitrate and atenolol in the treatment of stable exertional angina. Cardiology. 1991;79(Suppl):19-26.
16. Yusuf S, Wittes J, Friedman L. Overview of results of randomized clinical trials in heart disease. I. Treatments following myocardial infarction. JAMA. 1988;260:2088-93.
17. Rehnqvist N, Hjemdahl P, Billing E, et al. Effects of metoprolol vs verapamil in patients with stable angina pectoris. The Angina Prognosis Study in Stockholm (APSIS). Eur Heart J. 1996;17:76-81.
18. Subramanian VB, Bowles MJ, Davies AB, et al. Calcium channel blockade as primary therapy for stable angina pectoris. A double-blind placebo-controlled comparison of verapamil and propranolol. Am J CardioI. 1982;50:1158-63.
19. Haasenritter J, Bosner S, Vaucher P, et al. Ruling out coronary heart disease in primary care: external validation of a clinical prediction rule. Br J Gen Pract. 2012;62:e415-21.
20. Furberg CD, Psaty BM, Meyer V. Nifedipine. Dose-related increase in mortality in patients with coronary heart disease. Circulation. 1995;92:1326-31.
21. Pepine CJ, Handberg EM, Cooper-DeHoff RM, et al. A calcium antagonist vs a noncalcium antagonist hypertension treatment strategy for patients with coronary artery disease. The International Verapamil-Trandolapril Study (INVEST): a randomized controlled trial. JAMA. 2003;290:2805-16.
22. Steffensen R, Grande P, Pedersen F, et al. Effects of atenolol and diltiazem on exercise tolerance and ambulatory ischaemia. Int J Cardiol. 1993;40:143-53.
23. Wijns W, Kolh P, Danchin N, et al. Guidelines on myocardial revascularization. Eur Heart J. 2010;31:2501-55.
24. Tardif JC, Ford I, Tendera M, et al. Efficacy of ivabradine, a new selective I(f) inhibitor, compared with atenolol in patients with chronic stable angina. Eur Heart J. 2005;26:2529-36.
25. Fox K, Ford I, Steg PG, et al. Ivabradine for patients with stable coronary artery disease and left-ventricular systolic dysfunction (BEAUTIFUL): a randomised, double-blind, placebo-controlled trial. Lancet. 2008;372:807-16.
26. Timmis AD, Chaitman BR, Crager M. Effects of ranolazine on exercise tolerance and HbA1c in patients with chronic angina and diabetes. Eur Heart J. 2006;27:42-8.
27. Jerling M. Clinical pharmacokinetics of ranolazine. Clin Pharmacokinet. 2006;45:469-91.
28. Chazov EI, Lepakchin VK, Zharova EA, et al. Trimetazidine in angina combination therapy-the TACT study. Am J Ther. 2005;12:35-42.
29. Fragasso G, et al. Short- and long-term beneficial effects of trimetazidine in patients with diabetes and ischemic cardiomyopathy. Am Heart J. 2003;146:E18.
30. Noman A, Ang DS, Ogston S, et al. Effect of high-dose allopurinol on exercise in patients with chronic stable angina: a randomised, placebo controlled crossover trial. Lancet. 2010;375:2161-7.
31. Wagner F, Gohlke-Barwolf C, Trenk D, et al. Differences in the anti-ischaemic effects of molsidomine and isosorbide dinitrate (ISDN) during acute and short-term administration in stable angina pectoris. Eur Heart J. 1991;12:994-9.
32. Antithrombotic Trialists' Collaboration. meta-analysis of randomised trials of antiplatelet therapy for prevention of death, myocardial infarction, and stroke in high risk patients. BMJ. 2002;324:71-86.
33. CAPRIE Steering Committee. A randomised, blinded, trial of clopidogrel versus aspirin in patients at risk of ischemic events (CAPRIE). CAPRIE Steering Committee. Lancet. 1996;348:1329-39.
34. Bhatt DL, Fox KA, Hacke W, et al. Clopidogrel and aspirin versus aspirin alone for prevention of atherothrombotic events. N Engl J Med. 2006;354:1706-17.
35. Wiviott SD, Braunwald E, McCabe CH, et al. Prasugrel versus clopidogrel in patients with acute coronary syndromes. N Eng J Med. 2007;357:2001-15.
36. Cannon CP, Harrington RA, James S, et al. Comparison of ticagrelor with clopidogrel in patients with a planned invasive strategy for acute coronary syndromes (PLATO): a randomized double-blind study. Lancet. 2010;375:283-93.
37. Pekkanen J, Linn S, Heiss G, et al. Ten-year mortality from cardiovascular disease in relation to cholesterol level among men with and without preexisting cardiovascular disease. N Engl J Med. 1990;322:1700-7.
38. Cannon CP, Braunwald E, McCabe CH, et al. Intensive versus moderate lipid lowering with statins after acute coronary syndromes. N Engl J Med. 2004;350:1495-1504.
39. Corti R, Fayad ZA, Fuster V, et al. Effects of lipid-lowering by simvastatin on human atherosclerotic lesions: a longitudinal study by high-resolution, noninvasive magnetic resonance imaging. Circulation. 2001;104:249-52.
40. Ridker PM, Cannon CP, Morrow D, et al. C-reactive protein levels and outcomes after statin therapy. N Engl J Med. 2005;352:20-8.
41. The Post Coronary Artery Bypass Graft Trial Investigators. The effect of aggressive lowering of low-density lipoprotein cholesterol levels and low-dose anticoagulation on obstructive changes in saphenous-vein coronary-artery bypass grafts. N Engl J Med. 1997;336(3):153-62.
42. Yusuf S, Sleight P, Pogue J, et al. Effects of an angiotensin converting-enzyme inhibitor, ramipril, on cardiovascular events in high-risk patients. The Heart Outcomes Prevention Evaluation Study Investigators. N Engl J Med. 2000;342:145-53.
43. Pitt B, Remme W, Zannad F, et al. Eplerenone, a selective aldosterone blocker, in patients with left ventricular dysfunction after myocardial infarction. N Eng J Med. 2003;348:1309-21.
44. Bonetti PO, Barsness GW, Keelan PC, et al. Enhanced external counterpulsation improves endothelial function in patients with symptomatic coronary artery disease. J Am Coll Cardiol. 2003;41:1761-8.
45. Mannheimer C, Eliasson T, Augustinsson LE, et al. Electrical stimulation versus coronary artery bypass surgery in severe angina pectoris: the ESBY study. Circulation. 1998; 97:1157-63.
46. Boden WE, O'Rourke RA, TeoKK, et al. The evolving pattern of symptomatic coronary artery disease in the United States and Canada: baseline characteristics of the Clinical Outcomes Utilizing Revascularization and Aggressive Drug Evaluation (COURAGE) trial. Am J Cardiol. 2007;99:208-12.
47. Frye RL, August P, Brooks MM, et al. A randomized trial of therapies for type 2 diabetes and coronary artery disease. N Engl J Med. 2009;360:2503-15.

23

Complications of Myocardial Infarction

Nishant Kumar, Ashok K Omar, Anumeha Omar, Mitu A Minocha, Sameer Shrivatava

INTRODUCTION

The early part of the 20th century will be known as era where coronary artery disease (CAD) was identified and seriously reported. Various literature in this early part of the century explained the course of disease and how to and when to safely discharge the patients. The later part of the century initially belonged to fibrinolytic drugs ("the magical clot buster medication as they were reported in public") and then later to primary percutaneous intervention that have drastically reduced the morbidity and mortality of the patient. In 1952, Levine and Long were the first who challenged the view that patient with acute myocardial infarction (AMI) required prolonged bed rest and suggested they could be shifted out of bed to chair in 2–7 days and discharged in 4 weeks. In 1974, a study published by J Frederick entitled "the course of acute myocardial infarction" that enlisted about 522 patients showed that patients who do not develop complication at the end of 4 days can be safely discharged at the end of 10th day and patients who developed complication had very high mortality. This provided a glimpse into the future and it remains true in the modern era too. Early primary percutaneous transluminal coronary angioplasty (PTCA) has indeed caused reduction in complication, but complicated MI have very high mortality. This chapter briefly covers all the complication associated with AMI and recent updates.

CARDIOGENIC SHOCK

It is serious complication of AMI[1] and carries a mortality rate of approximately 50% even with rapid revascularization and modern medical care with inotropes and mechanical support.[2-3] It was first described by James Herrick in 1912, following which over the decades several trials explaining the pathophysiology and methods to effectively bring down the mortality have been carried out. It is defined as a clinical syndrome of inadequate tissue (end organ) perfusion due to cardiac dysfunction. It is characterized by marked persistent (>30 minutes) hypotension with systolic blood pressure < 80 mm Hg, cardiac index (CI) < 1.8 L/min/m^2, and increased left ventricular (LV) filling pressure (pulmonary capillary wedge pressure > 18 mm Hg).[4]

The classical model for pathophysiology explained that low stroke volume following MI led to the activation of endogenous vasopressors such as norepinephrine and angiotensin II, which increased systemic vascular resistance at the expense of marked reduction in tissue perfusion. This classical model, however, fails to explain the high mortality of patient with cardiogenic shock (CS) despite normalization of CI.[5] This mechanism has been challenged by the fact that post-MI shocks are associated with relative vasodilation rather than vasoconstriction. This response is similar to systemic inflammatory response that is associated with elevated serum cytokine concentration, interleukin-6 (IL-6), which leads to induction of nitric oxide (NO) synthase and elevated level of NO. This induces inappropriate vasodilation with reduced systemic and coronary perfusion.[6] The focus has now shifted to advanced glycation end products (AGES), heterogeneous complex group of compounds that are formed mainly when reducing sugar reacts in a nonenzymatic way with amino acids in proteins, lipids, or DNA (Maillard reaction).

The deleterious effects of AGES in different tissues are attributed to their chemical, pro-oxidant, and inflammatory actions.[7] The biological effects of AGES are exerted by two different mechanisms: first independent of the receptor (damage of protein structure and extracellular matrix metabolism) and second involving the receptor for advanced glycation end products (RAGEs) (*See* Fig. 23.2).[8] The interaction of AGES with the receptor RAGE triggers the activation of the mitogen-activated protein kinases and the phosphatidylinositol-3 kinase pathways that will lead to the activation of the transcription factor nuclear factor kappa B (NF-kB). After activation, NF-kB translocates to the nucleus where it will activate the transcription of genes for cytokines, growth factors, and adhesive molecules, such as tumor necrosis factor alpha, IL-6, well-known inflammation promoters, and vascular cell adhesion molecule 1.[8-12] The role of AGES in CS has been recently studied[9] that suggested that there are two forms of RAGE, soluble form RAGE that neutralizes the ligand-mediated damage by acting as a decoy and is significantly higher in patients who survive CS whereas as the monocytic RAGEs were significantly higher in nonsurvivor when measured through western blotting. This perhaps provides us a glimpse into the future where we could have biochemical markers to predict the high short-term mortality and adjust our treatment modality to reduce it.

Cardiogenic shock complicates around 7% of AMI;[10] majority of them have ST-elevation myocardial infarction (STEMI); and patients with old age, anterior MI, hypertension, diabetes mellitus, renal failure, prior MI, multiple vessels CAD are at higher risk. Early reperfusion and medical stabilization with or without the inotropic support is still the cornerstone therapy for management of CS. The role of early revascularization is well established due to randomized SHOCK trial that showed 13% absolute increase in 1 year survival in the early revascularization arm when compared to medical management alone. Numerous other studies have confirmed these results, the survival advantage of early revascularization whether percutaneous coronary intervention (PCI) or coronary artery bypass grafting (CABG), in young or elderly. Thrombolytic therapy is less effective but indicated when PCI or CABG is impossible or delayed due to transport or when the MI and CS onset were within 3 hours.

This survival benefit was present as long as 48 hours after MI and 18 hours after onset of shock. Coronary artery bypass grafting in CS is commonly performed in patients with left main coronary artery (LMCA) disease, three-vessel diseases, and diabetes mellitus; the 30 days mortality were equivalent to patients undergoing PCI (42% vs. 45%). SHOCK trial recommended emergency CABG within 6 hours of randomization in patients with severe tricuspid valve disease (TVD), or LMCA disease and for moderate TVD investigator suggested for PCI of the infarct related artery (IRA) followed by delayed CABG for those who are stabilized. Based on SHOCK trial, the ACC/AHA STEMI guideline recommended for early revascularization by PCI or CABG selected patients 75 years or older with ST elevation or left bundle branch block (LBBB) who developed shock within 36 hours of MI and who are suitable for revascularization that can be performed within 18 hours of shock (class IIa).

The role of intra-aortic balloon pump counter-pulsation (IABP) has been a source of much controversy in recent past, first introduced and used by Kantrowitz in 1968, and became a routine in modern cardiac setup for management of CS. Recent studies like IABP SHOCK II study that randomly assigned 600 patients with CS complicating AMI to IABP group and no IABP group did not find significant reduction in mortality in patients with planned early PCI. Following this, the ESC guideline changed the level of recommendation for IABP use in CS from class I to class IIb. ACC/AHA guidelines also put IABP in class IIa. Left ventricular-assisted devices are perhaps the future, percutaneous ventricular-assisted devices (pVADs), tandem heart pVAD, and impella recover system are being studied, a recent meta-analysis of both these VADs with IABP in 100 patients with AMI complicated by CS, found that patients on VAD had higher CI but there was no difference in 30 days mortality.[11] Extracorporeal membrane oxygenation (ECMO) is now an important tool in management of patients suffering from refractory CS, offering several advantages, simple, and easy insertion via femoral route even during CPR providing both cardiac and respiratory support without the need for sternotomy, and it provides time to assess potential transplant patients. It can be used with IABP and can be used as "bridge to bridge" followed by long-term VADs or as bridge to allow to restore systemic perfusion. Extracorporeal membrane oxygenation has several limitations preluding its long-term use, including hemolysis, stroke, bleeding, infection, inadequate LV decompression, and patient immobilization. Newer, minimized extracorporeal life support systems like ELS system and cardiohelp have been developed allowing rapid insertion and facilitated inter-hospital transport. Earlier studies with LVAD support were not encouraging, but recent data from Society of Thoracic Surgeons National Cardiac Database[12] suggest that their use saves approximately 60% of patients with persistent shock after CABG.[13] Both ESC and ACC/AHA guideline recommended LVADs as class IIb (level of evidence C) for their use in patients with STEMI and CS not responding to standard treatment including IABP and as a bridge to transplantation (Figs 23.1A to C).

ARRHYTHMIC COMPLICATION OF MYOCARDIAL INFARCTION

The incidences of arrhythmias following AMI are very high; about 90% of patients develop them immediately after the event and in some 25% of them, such rhythm abnormalities manifest within the first 24 hours. The risk of serious arrhythmias such as ventricular fibrillation (VF) significantly declines thereafter. STEMI have higher incidence of arrhythmias than non-STEMI. The basic pathophysiology is generalized autonomic dysfunction that results in enhanced automaticity of the myocardium and conduction system. This can further augmented by electrolyte imbalances (e.g. hypokalemia, hypomagnesemia) and hypoxia. The damaged myocardium acts as substrate for re-entrant circuit due to changes in tissue refractoriness. There is an enhanced efferent sympathetic activity with resultant increase in circulating catecholamines from nerve ending in heart muscle that contributes in the development of peri-infarct arrhythmias. There is also an interruption in afferent and efferent limbs of sympathetic nervous system distal to the area of infarction that results in autonomic imbalance that promotes arrhythmias. Peri-infarction arrhythmias can be classified into following categories:

- Supraventricular tachyarrhythmias include sinus tachycardia, PAC, supraventricular tachycardia (SVT), atrial flutter, and atrial fibrillation (AF)
- Accelerated junctional rhythms
- Bradyarrhythmias include bradycardia and junctional bradycardia

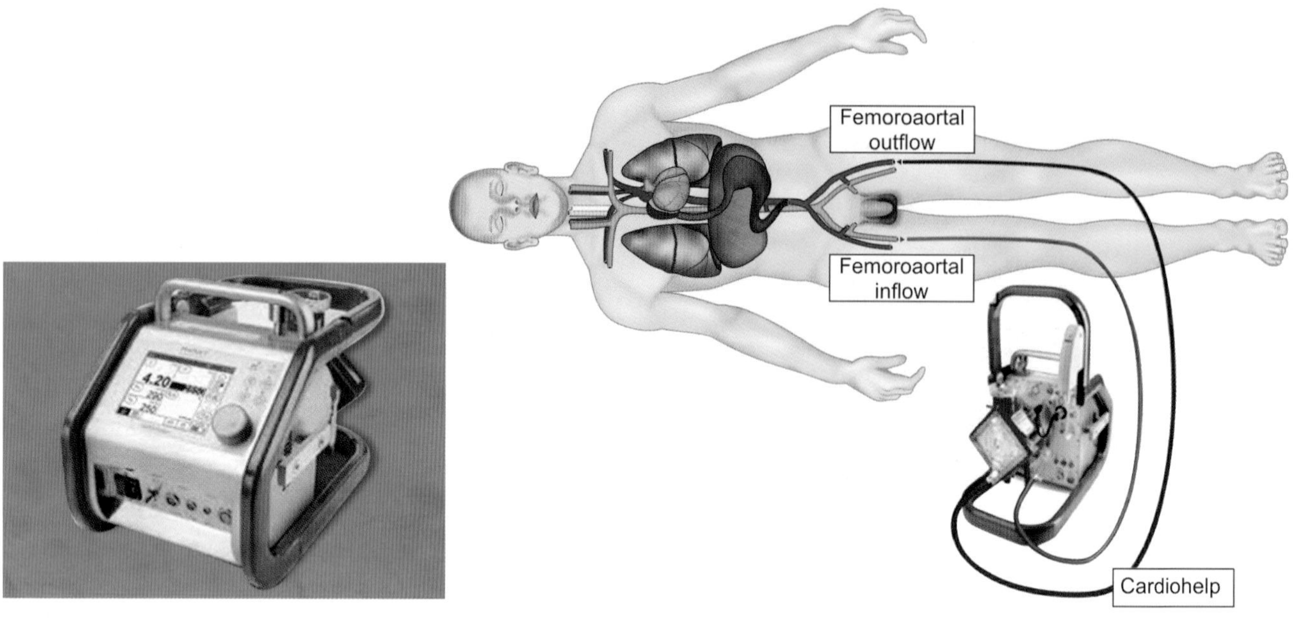

Fig. 23.1A Cardiohelp (Minimized extracorporeal life support)

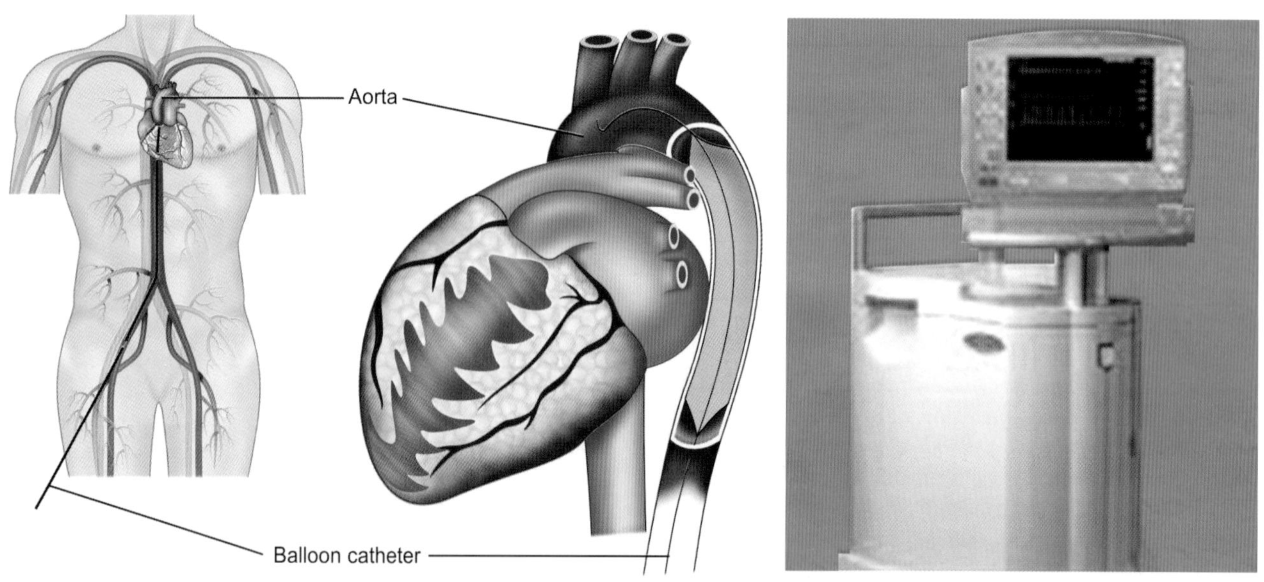

Fig. 23.1B Intra-aortic balloon pump (IABP)

- Atrioventricular (AV) blocks include first-degree heart block, second-degree heart block, and third-degree heart block
- Intraventricular block that includes LBBB, right bundle branch block (RBBB), and left anterior and posterior fascicular blocks
- Ventricular arrhythmias include premature ventricular contractions (PVC), accelerated idioventricular, ventricular tachycardia, and VF
- Reperfusion arrhythmias

Supraventricular Tachyarrhythmias

i. *Sinus tachycardia*: In setting of AMI, it is of utmost importance that the individual arrhythmias be identified and causing factors are corrected. Supraventricular tachyarrhythmias like sinus tachycardia can increase myocardial oxygen demand and by a decreased length of diastole compromise coronary flow and worsen coronary blood flow. Enhanced sympathetic activity can result in

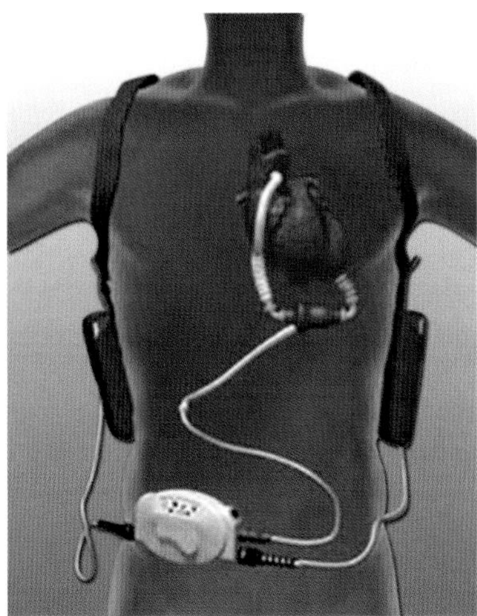

Fig. 23.1C Left ventricular assist device (LVAD)

transient hypertension or hypotension. Causative factor for persistent sinus arrhythmia includes:

- Pain
- Anxiety
- Hypovolemia
- Heart failure
- Hypoxia
- Anemia
- Pericarditis
- Pulmonary embolism.

Appropriate treatment strategies must be devised early, like managing heart failure with diuretics, oxygenation, administration of anti-inflammatory agents in case of pericarditis, and use of beta-blocker and nitroglycerin to relieve angina.

ii. Atrial fibrillation occurs in 8–22% of patients with AMI, onset within the first hour of AMI is suggestive of LV failure, atrial infarcts, or right ventricular (RV) infarcts. It is by far the most common supraventricular arrhythmia, the incidence of new onset AF during hospitalization was 6.3%[14] in a contemporary study. Patients with anterior AMI who develop AF have increased risk of stroke and have higher mortality. Atrial fibrillation commonly occurs with higher rates in elderly patients, and those with heart failure or pericarditis or factors causing elevated left atrial pressure. Nearly 30% of patients who are AMI survivors with LVEF < 40% develop AF over 2 years follow-up.[15] Treatment modality of new onset AF following AMI is based on hemodynamic status of the patient. Unstable patient with worsening hypotension and angina are best treated with synchronized electrical cardioversion with 200 J.

Ventricular rate control with intravenous (IV) amiodarone, IV beta blockers are used for patients who do not respond to electrical cardioversion or are hemodynamically stable. Less than 5% patients with AMI develop atrial flutter that is usually transient and is result of sympathetic overstimulation of the atria. The treatment strategy for atrial flutter is similar to AF, but ventricular rate control is less accomplished with drugs, therefore synchronized electrical cardioversion with 50 J, is generally preferred.

Role of anticoagulation in patients with AF with AMI: The role of anticoagulation in AF following AMI has been source of much debate. The recent ACC/AHA guidelines for STEMI tried to shed some light on this issue; it recommends anticoagulation with vitamin K antagonist to be provided to all patients with STEMI with AF who have a CHADS2 score ≥2, or have mechanical heart valve, venous thromboembolism, or hypercoagulable disorder (class I indication, level of evidence C). The duration of therapy with dual antiplatelet (DAPT) plus vitamin K antagonist should be minimized to the extent to limit bleeding, for patients who receive intracoronary stent; after initial therapy it is advisable to shift to vitamin K antagonist plus single antiplatelet. For patients treated with fibrinolysis alone, consider DAPT plus vitamin K antagonist for 14 days and then shift to single antiplatelet plus vitamin K antagonist.[16-19] The reason why 14 days is chosen as a benchmark for cessation of therapy in fibrinolysis group is because the role of DAPT beyond 14 days is not studied in this group or in those who do not receive intracoronary stent or who do not undergo reperfusion therapy. A study of 12,165 AF patients with MI or undergoing PCI showed within 1 year, MI or coronary death, ischemic stroke, and bleeding events occurred in 2,255 patients (18.5%), 680 (5.6%), and 769 (6.3%), respectively. Relative to triple therapy [oral anticoagulation (OAC) plus aspirin plus clopidogrel], no increased risk of recurrent coronary events was seen for OAC plus clopidogrel [hazard ratio (HR): 0.69, 95% confidence interval (CI): 0.48–1.00], OAC plus aspirin (HR: 0.96, 95% CI: 0.77–1.19), or aspirin plus clopidogrel (HR: 1.17, 95% CI: 0.96–1.42), but aspirin plus clopidogrel was associated with a higher risk of ischemic stroke (HR: 1.50, 95% CI: 1.03–2.20). Also, OAC plus aspirin and aspirin plus clopidogrel were associated with a significant increased risk of all-cause death (HR: 1.52, 95% CI: 1.17–1.99 and HR: 1.60, 95% CI: 1.25–2.05, respectively). When compared to triple therapy, bleeding risk was nonsignificantly lower for OAC plus clopidogrel (HR: 0.78, 95% CI: 0.55–1.12) and significantly lower for OAC plus aspirin and aspirin plus clopidogrel. It concluded in real-life AF patients with indication for multiple antithrombotic drugs after MI/PCI, OAC, and clopidogrel was equal or better on both benefit and safety outcomes compared to triple therapy.[20]

iii. Paroxysmal SVT occurs in <10% of patients with AMI; there is a consensus that adenosine can be safely used when hypotension is not present. In patients with clinically significant LV failure, IV diltiazem, or beta-blocker can be used. In patients who develop severe heart failure or hypotension, synchronized electrical cardioversion can be used.

Bradyarrhythmias

It is the most common arrhythmia in patients with inferior and posterior AMI, with incidence up to 40% observed with first 1–2 hours of AMI. Bradycardia and hypotension are result of stimulation of cardiac vagal afferent receptors that result in efferent cholinergic stimulation of the heart; this needs to be treated aggressively since clinically significant bradycardia may decrease cardiac output and hypotension may predispose to ventricular arrhythmias. In emergency situation (rate < 40 bpm with hypotension), atropine 0.6 mg may be given every 3–5 minutes to a maximum of 0.03–0.04 mg/kg. In setting of inferior MI with RV MI or hypovolemia atropine alone may not reverse the condition; volume correction is of importance in this circumstance. Atropine is equally ineffective in patients with denervated heart where external or transvenous pacing may be required. It is important to note that in early phase of AMI, resultant bradycardia is protective as it reduces myocardial oxygen demand. Isolated bradycardia does not increase acute mortality risk and therapy is unnecessary when patients have no adverse signs or symptoms.

Atrioventricular and Intraventricular Blocks

First-degree AV blocks (PR interval > 200 msec) occurs in 15% of patients with AMI, most commonly in inferior AMI, and does not require treatment (only continued cardiac monitoring may be required) in view of possible progression to higher block. Mobitz type I or Wenckebach AV block occurs in 10% of patients who have AMI, which accounts for 90% of all patients who have AMI with second-degree heart block. It is commonly associated with inferior AMI and does not necessarily require treatment. It does not affect the patients overall prognosis. Mobitz type II block occurs in 10% of all second-degree AV blocks and the overall rate following AMI is <1%. It is characterized by a wide QRS complex and mostly associated with anterior AMI. They are associated with poor prognosis, and overall progression to complete heart block is 10%. Atropine is less effective and helps in only 50% of cases and occasionally worsens the block. A temporary pacemaker is mostly required. Third-degree AV blocks [complete heart block (CHB)] accounts for 5–15% of AMI and occurs with anterior or inferior MI. In 70% of the cases, the block is supranodal or intranodal and the escape rhythm is usually stable with a narrow QRS, whereas rest may be have block below the His bundle, with a wide QRS and rate < 40 bpm, in inferior MI, CHB usually develops gradually progressing from first-degree or type I second-degree heart block and resolves within a few days without the need for temporary or permanent pacemaker. Mortality rate is approximately 15% unless a coexisting RV infarct is present, in which case the mortality rate is higher. Anterior MI with CHB carries a very high mortality rate. The cardiac arrhythmia's and risk stratification after myocardial infarction (CARISMA) trial that monitored patients with AMI and reduced LVEF found that high-degree AV block was the most powerful predictor of cardiac death.[21] Immediate treatment with atropine or transvenous pacing is indicated. These patients will eventually require a permanent pacemaker.

Ventricular Arrhythmia

i. Premature ventricular contractions was once considered an indicator of impending ventricular arrhythmias, but it is no longer true, on the converse primary VF often occurs without antecedent premature ventricular ectopy. Prophylactic suppression of PVCs has been associated with increased fatal bradycardia and is no longer recommended. It is advisable to pursue a conservative course to correct any electrolyte or metabolic abnormalities, and to identify and treat recurrent angina.
ii. Accelerated idioventricular rhythm is seen in 20% of patients with AMI. It is defined as a ventricular rhythm characterized by a wide QRS complex with regular escape rate faster than the atrial rate, but < 100 bpm. Atrioventricular dissociation is frequent and slow, and nonconducted P waves are seen that are unrelated to fast wide QRS rhythm. Episodes are short and terminate spontaneously and occur with equal frequency in anterior and inferior infarction. The mechanism might involve direct damage to sinoatrial node or AV node and depressed automaticity and/or an abnormal ectopic focus in the ventricle that takes over as the dominant pacemaker. It does not affect the patient prognosis and there is no evidence to show that in untreated cases there is an increase in VF or death. This rhythm does occur more frequently in patients who undergo early reperfusion but is neither a sensitive nor specific marker of reperfusion.

    Nonsustained ventricular tachycardia (NSVT) is defined as three or more consecutive ventricular ectopic beats at a rate of 100 bpm or greater and lasting <30 seconds. There is substantial risk of sudden hemodynamic collapse in patients with multiple runs of NSVT.

    Nonsustained ventricular tachycardia in immediate peri-infarction period (<48 hours) is not associated with increased mortality, and there is no evidence to suggest that usage of antiarrhythmic treatment in this period offers a morbidity or mortality benefit. Nonsustained ventricular tachycardia occurring beyond 48 hours in patients with LVEF < 40% poses an increased risk of sudden cardiac death. Electrolyte imbalance (serum potassium, serum magnesium) should be corrected and ongoing ischemia should be aggressively corrected.

iii. *Sustained ventricular tachycardia*: It is defined as three or more ventricular ectopic beats at a rate >100 bpm and lasting >30 seconds causing hemodynamic compromise. Myocardial scar is a most likely cause for monomorphic VT, whereas polymorphic VT may be most responsive measures directed against ischemia. Sustained VT is associated with 20% mortality rate after AMI.

Precipitating factors such as electrolyte imbalance, hypoxia, acid base balance, or medication should be corrected. Hemodynamic unstable polymorphic VT should be immediately treated with DC unsynchronized cardioversion 200 J whereas monomorphic VT will require synchronized discharge 100 J.

iv. *Ventricular fibrillation*: During the first hour of AMI, the incidence of VF is around 4.5% and decreases rapidly thereafter, 60% of episode occur within first 4 hours and 80% occur within first 12 hours. Secondary VF (occurring beyond 48 hours) is usually associated with pump failure and CS. Large infarcts, an intraventricular conduction delay, and an anteroseptal AMI are the factors associated with increased risk of secondary VF. Its conjunction with CS is associated with an in-hospital mortality rate of 40–60%. Immediate unsynchronized DC shock with 200–300 J is the treatment of choice. Each minute after onset of uncorrected VF is associated with 10% decrease in likelihood of survival. Antiarrhythmic agents like IV amiodarone and lidocaine facilitate successful electrical defibrillation and help prevent recurrence. They generally continued as constant IV infusion for 12–14 hours. Prophylactic usage of lidocaine has been studied; it is found to reduce the incidence of VF but is associated with increase mortality risk owing to asystolic and bradycardic events.[22] Beta-blocker, on the other hand, reduces the incidence of VF and death following an AMI.[23] Automated external defibrillator (AED) plays an important role in preventing sudden cardiac death, various committees have recommended that paramedical staff be trained and AED be installed at public places. Automated external defibrillator device training has now become an integral part of training of advanced cardiac life support, with this it is hoped that significant out of hospital death could be avoided and patients would be transported easily to nearby cardiac center for further management.

Role of AICD Following AMI

The 2012 ACCF/AHA/HRS guidelines for AICD implantation have recommended that patients who have LVEF ≤ 35% and who are at least 40 days post-MI and are in NYHA functional class II or III are class I candidates for AICD (level of evidence A).

Patients with LVEF < 40 post-MI with NSVT and inducible VF or sustained VT at electrophysiological study are also candidates for AICD (class I recommendation, level of evidence B). However, the recent ACC/AHA 2013 guideline for STEMI recommends AICD therapy before discharge for all those patients who develop sustain VT/VF beyond 48 hours after STEMI provided the arrhythmia is not due to transient or reversible ischemia, reinfarction, or metabolic abnormalities (level of evidence B).[24-26]

Mechanical Complications of MI

The three major mechanical complications of AMI are as follows:

1. Ventricular free wall rupture (VFWR)
2. Ventricular septal rupture
3. Papillary muscle rupture with severe mitral regurgitation.

Ventricular Free Wall Rupture (Fig. 23.2A)

It is the most serious complication occurring after AMI, and is usually associated with large transmural infarction and antecedent infarct expansion. It is associated with high mortality and accounts for 15–30% of death due to acute hemo-pericardium leading to cardiac tamponade. The overall incidence of VFWR ranges from 0.8% to 6.2%, there is decline in the incidence over the years due to better 24 hours blood pressure control, increased used of reperfusion strategy, beta-blocker, ACE inhibitor, and decreased usage of heparin. There was increased incidence of in-hospital mortality in data from National Registry of Myocardial Infarction (NRMI) among patients who received thrombolytic therapy (12.1%) than among patient who did not (6.1%). Thrombolysis in Myocardial Infarction Phase II (TIMI II) trial showed that 16% of patients died from cardiac rupture within 18 hours of therapy. The incidence was much lower in patients who underwent PTCA. Ventricular free wall rupture risk factor includes the following:

- Age above 70 years
- Female sex
- No previous MI

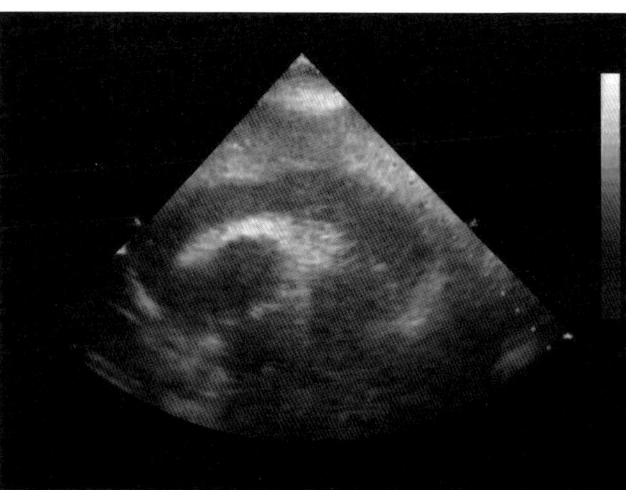

Fig. 23.2A Cardiac tamponade (Ventricular free wall rupture)

- Q wave in electrocardiography
- Hypertension during initial phase of AMI
- Corticosteroids or nonsteroidal anti-inflammatory drug usage
- Fibrinolytic therapy more than 14 hours after STEMI.

Ischemic preconditioning is protective from development of VFWR.

Becker et al. classified VFWR in three types

1. Type I—an abrupt slit-like tear that is frequently associated with anterior infarcts and that occurs early (within 24 hours).
2. Type II—an erosion of infarcted myocardium at the border between the infarcted and viable myocardium.
3. Type III—an early aneurysm formation correlated with older and severely expanded infarcts.

Thrombolytic therapy accelerates the occurrence of Becker type I and type II ventricular free wall rupture (VFWR) whereas in severely expanded infarction (type III), it decreases the incidence.

Myocardial rupture or perforation is often sealed with hematoma and adjacent pericardium leading to the formation of a pseudoaneurysm, which is often visualized as an aneurysmal outpouching that communicates with the LV cavity by means of a narrow neck. It can be differentiated from true aneurysm since its wall is composed of thrombus and/or hematoma and is devoid of myocardial element unlike a true aneurysm that has all the elements of the original myocardial wall and a relative wide base. Pseudoaneurysm may vary in size and risks for rupture.

The clinical presentation of VFWR may vary, it may be acute leading to severe chest pain, and abrupt electromechanical dissociation or asystole, hemodynamic collapse, and death. About one-third of patients have a subacute course wherein they present with syncope, hypotension, shock, arrhythmia, and recurrent chest pain.

Early diagnosis of VFWR and appropriate intervention is critical for patient's survival. A high index of suspicion is required in patients with AMI who have large infarcts, having shock and arrhythmia and developing abrupt electromechanical dissociation. Electrocardiography signs of impending VFWR include sinus tachycardia, intraventricular conduction defects, and persistent or recurrent ST elevation but are not specific. The diagnostic tool of choice is echocardiography; the key diagnostic finding that begins moderate-to-large pericardial effusion with echocardiographic finding of cardiac tamponade. The mortality rates are significantly higher in patients who develop electromechanical dissociation with moderate to severe pericardial effusion with tamponade compare to patients who do not develop tamponade, this group of patient should be followed closely since late rupture may still occur.[27] Absence of pericardial effusion has very high negative predictive value. The role of TEE is limited to patients with poor echo window or those who are on mechanical window.

The role of cardiac magnetic resonance imaging (MRI) has been studied by investigators in evaluation of post-MI pseudoaneurysm where the ventricular rupture is contained by adherent pericardial partition with a narrow neck, this is further complicated by rupture by heart failure and when pseudoaneurysm volume is large by thrombus and embolism. In 2005, Mousavi et al. reported that cardiac MRI is superior to TTE for diagnosis of ventricular aneurysm. Magnetic resonance imaging thus plays an important role as choice of investigation in such cases (Figs 23.2B and C).

Ventricular Septal Rupture (Fig. 23.3A)

The first reporting of post-MI VSD was about 100 year later than it was first described on autopsy in 1847.[28] It complicated about 1–3% of AMI,[29] occurring 3–8 days after index AMI

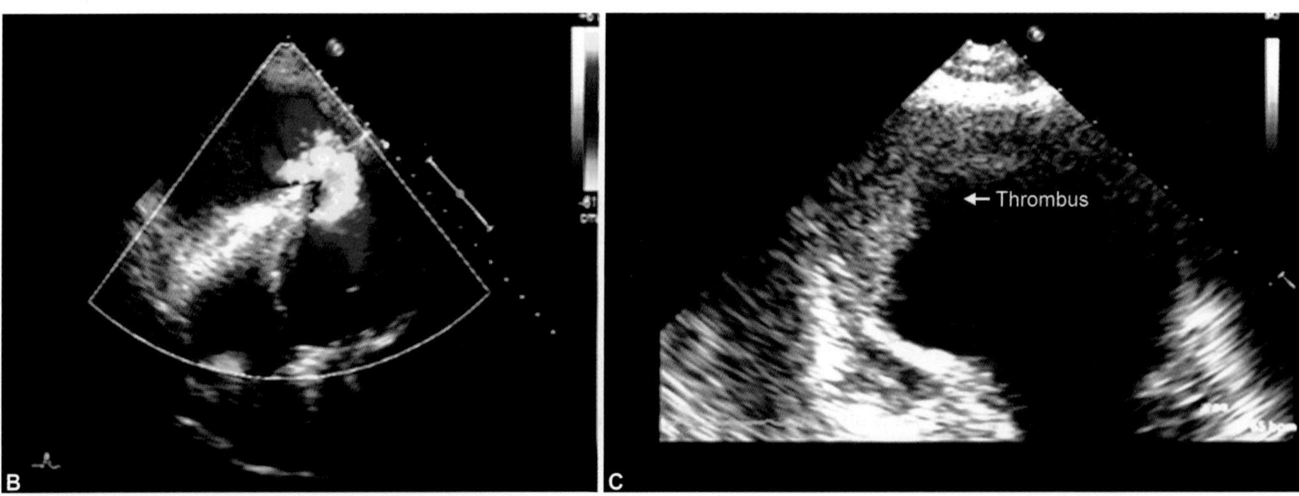

Figs 23.2B and C (B) Pseudoaneurysm; (C) Left ventricular aneurysm and thrombus

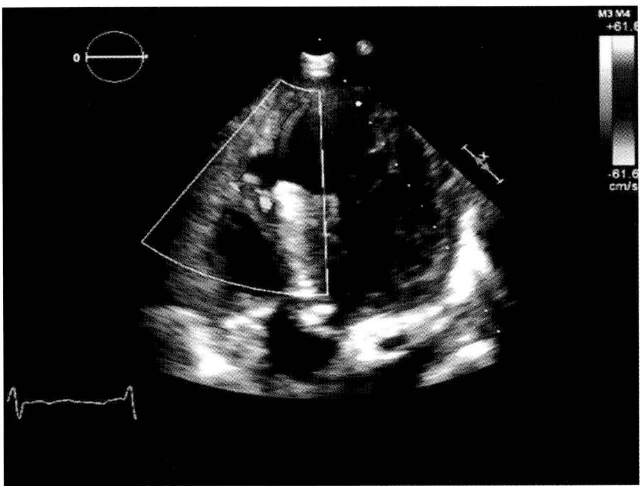

Fig. 23.3A Ventricular septal rupture

but may occur as early as in first 24 hours and, or as late as 2 weeks,[29] and carries a mortality rate of 50% in first week and 90% at 2 months with conservative medical management.[30] Early reperfusion strategies and adjunct medical therapy have significantly reduced the incidence to <1% of cases [0.2% in Global Utilization of Streptokinase and TPA for Occluded Coronary Arteries (GUSTO-I) trial].[31] Similar reports in reduction of incidence were reported in patients undergoing primary PCI. Yipes et al. reported that in 1,321 patients undergoing primary PCI the incidence was 0.23% versus 3% with no acute reperfusion therapy ($P = 0.0001$).[7]

Delayed hospital admission after infarction (>24 hours), undue physical activity in early postinfarct period, and recurrent angina correlate with development of VSD. Various other risk factors include age >60 years, female gender, no history of previous MI, and hypertension. They are common in patients with large anterior MI causing generally apical and simple VSD, and those occurring following inferior or posterior MI involve rupture of the basal and inferior posterior septum are mostly complex with serpiginous tunnels transversing through interventricular septum with multiple orifices. Intramural extension with dissection of interventricular septum or rarely the RV free wall may also occur.[31]

Chest pain, shortness of breath, hypotension, heart failure leading to shock within hours and days are symptoms of VSR complicating MI. Onset of new, loud, and harsh holo systolic murmur loudest at lower left sternal border and associated palpable systolic thrill with RV and LV S3 gallop are present in 50% of cases. Early diagnosis with TTE with Doppler interrogation reveals a high velocity, left to right ventricular shunt, and establishes the diagnosis. It is also helpful in:

- Defining the site and size of septal rupture
- Assess the LV and RV function
- Estimate the RV systolic pressure
- Quantify the left to right shunt.

Transesophageal echocardiogram (TEE) may be required in assessment of complex VSD. The use of real-time three-dimensional (3D) TEE provides a detailed assessment of the defect orifice and guide in closure procedure. Coronary catheterization quantifies the degree of left to right shunt and visualizes the coronary artery.

Early surgery is still the gold standard for the treatment of post-MI VSD. Acute surgery is technically complicated by friable myocardial tissue; various retrospective studies have suggested that better results are obtained in patients in whom surgery was delayed by 6 weeks since myocardial fibrosis had occurred and it permits a better hold of the suture and a more secure and long-lasting closure. However, the apparent favorable outcome in delayed surgical group reflects a selection bias with hemodynamically stable patients with small defects self-selecting by surviving to relative low-risk surgery. Surgery when delayed in hemodynamically stable patients has catastrophic consequences, and multiple studies have supported rapid interventions.[32,33] The recent ACC/AHA 2013 guidelines for STEMI support this view and advise emergency surgical repair even in hemodynamically stable patients, because the rupture site can expand abruptly, resulting in sudden hemodynamic collapse in previously stable patients. The in-hospital mortality, though lower than conservative modality, was still high (47%) in GUSTO-I trial. Residual shunt persists in 10–37% of cases after surgery due to overlooked additional defect or development of new VSD, and 11% of these patient require further surgical procedure. The long-term prognosis of patients who survive the acute 30 days postoperative period is, however, good. Transcatheter closure of VSD was initially carried out in patients who were deemed to be too high risk for surgical repair due to their recent post-MI status, advanced age, severe CAD, hemodynamic instability, and added comorbidity. They were also used in patients with residual VSD. Initial reports by Lock et al. in 1998 using Rashkind double umbrella,[34] various other devices have been used and reported like Clamshell occluder (USCI Angiographics, Tewksbury, MA), the Cardioseal (NMT medical boston, MA), and the Amplatzer septal occluder (AGA Medical Corporation). Outcomes using Amplatzer device have been reported in 11 series with a total of 130 patients of whom 64 were treated in acute phase of AMI (within 14 days from index infarction event), and in the remaining 66 patients the procedures were performed at least 14 days after infarction. The overall success rate was 85% (95% CI for mean 81–90%) with no difference between acute and subacute/chronic phase patients. The 30-days survival was 34% in acute phase compared to 81% in subacute chronic group. As for surgical repair, if a transcatheter procedure is technically feasible, it is advised not to delay it because secondary complication may ensue and impair subsequent prognosis even if VSD is corrected.

Complications after device implantation are as follows:

- Transient complete AV block (role of permanent proton pump inhibitor unclear)

- Ventricular tachycardia, VF, or AF
- Contrast medium nephropathy
- Device migration
- Residual shunting.

The role of transcatheter device in the treatment of post-MI VSD is expanding; they may provide as a bridge to urgent surgery or permit deferral of surgery until peri-VSD tissue has strengthened. Anatomically suitable patients will undergo definite correction with transcatheter device with increasing evidence.

Papillary Muscle Rupture with Severe Mitral Regurgitation (Fig. 23.3B)

It is a catastrophic mechanical complication following AMI and accounts for 5% of early death.[35] It may result in acute mitral regurgitation, acute pulmonary edema, and/or CS.[36] The posteromedial papillary muscle is more likely to rupture (6–12 times) compared to anteriolateral blood supply; this difference is due to the fact that while the later has dual blood supply (LAD and LCx), the former has single supply from the posterior descending artery. The diagnosis can be established with physical finding of new onset holosystolic murmur in patients with AMI, the murmur may be soft or even absent if there is an abrupt rise of left atrial pressure, which lessens the pressure gradient between the left atrium and LV as in acute MR. The murmur is best heard in lower left sternal border and may be uncommonly associated with a thrill. S3 and S4 gallop can be expected. The standard diagnostic tool is ECG with color Doppler imaging initial screening can be carried out with TTE followed by TEE or 3D TEE if suspicion of papillary muscle rupture is high. TTE has a sensitivity of 65–85%,[37] a flail segment of mitral valve, and a severed papillary muscle or chorda can be frequently seen moving freely within the left ventricular cavity. In few cases, the ruptured head does not prolapse into the left atrium, feature reported in 35% of the cases[38] then the diagnosis can be established by TEE. Emergency surgical intervention is the treatment of choice; surgical mortality has drastically reduced since it was first performed in 1965 from 18% to 8.7% particularly when associated with CABG.[39] Long-term outcome of patients after surgery is similar to MI without papillary muscle rupture. These observations only emphasize the importance of prompt diagnosis and an aggressive therapeutic approach.[39]

Pericarditis (Early and Late)

The aggressive use of reperfusion therapy has significantly reduced the incidence of acute pericarditis.[40] Early pericarditis complicates about 10% of MI, most of them are transmural infarcts and occur within 1–4 days. It is important to make distinction with acute stent thrombosis or reinfarction. Pain during supine position and its radiation to the trapezius and presence of pericardial friction rub provide some clue. Diagnosis can be further confirmed by presence of pericardial effusion in TTE. Magnetic resonance imaging shows contrast uptake in the pericardium. Late pericarditis occurs usually 1–8 weeks after MI (Dressler's syndrome) in 1–3% of patients with AMI and is usually associated with systemic feature of malaise, fever, and increased inflammatory markers. Aspirin is the drug of choice. Nonsteroidal anti-inflammatory drugs and corticosteroids are contraindicated in early pericarditis as they interfere with healing of infarcted myocardium; however, they can be used if the duration of MI is >4 weeks.

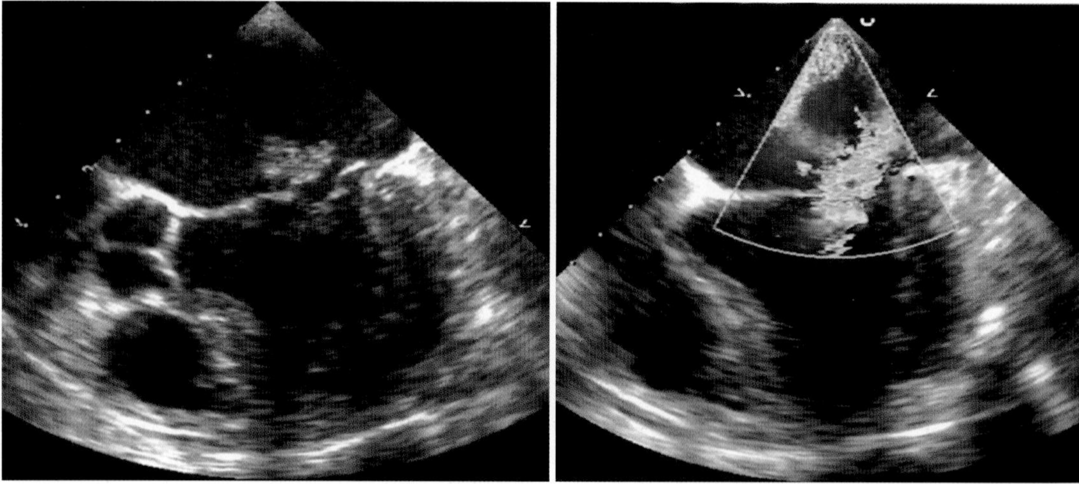

Fig. 23.3B Papillary muscle rupture with severe magnetic resonance

Embolic Complication

About 2% of patient with AMI develop embolic complications. It is not unlikely to have patient with an embolic event seeking treatment to begin, diagnosed as having recent silent AMI. Risk factors include large anterior MI and LV aneurysm. It usually occurs 10 days after the index event. Initial treatment with LMWH followed by vitamin K antagonist is recommended.

CONCLUSION

Complications following AMI have catastrophic result and lead to prolonged hospitalization, increased financial burden to the patient, and increased morbidity and mortality. Early diagnosis and appropriate treatment can significantly bring down the mortality associated with MI. Complications associated with MI provide significant challenge to treating physicians, cardiologist, and surgeons. With newer treatment modalities and better understanding of the basic pathophysiological processes involved and advanced surgical technique, this challenge can be met. The present century will be remembered for this.

REFERENCES

1. Sanborn T, Feldman T. Management strategies for cardiogenic shock. Curr Opin Cardiol. 2004;19(6):608-12.
2. Stegman B, Newby L, Hochman J, et al. Post-myocardial infarction cardiogenic shock is a systemic illness in need of systemic treatment. Is therapeutic hypothermia one possibility? J Am Coll Cardiol. 2012;59(7):644-7.
3. Iakobishvili Z, Hasdai D. Cardiogenic shock: treatment. Med Clin N Am. 2007;91(4):713-27.
4. Braunwald Textbook of Cardiology; 9th edn, Chapter 55.
5. Lim N, Dubois MJ, De Backer D, et al. Do all nonsurvivors of cardiogenic shock die with a low cardiac index? Chest. 2003;124(5):1885-91.
6. Prondzinsky R, Lemm H, Swyter M, et al. Intra-aortic balloon counterpulsation in patients with acute myocardial infarction complicated by cardiogenic shock: the prospective, randomized IABP Shock Trial for Attenuation of Multiorgan Dysfunction Syndrome. Crit Care Med. 2010;38(1):152-60.
7. Brownlee M, Vlassara H, Cerami A. Nonenzimatic glycosilation and the pathogenesis of diabetes complications. Ann Intern Med. 1984;101:527-37.
8. Ahmed, N. Advanced glycation endproductsosilation and the pathogenesis of diabetes comp. Ann Intern Clin Pract. 2005;67: 3-21.
9. Selejan SR, Pöss J, Hewera L, et al. Role of receptor for advanced glycation end products in cardiogenic shock. Crit Care Med. 2012;40(5):1513-22.
10. Aissaoui N, Puymirat E, Tabone X, et al. Improved outcome of cardiogenic shock at the acute stage of myocardial infarction: a report from the USIK 1995, USIC 2000, and FAST-MI French Nationwide Registries. Eur Heart J. 2012;33(20);2535-43.
11. Cheng JM, den Uil CA, Hoeks SE, et al. Percutaneous left ventricular assist devices vs. intra-aortic balloon pump counterpulsation for treatment of cardiogenic shock: a meta-analysis of controlled trials. Eur Heart J. 2009;30(17):2102-8.
12. Garatti A, Russo C, Lanfranconi M, et al. Mechanical circulatory support for cardiogenic shock complicating acute myocardial infarction: an experimental and clinical review. ASAIO J. 2007;53(3):278-87.
13. Hernandez AF, Grab JD, Gammie JS, et al. A decade of short-term outcomes in post cardiac surgery ventricular assist device implantation: data from the Society of Thoracic Surgeons' National Cardiac Database. Circulation. 2007;116(6):606-12.
14. Lopes RD, Elliott LE, White HD, et al. Antithrombotic therapy and outcomes of patients with atrial fibrillation following primary percutaneous coronary intervention: results from the APEX-AMI trial. Eur Heart J. 2009;30:2019 30:2.
15. Bloch Thomsen PE, Jons C, Raatikainen MJP, et al. Long-term recording of cardiac arrhythmias with an implantable cardiac monitor in patients with reduced ejection fraction after acute myocardial infarction: the Cardiac Arrhythmias and Risk Stratification After Acute Myocardial Infarction (CARISMA) study. Circulation. 2010;122:1258.
16. You JJ, Singer DE, Howard PA, et al. Antithrombotic therapy for atrial fibrillation: Antithrombotic Therapy and Prevention of Thrombosis, 9th ed: American College of Chest Physicians Evidence-Based Clinical Practice Guidelines. Chest. 2012;41:4.
17. Vandvik PO, Lincoff AM, Gore JM, et al. Primary and secondary prevention of cardiovascular disease: Antithrombotic Therapy and Prevention of Thrombosis, 9th edn: American College of Chest Physicians Evidence-Based Clinical Practice Guidelines. Chest. 2012;141:637S-68S.
18. Lip GYH, Huber K, Andreotti F, et al. Antithrombotic management of atrial fibrillation patients presenting with acute coronary syndrome and/or undergoing coronary stenting: executive summary: a Consensus Document of the European Society of Cardiology Working Group on Thrombosis. Eur Heart J. 2010;31(11):1311-8.
19. Faxon DP, Eikelboom JW, Berger PB, et al. Consensus document: antithrombotic therapy in patients with atrial fibrillation undergoing coronary stenting: a North-American perspective. Thromb Haemost. 2011;106:572-84.
20. Lamberts M, Gislason GH, Olesen JB, et al. Oral anticoagulation and antiplatelets in atrial fibrillation patients after myocardial infarction and coronary intervention. J Am Coll Cardiol. 2013;62(11):981-9.
21. *http://reference.medscape.com/medline/abstract/20837897*
22. *http://reference.medscape.com/medline/abstract/3047448*
23. *http://reference.medscape.com/medline/abstract/634283*
24. Wever EF, Hauer RN, van Capelle FL, et al. Randomized study of implantable defibrillator as first-choice therapy versus conventional strategy in postinfarct sudden death survivors. Circulation. 1995;91:2195-203.
25. Siebels J, Kuck KH. Implantable cardioverter defibrillator compared with antiarrhythmic drug treatment in cardiac arrest survivors (the Cardiac Arrest Study Hamburg). Am Heart J. 1994; 127:1139-44.
26. Connolly SJ, Hallstrom AP, Cappato R, et al. for the AVID, CASH and CIDS studies: Antiarrhythmics vs Implantable Defibrillator study: Cardiac Arrest Study Hamburg: Canadian Implantable Defibrillator Study. Meta-analysis of the implantable cardioverter defibrillator secondary prevention trials. Eur Heart J. 2000;21:2071–21.

27. http://reference.medscape.com/medline/abstract/20975001
28. Sager RV. Coronary thrombosis: perforation of the infarcted interventricular septum. Arch Intern Med. 1934;53:140-52.
29. Topaz O, Taylor AL. Interventricular septal rupture complicating acute myocardial infarction: from pathophysiologic features to the role of invasive and noninvasive diagnostic modalities in current management. Am J Med. 1992;93:683-8.
30. Edwards BS, Edwards WD, Edwards JE. Ventricular septal rupture complicating acute myocardial infarction: identification of simple and complex types in 53 autopsied hearts. Am J Cardiol. 1984;54:1201-5.
31. Crenshaw BS, Granger CB, Birnbaum Y, et al. Risk factors, angiographic patterns, and outcomes in patients with ventricular septal defect complicating acute myocardial infarction. GUSTO-I (Global Utilization of Streptokinase and TPA for Occluded Coronary Arteries) Trial Investigators. Circulation. 2000;101: 27-32.
32. Giombolini C, Notaristefano S, Santucci S, et al. Transcatheter closure of postinfarction ventricular septal defect using the Amplatzer atrial septal defect occluder. J Cardiovasc Med. 2008;9:941-5.
33. Held AC, Cole PL, Lipton B, et al. Rupture of the interventricular septum complicating acute myocardial infarction: a multicenter analysis of clinical findings and outcome. Am Heart J. 1988;116: 1330-6.
34. Lock JE, Block PC, McKay RG, et al. Transcatheter closure of ventricular septal defects. Circulation. 1988;78:361-8.
35. Nishimura RA, Schaff HV, Shub C, et al. Papillary muscle rupture complicating acute myocardial infarction: analysis of 17 patients. Am J Cardiol. 1983;51:373-7.
36. Sanders RJ, Neubuerger KT, Ravin A. Rupture of papillary muscles: occurrence of rupture of the posterior muscle in posterior myocardial infarction. Dis Chest. 1957;31:316-23.
37. Czarnecki A, Thakrar A, Fang T, et al. Acute severe mitral regurgitation: consideration of papillary muscle architecture. Cardiovasc Ultrasound. 2008;6:5.
38. Moursi MH, Bhatnagar SK, Vilacosta I, et al. Transesophageal echocardiographic assessment of papillary muscle rupture. Circulation. 1996;94:1003.
39. Russo A, Suri RM, Grigioni F, et al. Clinical outcome after surgical correction of mitral regurgitation due to papillary muscle rupture. Circulation. 2008;118:1528-34.
40. Imazio M, Negro A, Belli R, et al. Frequency and prognostic significance of pericarditis following acute myocardial infarction treated by primary percutaneous coronary intervention. Am J Cardiol. 2009;103:1525-9.

24

Heart Lung Machine for CABG: Should it be Relegated to Archives?

Rajesh Chauhan, Sanjay Gupta

INTRODUCTION

A series of scientific innovations initiated by Gibbon, Lillihei among others led to the development of heart lung machine, empowering medical science to gain control over the intricacies of circulation. Soon complicated corrective cardiac surgical procedures started being done by the cardiac surgeons, ably supported by anesthesiologists, owing to the development of monitoring systems to guide complicated surgical procedures safely. A chance shot of dye injected through the right coronary artery while doing aortogram in a case of rheumatic heart disease revealed the first coronary angiogram, which was later used in visualizing blocks in the coronary arteries, a feature of coronary artery disease. Consequently, medical science identified the cause behind an acute disabling chest pain, arising because of a decrease in the oxygenated blood supply to the myocardium, evoking symptoms of angina. This disease had become number one cause of death in the United States, which triggered a growing interest supported by a huge amount of money allocated in developing technologies that would assist medical scientists in seeking newer opportunities in the treatment, unknown until then.

Surgical techniques offered for the treatment of coronary artery disease witnessed an era of performing it on beating heart with limitations, which was later overcome by conducting it on the cardiopulmonary bypass (CPB). This procedure stood the test of time and became the gold standard technique. It gained popularity worldwide and became the standard of patient care in the treatment of coronary artery disease practiced for over three decades. This happened amidst developments in cardiology with the introduction and rapid advancement of the procedures for treating coronary artery disease through a percutaneous route from a peripheral artery. With this emerged the percutaneous transluminal coronary angioplasty (PTCA). The resurgence of off-pump bypass grafting took place in the mid-90s to counter the growing influence of PTCA as well as the shortcomings of doing it on CPB, well supported by the industry through the development of supportive devices and surgical instruments. Complete revascularization off-pump started being reported increasingly that was considered to be difficult. Thereafter, a stage was reached when almost all coronary bypass procedures were being performed off-pump in a large number of centers all over the world. In these centers, on-pump bypass grafting was restricted to conducting procedures combined along with valve repair/replacement or conversion of an off-pump procedure following unfavorable hemodynamics. At Fortis Escorts Heart Institute, New Delhi, off-pump bypass grafting has become the standard of care. Should it then be considered this as an end to the practice of performing coronary artery bypass grafting (CABG) on CPB, with the heart lung machine and perfusionists available on standby?

Does the literature on off-pump bypass so overwhelmingly favor it that the time has come to relegate heart lung machine to archives? To relegate heart lung machine to archives would mean that there may be no need to have heart lung machine even in the operating room and by no means there would be likelihood of it required at any time during the procedure. Local practices in hospitals, while effectively following the standard of care, can follow newer techniques, if the result is comparable or much above expectations of a standard operating procedure. With revolutionary changes taking place in the surgical techniques in the treatment of coronary artery disease, it seems pertinent at this stage to solve the crucial debate by reviewing the pros and cons of each procedure, off-pump and on-pump bypass, with comprehensive review of the literature available on the subject. We see no reason to defend the statement and suffice to say that its mere availability and presence of "Perfusionist" that enables the surgeon to carry out procedures is difficult to comprehend otherwise. Off-pump bypass grafting that has become more popular because of economic reasons requires close scrutiny. The inference in the end justifies the decision based on scientific evidences, in a world that is changing to newer technologies. Surely technology should stay if it holds promise and gives the best and most favored results under all circumstances.

THE HISTORY OF CORONARY ARTERY BYPASS GRAFTING

The search to find the treatment to ameliorate the disabling and life-threatening complications of the disease led to its treatment based on the principle of increasing blood supply beyond the block. This was proved in experimental studies at the dawn of twentieth century, by Alexis Carrel in 1910 by a series of experiments in the canines by creating "complimentary circulation" in the diseased coronary arteries. His vision could not take shape due to the lack of technology, not until 1945, when Arthur Vineberg introduced the "Vineberg Procedure" where he implanted the left internal thoracic artery (LITA) into the myocardium. Some success of the procedure was noted in follow-up studies, but the procedure has largely been abandoned. It was followed by a successful anastomosis of left anterior descending (LAD) coronary artery with LITA performed on beating heart by Spencer in United States in year 1964.[1] After series of works done by Murray, Goetz, Kolesov reported his first clinically successful CABG on beating heart and published his paper in 1967. He for the first time used direct coronary anastomosis involving suture technique and grafted LITA to the left circumflex coronary artery in a patient. He also designed magnifying glasses and scissors to work with precision during surgical anastomosis and considered beating heart bypass grafting safer than on-pump that was associated with global inflammatory phenomenon and was fraught with dangers. Favalro used saphenous venous graft in 1967 that proved its versatility as an aortocoronary graft as longer lengths of conduit became available in each subject. This gave birth to the modern day coronary bypass surgery.[1] Thus, it started the newly celebrated procedure of performing CABG, initially restricted to easily approachable vessels on the heart. Vessels on the anterior surface of the heart, mainly the LAD artery and the right coronary artery, were grafted using arterial conduits with the left and the right internal thoracic arteries. As it was impossible to maintain safe hemodynamics for diseased vessels on the lateral wall and vessels on the inferior wall, the procedure was restricted to certain selected patients. With the development of heart lung machine and perfusion technology, the procedure started being done on CPB. The advantages offered by the procedure was a reason enough to be considered as a major advancement in the treatment of coronary artery disease, as the arrested heart on pump could be turned around to visualize and complete the anastomosis without affecting perfusion pressures of the patient. Thus, it provided a motionless, bloodless operating field and the surgeon was able to visualize clearly the edge of the vessels during anastomosis. This helped greatly to perform excellent quality of grafting and for the first time it became possible to perform complete revascularization of all the vessels leading to the onset of multivessel grafting. It showed classical improvement in graft patency and the technique spread rapidly throughout the world. Millions of people were to be benefitted by the procedure. By the end of 80s, the practice of coronary bypass surgery reached Indian hospitals. Major improvement in the strategies employed in myocardial preservation had begun and much work was done on the subject by Buckberg and his research group, later refined and modified by Calafiore among other. The introduction of a standard blood cardioplegia done by mixing crystalloid solution in a ratio of 4:1 using double-headed roller pump and the temperature control by passing it through heat exchanger became the standard of care during aortic cross-clamp. This was a new advance over off-pump bypass grafting that also continued under favorable situation by a group of surgeons.

Meanwhile, the developments in the field of cardiology kept at pace and saw rapidly evolving technique of balloon dilatation of discrete lesions in the coronary arteries known as percutaneous transluminal angioplasty (PTCA) done through one of the peripheral arteries. It was first performed in 1977 by Andreas Gruentzig at Zurich, Switzerland. By mid-1980s, PTCA was an accepted procedure in the treatment of coronary artery disease and the practice spread rapidly throughout the world. Development of coronary stent, a device placed after balloon dilatation and repositioned permanently after dilatation with balloon, was a further refinement of the technology. PTCA was a simple, easy to learn, and almost as effectively executed by all cardiologists required a shorter stay, and was less invasive. The prevention of acute closure due to thrombosis was suitably prevented by antithrombotic drugs like aspirin and clopidogrel and the transformation was complete. This development opened up new vistas for offering safe modality of treating coronary artery disease. Its popularity grew well supported by results and soon multivessel angioplasty started being performed. Percutaneous interventions started to threaten the position of CABG, which until then had been the only modality available. With this, its monopoly as the modality of treatment for three decades started to wane, reaching its nadir in 2004. At this time, lowest volumes of coronary bypass surgery were recorded in Society of Thoracic Surgeons (STS) National Database. These trends of drop in the volume of surgical records were seen increasingly between 2001 and 2004 that returned to basal levels in terms of volumes by 2007, almost same as in the year 2000. Year 2004 was also the peak time of doing off-pump CABG (OPCABG). Between 2001 and 2004, there was a rise in percutaneous coronary interventions. STS National Database has a record of over 4.5 million surgical records that have undergone cardiac surgical procedures and have been subgrouped into various categories of which coronary artery bypass forms an important group. *Off-pump bypass has peaked to between 20% and 25% of all coronary bypass grafting surgeries performed in the United States, relegating 75–80% procedures still on-pump.* In the United States, "The Society of Thoracic Surgeons (STS) established the National Database (NDB) for Cardiac Surgery" in 1989. STS NDB is a "gold standard" worldwide for process and outcomes analysis related to cardiothoracic surgery.

Off-Pump Bypass Grafting

To remain on the competitive edge, with growing technologies in the field of cardiology, which was to grow far ahead of their surgical compatriots in the times to come, the method of doing coronary bypass grafting got a new impetus in mid-1990s with resurgence of the procedure due to the availability of cardiac stabilizers and intraluminal shunts. Changing over from the on-pump CPB grafting to off-pump bypass grafting grew slowly with the passage of time. As there were increasing number of papers claiming extracorporeal circulation as a cause of stimulation of inflammatory cascade and organ dysfunction, the practice of off-pump bypass was widely accepted, especially in the growing economies across the world.

Off-pump bypass grafting in the initial phase was more invasive and was being done after complete midsternotomy. But with miniaturization of the retractors and modification of surgical instruments, the surgical procedure became more direct with a small incision made in front of the vessel to be grafted, making the procedure less invasive. Thus, minimally invasive direct coronary artery bypass surgery (MIDCAB) performed through the:

1. Anterior midthoracotomy route from the edge of sternum between the ribs on the left side, or
2. Ministernotomy route

MIDCAB was restricted to vessels in the anterior wall. The conduit of choice was the LITA that was used to anastomose the LAD coronary artery. It was feasible to keep patients hemodynamically stable for short periods. The procedure enjoyed a short popularity phase as it was soon replaced by PTCA.

Off-pump bypass could also be accomplished through the lateral thoracotomy route (ThoraCAB) for target vessels on the lateral wall, saphenous venous graft being the conduit used commonly with proximal end anastomosed to the descending aorta. The procedure required use of a double lumen tube for one lung anesthesia at the time of grafting. ThoraCAB has been performed safely with good results.[2] It became possible to perform multivessel grafting off-pump with the introduction of tissue stabilizers and intraluminal shunts.

Off-Pump Versus On-Pump Bypass Grafting: Review of Literature

Morbidity and Mortality

The completion of revascularization resulted in excellent patency of grafts. Despite rapid development that was taking place in perfusion technology, a number of complications were being increasingly noted like the development of inflammatory markers causing multiorgan dysfunction presenting as coagulopathy, respiratory failure, myocardial dysfunction, renal failure, and neurocognitive defects.[3,4]

Cerebral Strokes

Evidence of calcium on X-ray chest, aortic knob calcification, is an important predictor of atheromatous disease.[5] This is also known by directly feeling the aorta, or confirmed with epiaortic ultrasonography to detect ascending aorta atheromas that can alter surgical strategies.[6] Intraoperative transesophageal echocardiography is also known to alter surgical strategies on finding atheromatous disease in the ascending aorta.[5,7,8]

Aortic manipulation must be avoided when there is extracoronary vasculopathy or arteriopathy in order to avoid cerebrovascular accidents; the use of side clamping during off-pump surgery evens out this risk with on-pump patients, while the use of total arterial revascularization promotes "anaortic technique" known to decrease embolization of calcium and atheromas in elderly and octogenarians.[9,10] Aortic side clamping avoidance results in significant reduction in solid microemboli.[11] The incidence of embolization occurs during application, insertion, and removal of each device from ascending aorta, clampless devices, Encore and Heartstring. The proportions of emboli were noted to be significantly high in side clamp group (23%) versus 6% and 1% in Encore and Heartstring groups.[11] Heartstring device[12] should be used if proximal anastomosis is required as it provides no touch technique to aorta. The study also found that off-pump bypass grafting is superior with regard to risk-adjusted outcomes. Strokes rates are similar in on-pump CABG (ONCABG) versus or when partial aortic cross-clamping is applied in OPCABG.[12] When saphenous grafts are used in off-pump bypass grafting, use of side biting clamp is a necessary concomitant. Few surgeons follow anaortic technique only in heavily calcified ascending aorta wherein the risk of stroke is very high.

The elderly patients were benefitted with off-pump surgery as it was associated with decreased morbidity and mortality and with a decreased incidence of cerebral strokes.[13] Fewer complications were observed while using bilateral skeletonized internal thoracic artery graft in diabetic patients on the left system versus a single internal thoracic artery. At midterm, there was a significant reduction in overall death, cardiac death, and cardiac events.[14] Total arterial revascularization with no touch aortic technique using bilateral internal thoracic artery was safe with low mortality in patients with triple vessel disease. Best results with lesser cardiac events were obtained when bilateral internal thoracic artery was combined with right gastroepiploic graft to the right coronary artery.[15]

Off-pump surgery has major role in patients in high-risk group comprising elderly patients ≥80 years and patients with peripheral vascular disease as it was associated with an absolute risk reduction in stroke rate when compared with on-pump isolated CABG.[16,17]

Hammon et al. have shown that it is the surgical technique that is primary cause of brain insults in CABG patients. Incidence of cognitive defects in CABG patients is significantly reduced by following surgical strategies that minimize aortic manipulation. A single-stage clamp to do distal grafting and proximals has results that were not significantly different from those patients having OPCABG.[18]

Again, there were economic reasons also for doing the procedure, as has been reported in numerous papers. Off-pump surgery could also be done in a shorter duration enabling operating on a larger number of patients except that its training requires a greater learning curve.[19]

OPCABG: Hemodynamic Monitoring Challenges and the Newer Technologies

These newer techniques ably supported by anesthesiologists who rapidly adapted to the new demands and helped the surgeons in the early days of off-pump bypass grafting. This they did by decreasing the heart rates using infusion of short-acting beta-blockers and also maintaining mean arterial pressures to near baseline levels with alpha-adrenergic stimulants chiefly norepinephrine infusion in low doses. At these heart rates, ambidextrous cardiac surgeons were able to see the edges of the small arteriotomy in the target coronary vessels to successfully complete coronary anastomosis. The conduit used most commonly was the LITA anastomosed to LAD artery lying on the anterior surface of the heart. Positioning the heart requires a gentle manipulation with a tilt and forward movement, with pericardial suture and a sponge behind and on the lateral surface of the heart. The blood loss during the surgery was inevitable requiring volume replacement. As the number of grafts generally was restricted to one or two, patients were kept hemodynamically stable by replacing blood loss with intravenous fluids, judicious use of inotropic supports and sometimes blood transfusion. Later on the instruments, which were to be introduced and used, were the devices that stabilized the heart by producing segmental hypokinesia or akinesis using vacuum suction devices, which result in near-baseline hemodynamics when compared with deep pericardial retraction sutures.[20] These devices were octopus, a tissue stabilizer, and starfish, a vacuum suction device, used to lift the heart close to or at the apex. Octopus was used to stabilize the target vessel and hold it still. Use of these means has at times caused severe bruises on the myocardial surface and become a cause of blood loss. It is imperative to be cautious and gentle to avoid myocardial injury as it can lead to a life-threatening complication. Octopus is fixed at one end on the sternal retractor with a one-handed attachment of clamp and the other end made up of flexible arm holds the portion of the vessel to be grafted. Starfish is also used similarly. With the availability of these devices, cardiac surgeons were able to reach almost all areas around the heart with suitably adjusted hemodynamics. The Trendelenburg position with tilt toward the operating surgeon so as to not compromise visualization of the surgeon assisting across the operating table helped in stabilizing hemodynamics. Greater changes in hemodynamics are expected when the heart is positioned to expose vessels on the lateral wall.[20-22] OPCABG without stabilization of hemodynamics may invariably end on CPB. The hemodynamic insults are due to direct compression and geometrical distortion with deep pericardial sutures.[20] Displacement of the beating heart and immobilization causing compression of the heart may interfere with coronary blood flow resulting in myocardial ischemia[23,24] and may be closely associated with hemodynamic collapse.[25] With the introduction of intraluminal shunts, operating conditions improved with less blood loss and clear view of the target vessel. This is done during OPCABG to clearly see the edges of the vessel to do the distal anastomosis. Placement of intraluminal shunts can decrease ischemia by promoting blood flow across the open end of the target vessel, protects it from myocardial ischemia, and prevent left ventricular dysfunction.[23,26-28] Intracoronary shunts can be a cause of acute graft failure as it may cause intraluminal injury damaging the intima.[29] External shunts have been used to perfuse the coronary distal to the arteriotomy site.[30] Temporary coronary occlusion can also contribute to regional myocardial ischemia and hemodynamic instability (Fig. 24.1).

Positioning of Heart, Hemodynamic Insults, and Shifting of Strategies

Positioning of the heart with octopus in position decreases the myocardial contractility, affecting the filling pressures of right side as well as left side of the heart. Positioning the heart is always associated with reduction in mean arterial pressures, cardiac output, stroke volume and left ventricular end-diastolic pressures by direct compression (Figs 24.2 to 24.4). Attempt is made to maintain hemodynamic parameters toward baseline without compromising visualization of the target vessel and vice versa. This may be a difficult maneuver and second attempt in repositioning is usually successful. This may require judicious use of inotropic support; fluid infusion in Trendelenburg position may limit the changes and prevent intraoperative conversion to on-pump bypass,[31] but the use of intra-aortic balloon in 11% patients, 55/500 patients, is high and is indicative of hemodynamic instability in a study.[21] A complete understanding of the hemodynamics of the patient is important to avoid circulatory collapse induced by displacement of the heart.[32] Care is taken to avoid operative strategies designed to minimize severe

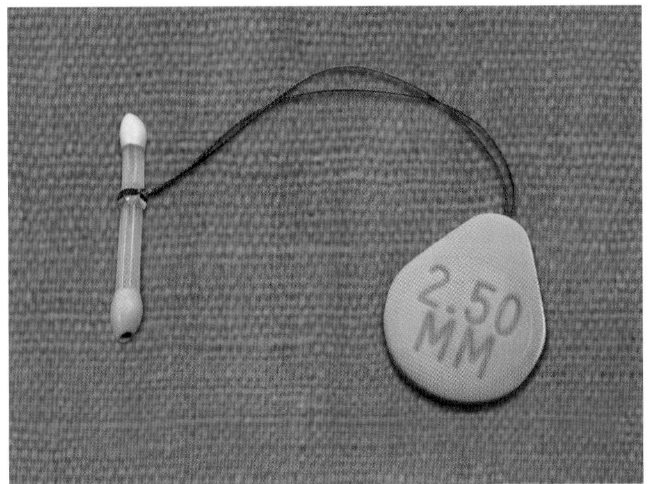

Fig. 24.1 Intraluminal shunt, size 2.5 mm, opening of the shunt is seen clearly

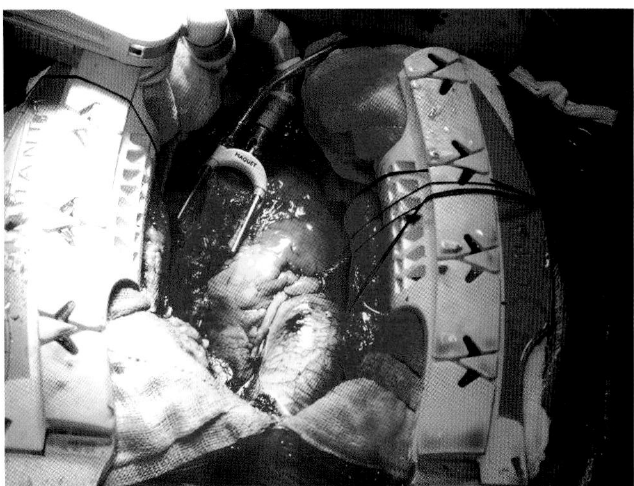

Fig. 24.3 Heart positioned for grafting of left anterior descending coronary artery, size minimum displacement

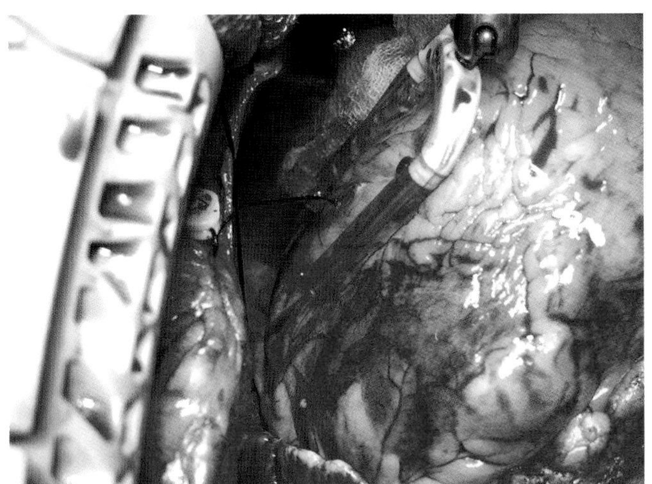

Fig. 24.2 Heart positioned for revascularization of obtuse marginal branch, held with Octopus

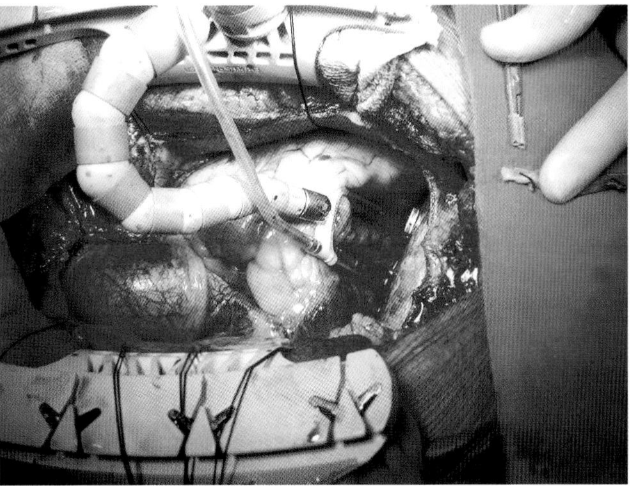

Fig. 24.4 Heart positioned for grafting of posterior descending coronary artery, *note* compression of right ventricle

compression of the right ventricle with very little need for pharmacological and mechanical support.[33] Undesirable compression of the right ventricle during positioning may cause signs of right ventricular outflow tract obstruction that may be associated with decrease in mean arterial pressure, cardiac output, and increasingly unresponsiveness to strategies used for stabilizing hemodynamics like Trendelenburg position of operating table and inotropic supports. It is imperative to recognize early signs of failing heart and try to alter pressure dynamics on the heart to be able to continue revascularization with stable hemodynamics. More often, the changed strategies help in stabilizing the hemodynamics. These include giving rest to the heart, judicious use of inotropes, nitroglycerine, vasopressors, and intra-aortic balloon pump (IABP). Leaving the heart in situ may present release phenomenon of inotropes trapped on right side of the heart resulting in tachycardia with rise in right- (pulmonary arterial pressure) and left-sided (systemic blood pressure) filling pressures, with or without ST segment shifts. Manifestations of subendocardial ischemia reflect prominently under adverse circumstances. Heart looks visibly distended with depressed contractility, confirmed with transesophageal echocardiography monitoring. On leaving the heart, hemodynamic stabilization continues over several minutes. A failing heart heading for conversion to on-pump may be the only viable strategy left to complete coronary artery grafting. Strategy of stabilizing with IABP might have been already late by then. An experienced team understands the dynamics of unstable hemodynamics. It avoids getting trapped into emergency conversion to on-pump. Decreasing the compression even marginally can result in significant improvement in cardiac output and mean arterial pressures. Monitoring beat-to-beat arterial waveforms on the monitor may be the best indicator of hemodynamic status. *A major responsibility of maintaining favorable hemodynamics until completion of coronary revascularization falls in the domain of the anesthesiologist; otherwise every off-pump bypass has the potential of conversion to on-pump procedure.*

Continuous transesophageal echocardiographic monitoring has become a valuable and often used device to monitor the dynamics. It has been shown to modify surgical plan while guiding hemodynamics, as a sole guiding tool in 23.53% of events, supportive of other monitoring modalities in 76.46% of events.[7] New changes in contractility and increasing valvular regurgitation may forewarn an impending crisis requiring an urgent change in position and pressure dynamics on the heart in order to be able to continue surgical anastomosis with more favorable hemodynamics. Visualization of arterial waveform pattern can give added information with continuous ST segment analysis, heart rate pattern, arrhythmias, and may continuously guide the hemodynamics. Off-pump surgery has been known to offer hypercoagulable state with activation of acute phase clotting factors that follows postoperatively unlike on-pump patients as has been suggested by Kurlansky.[34] With the rise in procoagulant activity, Mariani et al. have advised an aggressive anticoagulant regimen in all off-pump patients.[35] Since then, restarting of antiplatelets in the immediate postoperative period has become a common place.

Off-Pump Versus On-Pump Bypass Grafting: Morbidity Data (Effect on Low Ejection Fraction Patients, High-Risk Group Patients, Female Patients Ventilation, Blood Transfusion, Intensive Care Unit Stay, and Hospital Stay)

The STS National Database OPCABG was also reported to have significantly reduced adjusted morbidity and mortality with an ejection fraction <0.30.[36] In women, OPCABG offered reduced early morbidity and mortality as compared with on CPB that was associated with higher rates of death, strokes, myocardial infarction, and major adverse cardiac events (MACEs).[37] This study was negated in a meta-analysis of 10 randomized trials which concluded that off-pump bypass did not significantly reduce 1-year mortality, myocardial infarction, and revascularization vis-à-vis on-pump.[38]

Patients of coronary artery disease with left main disease, considered hemodynamically unstable, also had reduced morbidity and mortality.[39] Off-pump bypass has been reported to reduce early mortality in high-risk group patients.[40] Bonatti et al found that OPCAB surgery results were predictable based on a EuroSCORE and were safe for low risk group (EuroSCORE ≤ 5) but major complications seemed to occur preferentially in high risk group (EuroSCORE > 5) which included significant use of blood transfusion, intra-aortic balloon pump insertion, renal failure, and ICU length of stay.[41]

Others have come with just opposite results claiming that although off-pump surgery offered good early results with lower incidence of atrial fibrillation, blood transfusion, and less ventilator dependence but after a few years required repeat reoperative procedure and major vascular accidents in high-risk groups.[42] Transfusion of red blood cells, fresh frozen plasma, and platelets have been shown to increase the incidence of vasoplegia after cardiac surgery.[43]

In a high-risk group that included female patients with pre-existing renal failure and reoperations, off-pump bypass surgery was associated with less morbidity, blood transfusions, stroke, renal failure, pulmonary complications, reoperations, atrial fibrillation, and gastrointestinal complications with reduction in operative mortality, also in comparison with conventional on-pump bypass. Conversely, on-pump bypass was associated with higher mortality in reoperations in female patients and elderly patients above 75 years.[44]

Off-Pump and On-Pump Revascularization, Extent of Disease and Mortality: Is There a Relationship Between These Factors?

Incomplete revascularization, if restricted to only one diseased vessel, which was noted more in off-pump surgery patients, had no significant effect on survival between off-pump and on-pump patients. But leaving two vascular segments without a graft increased long-term mortality.[45] The early benefit of reduced mortality with OPCABG was not continued to the late term due to *incomplete revascularization* found more often in OPCABG.[46]

It is being repeatedly reported that off-pump may be associated with *incomplete revascularization* that was noted as an independent risk factor with effects being more distinct in those patients with low left ventricular ejection fraction (LVEF) and less noticeable in patients with normal LVEF. It is imperative to ensure complete revascularization in patients with low ejection fraction. Lower incidence of in-hospital mortality, cardiac mortality, and major accidents of cardiac and cerebrovascular accidents (MACCE) were observed in patients who had complete revascularization.[47] Despite receiving lesser number of grafts versus on-pump patients and having incomplete revascularization, the two groups had comparable results.[48] The details on Surgical Management of Arterial Revascularization (SMART) Trial at Emory University described the index of completeness of revascularization (ICOR),[37] and has been defined as the number of grafts performed versus grafts planned on the basis of preoperative coronary angiogram. The ICOR was shown to be identical in OPCABG and ONCABG.

Complete revascularization was possible with off-pump bypass using total arterial revascularization. CPB avoidance decreased postoperative ventilation, ICU stay, and hospital stay.[49,50] Along with these advantages, off-pump surgery could be done in multivessel disease as well and was economical.[49,51,52] It was possible to do reoperative procedures off-pump through anterior thoracotomy. MIDCAB procedure and majority patients did not require homologous blood transfusion with an overall short stay in hospital.[53,54]

International Society for Minimally Invasive Cardiothoracic Surgery (ISMICS): Conclusion (Year 2004)

The ISMICS consensus conference on OPCAB versus ONCAB in the year 2004 concluded that it supported OPCAB as a safe alternative to ONCAB with similar mortality and quality of life and a decreased risk of perioperative morbidity including duration of mechanical ventilation, ICU and hospital stay. The conference also revealed an overall mortality benefit for high-risk patients with OPCABG: EuroSCORE >5, left ventricular dysfunction, and atherosclerotic aortic disease and so have special role in elderly patients undergoing CABG.[19]

Off-Pump and On-Pump Bypass Surgery in Patients with Left Ventricular Dysfunction and Diabetic Patients

In patients that were offered isolated coronary artery bypass grafting with Ischemic left ventricular dysfunction, LVEF ≤ 0.30, it was noted that ventricular tachycardia and ventricular fibrillation were independent predictors of mortality, absolving cardiopulmonary bypass as an independent risk predictor of mortality while exonerating other associated risk factors.[55]

Preoperative use of *IABP* in hemodynamically unstable patients undergoing off-pump surgery was associated with shorter stay in the ICU, decreased need of postoperative dialysis, acute heart failure, and reduced postoperative mortality as compared to off-pump alone patients where IABP was not used.[56]

Off-pump coronary grafting was also found to be superior *in diabetic patients* with lower 30-day mortality as compared to on-pump patients, with lower postoperative neurologic complications (1.7% vs. 5.4%), and less frequent need for hemofiltration (3.4% vs. 10.4%); 6-month mortality rate was lesser (2.3% vs. 8.8%), and also 1-year mortality rate significantly lower (4.0% vs. 10.6%). Thus, in terms of postoperative complications and early and mid-term survival, OPCABG is superior to ONCABG in diabetic patients.[57]

MIDCAB has been proved to benefit out of proportion in diabetic patients with isolated lesion of LAD with the use of LITA as graft to LAD.[58] In a study in 411 patients who underwent MIDCAB procedure, 63 were diabetic patients and 348 were nondiabetic patients. Isolated proximal stenosis or an occlusion of the LAD was present in 262 patients, whereas 149 had multivessel disease. Incidence of myocardial infarction was higher in diabetic patients, with rates of subsequent revascularization similar during follow-up. In patients with multivessel disease, the 3-year cardiac mortality was significantly higher in diabetic patients as compared to nondiabetic patients. There was no significant difference in 3-year mortality between diabetic and nondiabetic patients in isolated disease of LAD.

Off-Pump Bypass and Conversion to On-Pump

The data from STS National database over a period of three and half years[36] indicates that there was a 5.2% risk of conversion to on-pump bypass grafting in patients who were undergoing reoperative procedure or were in cardiogenic shock.[59] *This conversion rate is high as the risk is associated with higher morbidity and mortality.*[60,61] *The outcome of emergency conversion to on-pump while pursuing off-pump procedure remains worse in comparison to nonconverted patients and had higher mortality, frequent sternal infections, hemorrhage during reoperations, respiratory failure, and sepsis.*[61]

In a meta-analysis of organ damage, following conversion to on-pump, Mukherjee et al. state that "emergency conversion is a result of cardiorespiratory instability or cardiac arrest which can occur during off-pump bypass grafting. *The systematic review of literature suggests that between 1.1% and 15.6% of patients in whom off-pump is attempted will subsequently require conversion to cardiopulmonary bypass.*"[62] They also stated that it was essential to establish prevention and treatment protocols for off-pump bypass grafting, as there is always a risk of conversion to pump and a detailed discussion done while taking informed consent.[62] Conversion to pump was associated with a rise in mortality, and complications include stroke, myocardial injury, bleeding, renal failure, wound infection, IABP requirement, transfusion, and respiratory and gastrointestinal complications.[62]

Patel et al. have mentioned that conversion to on-pump as an emergency is unpredictable.[63] End points for emergency conversion were hemodynamic compromise, hemorrhage, ischemic episodes, and cardiac arrest. Reasons quoted for conversion were hypotension 76%, bradycardia 2%, hemorrhage 8%, ventricular fibrillation 8%, aortic dissection 2%, and graft occlusion 4%. The average time taken to establish CPB was 7.6 minutes in patients requiring internal cardiac massage following cardiac arrest (median 3–16 minutes). In converted group versus nonconverted group in hospital mortality was 12% versus 1.47%, stroke

6% versus 1.1%, renal failure 6% versus 1.23%, deep sternal wound infection 8% versus 1.54%, and respiratory failure 24% versus 3.75%, an eightfold increase in mortality. [63] Edgerton et al. found that there was significantly no difference between mortality rate of electively converted group (n 1/24) and the ONCABG group 6.1% versus 2.7%; but patients who had urgent-emergent conversions had a 12-fold increase in mortality than the ONCABG group.[64]

So much importance has been given to on-pump conversion that since 2002, conversion to on-pump bypass grafting is being noted under a separate heading by STS National Database. Prior to 2000, this category was analyzed under on-pump bypass grafting group.

Off-Pump Bypass Grafting in Acute Coronary Syndrome

In a large-scale study with acute coronary syndromes, off-pump bypass was associated with lower rates of bleeding and non-Q wave myocardial infarctions and required early reinterventions, but at 1 year there were no major differences in two groups: off-pump and on-pump.[65]

Rastan et al. have reported lower mortality with significant benefit in terms of less drainage loss, less transfusion requirement, less inotropic support, shorter ventilation time, lower stroke rate, and shorter ICU stay, while avoiding cardioplegic arrest in patients with acute coronary syndromes undergoing off-pump bypass with cardioplegic arrest versus beating heart bypass grafting (including both ONCABG and beating heart on CPB).[66] The role of cell saver in off-pump was found to be useless in most cases. Careful surgical hemostasis is essential to limit hypovolemia.[67]

Off-Pump Bypass in Patients with Renal Disease

It is known that cardiovascular disease is an important cause of death in patients with end-stage renal disease. In a follow-up study for 39 months on the effect of performing CABG on-pump and off-pump in patients with end stage renal disease, it was shown that although off-pump shows reduced mortality when compared with conventional on cardiopulmonary bypass CABG, the long term survival was better when revascularization was done on bypass as compared to the off-pump group. This was related to complete revascularization that was possible in patients offered CABG on CPB. These patients also received more number of grafts 3.3 ± 0.9 versus 2.4 ± 1.0 in patients with off-pump group.[68]

OPCABG was found to be a favored procedure with surgeons when the graft numbered 1–3 and ONCABG when numbering 4–7 and was associated with reduced adjusted risk outcomes with OPCABG then with ONCABG.[69] As 5-year survival has been found to be markedly improved despite significant increase in perioperative blood loss and increased blood transfusion rates with OPCABG, discontinuation of clopidogrel cannot be recommended.[70]

On- or Off-Pump Bypass Surgery and Heart Failure

Atrial natriuretic peptide (ANP) and brain natriuretic peptide (BNP) hormones are secreted from the heart in heart failure. Both ANP and BNP were noted to have a similar rise in early postoperative period in both off-pump and on-pump bypass patients representing ischemia, though the rise of cardiac enzymes were significantly lesser in off-pump bypass patients. Careful monitoring and management is warranted in off-pump patients also in the immediate postoperative.[71]

Long-term Off-Pump Surgery Performed Between 1969 and 1985

In a follow-up study of 264 out of 733 cases that underwent off-pump bypass from years 1969 to 1985 after an initial mortality of 4.5% up to 1972, fell after 1972 to 1.3%. Use of Internal thoracic artery as a conduit was first reported in the year 1973 and ever since has been used increasingly. A follow-up of over 34 years showed open saphenous venous graft in 64.3% (18/24) patients and functioning LITA in 92.2% (59/64) patients. Possible reasons for performing off-pump bypass were avoiding the inflammatory response syndrome associated with on-pump bypass grafting but it was economical too.[72] Further follow-up of these patients shows that mean survival of patients receiving LITA graft was 23.7 years versus 17 years for patients receiving saphenous grafts. Forty of seventy-four patients still alive in 2003 did not require any invasive treatment.[73]

Status of Off-Pump and On-Pump Bypass Grafting from STS National Database and SCTS Database

The experience gained from the publication of the results of long term follow-up of series of cases done on beating heart in gone by era, has led to the resurgence of off-pump bypass surgery. Simultaneous innovative developments that took place in the medical industry led to the development of devices that made it possible to perform coronary artery bypass grafting on beating heart off-pump but required highly trained skillful surgeons and motivated team. Now it has become one of the standard surgical techniques to perform coronary artery bypass surgery. Despite almost two decades since it began, it is interesting to note that in 2007 20.4% of all primary CABG cases in the STS National Database were performed with off-pump techniques and by

2011 STS National Database of CABG in the United States and Society for Cardiothoracic Surgery (SCTS) in Great Britain and Ireland has recorded a marginal increase up to 20–25% of total bypass procedures.[74] This indicates that larger volumes up to 80% bypass surgeries are still being performed on-pump. Sure enough if such large volumes are being done on-pump, there must be strong scientifically proven reasons. "The European Association for Cardio-Thoracic Surgical (EACTS) Database Report 2010 provides data of isolated CABG from contributing countries (with no contribution from India). The proportion of off-pump bypass from contributor countries varied from 0.8% to over 91.4% overall 21%, mortality of 1.4% versus 2.9% when performed on-pump. Cause of decline in mortality has been reported to be uncertain. The mortality for octogenarians is nearly 7-times higher than patients under 56 years age. The median grafts used were 3. Mortality with only saphenous venous grafts has been noted to be 6.3%, single arterial graft 2.1%, with more than one arterial grafts it was the least at 1.3%."[75]

DISCUSSION

The major complications that were reported of on-pump surgery were as a result of stimulation of inflammatory cascade leading to coagulopathy, respiratory failure, myocardial dysfunction, renal failure, and neurocognitive dysfunction.[3,4] It is also known that systemic inflammatory response syndrome is a feature of tissue trauma and is a part of every surgical procedure.

To lay at rest the controversy about the suitability of the two procedures, studies clearly indicate that off-pump surgery is highly recommended in high-risk cases and elderly patients ≥80 years or patients with evidence of extra vasculopathy—peripheral vascular disease.[16,17] In these patients, aortic manipulation that is a feature of on-pump bypass is associated with high incidence of cerebral strokes and serious neurocognitive dysfunctions. It has been found by Calafiore and others that there is significant reduction in the incidence of strokes and cerebrovascular accidents in the immediate postoperative period, a major devastating complication, if aortic manipulation is avoided. Application of side biting aortic clamp to do proximal anastomosis on ascending aorta would even out the advantage of off-pump versus on-pump surgery.[9,10]

Use of total arterial revascularization that offers "clampless" coronary artery bypass surgery or minimizing aortic manipulation with devices like Encore and Heartstring to complete proximal anastomosis on ascending aorta reduces the risk of strokes.[11,12,15] Unfortunately, these techniques are not routinely practiced in most centers unless the ascending aorta is severely calcified. Kinoshita et al. have shown that at mid-term there was significant reduction in overall death, cardiac death, and cardiac events.[14] Puskas et al. have suggested that off-pump surgery could also be done in shorter time enabling larger number of bypass procedures except its training that requires a greater learning curve and is especially indicated in high-risk patients.[19] There is no study which reports that the off-pump surgery results are significantly superior to on-pump surgery in low-risk cases.

In fact, incomplete revascularization is frequently noted in off-pump bypass surgery.[46] Lower incidence of in-hospital mortality, cardiac mortality, and MACCE was observed in patients who had complete revascularization.[47] Few studies have shown, especially in patients with end-stage renal disease, that it is the completeness of revascularization which is possible only in on-pump procedure that is important. The long-term results were better in these patients when the procedure was done on-pump than off-pump.[68] Hu S et al. have reported early benefits of off-pump bypass grafting are lost with reoperative procedures within a few years with increased financial burden.[42]

The major advancement of on-pump coronary artery bypass surgery was that the surgeon could rotate the cold, arrested heart in all direction with comfort. It became possible to do quality grafting in a bloodless field with clearly seen margins of the vessels with corneal loops. Multivessel grafting had become possible with on-pump surgery. It was clearly advancement over restricted number of grafting that was performed in 60s when case selection was an important issue. The advances in coronary artery bypass surgery were results of improved perfusion technology, myocardial protection, and above all technological advances and refinements in monitoring systems. While the knowledge gained during this period was used with further refinements, introduction of new technologies resulted in the resurgence of off-pump bypass surgery.

Studies have concluded that there is significant reduction in operating time, blood loss, postoperative ventilation period, and the stay in the ICU and hospital is more economical.[49-52] On-pump conversion to off-pump bypass surgery is one of the major complications of the procedure. It is associated with higher mortality, frequent sternal infections, and hemorrhage during reoperations, respiratory failure and sepsis, IABP, and gastrointestinal complications.[61,62] A recent systematic review of literature has suggested that between 1.1% and 15.6% of patients in whom off-pump revascularization is attempted will require conversion to on-pump.[62] At this crucial juncture, it is availability of heart lung machine and the perfusionist that can help complete the procedure albeit with an increased morbidity and mortality, which is 8 times compared to nonconverted group and 12 times when compared to elective revascularization on CPB.[63,64] When there is a possibility of conversion to on-pump, the team banks completely on the system for salvaging the life. Mukherjee et al. have advised that this complication is acute that needs to be addressed while taking informed consent and it is important to lay down prevention and treatment protocols for conversion.[62] Since 2002, conversion of on-pump has been separately grouped in STS National Database registry of surgical records.

There is an increased need to treat heart failure in the immediate postoperative period to patients who have undergone on-pump and off-pump revascularization as there is evidence of rise in brain natriuretic peptide secretions, which indicates intraoperative ventricular distension.[71] According to Livesay et al. "Newer technique should not take away conventional wisdom in selecting operating techniques which ensure appropriate myocardial revascularization."[76]

CONCLUSION

In the end, local practices and quality control should decide the best procedure that should be performed. Off-pump bypass is an evolving procedure and practices need to be evolved to prevent crisis of emergency conversion of on-pump that is associated with high mortality. The need and importance of heart lung machine cannot be over emphasized. On-pump and off-pump surgeries are mutually complimentary and supportive of each other. Performing off-pump bypass grafting in the absence of or a malfunctioning "Heart Lung Machine" and a trained Perfusion technologist should be categorized as medical negligence as it imposes a risk of adverse cardiac events causing increased morbidity and mortality with increased cost and hospital stay. When indicated, a trained perfusion team along with experienced cardiac anesthesiologists can greatly mitigate the complications of emergency conversion to on-pump procedure. There is also a need to develop a National Database of Coronary Artery Bypass Grafting in the Indian perspective, for off-pump and on-pump bypass grafting, which will lay a standard of care and create national averages of the results. This will be a considerate step towards creating a benchmark in healthcare while performing CABG on prospective patients.

REFERENCES

1. Buxton BF, Galvin SD. The history of arterial revascularization: from Koselov to Tector and beyond. Ann Cardiothorac Surg. 2013;2(4):419-26.
2. Srivastava SP, Patel KN, Skantharaja, et al. Off-pump complete revascularization through a left lateral thoracotomy (ThoraCAB): the first 200 cases. Ann Thorac Surg. 2003;76(1):46-9.
3. Jerrold HL, Tanaka KA. Inflammatory response to cardiopulmonary bypass. Ann Thorac Surg. 2003;75(2):S715-S720.
4. Taylor KM. Central nervous system effects of cardiopulmonary bypass. Ann Thorac Surg. 1998;66(5) supplement 1:S20-S24.
5. Trehan N, Mishra M, Dhole S, et al. Significantly reduced incidence of stroke during coronary artery bypass grafting using transesophageal echocardiography. Eur J Cardiothorac Surg. 1997;11(2):234-42.
6. Rosenberger P, Shernan SK, Loeffler M, et al. The influence of epiaortic ultrasonography on intraoperative surgical management in 60511 cardiac surgical patients. Ann Thorac Surg. 2008;85(2):548-53.
7. Mishra M, Chauhan R, Sharma KK, et al. Real-time intraoperative transesophageal echocardiography-how useful? Experience of 5,016 cases. J Cardiothorac Vasc Anesth. 1998;12(6):625-32.
8. Sharony R, Grossi EA, Saunders P, et al. Propensity matches analysis of off-pump coronary artery bypass grafting in patients with atheromatous aortic disease. J Thorac Cardiovasc Surg. 2004;127(2):406-13.
9. Calafiore AM, Mauro Michele Di, Giovanni T, et al. Impact of aortic manipulation on incidence of cerebrovascular accidents after surgical myocardial revascularization. Ann Thorac Surg. 2002;73(5):1387-93.
10. Edelman JJ, Yan TD, Vallely MP. Anaortic off-pump coronary artery bypass grafting. The criterion standard for minimization of neurologic injury. J Thorac Cardiovasc Surg. 2012;143(1):251-2.
11. Wolf LF, Abu-Omar Y, Choudhary BP, et al. Gaseous and solid microembolization during proximal aortic anastomosis in off-pump coronary surgery: the effect of an aortic side-biting clamp and two clampless devices. J Thorac Cardiovasc Surg. 2007;133(2):485-93.
12. Emmert MY, Seifert B, Wilhelm M, et al. Aortic no touch technique makes the difference in off-pump coronary artery bypass grafting. J Thorac Cardiovasc Surg. 2011;142(6):1499-1506.
13. Raja SG. Myocardial revascularization for the elderly: current options, role of off-pump coronary artery bypass grafting and outcomes. Curr Cardiol Rev. 2012;8(1):26-36.
14. Kinoshita T, Asai T, Nishimura O, et al. Off-pump bilateral versus single skeletonized internal thoracic artery grafting in patients with diabetes. Ann Thorac Surg. 2010;90(4):1173-9.
15. Kim WS, Lee J, Lee YT, et al. Total arterial revascularization in triple vessel disease with off-pump and aortic no-touch technique. Ann Thorac Surg. 2008;86(6):1861-5.
16. Cavallaro P, Itagaki S, Seigerman M, Chikwe J. Operative mortality and stroke after on-pump vs off-pump surgery in high-risk patients: an analysis of 83,914 coronary bypass operations. European Journal of Cardiothorac Surgery. 2014;45:159-64.
17. Masuda M, Morita S, Tomita H, et al. Off-pump CABG attenuates myocardial enzyme leakage but not postoperative brain natriuretic peptide secretion. Ann Thorac Surg. 2002;8(3):139-44.
18. Hammon JW, Stump DA, Butterworth JF, et al. Single aortic clamp improves 6-month cognitive outcome in high-risk coronary bypass patients: the effect of reduced aortic manipulation. J Cardiothorac Vasc Surg. 2006;131(1):114-21.
19. Kerendi F, Morris Cullen D, Puskas JD. Off-pump coronary bypass for high-risk patients: only in expert centers? Curr Opin Cardiol. 2008;23:573-8.
20. Sepic J, Wee JO, Soletsz EG, et al. Cardiac positioning using an apical suction device maintains beating heart hemodynamics. Heart Surg Forum. 2002;5:279-84.
21. Mishra M, Malhotra R, Mishra A, et al. Hemodynamic changes during displacement of the beating heart using epicardial stabilization for off-pump coronary artery bypass graft surgery. J Cardiothorac Vasc Anesth. 2002;16:685-90.
22. Mueller XM, Chassot PG, Zhou J, et al. Hemodynamics optimization during off-pump coronary artery bypass: the "no compression" technique. Eur J Cardiothorac Surg. 2002;22(2):249-54.
23. Gandra SM, Rivetti LA. Experimental evidence of regional myocardial ischemia during beating heart coronary bypass: prevention with temporary intraluminal shunts. Heart Surg Forum. 2002;6:10-18.

24. Grundeman PF, Borst C, van Herwaarden JA, et al. Vertical displacement of the beating heart by the octopus tissue stabilizer: influence on coronary flow. Ann Thorac Surg. 1998;65(5):1348-52.
25. Vassiliades TA, Nielsen JA, Longquist JL. Hemodynamic collapse during off-pump coronary artery bypass grafting. Ann Thorac Surg. 2002;73(6):1874-9.
26. Rivetti LA, Gandra SM. An intraluminal shunt for off-pump coronary artery bypass grafting: report of 501 consecutive cases and review of the technique. Heart Surg Forum. 1998;1:330-36.
27. Rivetti LA, Gandra SM. Initial experience using an intraluminal shunt during revascularization of the beating heart. Ann Thorac Surg. 1997;63:1742-7.
28. Luccheti V, Capasso F, Caputo M, et al. Intracoronary shunt prevent left ventricular function impairment during beating heart revascularization. Eur J Cardiothorac Surg. 1999;15:255-9.
29. Izutani H, Gill IS. Acute graft failure caused by an intracoronary shunt in minimally invasive direct coronary artery bypass grafting. J Thorac Cardiovasc Surg. 2003;125:723-4.
30. Arai H, Yoshida T, Izumi H, et al. External shunt for off-pump coronary artery bypass grafting: distal coronary artery perfusion catheter. Ann Thorac Surg. 2000;70(2):681-2.
31. Soltoski P, Salerno T, Levinsky L, et al. Conversion to cardiopulmonary bypass in off-pump coronary artery bypass grafting: its effect on outcome. J Card Surg. 1998;13:328-34.
32. Giuseppe F, Latrofa ME, Pasquale T, et al. Hemodynamics in off-pump surgery: normal versus compromised preoperative left ventricular function. Eur J Cardiothorac Vasc Surg. 2005;27(3):488-93.
33. Hart JC. Maintaining hemodynamic stability and myocardial performance during off-pump coronary artery bypass surgery. Ann Thorac Surg. 2003;75(2):S740-S744.
34. Kurlansky PA. Is there a hypercoagulable state after off-pump coronary artery bypass surgery? What do we know and what can we do? J Thorac Cardiovasc Surg. 2003;126(1):7-10.
35. Mariani AM, Gu J, Boonstra PW, et al. Procoagulant activity after off-pump coronary operation: is the current anticoagulation adequate? Ann Thorac Surg. 1999;67(5):1370-75.
36. Keeling BW, Mathew WL, Slaughter MS, et al. Off-pump and on-pump coronary revascularization in patients with low ejection fraction: a report from the Society of Thoracic Surgeons National Database. Ann Thorac Surg. 2013;96(1):83-9.
37. Puskas John D, Williams WH, et al. Off-pump coronary artery bypass grafting provides complete revascularization with reduced myocardial injury, transfusion requirements, and length of stay: a prospective randomized comparison of two hundred unselected patients undergoing off-pump versus conventional coronary artery bypass grafting. J Thorac Cardiovasc Surg. 2003;125(4):797-808.
38. Zheng-Zhe Feng, Jian Shi, Xue-Wei Zhao, et al. Meta-analysis of on-pump and off-pump coronary arterial revascularization. Ann Thorac Surg. 2009;87(3):757-67.
39. Murzi M, Caputo M, Aresu G, et al. On-pump and off-pump coronary artery bypass grafting in patients with left main stem disease; a propensity score analysis. J Thorac Cardiovasc Surg. 2012;143(6):1382-8.
40. Lemma MG, Coscioni E, Tritto FP, et al. On-pump versus off-pump coronary artery bypass in high risk patients: operative results of prospective randomized trial (on-off study). J Thorac Cardiovasc Surg. 2012;143(3): 625-31.
41. Riha M, Danzmayr M, Nagele G, et al. Off-pump coronary artery bypass grafting in EuroSCORE high and low risk patients. Eur J Cardiothorac Surg. 2002;21(2):193-8.
42. Hu S, Zheng Z, Yuan X, et al. Increasing long term major vascular events and resource consumption in patients receiving off-pump coronary artery bypass: a single center prospective observational study. Circulation. 2010;121(16):1800-8.
43. Alfirevic A, Meng X, Douglas J, et al. Transfusion increases the risk of vasoplegia after cardiac operations. Ann Thorac Surg. 2011;92(3):812-9.
44. Mack MJ, Pfister A, Bachand D, et al. Comparison of coronary artery bypass surgery with and without cardiopulmonary bypass in patients with multivessel disease. J Thorac Cardiovasc Surg. 2004;127(1):167-73.
45. Synnergren MJ, Ekroth R, Oden A, et al. Incomplete revascularization reduces survival benefit of coronary artery bypass grafting: role of off-pump surgery. J Thorac Cardiovasc Surg. 2008;136(1):29-36.
46. Jarral OA, Srdjan Saso, Athanasiou T. Off-pump coronary artery bypass in patients with left ventricular dysfunction: a meta-analysis. Ann Thorac Surg. 2011;92(5):1686-94.
47. Yi G, Youn Y-M, Joo H-C, Hong S, Yoo K-J. Association of incomplete revascularization with long-term survival after off-pump coronary artery bypass grafting. J Surg Res. 2013;185(1): 166-73.
48. Robertson MW, Buth KJ, Stewart KM, et al. Complete revascularization is compromised in off-pump coronary artery bypass grafting. J Thorac Cardiovasc Surg. 2013;145(4):992-8.
49. Muneretto C, Bisleri G, Negri A, et al. Off-pump coronary artery bypass surgery technique for total arterial myocardial revascularization: a prospective randomized study. Ann Thorac Surg. 2003;76(3):778-83.
50. Pandey R, Grayson AD, Pullan DM, et al. Total arterial revascularization: effect of avoiding cardiopulmonary bypass on in-hospital mortality and morbidity in a propensity-matched cohort. Eur J Cardiothorac Surg. 2005;27(1):94-8.
51. Mishra YK, Mishra M, Malhotra R, et al. Evolution of off-pump coronary artery bypass grafting over 15 years: a single-institution experience of 14,030 cases. Innovations (Phila). 2005;1(2):88-91.
52. Mishra YK, Collison SP, Malhotra R, et al. Ten-year experience with single-vessel and multivessel reoperative off-pump coronary artery bypass grafting. J Thorac Cardiovasc Surg. 2008;135(3):527-32.
53. Trehan N, Mishra YK, Malhotra R, et al. Off-pump redo-coronary artery bypass grafting. Ann Thorac Surg. 2000;70(3):1026-9.
54. Mishra Y, Mehta Y, Mittal S, et al. Mammary coronary artery stenosis without coronary artery bypass through minithoracotomy: one year clinical experience. Eur J Cardiothorac Surg. 1998;14(Supplement 1):S31-S37.
55. Al-Ruzzeh S, Athanasiou T, George S, et al. Is the use of cardiopulmonary bypass surgery an independent predictor of operative mortality in patients with left ventricular dysfunction? Ann Thorac Surg. 2003;76(2):441-51discussion 451-2.
56. Shi M, Huang J, Pang L, et al. Preoperative insertion of intra-aortic balloon pump improved the prognosis of high-risk patients undergoing off-pump coronary artery bypass grafting. J Int Med Res. 2011;39(4):1163-8.
57. Renner A, Zittermann A, Aboud A, et al. Coronary revascularization in Diabetic patients. Ann Thorac Surg. 2013;96(2):528-34.
58. Lichtenberg A, Klima U, Max-Pichlmaier HP, et al. Impact of diabetics on outcome following isolated minimally invasive bypass grafting of the left anterior descending artery. Ann Thorac Surg. 2004;78(1):129-34.
59. Hirose H, Amano A. Routine off-pump coronary artery bypass: reasons for on-pump conversion. Innovations (Phila). 2005 Fall; 1(1):28-31.

60. Calafiore AM Mauro MD, Canosa C, et al. Myocardial revascularization with and without cardiopulmonary bypass: advantages, disadvantages and similarities. Eur J Cardiothorac Surg. 2003;24(6):953-60.
61. Hemli JM, Patel NC, Subramanian VA. Increasing surgical experience with off-pump coronary surgery does not mitigate the morbidity of emergency conversion to cardiopulmonary bypass. Innovations (Phila). 2012;7(4):259-65.
62. Mukherjee D, Rao C, Ibrahim M, et al. Meta-analysis of organ damage after conversion from off-pump coronary artery bypass procedures. Ann Thorac Surg. 2011;92(2):755-61.
63. Patel NC, Patel NU, Loulmet DF, et al. Emergency conversion to cardiopulmonary bypass during attempted off-pump revascularization results in increased morbidity and mortality. J Thorac Cardiovasc Surg. 2004;128(5):655-61
64. Edgerton JR, Dewey TM, Magee MJ, et al. Conversion in Off-Pump coronary artery bypass grafting: an analysis of predictors and outcomes. Ann Thorac Surg. 2003;76(4):1138-43.
65. Ben-Gal Y, Stone GW, Smith CR, et al. On-pump versus off-pump surgical revascularization in patients with acute coronary syndromes: analysis from the acute catheterization and urgent intervention Triage Strategy Trial. J Thorac Cardiovasc Surg. 2011;142(2):e33-39.
66. Rastan AJ, Eckenstein JI, Hentschel B, et al. Emergency coronary artery bypass *graft* sur*gery for acute* coronary syndrome: beating heart versus conventional cardiac arrest strategies. Circulation. 2006;114(1 Suppl):I477-85.
67. Tan NL, Corbineau H, Phu BD, et al. Is cell saver necessary in coronary artery bypass surgery? Asian Cardiovasc Thoracic Ann. 2012;20(5):539-43.
68. Dewey TM, Herbert MA, Prince SL, et al. Does coronary artery bypass graft surgery improve survival among patients with end stage renal disease? Ann Thorac Surg. 2006;81(2):591-8.
69. Lattouf OM, Puskas JD, Thourani VH, et al. Does the number of grafts influence surgeon choice and patient benefit of off-pump over conventional on-pump coronary artery revascularization in multivessel coronary artery disease? Ann Thorac Surg. 2007;84(5):1485-94.
70. Bittner HB, Lehman S, Rastan A, et al. Impact of clopidogrel on bleeding complications and survival in off pump coronary artery bypass grafting. Interact Cardiovasc Thorac Surg. 2012;14(3): 273-7.
71. Masuda M, Morita S, Tomita H, et al. Off-pump CABG attenuates myocardial enzyme leakage but not postoperative brain natriuretic peptide secretion. Ann Thorac Surg. 2002;8(3): 139-44.
72. Ankeny JL. Off-pump bypass surgery: the early experience. Texas Heart Inst J. 2004;31(3):210-13.
73. Ankeney JL, Goldstein DJ. Off-pump bypass of the left anterior descending coronary artery: 23- to 34-year follow-up. J Thorac Cardiovasc Surg. 2007;133(6):1499-1503.
74. Societies of Thoracic Surgeons National Adult Cardiac Database: Spring Report 2008. Duke Clinical Research Institute, Durham, NC (June 2008).
75. Bridgewater B, Gummert J. Isolated CABG. Fourth EACTS Adult Cardiac Surgical Database Report: Towards global benchmarking. Peter KH Walton and Robin Kinsman, Dendrite Clinical Systems Ltd.
76. Livesay JA. The benefits of off-pump coronary bypass. A reality or an illusion? Texas Heart Inst J. 2003;30(4):258-60.

25

Coronary Artery Bypass Graft in Awake: A Reality Check

KK Sharma, Devesh Dutta

INTRODUCTION

Coronary artery bypass graft (CABG) operation in awake patient without endotracheal anesthesia was first performed in October 1998 with high thoracic epidural anesthesia (TEA) block by Dr Haldun Karagoz of Guven Hospital in Ankara, Turkey.[1] Since then, similar cases have been reported in the literature in an attempt to decrease the invasiveness of the CABG procedure.[2,3]

General anesthesia (GA) remains the preferred anesthetic technique for CABG. Efforts to reduce anesthetic or surgical mortality and morbidity during open heart surgery have continually evolved and new strategies in cardiac anesthesia now enable immediate extubation (ultra-fast-track anesthesia). The perioperative use of high TEA as an adjunct to GA has been shown to be beneficial in patients with coronary artery disease. As patients referred for CABG increasingly show severe comorbidities, this has led to developments in cardiac surgery focusing on minimizing the invasiveness of the procedure by revascularization on beating heart without cardiopulmonary bypass and by reducing surgical trauma using smaller surgical incisions. Progress in minimally invasive cardiac surgery has led to the invention of minimally invasive technique like high TEA as the sole technique in a conscious patient known as awake coronary artery bypass (ACAB) grafting. Despite the various documented benefits of TEA, anesthesiologists are reluctant to use it in cardiac surgical patients because of fear of development of symptomatic epidural hematoma.[4,5]

It appeared that patients who had undergone surgery under regional anesthetic techniques like endoscopic transurethral prostrate surgery were quite willing to undergo cardiac surgery under TEA. In addition, the fear of "not waking up" after surgery is a main concern and the possibility of staying awake during surgery seemed very attractive. Careful psychological assessment of the patient's suitability and acceptance for "awake" cardiac surgery is important as it is for other types of surgeries and not everyone may be suited for this technique. ACAB is specially good for patients with severe lung and liver disease, past history of stroke/unconsciousness and in patients who are at high risk of GA. There were no definite criteria other than the prerequisites outlined previously and the anesthesiologist can decide about the suitability of the patient for the regional technique apart from consideration of left ventricular function.

ADVANTAGES OF AWAKE CORONARY ARTERY BYPASS[6]

- *Avoidance of endotracheal intubation*—Hemodynamic responses to tracheal intubation, suction of the endotracheal tube, and extubation may lead to myocardial ischemia and pose a potential risk in patients with coronary artery disease.[7,8] Endotracheal intubation has been shown to cause mucosal injury, reduced mucociliary function, bypassing of upper airway defenses, and reduced effectiveness of cough later. In addition to these adverse effects of GA, endotracheal intubation has been shown to play an important role in causing pulmonary infection in intubated and mechanically ventilated patients.[9] All these complications and side effects can be negated by avoiding intubation. Overcoming any factors contributing to increased incidence of nosocomial pulmonary infection may benefit patients particularly in those with cardiac implants. These complications could partially be avoided by using supraglottic devices like a laryngeal mask airway with some limitations.
- *Cerebral function monitoring*—A conscious patient can surrogate as a cerebral function monitor while undergoing ACAB. Despite advances made in neurological monitoring no final word can be said about the safety and efficacy of conventionally used cerebral function monitors. One of the benefits of performing ACAB is the ability to monitor the cerebral, motor, and sensory functions, with the patient himself offering necessary

details. Chakravarthy et al.[10] have reported that patient may get irritated during phases of hypotension that could be reversed by restoration of arterial pressure. The same authors[11] have reported a case of carotid endarterectomy, when the patient became unresponsive during clamping of "culprit" internal carotid artery, which was reversed by declamping. So, ACAB provides ready access to assessment of cerebral function in most of the patients.

- *Advantage of sympathetic block*—Documented benefits of TEA are hemodynamic stability,[12] superior intra- and postoperative analgesia, reduced oxygen demand, optimization of coronary blood flow,[13] improved pulmonary function,[14,15] early extubation,[11] attenuation of stress response, and decreased neurocognitive dysfunction.[16]

It is not known whether these potential advantages translate to clinical benefits or not; large-scale multicentric studies are needed to arrive at conclusive evidence.

DISADVANTAGES OF AWAKE CORONARY ARTERY BYPASS[7]

- *Patient admission a day prior to surgery*—Admitting the patient a day before the surgery for the sake of performing epidural catheterization thus increasing the average length of stay is a limitation. However, this is not a concern in institutes where patients for cardiac surgery are routinely admitted to the hospital a day prior to surgery. In centers where patients are admitted only on the day of surgery, epidural catheters can be inserted 4–5 hours before the time of probable heparinization, and the technique of avoiding GA may be practiced. Admission of patient a day prior to surgery is not required in order to perform epidural catheterization. There is evidence to show that it can be safely undertaken at least 1 hour prior to heparinization.[17]
- *Temporary neurologic deficits (TND)*—Although various authors have described TND during regional blocks,[18,19] the incidence of TND associated with TEA appears to be very low. Chakravarthy et al.[20] have reported incidence of 1.2% of TND in their series of 3057 cases of TEA in cardiac surgical patients over a period of 15 years. There are many other studies showing occurrence of TND after neuraxial anesthesia with an average incidence of 0% to 0.08%.[21,22]
- *Permanent neurologic injury*—With occasional reports of symptomatic epidural hematomas in cardiac surgical patients,[5,6] various mathematically calculated incidences became redundant.[23] The risk of catheter-related epidural hematoma in cardiac surgery is comparable to the risk of epidural hematoma after the use of epidural catheters for general surgery.[24,25] Based on analysis by Hemmerling et al.[26] the risk of catheter-related epidural hematoma is 1 in 5493 with a 95% confidence interval (CI) of 1/970-1/31114 in expert hands.
- *Epidural space infection*—Though epidural space infection is a potential complication of TEA, in cardiac surgery there appears to be no reports of it in the literature.
- *Unprotected airway*—Cardiac surgeons and anesthesiologist commonly refrain from practicing ACAB for the fear of performing surgery in a patient with unprotected airway. Intubation during emergency may be delayed because of presence of drapes. Since the cranial nerves are not blocked by TEA, upper airway reflexes and cough reflex are intact. However, in the light of many studies the fear of carrying out surgery in spontaneously breathing patient is more theoretical.[27,28]
- *Transesophageal echocardiography (TEE) monitoring is not possible*—TEE probe cannot be inserted in spontaneously breathing patient. Inability to perform TEE during cardiac surgery is a real limitation of ACAB. This can be overcome by performing epicardial echocardiography when valve function and wall motion abnormalities have to be assessed intraoperatively.
- *Excessive movement of heart and great vessels*—Spontaneously breathing patient may cause discomfort to the surgeons by excessive movement of heart and great vessels. This can be minimized to a great extent by routine use of noninvasive pressure support ventilation through the face mask.
- *Phrenic nerve palsy*—Although diaphragmatic paralysis due to spillover block of phrenic nerve is a rare complication of TEA, it can be treated without adverse outcomes. Administering the local anesthetic agent as an infusion seems effective to prevent this problem.
- *Influence of ACAB on neurocognitive functions*—Psychological aspects of ACAB are not fully studied. Yet a study by Chakravarthy et al. showed no increase in the incidence of neurocognitive dysfunction in ACAB patients compared to the patients who underwent conventional off-pump coronary artery bypass (OPCAB) under GA. Reduction in stress-related neurocognitive dysfunction during CABG has been demonstrated with concomitant use of TEA.[29]
- *Abdominal distention*—Gastric distension may result due to continuous positive airway pressure ventilation in patients who are deeply sedated. It is common to see this complication in obese individuals undergoing continuous positive airway pressure therapy.
- *Patient discomfort*—Patient may not be able to lie still for such long a period and cough reflex cannot be suppressed.

CURRENT STATUS

The issue of avoiding GA with endotracheal intubation is said to offer more risks with little advantage while exposing the patient to risks that he would not otherwise be incurring (epidural hematoma, pneumothorax in a spontaneously breathing patient, etc.) and therefore the issue of coronary artery surgery without endotracheal GA remains controversial.

The proponents of TEA suggest that epidural use should be encouraged. It is premature to comment whether ACAB will survive the test of time, but it is prudent to perceive ACAB as a new technique that requires standardization.

Awake cardiac surgery is not yet accepted clearly. To determine the safety of this technique in comparison with OPCAB under GA, many more patients and multicentric studies are needed. In addition, future studies should focus on the impact of awake cardiac surgery on cognitive assessment and recovery and its relation to neurohormonal responses during surgery.[30] Owing to unresolved problems with on-pump awake cardiac surgery, especially temperature management and apnea at the beginning of extracorporeal circulation, OPCAB seems to be the main domain for this technique. However, it should be in the armamentarium of cardiac anesthesiologist even if for the sake of saying that "I can do it when required."

REFERENCES

1. Karagoz H, Sonmez B, Bakkaloglu B, et al. Coronary artery bypass grafting in the conscious patient without endotracheal general anesthesia. Am Thorac Surg. 2000;70:91-6.
2. Stritesky M, Semrad M, Kunstyr J, et al. On-pump cardiac surgery in a conscious patient using a thoracic epidural anesthesia—an ultra fast track method. Bratisl Lek Listy. 2004;105:51-5.
3. Karagoz HY, Kurtoglu M, Bakkaloglu B, et al. Coronary artery bypass grafting in the awake patient: three years' experience in 137 patients. J Thorac Cardiovasc Surg. 2003;125:1204-7.
4. Chakravarthy M, Jawali V, Manohar M, et al. Conscious off-pump coronary artery bypass surgery. Indian Heart J. 2005;57:49-53.
5. Sharma S, Kapoor MC, Sharma VK, et al. Epidural hematoma complicating high thoracic epidural catheter placement intended for cardiac surgery. J Cardiothorac Vasc Anesth. 2004;18:759-62.
6. Ho AM, Chung DC, Joynt GM. Neuraxial blockade and hematoma in cardiac surgery. Chest. 2000;117:551-5.
7. Jawali V. Awake cardiac surgery: where does it stand today? Medicine Update. 2010;20:283-6.
8. Paulissian R, Salem MR, Joseph NJ, et al. Hemodynamic responses to endotracheal extubation after coronary artery bypass grafting. Anesth Analg. 1991;73:10-5.
9. Mikawa K, Nishina K, Takao Y, et al. Attenuation of cardiovascular responses to endotracheal extubation: comparison of verapamil, lidocaine and verapamil and lidocaine combination. Anesth Analg. 1997;85:1005-10.
10. Bauer TT, Torres A, Ferrer R. Biofilm formation in endotracheal tubes. Association between pneumonia and the persistence of pathogens. Monaldi Arch Chest Dis. 2002;57:84-7.
11. Chakravarthy M, Jawali V, Manohar M, et al. Conscious off pump coronary artery bypass surgery—an audit of our first 151 cases. Ann Thorac Cardiovasc Surg. 2005;11:93-7.
12. Chakravarthy M, Jawali V, Manohar MV, et al. Combined carotid endarterectomy and off-pump coronary artery bypass surgery under thoracic epidural anesthesia without endotracheal GA. J Cardiothorac Vasc Anesth. 2006;20:850-2.
13. Liem TH, Hasenbos MA, Booij LH, et al. Coronary artery bypass grafting using two different anesthetic techniques: Part 2: Post-operative outcome. J Cardiothorac Vasc Anesth. 1992;6:156-61.
14. Blomberg S, Emanuelsson H, Kvist H, et al. Effects of thoracic epidural anesthesia on coronary arteries and arterioles in patients with coronary artery disease. Anesthesiology. 1990;73:840-7.
15. Stenseth R, Bjella L, Berg EM, et al. Effects of thoracic epidural analgesia on pulmonary function after coronary artery bypass surgery I: haemodynamic effects. Acta Anaesthesiol Scand. 1994;38:826-33.
16. Arom KV, Flavin TF, Emery RW, et al. Safety and efficacy of off-pump coronary artery bypass grafting. Ann Thorac Surg. 2000;69:704-10.
17. Royse C, Royse A, Soeding P, et al. Prospective randomized trial of high thoracic epidural analgesia for coronary artery bypass surgery. Ann Thorac Surg. 2003;75:93-100.
18. Pastor MC, Sanchez MJ, Casas MA, et al. Thoracic epidural analgesia in coronary artery bypass graft surgery: seven years' experience. J Cardiothorac Vasc Anesth. 2003;17:154-9.
19. Auroy Y, Narchi P, Messiah A, et al. Serious complications related to regional anesthesia. Anesthesiology. 1997;87:479-86.
20. Schneider M, Ettlin T, Kaufman M, et al. Transient neurologic toxicity after hyper baric sub arachnoid anesthesia with 5% lidocaine. Anesth Analg. 1993;76: 1154-7.
21. Chakravarthy M, Nadiminti S, Krishnamurthy J, et al. Temporary neurologic deficits in patients undergoing cardiac surgery with thoracic epidural supplementation. J Cardiothorac Vasc Anesth. 2004;18:512-20.
22. Chakravarthy M, Jawali V, Manohar M, et al. Conscious off pump coronary artery bypass surgery in a patient with end stage renal failure using thoracic epidural anaesthesia as the sole anaesthetic. Anaesth Clin Pharmacol. 2005;21:217-20.
23. Giebler RM, Scherer RU, Peters J. Incidence of neurologic complications related to thoracic epidural catheterization. Anesthesiology. 1997;86:55-63.
24. Horlocker TT, Wedel DJ, Benzon H, et al. Regional anesthesia in the anticoagulated patient: defining the risks (the second ASRA Consensus Conference on Neuraxial Anesthesia and Anticoagulation). Reg Anesth Pain Med. 2003;28:172-97.
25. Bateman BT, Mhyre JM, Ehrenfeld J, et al. The risk and outcomes of epidural hematomas after perioperative and obstetric epidural catheterization: a report from the multicenter perioperative outcomes group research consortium. Anesth Analg. 2013;116:1380-5.
26. Volk T, Wolf A, Van Aken H, et al. Incidence of spinal haematoma after epidural puncture: Analysis from the German network for safety in regional anaesthesia. Eur J Anaesthesiol. 2012;29:170-6.
27. Hemmerling TM, Cyr S, Terrasini N. Epidural catheterization in cardiac surgery: The 2012 risk assessment. Ann Card Anaesth. 2013;16:169-77.
28. Karagoz HY, Kurtoglu M, Bakkaloglu B. Coronary artery bypass grafting in the awake patient: three years' experience in 137 patients. J Thorac Cardiovasc Surg. 2003;125:1204-7.
29. Chakravarthy M, Thimmangowda P, Krishnamurthy J, et al. Thoracic epidural anesthesia in cardiac surgical patients: a prospective audit of 2,113 cases. J Cardiothorac Vasc Anesth. 2005;19:44-8.
30. Royse C, Royse A, Soeding P, et al. Prospective randomized trial of high thoracic epidural analgesia for coronary artery bypass surgery. Ann Thorac Surg. 2003;75:93-100.

26

Surgery on Aorta: Current Status and Desires of a Surgeon

Ajay Kaul

INTRODUCTION

Open surgical repair of aortic aneurysm has evolved significantly over the last decade. At some high volume centers, morbidity and mortality has come down significantly. The morbidity and mortality remains high in patients with extensive aneurysms, prior aortic surgery and in patients with comorbid conditions.

Hybrid repair is an appealing technique, not only for simple cases but also for complex lesions. Hybrid repair may be particularly advantageous in patients with previous thoracic surgery, where a redo left-sided thoracotomy may be associated with major bleeding. By avoiding thoracic aortic cross-clamping, hybrid repair is also useful in patients with poor cardiac function and valvular heart disease.

The occurrence of life-threatening complications specific to hybrid procedures, especially related to the visceral grafts such as bowel infarction, pancreatitis and renal artery thrombosis are a cause for concern.

Aortic surgery and interventions are continuously evolving. There is a need for surgeons to be updated, on both the state-of-the-art open and endovascular procedures.

HISTORY

The role of allograft replacement in the descending thoracic aneurysm was introduced by Lam and Aram in the year 1951.[1]

The introduction of cardiopulmonary bypass by Cooley and DeBakey in 1956, revolutionized the cardiovascular surgery and subsequently used for the ascending aortic replacement.[2] Aortic allograft was used for replacement of ascending aorta by them.[3]

Dacron was introduced by DeBakey. In 1968, Bentall and De Bono performed a procedure consisting of replacement of ascending aneurysm along with replacement of aortic valve and reimplantation of the coronary arteries, using mechanical valve with a Dacron conduit.[4]

Orthotopic aortic homograft implantation was done by Ross and Barratt-Boyes, in 1962 and 1964 respectively.[5-7]

Recently, minimally invasive techniques have been developed for the descending thoracic aortic aneurysm repair. In 1994, Dake et al. performed first endovascular repair of thoracic aortic aneurysm.[8] The thoracic aortic stent graft was given green signal by US Food and Drug Administration (FDA) in March 2005.[9]

DEFINITION

An aneurysm is a localized or diffuse dilatation of an artery with a diameter of at least 50% greater than the normal size of the artery.

A blood vessel has three layers—(1) the intima (inner layer made of endothelial cells), (2) media (contains muscular elastic fibers), and (3) adventitia (outer connective tissue). Aneurysms are either true or false.

True Aneurysm

It involves all the three layers, and the aneurysm is contained inside the endothelium.

False or Pseudoaneurysm

It involves the outer layer and is contained by the adventitia. Aneurismal degeneration that occurs in the thoracic aorta is termed as thoracic aneurysm (TA).

Aneurysms that coexist in both segments of the aorta (thoracic and abdominal) are termed thoracoabdominal aneurysms (TAA).

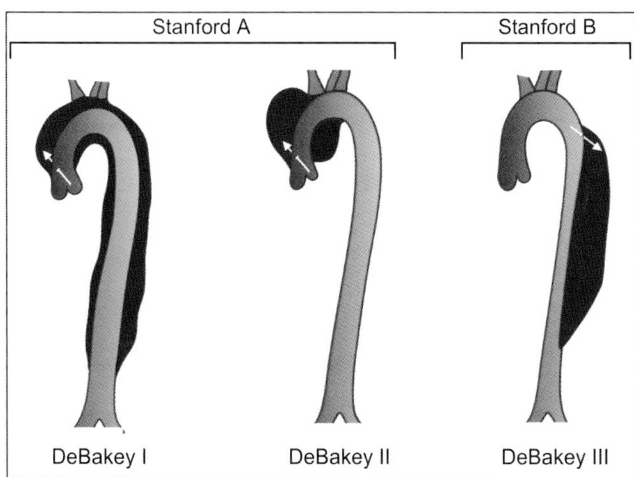

Fig. 26.1 Classification of aortic dissections

Aortic Dissection (Fig. 26.1)

It is initiated by intimal tear and is contained by the media, leading to creator of a true and a false lumen. An intimal tear causes separation of the walls of the aorta and a false passage for blood develops between the layers of the aorta.

The dissection may extend into the branches of the aorta in the chest or abdomen, and subsequently can come malperfusion, ischemia, or occlusion-related problems. The aortic sinus, valve and coronary arteries can also be involved by proximal of the dissection.

A *chronic dissection* is the one that is diagnosed more than 2 weeks after the onset of symptoms.

Aortic dissection should not be termed as dissecting aneurysm unless there is aneurysmal enlargement of the aorta.

On the basis of shape, aortic aneurysm can be broadly classified as saccular or fusiform.

A fusiform (also known as true) aneurysm is consisting of circumference of the wall with symmetrical dilatation.

A saccular aneurysm does not involve the entire circumference, rather formed by localized outpouching of the aortic wall.

Classification

Two classifications are used:

- *The Stanford classification*:
  - Type A involves ascending aorta (DeBakey types I and II).
  - Type B does not involve the ascending aorta (DeBakey type III).
- *The DeBakey classification*:
  - *Type I*: Aorta, aortic arch, and descending aorta (30%).
  - *Type II*: Ascending aorta only (20%).
  - *Type III*: Descending aorta distal to left subclavian (50%).

If Acute dissection is diagnosis within 14 days of onset. Anything of longer duration is termed chronic dissection.

ETIOLOGY

- Atherosclerotic (degenerative) aneurysm is the most common cause
- Chronic aortic dissection
- Chronic traumatic aortic transection
- Annuloaortic ectasia
- Aortitis: Granulomatous or syphilis.

INDICATIONS FOR SURGERY OR INTERVENTION

- *Aortic size*: Ascending aortic diameter more than or equal to 5.5 cm or twice the diameter of the normal contiguous aorta.

  Descending aortic diameter more than or equal to 6.5 cm (subtract 0.5 cm from the cut-off measurement in the presence of Marfan syndrome, family history of aneurysm or connective tissue disorder, bicuspid aortic valve, aortic stenosis, dissection and a patient undergoing another cardiac operation). Growth rate is more than or equal to 1 cm/year.
- Symptomatic aneurysm
- Traumatic aortic rupture
- Acute type B aortic dissection with associated rupture, leak or distal ischemia
- Pseudoaneurysm
- Large saccular aneurysm
- Mycotic aneurysm
- Aortic coarctation
- Bronchial compression by aneurysm
- Aortobronchial or aortoesophageal fistula.

Imaging Studies

Chest Radiograph

- In the case of ascending aortic aneurysms, chest X-rays may reveal a widened mediastinum, however, the aneurysms may also be completely obscured by the heart, and the chest X-ray may appear normal.

Echocardiography

- Transthoracic echocardiography demonstrates the aortic valve and proximal aortic root. It may help to detect aortic insufficiency and aneurysms of the sinus of Valsalva.

- Transesophageal echocardiography is more specific and sensitive than transthoracic echocardiography. Images show the aortic valve, ascending aorta, and descending thoracic aorta, but they are limited in the area of the distal ascending aorta, transverse aortic arch, and upper abdominal aorta.
- Transesophageal echocardiography can help to accurately differentiate aneurysm and dissection, but the images must be obtained and interpreted by skilled personnel.
- Ischemia may be evaluated using dipyridamole-thallium or dobutamine echocardiography scans.

Ultrasonography

- Infrarenal abdominal aortic aneurysms may be visualized using ultrasonography.
  Carotid ultrasound in patients with a history of transient ischemic attacks, or cerebrovascular accidents to evaluate carotid disease.
- *Intraoperative intravascular ultrasound (IVUS)* can be very much helpful in understanding anatomy and simultaneously placement of the endovascular stent.
- *Intraoperative epiaortic ultrasound* provides detail about aortic atherosclerotic disease or thrombus.
- *Aortography* images can help define the extent of the aneurysm, and simultaneously involvement or stenosis of the branch vessels. It also helps ostia take off. In elderly it also helps to evaluate coronary artery anatomy and pathology.
- Disadvantages include the use of nephrotoxic contrast and radiation. The risk of aortography includes embolization from laminated thrombus and carries a 1% stroke risk.

Computed Tomography Scan

- Contrast enhanced computed tomography (CT) scans are the most widely occupied means to localize the aneurism. At the same time it also says about the size, extent, involvement of the branch vessels and relationship with the surrounding structures. It is also helpful in diagnosing minal thrombus, intramural hematoma, free rupture, and contained rupture with hematoma.
- A spiral CT scan with 1 mm cuts and three-dimensional reconstruction with the ability to make centerline measurements is crucial to stent graft planning.
- Aortic size on imaging is widely used to guide clinical decision making. Double-oblique measurement is recommended.[10]
- CT angiography may create multiplanar reconstructions and cines. This requires nephrotoxic contrast and radiation, but the procedure is noninvasive.

Magnetic Resonance Imaging

- Magnetic resonance imaging (MRI) and magnetic resonance angiography have the advantage of avoiding nephrotoxic contrast and ionizing radiation compared to CT scans.
- MRI accurately demonstrates the location, extent, and size of the aneurysm. However, they are more time consuming, less readily available, and more expensive than CT scans.

Medical Therapy

Systemic hypertension probably contributes to the formation of aneurysms and certainly contributes to expansion and rupture.

Cessation of smoking is recommended.

For acute aortic dissections, the first-line treatment of hypertension is with a short-acting beta-blocker (e.g. esmolol). Beta blockade decreases the force of contraction. It also decreases the heart rate and the inotropic effect and reduces the likelihood of propagation of the dissection.

Surgical Therapy

Collagen impregnated Dacron tube grafts are used for most of the aortic aneurysm replacements. These grafts do not require preclotting and the ingrowth forms a pseudoendothelial layer, thus minimizing the risk of embolization.

Ascending Aortic Aneurysms

Determinants for the surgery of ascending aortic aneurysms are involvement of the aortic valve, annulus, sinuses of Valsalva, sinotubular junction and coronary orifices.

The choice of operation depends on the surgeon's experience and preference.[11]

Simple Supracoronary Dacron Tube Graft

Patients with normal aortic valve leaflets, annulus, and sinuses of Valsalva are replaced with a Dacron tube from the sinotubular junction to the origin of the innominate artery, with the patient under cardiopulmonary bypass.

Aortic Valve Disease

If the aortic sinuses and annulus are normal, Wheat procedure is performed. In this, aortic valve is replaced separately and the ascending aortic aneurysm is replaced with a supracoronary synthetic graft, leaving the coronary arteries intact.

Sinus of Valsalva Aneurysms

Valve sparing aortic root replacement can be used for normal aortic valve leaflets and aortic insufficiency due to dilated sinuses.[12]

There are two valve-sparing procedures:
1. The remodeling method
2. The reimplantation method.

Abnormal Aortic Valve and Aortic Root

For abnormal aortic valve and aortic root aneurysm Bentall procedure or Cabrol procedure is performed. This requires aortic root replacement (ARR).

The valved conduit, consisting of mechanical valve and Dacron graft, along with coronary reimplantation can be used for aortic root replacement in young patients who can undergo anticoagulation with reasonable safety.[13,14]

Stentless porcine roots, aortic homografts, and pulmonary autografts (Ross procedure) is used for elderly patients, women of childbearing age, and patients with contraindications to warfarin.

Reduction Aortoplasty

The wrapping of ascending aorta with a prosthetic graft can be done for elderly patients who cannot undergo a complex operational procedure.

Marfan Syndrome

In tube graft replacement alone may not be sufficient for the patient of Marfan syndrome, because of abnormal aorta, so they must undergo a valve sparing aortic root replacement or a complete aortic root replacement.

Endocarditis

Aortic root replacement with a homograft is ideal especially for aortic root abscess.

OPERATIVE PROCEDURE

Monitoring of central venous pressure, pulmonary artery pressure and systemic pressure is required. Nasopharyngeal and bladder temperature are also monitored. It is essential to perform transesophageal echocardiography in the operation theater before the surgical procedure, to reconfirm the anatomy and the cardiac function.

Ascending Aortic Replacement

Arterial cannulation is done either through the arch of aorta or the femoral artery. For venous drainage, the right arterial cannulation is done and cardiac pulmonary bypass is established. Cardioplegia is given after cross clamping the aorta just below the innominate artery. The aorta is opened at the sinotubular junction. An appropriate size Dacron tube graft is anastomosed using 5.0 prolene. This may be reinforced using Teflon felt.

Valve Sparing Aortic Root Replacement

In this procedure, it is very important to inspect the aortic valve for any pre-existing pathology. If found suitable, a carefully selected size of Dacron tube is used to allow co-optation of aortic valve with no aortic regurgitation. Sutures are placed along the subannular plane and then passed through the Dacron tube. The proximal suture line is thus secured. The aortic valve is now inside the tube graft and should be checked for regurgitation. Next, the subcoronary suturing is performed using 5.0 prolene. The valve is again tested for any incompetence. The coronary ostia are implanted on the graft and the distal end of the graft sutured.

Aortic Root Replacement

The aortic valve is removed and the annulus sized. An appropriate size of mechanical conduit or homograft is prepared. The coronary ostia are carefully mobilized. The proximal suture line passes through the annulus and the conduit. Next the coronary ostia are implanted followed by distal suture line. Cabrol procedure is rarely performed these days.

Aortic Arch Replacement

This is one of the most complex operations. Deep hypothermic circulatory arrest (DHCA) is used to perform reanastomosis of neck vessels. Additional cerebral protection is provided by antegrade cerebral perfusion.

Monitoring of central nervous system function includes
- Electroencephalography (EEG) monitoring
- Somatosensory potential monitoring
- Cooling to 18–20°C
- Trendelenburg position
- Mannitol
- CO_2 flooding
- Packing patients head in ice
- Thiopental and steroids
- Antegrade and retrograde cerebral perfusion.

OPERATIVE STEPS

Arterial cannulation may be performed through femoral artery, right axillary artery and ascending aorta. Cannulation of right atrium is done for venous drainage. Cardiopulmonary bypass is thus established and the patient cooled to 18–20°C. Antegrade cerebral circulation is used to minimize brain injury. This usually gives the surgeon about 30 minutes of safe circulatory arrest. Carbon dioxide is flooded in the operating field to reduce air embolism. Individual perfusion catheters can also be placed in the neck vessels for antegrade perfusion. The three lead vessels may be anastomosed individually or as an island on the Dacron graft.

Hybrid Procedures

Hybrid operating rooms with advanced imaging facility is required. Different hybrid procedures have been standardized according to the location of the most proximal placement of the endograft in relation to the arch vessels.

Criado Classification

Zone 0 pathology involves all aortic arch vessels and requires revascularization of at least the innominate artery and left common carotid artery (CCA), and possibly the left subclavian artery (LSA). Reimplantation of LSA is important in the case of symptoms of left arm ischemia, functional left internal mammary arterial bypass graft, or dominant left vertebral artery circulation. Operation involves a median sternotomy and the use of a bifurcated or trifurcated graft from the ascending aorta to the arch vessels. Following revascularization, a stent-graft is then implanted either in an antegrade or retrograde fashion.

Zone 1 placement, commonly avoids a median sternotomy. A right CCA to left CCA bypass, prior to endograft placement is performed. Depending on the quality of angiographic resources in the operating room, this procedure may be performed in a single stage if a dedicated angiographic suite is available.

Partial or complete coverage of the LSA is required in Zone 2 landing thorough assessment of the carotid, vertebral and circle of Willis circulations should be preoperatively performed,[15,16] and if circulation is adequate only then should LSA be covered.

A major concern in arch surgery is neurologic injury, patient with a history of stroke should undergo a brain CT scan.

DESCENDING THORACIC AND THORACOABDOMINAL ANEURYSM

Aneurysm repair is possible both by open and endovascular techniques.[17-21] It is important to look for comorbidities such as patients' age, life expectancy, aortic diameter and extent of aneurysm.

Stent graft repair of descending thoracic aneurysm should be performed if the predicted operative risk is lower than the open surgical method.

Operative Steps

A left thoracotomy or thoracoabdominal incision is made. Proximal aortic clamp is placed just proximal or distal to the LSA. Distal clamp is placed between T4 and T7. This reduces the chances of ischemia to the spinal cord, abdominal visceral and the kidneys. Proximal anastomosis is performed and when complete, the proximal clamp is released and applied on the tube graft. The distal cross clamp is moved sequentially down to allow visceral and renal perfusion. Important intercostal vessels are reimplanted on the graft if required. Sometimes direct catheters may be placed in renal and visceral arteries to allow continuous perfusion. If the distal aneurysm extends to the bifurcation, the visceral and renal arteries are reimplanted on the tube graft.

Measures to reduce spinal cord injury include cerebrospinal fluid drainage, reimplantation of intercostal arteries, partial bypass, and mild hypothermia. Left atrial femoral bypass is established with a Bio-Medicus circuit, and the patient is cooled to 32–34°C (89.6–93.2°F).

Endovascular Stent Grafting Techniques

The arterial access is most commonly through the femoral or iliac arteries. These are free of calcium, lack tortuosity and are adequately sized typically more than 8 mm. If femoral access is not possible then retroperitoneal dissection can give access via common iliac arteries. There should be a proximal 2 cm landing zone beyond the LSA and distally sufficient landing zone prior to iliac artery. It requires experience to treat thoracoabdominal aneurysms using custom built fenestrated and branched stent grafts. Such grafts require precise tailoring according to the patient's anatomy. The making of this device can delay the operation. However, recent availability of standardized multi-branched endografts has reduced the delay as these grafts can be placed in 90% of the patient population.

PARAPARESIS OR PARAPLEGIA

Paraplegia is a serious complication. There are various ways to reduce the incidence of this complication.

- Preoperative angiogram to localize and reimplant the major blood supply of spinal cord on the graft
- Motor evoked potential is used to assess spinal cord ischemia and identify critical segmental arteries for spinal cord perfusion

- Cerebrospinal fluid drainage is performed to increase spinal cord perfusion pressure during aortic cross-clamping.

The incidence of spinal cord injury is less with endovascular stent grafting than with open repair but exists with both types of surgical treatment.

Paraplegia is a matter of concern after endovascular stent grafting especially in patients with anticipated endograft coverage of T9–T12, coverage of the long segment of the thoracic aorta, compromised collateral pathways, prior infrarenal AAA repair, and symptomatic spinal ischemia.[22,23] It is important to use the following measures of—cerebrospinal fluid drainage. Motor evoked potential monitoring and increasing mean arterial pressure with pressors.

Postoperative Care

It depends on the type of surgery performed.

- The signs of coronary ischemia should be carefully observed in the postoperative period of Bentall procedure
- Aortic insufficiency is a major concern in case of David's operation
- In case of arch repair, neurological status should be addressed properly
- In case of elephant trunk repair, paraplegia is a major concern as telescoped sleeve in the descending aorta may obstruct critical spinal vessels
- Repair of descending and thoracoabdominal aorta carries a risk of paraplegia
- Acute postoperative renal dysfunction is another concern and may be due to extended ischemic cross-clamping or to hypothermic circulatory arrest
- Endovascular stented patients are often extubated early with a decreased stay in ICU and hospital stay.

REFERENCES

1. Lam CR, Aram HH. Resection of the descending thoracic aorta for aneurysm; a report of the use of a homograft in a case and an experimental study. Ann Surg. 1951;134(4):743-52.
2. Cooley DA, De Bakey ME. Resection of entire ascending aorta in fusiform aneurysm using cardiac bypass. J Am Med Assoc. 1956;162(12):1158-9.
3. De Bakey ME, Crawford ES, Cooley DA, Morris GC. Successful resection of fusiform aneurysm of aortic arch with replacement by homograft. Surg Gynecol Obstet. 1957;105(6):657-64.
4. Deterling RA, Bhonslay SB. An evaluation of synthetic materials and fabrics suitable for blood vessel replacement. Surgery. 1955;38(1):71-91.
5. Bentall H, De Bono A. A technique for complete replacement of the ascending aorta. Thorax. 1968;23(4):338-9.
6. Ross DN. Homograft replacement of the aortic valve. Lancet. 1962;2:487.
7. Barratt-Boyes BG. Homograft aortic valve replacement in aortic incompetence and stenosis. Thorax. 1964;19:131-50.
8. Dake MD, Miller DC, Semba CP, Mitchell RS, Walker PJ, Liddell RP. Transluminal placement of endovascular stent-grafts for the treatment of descending thoracic aortic aneurysms. N Engl J Med. 1994;331(26):1729-34.
9. US Food and Drug Administration (FDA). (2005). FDA Approves First-of-Kind Device to Treat Descending Thoracic Aneurysms. [online] Available from *http://www.fda.gov/NewsEvents/Newsroom/PressAnnouncements/2005/ucm108424.htm*. [Accessed May, 2015].
10. Mendoza DD, Kochar M, Devereux RB, Basson CT, Min JK, Holmes K, et al. Impact of image analysis methodology on diagnostic and surgical classification of patients with thoracic aortic aneurysms. Ann Thorac Surg. 2011;92(3):904-12.
11. Ergin MA, Spielvogel D, Apaydin A, Lansman SL, McCullough JN, Galla JD, et al. Surgical treatment of the dilated ascending aorta: when and how? Ann Thorac Surg. 1999;67(6):1834-9.
12. Patel ND, Williams JA, Barreiro CJ, Bethea BT, Fitton TP, Dietz HC, et al. Valve-sparing aortic root replacement: early experience with the De Paulis Valsalva graft in 51 patients. Ann Thorac Surg. 2006;82(2):548-53.
13. Cabrol C, Pavie A, Mesnildrey P, Gandjbakhch I, Laughlin L, Bors V, et al. Long-term results with total replacement of the ascending aorta and reimplantation of the coronary arteries. J Thorac Cardiovasc Surg. 1986;91(1):17-25.
14. Kouchoukos NT, Marshall WG, Wedige-Stecher TA. Eleven-year experience with composite graft replacement of the ascending aorta and aortic valve. J Thorac Cardiovasc Surg. 1986;92(4):691-705.
15. Criado FJ, Barnatan MF, Rizk Y, Clark NS, Wang CF. Technical strategies to expand stent-graft applicability in the aortic arch and proximal descending thoracic aorta. J Endovasc Ther. 2002;9(2):II32-8.
16. Schoder M, Lammer J, Czerny M. Endovascular aortic arch repair: hopes and certainties. Eur J Vasc Endovasc Surg. 2009;38(3):255-61.
17. US Food and Drug Administration (FDA). (2008). Talent™ Thoracic Stent Graft System-P070007. [online] Available from *http://www.fda.gov/MedicalDevices/ProductsandMedicalProcedures/DeviceApprovalsandClearances/Recently-ApprovedDevices/ucm074063.htm*. [Accessed May, 2015].
18. Sweet MP, Hiramoto JS, Park KH, Reilly LM, Chuter TA. A standardized multi-branched thoracoabdominal stent-graft for endovascular aneurysm repair. J Endovasc Ther. 2009;16(3):359-64.
19. Reilly LM, Chuter TA. Reversal of fortune: induced endoleak to resolve neurological deficit after endovascular repair of thoracoabdominal aortic aneurysm. J Endovasc Ther. 2010;17(1):21-9.
20. Ullery BW, Cheung AT, Fairman RM, Jackson BM, Woo EY, Bavaria J, et al. Risk factors, outcomes, and clinical manifestations of spinal cord ischemia following thoracic endovascular aortic repair. J Vasc Surg. 2011;54(3):677-84.
21. Baril DT, Carroccio A, Ellozy SH, Palchik E, Addis MD, Jacobs TS, et al. Endovascular thoracic aortic repair and previous or concomitant abdominal aortic repair: is the increased risk of spinal cord ischemia real? Ann Vasc Surg. 2006;20:188-94.
22. Böckler D, Kotelis D, Kohlhof P, von Tengg-Kobligk H, Mansmann U, Zink W, et al. Spinal cord ischemia after endovascular repair of the descending thoracic aorta in a sheep model. Eur J Vasc Endovasc Surg. 2007;34:461-9.
23. Carroccio A, Marin ML, Ellozy S, Hollier LH. Pathophysiology of paraplegia following endovascular thoracic aortic aneurysm repair. J Card Surg. 2003;18:359-66.

27

Preoperative Anesthetic Considerations for Adult Cardiac Patient Undergoing Noncardiac Surgery

Anil Karlekar

Over the years, a phenomenal improvement in understanding of disease processes, better diagnostic and therapeutic facilities and their wider reach in areas hitherto inaccessible, have predictably seen a rise in life expectancy. While on one hand, higher life expectancy has meant that number of high-risk patients presenting for surgical interventions are on the rise, the reverse is also true: enhanced anesthetic safety over years has also contributed to better outcomes and in a way added to the improved longevity.

THE CHALLENGE

The World Health Organization has estimated that 230 million major surgical operations are undertaken annually.[1] Despite the improved patient management, however, noncardiac surgery is associated with significant morbidity and mortality. Major adverse cardiac and cerebrovascular events (MACCE, see Table 27.1) represent the most common cause of serious perioperative morbidity and mortality. The occurrence of cardiac or cerebrovascular events may be infrequent, reportedly 1–7%, but when they happen, they are potentially life threatening. Cardiac events comprise the most common cause of perioperative mortality and morbidity. Recently, Sabaté[2] has reported 4.3% incidence of MACCE and one death out of 10 patients who developed MACCE during the hospital stay, in a study of over 3300 patients undergoing noncardiac surgery. Earlier, Canadian province of Ontario has reported 1.3% mortality in the 30-day postoperative period of intermediate to high-risk non-cardiac surgical patients in the decade ending 2004.[3] Extrapolating the Canadian statistics to the world, 2 million patients annually are at risk of sustaining a major adverse cardiac event.

A 1995 review of major published series reveals what we consider obvious today: underlying cardiovascular disease does significantly impact perioperative morbidity and mortality.[4] Among unselected patients over 40 years of age, MI was reported in 1.4% and cardiac death in 1%, with some selection criteria MI was reported in 3.2% and cardiac death in 1.7%, while among those selected to undergo preoperative thallium scintigraphy preoperatively, the incidence of MI and death was even higher, 6.9% and 3.2% respectively.[5] The conclusion: incidence of MI and cardiac death varied with the risk associated with the population studied.[6] Depending on the type of surgery and patient age, the prevalence of various cardiovascular diseases in patients undergoing noncardiac surgery ranges from 5% to 70%, being highest in patients older than 70 years undergoing major vascular surgery.

What makes the cardiac patients undergoing noncardiac surgery vulnerable for adverse cardiac events? Surgery and anesthesia involve manipulation of body tissues and disruption of many physiological functions. The manipulation and disruption leads to activation of stress response essentially meant to defend body by improving wound healing, coagulation and humoral immunity. The release of various stress hormones may cause increased myocardial oxygen demand and disturb the delicate balance leading to ischemia. Patients with underlying cerebrovascular disease (e.g. peripheral artery disease, stroke) have an increased risk of perioperative cardiac complications for two reasons:

1. Patients with cerebrovascular disease have higher incidence of CAD[7,8] and
2. Systolic dysfunction.[9]

Certain accompaniments of surgery like volume shifts, blood loss and enhanced myocardial oxygen demand due to changes in heart rate and blood pressure besides overall increased hypercoagulability, predispose patients to myocardial ischemia.[10]

The burden of cardiovascular diseases is forever increasing; the Indian subcontinent particularly appears to be ahead of others. Cardiovascular disease will be the

Table 27.1 Definition of MACCE[75]

MACCE	Definition
Non-fatal cardiac arrest	An absence of cardiac rhythm or presence of chaotic rhythm requiring any component of basic or advanced cardiac life support
Acute myocardial infarction	Increase and gradual decrease in troponin level or a faster increase and decrease of creatine kinase isoenzyme as markers of myocardial necrosis in the company of at least one of the following: ischemic symptoms, abnormal Q-waves on the ECG, ST-segment elevation or depression; or coronary artery intervention (e.g. coronary angioplasty) or a typical decrease in an elevated troponin level detected at its peak after surgery in a patient without a documented alternative explanation for the troponin elevation
Congestive heart failure	New in-hospital signs or symptoms of dyspnea or fatigue, orthopnea, paroxysmal nocturnal dyspnea, increased jugular venous pressure, pulmonary rales on physical examination, cardiomegaly, or pulmonary vascular engorgement
New cardiac arrhythmia	ECG evidence of atrial flutter, atrial fibrillation, or second- or third-degree atrioventricular conduction block
Angina	Dull diffuse substernal chest discomfort precipitated by exertion or emotion and relieved by rest or Nitroglycerin
Stroke	Embolic, thrombotic, or hemorrhagic event lasting at least 30 minutes with or without persistent residual motor, sensory, or cognitive dysfunction; if the neurological symptoms continue for >24 h, a person is diagnosed with stroke, and if lasting <24 h the event is defined as a transient ischemic attack
Cardiovascular death	Any death, unless an unequivocal non-cardiovascular cause could be established
Cerebrovascular death	A death caused by cerebrovascular disease

largest cause of death and disability by 2020 in India. It has been forecasted that 2.6 Million people will die from coronary artery disease (CAD), which constitutes 54% of all cardiovascular disease deaths. Approximately half of these deaths will occur in young and middle-aged individuals, making the impact on society and the economy even more significant[11] with these frightening figures, it is obvious that we should brace ourselves to manage higher percentage of cardiac patients presenting for noncardiac surgery.

Patients with cardiac disease presenting for noncardiac surgery pose considerable challenge to the anesthesiologist. Interestingly, it is not the anesthetic management per se that is a matter of debate, what is mired in controversy and often generates strong diverse views among caregivers is the preoperative workup and preparation of a cardiac patient for noncardiac surgery: what investigations and testing should the patient be subjected to? And once evaluated and diagnosed, what therapeutic measures be undertaken to optimize the cardiac status? This chapter is largely focused on preoperative concerns of anesthesiologists, since ultimately it is the anesthesiologist who has to manage the case perioperatively!

Anesthesiologists objective is optimize a cardiac patient to be able to withstand the wide variations in physiologic, biochemical, rheological, hemodynamic, metabolic, and respiratory parameters apart from temperature and fluid shifts, pharmacological load of host of anesthetic and non-anesthetic medications, stress response and hypercoaguable state that generally accompany the surgery. An all round challenge indeed!

CARDIAC CLEARANCE AND FITNESS FOR SURGERY

The problem often starts with a request from the surgeon and/or anesthesiologist forwarded to a cardiologist for a vaguely defined, understood and agreed task of 'cardiac clearance and fitness for surgery and anesthesia' for a given patient. The responses could be as varied as a direct telephonic clearance given by one cardiologist to a full battery of investigations including stress testing and coronary angiography by another, depending on their understanding of the patient and the problems.

What the anesthesiologists and surgeons should actually seek from the cardiologist are if the patient has any hitherto unknown cardiac problem that may have been missed or in a known cardiac patient, if the cardiac status can be further optimized prior to the procedure. Anesthesiologists should neither seek a 'fit to undergo surgery' opinion by the cardiologists nor should the cardiologists themselves give such a 'clearance'. The cardiologists should refrain from making specific recommendations like 'fit for GA or spinal anesthesia', as they may not be familiar with nuances of the anesthetic techniques, effects of variety of anesthetic drugs on hemodynamics or surgery specific perturbations in homeostasis. It will be worthwhile remembering that 'Revised Cardiac Risk Index' (RCRI) predicts a 0.5% incidence of untoward events in patients with no risk factors at all! At best, one could only predict only a likelihood! *Ideally, the team comprising of surgeon, anesthesiologist and cardiologist should jointly do a risk stratification for the given patient and offer the best option in a given situation in their joint communication to the patient and/or family.*

GETTING STARTED: UNEARTHING THE 'CARDIAC LOAD'

Among patients presenting for noncardiac surgery, the anesthesiologist may have to encounter any of the following situations:

- A known cardiac patient who is:
  - On medical therapy only
  - Or may have had or may warrant fresh interventional or surgical treatment; could have been optimally or partially cured or be having recurrence of the same disease entity
  - Though over years, though globally cardiac transplants have reached a plateau and ventricular assist devices (VADs) are on the rise, in India, the cardiac transplant programs appears to be picking up and anesthesiologists will have to equip themselves to manage such cases.[12]
- Apparently not a known cardiac patient:
  - Someone unaware of presence of any cardiac disease or
  - A patient who may have deliberately chosen to ignore his symptoms.

In view of higher incidence of adverse perioperative cardiac events in 'high-risk' patients undergoing noncardiac surgery, it appears prudent to stratify risk for each patient and manage accordingly. Thus, anesthesiologist is faced with the daunting task of 'unearthing' a probable cardiac ailment in a hitherto undiagnosed patient or evaluating a known cardiac patient, assigning the risk, optimizing patient's clinical status, regulate medications perioperatively, help decide appropriate timing at least for elective surgery, administer appropriate anesthesia, ensure safe and uneventful recovery and thus a perfect outcome.

Various guidelines[13] have highlighted the impact of nature of the proposed surgery and its urgency, presence of other comorbidities and functional reserve of the patient on the incidence of perioperative adverse cardiovascular event, apart from presence of a cardiac ailment itself. The risk stratification of a cardiac patient presenting for noncardiac surgery thus includes consideration for the type of surgery and comorbidities if any, in addition to the evaluation of cardiac status. Following three elements form the basis of such evaluation:

1. *Patient specific clinical variables (Table 27.2)*
   Cardiac diseases: Coronary artery disease, valvular heart disease, congenital heart disease, other cardiac diseases like heart failure, hypertension, etc.
   Age: Geriatric group is particularly vulnerable
   Peripheral vascular disease,
   Diabetes mellitus,
   Renal insufficiency
   Pulmonary diseases like chronic obstructive airway disease, obstructive sleep apnea, etc.
2. *Functional capacity* or effort tolerance of the patient (Table 27.3).
3. *Surgery specific risk*: Certain operative procedures like peripheral vascular surgery have higher incidence of adverse cardiac events, morbidity and mortality while others like cataract surgery are associated with very little risk of an adverse cardiac event (Table 27.4).

Table 27.2 Patient-specific clinical variable

Clinical conditions that warrants intensive management since risk is high if undertaken for surgery without optimization
Unstable coronary syndromes, like unstable angina, severe angina or MI
Decompensated heart failure
Significant arrhythmia like high grade AV block, symptomatic ventricular arrhythmia, supraventricular arrhythmia with heart rate >100 beats per minute, symptomatic bradycardia
Severe valvular heart disease, like aortic stenosis, mitral stenosis
Clinical conditions that warrant careful assessment
History of ischemic heart disease
History of cerebrovascular disease
History of heart failure
Diabetes mellitus
Renal insufficiency
Obesity
Sleep apnea
Age more than 65 years
Uncontrolled hypertension

Table 27.3 Functional status

Functional status or effort tolerance can be expressed in Metabolic Equivalents or MET

1 MET = 3.5 mL of oxygen uptake/kg/minute and is the oxygen requirement at rest in sitting position

In clinical practice, simple questions to patients can give fairly good idea of functional status:

- If patient can eat, dress, use toilet on his own, walk indoors in the house, and on level ground at a pace of approx 3.2 to 4–8 km an hour apart from doing light domestic work can be considered to be meeting 1 MET requirement
- If a patient can climb a flight of stairs, walk level ground at 6 km an hour, engage in little heavy work in the house or is able to play light sports can be considered to be meeting 4 METs requirement
- If a patient can participate in strenuous sports like swimming can be said to be meeting 10 METs requirement

Patients who are unable to meet 4 MET requirement during normal activity have higher risk of adverse perioperative cardiac events[76,77]

Systematic Approach to a Patient Having Cardiac or Suspected Cardiac Disease Presenting for Noncardiac Surgery: (See Algorithms)

1. *Urgency of surgery:* One may have to proceed with emergency surgery irrespective of risk assessment and recommendations therein, without any additional preoperative assessment or treatment depending on patient condition except for what may be required as optimization for emergency surgery.
2. *The triad of clinical status:* For all elective surgery cases a methodical approach to assess a patient's clinical status, risk stratification and optimization where necessary, should be undertaken. As mentioned earlier, further workup of the patient would depend on the three elements namely the type of contemplated surgery, functional capacity and clinical variables. A *low risk surgery* generally does not need elaborate risk stratification and additional cardiac testing, and can be performed safely. A direct interaction with patient to assess *functional capacity* usually suffices to decide if patient scheduled for low to intermediate risk surgery could be done without elaborate further

Table 27.4 Surgery-specific cardiac risk

Risk	Surgery
High risk Reported risk of cardiac death or nonfatal myocardial infarction [MI] often greater than 5%	Aortic-open or other major vascular surgery Peripheral artery surgery
Intermediate risk Reported risk of cardiac death or nonfatal myocardial infarction [MI] 1–5%	Carotid endarterectomy Head and neck surgery Intraperitoneal and intrathoracic surgery Orthopedic surgery Prostate surgery
Low risk Reported risk of cardiac death or nonfatal myocardial infarction [MI] less than 1%	Ambulatory surgery Endoscopic procedure Superficial procedure Cataract surgery Breast surgery
Emergency surgery In emergency surgery, cardiac complications are 2–5 times more likely	
Institution/surgeon/anesthesiologist specific The incidence of perioperative cardiac events will undoubtedly be have an undetermined impact of the institution and the competence of surgical team	

Source: Based on ACC/AHA 2007 guidelines on perioperative cardiovascular evaluation and care for noncardiac surgery: a report of the American College of Cardiology/American Heart Association Task Force on Practice Guidelines with few modifications[5]

testing, since those who can generate 4 METs (Metabolic Equivalent of Task, see Table 27.3) or more would usually stand the procedure well. This premise would usually hold good even for those who may have some cardiac disease since good exercise tolerance in general would indicate a compensated and stable cardiac status. It is the *clinical variables*, which need a detailed and considered approach, an area where the much desired agreement between surgeon, anesthesiologist and surgeon is usually conspicuous by its absence! Let us unfold the facts that lie beneath *clinical variables*.

Patient History

Detailed history taking is an absolutely essential. Every effort should be made to elicit history related to cardiorespiratory system like complaints of breathlessness, effort tolerance, angina, palpitations and sudden blackout. Pointed questions regarding patients' functional status must be asked to ascertain whether patient can undertake physical activity of 4 METs or not. History of pain in lower limbs on walking must be probed further and investigated for presence of peripheral vascular disease.

A healthy looking individual with no history suggestive of involvement of any cardiovascular and respiratory system with good functional reserve and scheduled for an intermediate to low-risk surgery, should need minimum preoperative workup.

Physical Examination

Physical examination should include pulse rate and contour, rhythm, blood pressure measurement, peripheral pulsations, presence of bruit, auscultations of lungs for crepitations and rhonchi, precordial palpation and auscultation, abdominal palpation and examination of limbs for the presence of edema. Important findings deciding future course of action would be signs of heart failure, aortic stenosis or uncontrolled hypertension.

Certain clinical predictors derived from history and physical examination and described below warrant further evaluation and aggressive management.

Recent myocardial infarction or severe angina: In the past, management was based on the observations that patients undergoing noncardiac surgery had higher chances of reinfarction or cardiac death if surgery was performed within 3 months of MI, when compared to time periods of 3–6 months or more than 6 months when it was least. With preoperative optimization and aggressive monitoring coming in place, a study done between 1977 and 1982, revealed overall lower rates, though the pattern of lower incidence if farther away from MI, was similar (Table 27.5).[14]

Currently, the management of Acute Coronary Syndromes (ACS) having changed with aggressive reperfusion and revascularization strategies being practiced, the risk stratification for coronary artery disease (CAD) admittedly deserves a review, though consensus is elusive. Patients not fully revascularized following MI should undergo stress test. If the stress test does not indicate ischemic myocardium at risk, the likelihood of reinfarction is low after noncardiac surgery. Those with positive stress test will be advised coronary angiography and revascularization, irrespective of a proposed elective noncardiac surgery. Though there is paucity of clinical trials to advise firm guidelines, it appears reasonable to defer elective surgery for at least 4–6 weeks after MI.[15]

Recent percutaneous intervention (PCI):[15,16] With rise in incidence of CAD, the number of patients undergoing PCI is also increasing every year. It is estimated that 5% of patients after PCI will present within first year for noncardiac surgery. The timing of surgery for patients with recent PCI continues to be debated and so is the management of antiplatelet therapy for such patients. Continued antiplatelet therapy increases the risk of surgical bleeding while interruption is fraught with the consequence of stent thrombosis. While bare metal stents (BMS) do successfully prevent abrupt vessel closure by circumventing elastic recoil and negative vessel remodeling, they fail to prevent, in fact they stimulate neointimal hyperplasia. Drug eluting stents (DES) are coated with drugs like sirolimus and paclitaxel which inhibit smooth muscle cell proliferation. Till the time exposed surfaces of stents are covered with endothelium, there is always a danger of stent thrombosis due to formation of platelet rich microthrombi. The process of endothelialization of metal stents occurs rapidly and may complete in 2–6 weeks

Table 27.5 Differences in predicted incidence of reinfarction in patients undergoing noncardiac surgery after suffering a myocardial infarction as a function of time interval between the MI and surgery, in two groups of studies, one conducted in eighties and other recent ones

Time interval between MI and surgery	Older studies	Later studies	Current
>6 months old	5%		Acute reperfusion and revascularization would change the incidence, available data insufficient
3–6 months	15–25%	2.3%	
<3 months	36%	5.7%	

while that of DES may take months. It is for this difference in time taken for endothelialization that dual antiplatelet therapy is recommended for a minimum of 1 month for BMS implantation and minimum of 1 year for DES implantation.[17] Bioabsorbable coronary stents as they become common place may change the way we look at these time intervals in very near future.

Stent thrombosis is a devastating complication with up to 45% mortality; the factors contributing to increased stent thrombosis in perioperative period are incomplete endothelialization of stent and stress response triggering a hypercoagulable state mediated through increased release of procoagulant factors, decreased fibrinolysis, and cytokines causing platelet activation. In addition, abrupt and premature discontinuation of antiplatelet therapy causes a rebound increase in cyclooxygenase and thromboxane also leading to platelet activation. The reported incidence of adverse cardiac events in patients undergoing noncardiac surgery with either BMS or DES at different time intervals between stent implantations and noncardiac surgery as depicted in Table 27.6, demonstrates that timing of surgery plays a very significant role.[18,78]

Chassot estimated that surgical blood loss increases 2.5–20% for aspirin and 30–50% for clopidogrel perioperatively with 30% increased need for transfusions but no bleeding related mortality, except during intracranial surgery.[19] Vicenzi concluded that in many patients with recently implanted stents, the risk of surgical bleeding may be outweighed by the benefit of continued antiplatelet therapy.[20] The search for an ideal antiplatelet agent particularly in terms of reversibility for better control of their effect in case the patient has bleeding, continues. Ticagrelor (reversible, oral route), cangrelor (reversible, intravenous route) and elinogrel (reversible, both oral and intravenous route) are recent additions to the $P2Y_{12}$ inhibitor class of drugs and hold lot of promise not only for reliability of their intended action but also for reversibility when so desired.[21]

Aspirin: POISE-2 Trial

Perioperative ischemic evaluation 2 (POISE-2), a randomized controlled multicenter international double-blinded trial,[22] conducted between 2010 and 2013 enrolling 10,010 patients from 135 hospitals spread over 23 countries, was designed to attempt clear uncertainty over risks and benefits associated with perioperative use of aspirin in at-risk patients undergoing noncardiac surgery; the results having been published in April 2014 issue of NEJM. Aspirin, apart from other measures, has been advocated for attenuating risk of cardiovascular complications. That patients receiving aspirin perioperatively are likely to bleed more is well known and accepted, though its quantum and impact on outcome, directly in the form of hemodynamic instability or related to excess transfusion of blood/blood products versus cardiovascular protection aspirin offers has been a matter of debate among clinicians.

The conclusion of the study: *'Administration of aspirin before surgery and throughout the early postsurgical period had no significant effect on the rate of composite of death or nonfatal myocardial infarction but increased the risk of major bleeding'* has, not unexpectedly, prompted many clinicians to question the methodology employed in the study. In the Focussed Review 'Perioperative Aspirin Management after POISE-2: Some Answers, but Questions Remain,' Gerstein and colleagues[23] have attempted to answer the questions that seem to have been raised by results of POISE-2 trial. While looking for possible reasons why aspirin use failed to protect at-risk patients against cardiovascular complications, it appears that low-risk patients outnumbered at-risk patients in the study, like 2/3rd of patients in aspirin group did not meet primary or secondary cardiovascular risk prevention criteria; those included were for high-risk surgery (rather than having risks related to cardiovascular system), and among that category too, vascular surgeries were just 4.9%, thus *masking possible advantages of aspirin*! In addition, 9.5% patients in aspirin group received NSAIDs concurrently that could have caused aspirin resistance. Patients undergoing carotid endarterectomy and those having undergone recent coronary stenting were also excluded from the study.

Aspirin, for more than two decades, has enjoyed the position of first line antiplatelet medication in the prevention of cardiovascular diseases partially due to its unique mode of action, not shared by other agents, and its reliable pharmacological efficacy.[24] Table 27.7 sums up the current usage of aspirin.

Table 27.6 Incidence of adverse cardiac events in noncardiac surgery patients after stent placement

	<30 days	31–90 days	>90 days	0–90 days	91–180 days	181–365 days	>1 year	Elective surgery	Emergent surgery
BMS[14]	10.5%	3.8%	2.8%					4.4%	11.7%
DES[15]				6.4%	5.7%	5.9%	3.3%	4.7%	17.9%
Conclusion[75]	Longer the surgery was delayed after stent placements, lower the adverse events!							More adverse events during emergency surgery	

Table 27.7 Current usage of aspirin

	Indications	Evidence in favor
1.	Primary (aims to prevent disease before it occurs) prevention of stroke, coronary artery disease and malignancy	Has not been robust
2.	Secondary (aims to reduce the impact of a disease after it has already occurred) prevention of cardiovascular disease	Enough to recommend use indefinitely of aspirin unless the risk of bleeding outweighs benefits
3.	As a component of 'Dual Antiplatelet Therapy (DAT)' following coronary artery stenting to prevent in-stent thrombosis	Enough to recommend use in patients with stents for durations determined by the type of stent
4.	For prevention of thrombo-embolism in patients with bioprosthetic valves or pericardial patch repair of ASD or for DVT prophylaxis'	Has not been robust
5.	Perioperatively to attenuate surgery induced hypercoagulability, aimed at preventing MACE in patients at high risk for such events	? The issue being debated!

The author recommends readers to refer to ACC/AHA guidelines (JACC 2014)[25] and two excellent articles in Current Opinion Anesthesiology June 2015, 'Aspirin in perioperative period; a review of the recent literature'[26] and 'Update on perioperative care of cardiac patient for noncardiac surgery',[27] all publications post-POISE-2 and citing the study, to help them decide whether to initiate aspirin preoperatively in a patient de novo, or to stop/continue among those already taking. However, author's recommendations are as follows:

- In general, since the risk of increased bleeding is considerable, *aspirin should not be prescribed* unless risk of thromboembolic complications outweighs the bleeding risk.
- In general, *do not initiate* perioperative aspirin therapy.
- VTE and pulmonary embolism (POISE-2 trial not sufficiently powered to assess the impact)
  - Primary prevention—most of other trials report aspirin offering protection, *may continue*
  - Secondary prevention—offers benefit, *continue.*
- *Discontinue* if prescribed solely for primary prevention.
- If prescribed for secondary prevention of
  - Cerebrovascular or coronary ischemic complications—*continue* if bleeding risk does not outweigh the risk of complication.
  - Following coronary artery stenting, intervening time interval and urgency of noncardiac to be considered:
    - Urgent surgery, within 6 weeks of PCI, irrespective of stent: *continue*
    - Elective surgery, since the recommendation is to *continue* (DAT, including aspirin) perioperatively, consider deferring timing of surgery where possible, types of stent being an important variable to decide the interval as mentioned below:

      Angioplasty : 14 days
      Bare metal stents : 30 days
      Drug-eluting stents : 365 days

      Already under review, recommendations likely to be revised in favor of shorter intervals.
  - Carotid revascularization: *continue.*
  - CHF: weigh against bleeding risk.
  - Neurosurgical and spinal procedures (discuss risk): *discontinue*; Endovascular interventions: *continue* as part of DAT.
  - Ophthalmic surgery: no consensus, not absolute contraindication.
  - CABG: *continue*
  - Peripheral vascular surgery: *continue.* (*Regional/neuraxial anesthesia not contraindicated*[28])
  - Transplant, Renal: *discontinue*; Liver: ? continue.
  - Orthopedics, Joint surgery: *discontinue*; Other surgeries: *continue.*
  - Urology: *May continue,* meticulous surgical hemostasis advised.

Role of Tests for Platelet Functions and Transfusions

It may be worthwhile mentioning that when faced with excessive bleeding in patients taking aspirin, particularly in neurosurgical setting, point of care tests[29] may help clinicians determine status of platelet function, but platelet administration[30] is not reported to affect outcomes.

Conclusion: For patients treated with plain old balloon angioplasty (POBA) elective surgery should be deferred for 2 weeks, with bare metal stent, it may be safe to stop antiplatelet therapy 4–6 weeks after implantation, but those treated with drug eluting stent, antiplatelet therapy should be continued for at least 3–6 months, preferably longer, even if surgery is to be performed except in closed cavity surgery like cranium or posterior chamber of eye. The noncardiac surgery of patients with stents should preferably be undertaken in a setup where facilities of PCI are available in case any urgent intervention is required.

Heart failure, decompensated or compensated: Heart failure is undoubtedly the most commonly encountered cardiac complication in noncardiac surgery perioperatively, the incidence being 1–6% after major surgery and 6–25% among patients with prior history of heart failure, ischemic heart disease or valvular disease. Heart failure carries a greater perioperative risk than ischemic heart disease.[31] Risk is higher in patients with diabetes mellitus, renal dysfunction and high risk surgery like vascular surgery.[32-34] While the association between presence of heart failure and postoperative cardiac complications is undisputed, few issues like influence of etiology of heart failure (ischemic cardiomyopathy, diastolic dysfunction) and optimum interval between its detection and surgery, remain unresolved.

Postoperative pulmonary edema without any prior cardiac history is a separate entity, reported in 0.1% of all anesthetics administered, associated with laryngeal spasm, commonly seen in young healthy individuals after minor surgeries and has been called 'negative pressure pulmonary edema', but remains poorly understood. Chances of recovery are excellent and other associations are cases of pneumonectomy, lung transplants, or those operated in lateral positions.[35]

What remains undisputed is that patients scheduled for noncardiac surgery should be assessed to rule out presence of heart failure by careful history, physical examination, and exercise tolerance and where necessary by direct assessment of cardiac function at rest or stress.[24]

The ACC/AHA guidelines leave the final decision about employing echocardiography to assess cardiac function on the presence of risk factors (none to one or more) and to the discretion of physician with the phrase 'if likely to alter management'. In the Indian scenario, as discussed elsewhere too, other factors like high incidence of DM and CAD, including the possibility of 'silent CAD', relatively low reach of education, generally sedentary lifestyle, apathy and indifference towards health consciousness and wellness, and combined with relatively low cost involved for such an evaluation, should play a significant role and a low threshold for ordering a noninvasive ECG and echocardiography at rest and/or stress may be justified. However, there are no studies to justify such an approach and is a matter of individual preference.

The 2007 ACC/AHA perioperative guidelines for noncardiac surgery recommended that heart failure should be treated before noncardiac surgery and even postponement of surgery is appropriate while this is being accomplished. Guidelines do not mention any specific treatment.

Beta-blockers have been commonly used in patients undergoing noncardiac surgery, particularly in those at high risk, to prevent cardiovascular events. However, studies evaluating their efficacy and safety in this setting have produced inconsistent results and some have shown that beta-blockers may cause harm, reporting higher incidence of stroke and death. While those already receiving beta-blockers should continue perioperatively, initiation of beta-blockade preoperatively is controversial, and in acute decompensated heart failure is generally deferred.[36]

Significant valvular disease: Among valvular lesions, aortic and mitral lesions are more likely to lead to adverse cardiac events and poor outcomes after noncardiac surgery.

Aortic stenosis (AS) has been identified as a major risk factor and apart from other etiopathologies, also appears to be a part of aging, and since patients with aortic stenosis can remain asymptomatic for a long time, AS should be specifically looked for in elderly population. The risk of cardiac complications in patients with aortic stenosis undergoing noncardiac surgery is to the tune of 10–30%.

Aortic stenosis causes obstruction to the forward flow resulting in concentric hypertrophy of left ventricle that eventually leads to reduction in compliance and diastolic dysfunction. Simultaneous fall in coronary flow reserve would cause mismatch between myocardial demand and coronary blood flow supply and thus may result in myocardial ischemia. Patients with aortic stenosis tolerate hypotension poorly as coronary flow will reduce even further and are particularly vulnerable to fall in systemic vascular resistance. Therefore, clinical deterioration can occur in patients with asymptomatic aortic stenosis during the hemodynamic stress associated with noncardiac surgery (as well as other states that require augmentation of cardiac output such as infection, anemia, or pregnancy). Many adverse events, by appropriate management, can be prevented if diagnosis of aortic stenosis was known preoperatively.

To conclude, patients with significant aortic stenosis are at increased risk for cardiac complications, including intraoperative hypotension, myocardial infarction, ischemia, heart failure, arrhythmias, and death. Severe aortic stenosis should preferably undergo valve replacement, conventional or Transcatheter Aortic Valve Implantation (TAVI) as indicated, prior to noncardiac surgery. In addition, patients with aortic stenosis have a bleeding tendency due to the presence of an acquired form of von Willebrand syndrome.

Mitral stenosis (MS): Patients with mitral stenosis should be assessed for functional severity of the stenosis, their exercise tolerance and presence of heart failure and a detailed echocardiographic study should usually suffice. Patients with mild to moderate MS tolerate noncardiac surgery well but those with severe MS (valve area < 1 cm^2) and with signs and symptoms of heart failure and pulmonary hypertension should be considered for prior optimization, if need be by intervention. The goals of management should be to preserve normal sinus rhythm, avoid tachycardia, and maintain good gaseous exchange and cautious volume infusion.

Mitral regurgitation (MR): The severity of MR should be assessed by clinical examination and echocardiography that should include measurement of jet area, left atrial area occupied by regurgitation jet, and left ventricular end diastolic diameter (>45 mm synonymous with severe MR). Heart failure may need optimization with digoxin and diuretics. These patients tolerate bradycardia poorly and vasodilation is advocated.

Aortic regurgitation (AR): Severity of AR should be assessed by clinical examination and echocardiography. Left ventricular dysfunction and heart failure may complicate AR. These patients tolerate bradycardia and diastolic hypotension poorly. Patients with AR generally tolerate noncardiac surgery and anesthesia well.

Patients with valve prosthesis will need special attention to antibiotics coverage for prevention of infective endocarditis and those with mechanical valves should have plan for anticoagulation perioperatively that would require discontinuation of oral anticoagulants few days prior to planned surgery, monitoring of INR and switching over to heparin in the interim.

Arrhythmias: They can be form a simple innocuous sinus arrhythmia to life-threatening ventricular fibrillation, be totally asymptomatic or can cause syncope to a cardiac arrest, and is probably most commonly faced and feared cardiac abnormality in operating rooms and critical care setting, yet probably most poorly understood and managed entity. Arrhythmias once detected should be properly evaluated, requiring at times, the expertise of a cardiology electrophysiologist and management initiated as a part of optimization of a patient undergoing noncardiac surgery.

Arrhythmias need to be treated to relieve symptoms, to prevent death and hemodynamic collapse in case of life-threatening rhythm disorders and to reduce other risks like that of stroke in atrial fibrillation. Conditions like syncope or near syncope in patients with high degree AV block or bradycardia, wide complex rhythms including sustained ventricular tachycardia, atrial fibrillation or flutter with rapid or slow rates should be fully investigated and optimized under supervision of a specialist. It is important to remember that all antiarrhythmic drugs have the potential to induce or aggravate monomorphic VT, torsades de pointes, ventricular fibrillation (VF), conduction disturbances, or bradycardia, and due precautions be taken.

Presence of Cardiac Implantable Electronic Devices (CIED) like pacemaker or implantable cardioverters-defibrillator in a patient scheduled for noncardiac surgery need very careful assessment and planning. Adverse outcomes related to CIED could be device malfunction, damage to device, lead-tissue interface damage, inappropriate delivery of intended therapies resulting in hemodynamic instability, life-threatening arrhythmias, myocardial tissue damage and myocardial ischemia and infarction. The preparation and management should consider following:[37]

- Ascertaining presence of CIED and dependence on the device
- Identifying indication for the device placement
- Identifying the make and manufacturer through patient records, an X-ray chest may help at times if no details are available
- Determining whether electromagnetic interference (EMI) is likely to occur during the planned procedure
- Determining whether CIED needs to be reprogrammed to an asynchronous mode
- Exploring the possibility of deploying a bipolar electro-cautery system or ultrasonic (harmonic) scalpel
- Availability of temporary pacing and defibrillator in the operating room
- Discuss the interference that a surgical procedure like lithotripsy may cause to CIED and planning the alternatives with surgeons
- Use of non-conductive gloves by OT personnel to avoid electrical counter shock delivered by the device
- Appropriate anesthetic management that should include review of drugs patients is taking and appropriateness of their perioperative administration
- Choosing appropriate anesthetic technique least likely to interfere with CIED
- Overall ennsuring hemodynamic stability
- Direct arterial pressure waveform monitoring may help resolve many rhythm related issues
- Avoiding placement of central venous lines that could adversely affect CIED functioning
- Ensuring normal electrolytes and metabolic parameters.

However, it may not be out of place to quote word of caution from G Alec Rooke 'Perioperative management of pacemakers and implantable cardioverter defibrillators is neither trivial nor easy. These devices are complicated, and there are too many exceptions to allow formulation of simple rules for straightforward management.[38]

To address the complexity of issue and to provide expertise, University of Washington has deployed a team of specially trained anesthesiologists who take full charge of patients with CIED from interrogating devices before surgery until postoperative care and claim improved outcome.[39]

Obesity, obstructive sleep apnoea (OSA): A 2009 American Heart Association (AHA) scientific advisory on obesity has commented that noncardiac surgery may have adverse outcome due to its association with cardiac and pulmonary diseases.[40] Heart failure and myocardial steatosis (lipid deposition) have been implicated as causative factors. OSA has been associated with pulmonary hypertension, deep vein thrombosis and pulmonary embolism. There can be overlap of signs and symptoms of cardiac origin with those of obesity (breathlessness, edema) making individual assessment more difficult. In conclusion, obese patients should be assessed and evaluated carefully.

Elderly on account of reduced functional reserves, frailty and vulnerability for hypothermia and infections and frequent association with other conditions like aortic stenosis and CAD should be evaluated thoroughly for any ST changes, hypertension and arrhythmia.

Cardiac risk reassessment: Although perioperative cardiac management of patients undergoing noncardiac surgery has improved over past decades, it has still not been possible to predict individual risk. The outcome is a complex interplay of preoperative risk factors, individual patient's responses to interventions, interaction of various pharmacological agents between them and with the patient and several intraoperative and postoperative factors. The preoperative management is directed at defining risks and targeting them to optimize where feasible. Such an exercise generally provides straightforward unambiguous answers in only few situations as mentioned in step 2, but in a vast majority further risk stratification is required. These risk stratification tools are used in decision making for further noninvasive cardiac testing, and eventual optimization.

Several risk scoring modules have been developed, some have become outdated, others have been suitably revised (like original Goldman to Lee's Revised Cardiac Risk Index, RCRI) and few new ones too have been added. Overall, one is left with lack of clarity as to which one to use and when? Priebe[41] has questioned the European Society of Cardiology guidelines[5] recommendation to use clinical risk indices for postoperative risk stratification and RCRI for perioperative risk stratification with a sound logic that cardiac indices have several limitations, like they are not individualized for a patient; definition and diagnosis of risk factors like angina, MI and heart failure vary and can be highly subjective and risk factors do not specify duration of the exposure to the risk factor that could reflect its severity. Further inclusion of objective information like functional capacity, BNP, CRP and echocardiographic LV assessment could be important in making the assessment patient specific."

Risk Stratification Tools are generally of two types:[42]

Risk scores: Factors that affect the outcome are identified and certain weightings given to each one of them based on statistical calculations; the sum of the weightings read as risk score reflects risk applicable to a group of patients but is not individualized for a patient. For example, Lee's Revised Cardiac Risk Index states that likelihood of adverse cardiac event is 0.5% if no risk factors were present, 1% if one risk factor was present, 2.4% if two risk factors were present or 5.4% if three or more risk factors were present; risk calculated is not individualized.

Risk prediction tool: In a prediction tool, patient specific data is entered into the model, and it displays the patient's individual risk. Risk Prediction tools are more accurate to predict risk but are cumbersome to use. However, it must be added that though risk scoring is more user-friendly, its use too is not common in day-to-day clinical practice.

Goldman's risk index[43] was introduced in late 70s, became a gold standard but has largely been replaced with Lee's Revised Cardiac Risk Index (RCRI) following multiple limitations like some of the factors becoming irrelevant as major changes in the perioperative management took place over last few decades.

Detsky risk index was introduced in 1986 with few modifications[44] to Goldman's original risk scoring index but is said to have insufficient power to identify significant coronary artery disease in patients at the lower end of the spectrum of clinical risk and in vascular patients.[45]

Revised cardiac risk index (RCRI): Recognized six most important predictors (certain types of high-risk surgery, ischemic heart disease, history of heart failure, history of cerebrovascular disease, diabetes mellitus on insulin and renal dysfunction) and then went on to predict the likelihood of a major adverse cardiac event (myocardial infarction, pulmonary edema, cardiac arrest, or complete heart block, excluding all cause mortality) depending on the presence of number of risk factors in a given patient undergoing noncardiac surgery. The reported rates of major cardiac complication with 0, 1, 2, or 3 or more of these factors were 0.5%, 1.3%, 4%, and 9%, respectively, in the derivation cohort and 0.4%, 0.9%, 7%, and 11%, respectively, among 1422 patients in the validation cohort.[46] Subsequent studies predicting adverse outcomes in cardiac patients undergoing noncardiac surgery using RCRI have reported higher rate of events possibly due to inclusion of instances of death, emergency cases, relatively sicker patients and doing Troponin test (more sensitive index than CPK MB) in the study.

RCRI probably remains the most frequently used scoring model, and has worked well to predict adverse cardiac events in cardiac patients undergoing noncardiac *nonvascular* surgery. RCRI may underestimate true risk, and it does not predict all-cause mortality, which in any case it was not meant to.[47] RCRI has been used in several studies to assess the role of additional testing and the value of interventions during preoperative evaluation.

Eagle criteria: Eagle and colleagues identified five clinical predictors (angina, ventricular ectopics requiring treatment, Q-waves, diabetics receiving therapy and age of 70 or above) in patients advised preoperative dipyridamole or thallium imaging for postoperative adverse cardiac events. Application of these criteria and subsequent additions to identify high-risk patients to evaluate them further by noninvasive testing is useful for high and intermediate-risk patients while low-risk patients stand to benefit little from the noninvasive testing.[48]

Fleisher and eagle:[49] Fleisher and Eagle in their review added one more factor, poor functional status, to the existing five of RCRI (ischemic heart disease, heart failure, high-risk surgery, diabetes mellitus, renal insufficiency) to ascertain usefulness of further testing in patients undergoing noncardiac surgery, including vascular surgery and recommended that further evaluation would add value if one or more risk factors were present.

National Surgical Quality Improvement Program (NSQIP) risk model was developed in two stages: initially the authors determined the incidence of intra or postoperative Myocardial Infarction (MI) or Cardiac Arrest (MICA) in over 200,000 patients and then through multivariate regression analysis identified 5 predictors for MICA, namely type of surgery, functional state, renal dysfunction, advanced age and ASA class. Subsequently a model was developed and tested on another 257,385 patients that confirmed its high predictive accuracy. The authors claim NSQIP outperforms RCRI.[50] A simple online calculator is available and also has an 'app' that can be [*http://www.qxmd.com/calculate-online/cardiology/gupta-perioperative-cardiac-risk*] used at bedside on a smartphone to calculate individual patient risk. It is noteworthy that this tool does not take into account the direct preoperative information on stress test, echocardiography, arrhythmia, heart failure, cerebrovascular event, aortic valve disease or coronary artery disease.

By clicking on the "submit" button below, you acknowledge that you have read, understand, and agree to be bound by the terms of the QxMD Online Calculator End User Agreement

Estimate risk of perioperative myocardial infarction or cardiac arrest.

Age	75
Creatinine	>1.5 mg/dL/133 μmol/L
ASA Class	ASA 3 ASA 1 = Normal healthy patient ASA 2 = Patients with mild systemic disease ASA 3 = Patient with severe systemic disease ASA 4 = Patient with severe systemic disease that is a constant threat to life ASA 5 = Moribund patients who are not expected to survive without the operation
Preoperative Function	Partially dependent
Procedure	Urology

Submit

Gupta Perioperative Cardiac Risk

Estimated risk of perioperative myocardial infarction or cardiac arrest: 0.91%

About this calculator

This risk calculator provides an estimate of perioperative cardiac risk for individual patients based on a model derived from a large sample (>400,000) of patients. This is intended to supplement the clinician's own judgment and should not be taken as absolute. Certain limitations exist such as absence of information on preoperative stress test, echocardiography, arrhythmia, and aortic valve disease. Unfortunately, known/remote coronary artery disease (except prior PCI and cardiac surgery) was also not controlled for in the multivariate analysis. In spite of the absence of these variables, the predictive ability of the calculator as measured by c-statistic was 0.88 (88%) much higher than previous models such as Revised Cardiac Risk Index.

The details of the methodology are provided in the published paper.

Citations

Gupta PK, Gupta H, Sundaram A, Kaushik M, Fang X, Miller WJ, Esterbrooks DJ, Hunter CB, Pipinos II, Johanning JM, Lynch TG, Forse RA, Mohiuddin SM, Mooss AN. Development and validation of a risk calculator for prediction of cardiac risk after surgery. Circulation 2011;124(4):381-7 Epub 2011 Jul 5.

The two snapshot views show parameters that need to be entered (left panel) and the estimated prediction of MICA (right panel).

ADDITIONAL TESTS

Resting Echocardiography

Resting transthoracic echocardiography does not offer any specific information in a suspected coronary artery disease patient unless an event like myocardial infarction has already taken place. Its main utility is in assessing valvular heart disease such as aortic or mitral stenosis and regurgitation and left ventricular systolic function.

Exercise Testing

Exercise stress testing is usually preferred since exercise tolerance is more informative than ECG changes. Pharmacological stress testing is required in patients who cannot exercise, and the available options are thallium radionuclide myocardial perfusion imaging or dobutamine echocardiography.

Authors of DECREASE II study concluded that preoperative stress testing can safely be omitted in intermediate risk group who have stable or no coronary artery disease and heart rate has been controlled by preoperative beta-blockers. Only six of their patients were managed with preoperative revascularization.

Current Recommendations

After careful evaluation of various risk stratification tools and the recommendations, what emerges is that there is no consensus on an approach to a cardiac patient undergoing noncardiac surgery to either predict the risk of an adverse cardiac event or to recommend further noninvasive tests to optimize patient's preoperative status. However, what is evident is that there are certain risk factors, which are common to most of risk stratification tools implying that they indeed impact the incidence and outcome. While most of the studies do not support routine extensive preoperative testing in apparently healthy individual, the same appears justifiable in presence of certain comorbidities, though evidence again is sketchy.[51] The standard recommendations are:

- To proceed with further testing if there are three or more clinical risk factors with poor functional reserve and scheduled for high-risk surgery.
- Less well established in patient with one clinical risk factor having good functional capacity and scheduled for intermediate-risk surgery.
- Less well established in patient with one clinical risk factor having good functional capacity and scheduled for vascular surgery.

Stress testing has a very high negative predictive value for postoperative cardiovascular events (90–100%) but a low positive predictive value (6–67%), thus *stress testing is more useful for reducing estimated risk when found negative or normal than for identifying patients at very high risk when reported positive or abnormal.*[52] In general, indications for performing noninvasive stress tests are restrictive. It may be worth remembering that these tests in any case primarily detect flow-limiting lesions but not non-flow-limiting plaques, frequently source of myocardial infarctions.[32]

Choice of Stress Tests[53]

Following choice of stress tests is available:

Exercise ECG test: Sensitivity 74%, specificity 69%.

Thallium: Sensitivity 83% specificity 49%.

Dobutamine Stress Echo (DSE): Sensitivity 85% specificity 70%.

Exercise ECG is usually the preferred test since exercise tolerance appears to be more important than ECG response. It can be combined with echocardiography or perfusion imaging which provides more information in specific situations like reversible wall defects, ischemia occurring at low rates, paced ventricular rhythm, preexcitation syndrome, LBBB, etc. Cardiopulmonary exercise testing to assess functional capacity has been attempted by combining exercise testing with respiratory gas analysis but a meta-analysis done in 2012 concluded that the findings were inconsistent.[54] Dobutamine echocardiography and thallium radionuclide myocardial perfusion imaging are alternatives for patients who cannot exercise sufficiently to reach target rates like those with joint diseases, claudication, etc. Thallium imaging is usually preferred in patients with known cardiac arrhythmias, since dobutamine can induce atrial or ventricular arrhythmias, while dobutamine stress testing is preferred in patients with bronchospastic diseases and carotid artery disease as dipyridamole can induce bronchospasm and can cause fall in blood pressure. Dobutamine appears safe in patients of aortic aneurysm. Dobutamine stress test has additional advantage that it also provides information about valvular anatomy and ventricular function during rest and exercise.

DSE appears to have limited utility in patients at very low risk[55] and in lower risk patients taking a beta-blocker[56] though it provides additional prognostic information in patients who had three or more clinical risk factors. Prognostic information that could also be correlated is in those patients who had involvement of 5 or more segments exhibiting more cardiac events (36%) than in those with limited stress-induced ischemia (3%).

Special care should be taken in those patients who have hypotension during DSE, since its occurrence is associated with higher incidence of adverse cardiovascular outcome (cardiac death, infarction, and ischemia) in the perioperative period.[57]

Globally Applicable Recommendations and Regional Concerns

Taking the argument of justification little further, despite lack of clinching evidence, we in this part of the world, the Indian subcontinent, should take into account the fact that most of the studies are performed on patients belonging to different geographical regions with marked differences in patients physique, predilection for certain cardiac diseases, genetic predisposition, environmental, cultural and life-styles, levels of education and health awareness and food habits. We may have to consider resources that govern availability of perioperative monitoring and therapeutic facilities in the hospitals and vast difference in socioeconomic status in the two populace. Recommendations for invasive testing are usually beyond controversy, despite known complications, since patients would have 'earned' them independent of the disease state requiring a noncardiac surgical intervention. However, uncertainty or reluctance to subject a patient to noninvasive testing is mainly due to concerns of additional economic burden in absence of tangible benefits. There is an additional consideration in third world countries like India; higher incidence of coronary artery disease among urban and even rural population has led cardiologists to routinely advise annual preventive check-up including provocative cardiac stress for public at large. The relatively affordable tests set against a high yield of positive results in asymptomatic subjects probably justifies carrying out same strategy to patients presenting for elective noncardiac surgery. Comparative cost of certain tests including noninvasive or minimally invasive tests like stress echocardiography or CT angiography is low when compared to western world. Considering value addition that such tests may offer to a populace that is not only genetically prone to coronary artery disease but even its reach to health and education is suboptimal, this author is inclined to recommend a lower threshold for ordering such tests at least in a select population. An adequately powered multicenter study comprising of Indian patients, is required to justify or refute a recommendation such as this, based solely on general perception and individual experience.

Our approach would be:

- *Evaluate the patient:* If surgery is urgent and can not be postponed, stabilize the patient as much possible and go ahead with surgery.
- Evaluate the patient for elective surgery. Take detailed history for past illnesses, present symptoms and carefully and painstakingly assess functional capacity. All patients with poor exercise tolerance should also be evaluated by a cardiologist and go through a similar exercise of evaluation and optimization.

  If patient has history of, or is currently having symptoms suggestive of any of the following, patient should be referred to a cardiologist for further evaluation and stabilization:

- Angina, or history suggestive of angina
- MI
- Ischemic heart disease (IHD) or history suggestive of IHD
- Heart failure, current or history of
- Significant arrhythmia
- Severe valvular disease
- Cerebrovascular disease
- Obesity
- Sleep apnea
- Physiological age of 70 years or more (subjective assessment on physician's discretion, even a 40+ patient with diabetes and/or hypertension and/or family history may be recommended a stress test)
- Diabetes mellitus, on insulin therapy or poorly controlled (HbA1c >8)
- Renal insufficiency (Serum creatinine of 2 mmol/dL or more).

The practice of declaring a patient as 'fit' or 'cardiac clearance given' by the cardiologist should be dispensed with as alluded to earlier. After careful evaluation, additional testing with probably a lower threshold for noninvasive/minimally invasive testing, and subsequent optimization, the cardiologist should simply assign a low or high risk for a likely adverse cardiac event to the patient. It would then be appropriate to discuss the *probability* with the patients and family jointly by the surgeon, anesthesiologist and cardiologist and plan a future course of action. Communication and consensus among the anesthesiologist, cardiologist and surgeon are crucial requisites, and they should, as a team, counsel the patient and family and obtain an informed consent.

OPTIMIZATION OF PATIENT STATUS WITH MEDICATIONS AND/OR INTERVENTIONS

The dilemma of which patient should be subjected to further interventional management continues well beyond ordering the tests themselves. Only a normal stress test probably has a straightforward answer to go ahead with the planned surgery. A mildly positive test can again generate a controversy since most of the studies do not support further invasive testing though the surgical team, mainly anesthesiologists, would feel uncomfortable going ahead with such borderline situation. Evidence, however, is in favor of only preoperative optimization with statins and beta-blockers. The dose and duration of such therapy before surgery again is a matter of patient's overall condition and pathophysiology of the contemplated surgery.

Beta-blockers

Dutch Echocardiographic Cardiac Risk Evaluation Applying Stress Echocardiography (DECREASE) series of studies have been undertaken to evaluate the effect of beta-blockers, statins and revascularization on postoperative adverse cardiac outcomes in cardiac patients. DECREASE series of studies with their findings are listed below. The studies generally have concluded that preoperative use of betablockers and statins reduce the incidence of adverse cardiac events in short as well as long-term while preoperative revascularization does not provide any additional protection.

DECREASE I found that perioperative beta-blockade with bisoprolol reduces cardiac death and MI significantly in short and long-term in high-risk patients undergoing noncardiac surgery reduces cardiac death and MI in the short- and long-term.

DECREASE II concluded that intermediate risk patients on the basis of clinical assessment and receiving bisoprolol to maintain resting heart rate at 60–65 beats per minute do not need preoperative echocardiographic cardiac stress testing.

DECREASE III elucidated the significant role of fluvastatin XL in reducing myocardial ischemia, MI and death high-risk patients undergoing major vascular surgery.

DECREASE IV showed that while bisoprolol significantly reduces cardiac death and MI, fluvastatin had a nonsignificant beneficial effect in intermediate-risk patients.

DECREASE V found that preoperative coronary revascularization in high-risk patients (with extensive stress-induced ischemia), did not contribute additional advantage if rates were already well controlled by prior administration of bisoprolol.[58]

While most of the studies do support the beneficial role of beta-blockers and statins taken preoperatively in reducing adverse cardiac events in patients undergoing noncardiac surgery, there are studies that have reported negative results as well. POISE study[59] has raised concerns about the use of beta-blockers perioperatively; the study reported reduced risk of cardiac death and MI but increased risk of stroke and overall death in patients given metoprolol. The study however has been criticized for high doses used and immediate preoperative timing of the beta-blocker, though the sheer size of the sample has impacted many meta-analyses that included the study and to a great extent the AHA/ACC focused update released in 2009. AHA/ACC guidelines recommend only one class I indication for perioperative beta-blocker therapy: continuation of beta-blockers in patients already taking beta-blockers.[60] European guidelines though recommend two more indications in addition for starting preoperative betablocker therapy: patients with known coronary artery disease or evidence of myocardial ischemia on stress testing and patients undergoing high risk surgery.[61] Both the guidelines recommend that the beta-blockers be started days to weeks in advance and the target heart rate should be 60–80 beats per minute and hypotension should be avoided. It is important that other causes of tachycardia be treated before starting beta-blockers.

Algorithm for preoperative cardiac risk assessment and management after Priebe (with permission)[41]

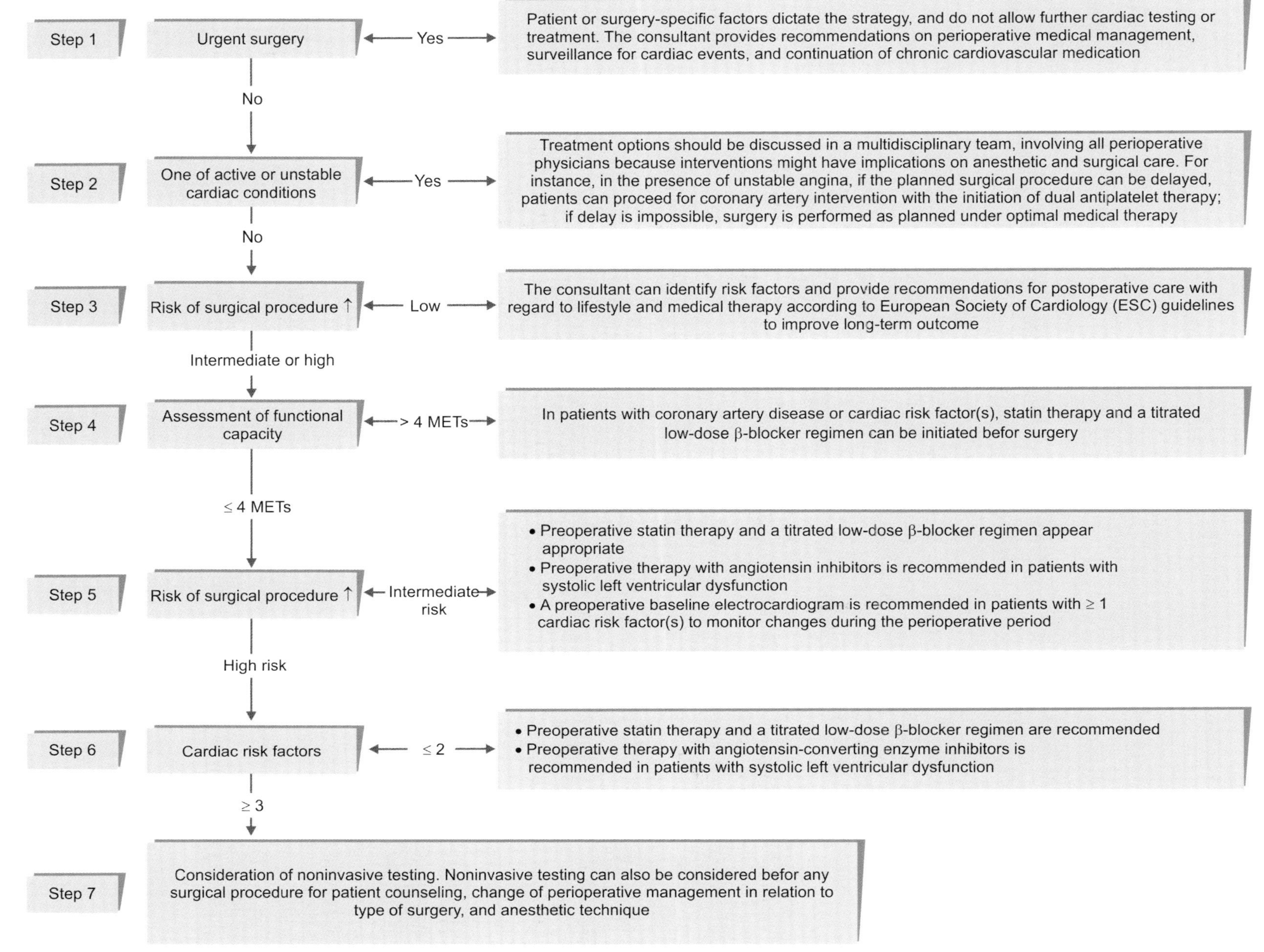

Step 1
Urgent surgery
Yes
Patient or surgery-specific factors dictate the strategy, and do not allow further cardiac testing or treatment. The consultant provides recommendations on perioperative medical management, surveillance for cardiac events, and continuation of chronic cardiovascular medication
No
Step 2
One of active or unstable cardiac conditions
Yes
Treatment options should be discussed in a multidisciplinary team, involving all perioperative physicians because interventions might have implications on anesthetic and surgical care. For instance, in the presence of unstable angina, if the planned surgical procedure can be delayed, patients can proceed for coronary artery intervention with the initiation of dual antiplatelet therapy; if delay is impossible, surgery is performed as planned under optimal medical therapy
No
Step 3
Risk of surgical procedure ↑
Low
The consultant can identify risk factors and provide recommendations for postoperative care with regard to lifestyle and medical therapy according to European Society of Cardiology (ESC) guidelines to improve long-term outcome
Intermediate or high
Step 4
Assessment of functional capacity
> 4 METs
In patients with coronary artery disease or cardiac risk factor(s), statin therapy and a titrated low-dose β-blocker regimen can be initiated befor surgery
≤ 4 METs
Step 5
Risk of surgical procedure ↑
Intermediate risk
• Preoperative statin therapy and a titrated low-dose β-blocker regimen appear appropriate
• Preoperative therapy with angiotensin inhibitors is recommended in patients with systolic left ventricular dysfunction
• A preoperative baseline electrocardiogram is recommended in patients with ≥ 1 cardiac risk factor(s) to monitor changes during the perioperative period
High risk
Step 6
Cardiac risk factors
≤ 2
• Preoperative statin therapy and a titrated low-dose β-blocker regimen are recommended
• Preoperative therapy with angiotensin-converting enzyme inhibitors is recommended in patients with systolic left ventricular dysfunction
≥ 3
Step 7
Consideration of noninvasive testing. Noninvasive testing can also be considered befor any surgical procedure for patient counseling, change of perioperative management in relation to type of surgery, and anesthetic technique

Suggested algorithm for preoperative evaluation of cardiac patient undergoing noncardiac surgery

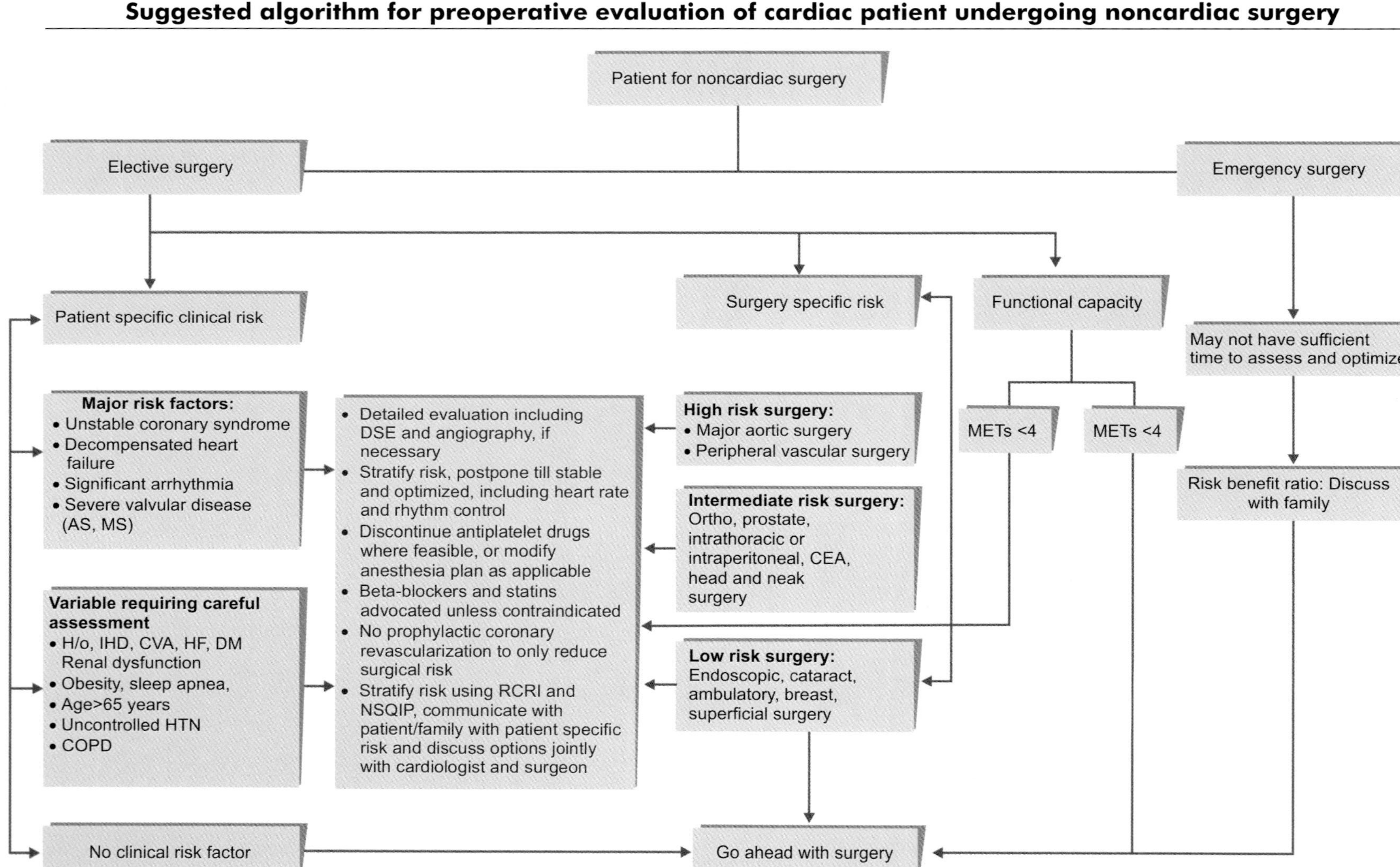

Statins

Statins, apart from their lipid lowering effect, have also been credited with pleiotropic effects that improve endothelial function and stabilize plaques. Statins have beneficial effects even if started one day before the surgery, though earlier the better.[62-66] Preoperative withdrawal of chronic statin therapy has been associated with adverse outcomes.[67,68]

Revascularization

What does one do when faced with a stress inducible myocardial ischemia? Only medical management may fail to provide sufficient cardioprotection, though studies have shown that preoperative prophylactic coronary revascularization too does not improve patient outcomes in this patient population.[69,70] However, following conditions merit serious consideration for preoperative revascularization as recommended by different guidelines (ACC/AHA and ESC):

- High-risk unstable angina or non-ST-elevation myocardial infarction,
- Acute ST-elevation myocardial infarction,
- Angina and left main or three-vessel disease, or
- Angina and two-vessel disease if this includes proximal left anterior descending (LAD) stenosis as well as left ventricular (LV) dysfunction or ischemia on stress testing.

Even when guidelines are followed, the proportion of patients subjected to revascularization is quite low, as is evident in three studies which included only symptomatic patients (2–11% patients underwent coronary angiography and only 0–2% underwent preoperative revasularization).[71-74]

In general, a very highly individualized approach is recommended. A patient should not be subjected to a prophylactic revascularization only to 'optimize prior to noncardiac surgery' unless the cardiac status on its own deserves the intervention. However, if a patient needs a revascularization, several factors like likely interval between intervention and noncardiac surgery, severity of patient's cardiac status and the disease, and patient preference would determine the timing and type of revascularization.[78]

Algorithms

Since the preoperative evaluation of a cardiac patient for noncardiac surgery is complex subject, an algorithmic approach may appear to be a simpler solution. Algorithms are difficult to write, appear easy to follow and yet do not find wider acceptability. Several algorithms have been written by various authors, two simpler examples are reproduced here one suggested by Priebe based on ESC and other practiced at author's institute.

REFERENCES

1. Weiser TG, Regenbogen SG, Thompson KD, Haynes AB, Lipsitz SR, Berry WR, et al. An estimation of the global volume of surgery: a modelling strategy based on available data. Lancet. 2008;372:139-44.
2. Sabaté S, Mases A, Guilera N, Canet J, Castillo J, Orrego C, et al. Incidence and predictors of major perioperative adverse cardiac and cerebrovascular events in non-cardiac surgery. BJA. 2011;107:879-90.
3. Wijeysundera DN, Austin PC, Beattie WS, Hux JE, Laupacis A. Outcomes and processes of care related to preoperative medical consultation. Arch Intern Med. 2010;170:1365-74.
4. Poldermans D, Bax J, Boersma E, et al. Guidelines for pre-operative cardiac risk assessment and peri-operative cardiac management in non-cardiac surgery: the Task Force for Preoperative Cardiac Risk Assessment and Peri-operative Cardiac Management in Non-cardiac Surgery of the European Society of Cardiology (ESC) and endorsed by the European Society of Anaesthesiology (ESA). Eur Heart J. 2009;30:2769-812.
5. Mangano DT, Goldman L. Preoperative assessment of patients with known or suspected coronary disease. N Engl J Med. 1995; 333:1750.
6. Devereaux PJ, Goldman L, Cook DJ, et al. Perioperative cardiac events in patients undergoing noncardiac surgery: a review of the magnitude of the problem, the pathophysiology of the events and methods to estimate and communicate risk. CMAJ. 2005; 173:627-34.
7. Criqui MH, Langer RD, Fronek A, Feigelson HS, Klauber MR, McCann TJ, et al. Mortality over a period of 10 years in patients with peripheral arterial disease. N Engl J Med. 1992;326:381-6.
8. Wong T, Detsky AS. Preoperative cardiac risk assessment for patients having peripheral vascular surgery. Ann Intern Med. 1992;116:743-53.
9. Kelly R, Staines A, MacWalter R, Stonebridge P, Tunstall-Pedoe H, Struthers AD. The prevalence of treatable left ventricular systolic dysfunction in patients who present with noncardiac vascular episodes: a case-control study. J Am CollCardiol. 2002;39:219-24.
10. Stampfer MJ, Grodstein F, Bechtel S. Postmenopausal estrogen and cardiovascular disease. Contemp Intern Med. 1994;6:47-56, 59.
11. India Disease incidence and Prevalence Report #CS 301IN - February 2012, *http://www.medtechinsight.com*)
12. Slininger KA, Haddadin AS, Mangi AA. Perioperative management of patients with left ventricular assist devices undergoing noncardiac surgery. J Cardiothorac Vasc Anesth. 2013;27:752-9.
13. Fleisher LA, Fleischmann KE, Auerbach AD, Barnason SA, Beckman JA, Bozkurt B, et al. 2014 ACC/AHA guideline on perioperative cardiovascular evaluation and management of patients undergoing noncardiac surgery: executive summary: a report of the ACC/AHA Task Force on Practice Guidelines. Circulation. 2014;130(24):2215-45.
14. Rao TL, Jacobs KH, El-Etr AA. Reinfarction following anesthesia in patients with myocardial infarction. Anesthesiology. 1983; 59:499-505.
15. Eagle KA, Berger PB, Calkins H, Chaitman BR, Ewy GA, Fleischmann KE, et al. ACC/AHA guideline update for perioperative cardiovascular evaluation for noncardiac

surgery--executive summary: a report of the American College of Cardiology/American Heart Association Task Force on Practice Guidelines (Committee to Update the 1996 Guidelines on Perioperative Cardiovascular Evaluation for Noncardiac Surgery). J Am Coll Cardiol. 2002;39:542-53.
16. Nuttall GA, Brown MJ, Stombaugh JW, Michon PB, Hathaway MF, et al. Time and cardiac risk of surgery after bare-metal stent percutaneous coronary intervention. Anesthesiology. 2008;109: 588-95.
17. Rabbitts JA, Nuttall GA, Brown MJ, Hanson AC, Oliver WC, Holmes DR, Rihal CS. Cardiac risk of noncardiac surgery after percutaneous coronary intervention with drug-eluting stents. Anesthesiology. 2008;109:596-604.
18. Grines CL, Bonow RO, Casey DE Jr, Gardner TJ, Lockhart PB, Moliterno DJ, O'Gara P, et al. Prevention of premature discontinuation of dual antiplatelet therapy in patients with coronary artery stents: A science advisory from the American Heart Association, American College of Cardiology, Society for Cardiovascular Angiography and Interventions, American College of Surgeons, and American Dental Association, with representation from the American College of Physicians. Circulation. 2007;115:813-8.
19. Chassot PG, Delabays A, Spahn DR. Perioperative antiplatelet therapy: The case for continuing therapy in patients at risk of myocardial infarction. Br J Anaesth. 2007;99:316-28.
20. Vicenzi MN, Meislitzer T, Heitzinger B, Halaj M, Fleisher LA, Metzler H. Coronary artery stenting and noncardiac surgery: A prospective outcome study. Br J Anaesth. 2006;96:686-93.
21. Oprea AD, Popescu WM. ADP-receptor inhibitors in the perioperative period: the good, the bad, and the ugly. J Cardiothorac Vasc Anesth. 2013;27(4):779-95.
22. Devereaux PJ, Mrkobrada M, Sessler DI, Leslie K, Alonso-Coello P, Kurz A, et al. POISE-2 Investigators. Aspirin in patients undergoing noncardiac surgery. N Engl J Med. 2014;370:1494-503.
23. Gerstein NS, et al. Perioperative Aspirin Management After POISE-2: Some Answer but Questions Remain. Anesth Anal. 2015;120:570-5.
24. Schrör K. Why we should not skip aspirin in cardiovascular prevention. Hamostaseologie. 2015;35(20150420). Ahead of print.
25. Fleisher LA, Fleischmann KE, Auerbach AD, Barnason SA, Beckman JA, Bozkurt B, et al. 2014 ACC/AHA guideline on perioperative cardiovascular evaluation and management of patients undergoing noncardiac Surgery: executive summary: a report of the American College of Cardiology/American Heart Association Task Force on Practice Guidelines. J Am Coll Cardiol. 2014;64:e77-e137.
26. Kibird MB. Aspirin in perioperative period: a review of the recent literature. Curr Opin Anesthesiol. 2015;28:349-55.
27. Khadimi K. Update on perioperative care of cardiac patient for noncardiac surgery. Curr Opin Anesthesiol. 2015;28:342-8.
28. Horlocker TT, Wedel DJ, Rowlingson JC, et al. Regional anesthesia in the patient receiving antithrombotic or thrombolytic therapy: American Society of Regional Anesthesia and Pain Medicine Evidence-Based guidelines (Third Edition). Reg Anesth Pain Med. 2010;35:64-101.
29. Beynon C, et al. Initial experiences with Multiplate for rapid assessment of anriplatelet agent activity in neurosurgical emergencies. Clin Neurol Neurosurg. 2013;115:2003-08.
30. Jaben EA, et al. Reversing the effects of antiplatelet agents in the setting of intracranial haemorrhage: a look at the literature. J Intensive Care Medicine. 2015;30:3-7.
31. Hammill BG, Curtis LH, Bennett-Guerrero E, et al. Impact of heart failure on patients undergoing major noncardiac surgery. Anesthesiology. 2008;108:559-67.
32. Goldman L, Caldera DL, Nussbaum SR, et al. Multifactorial index of cardiac risk in noncardiac surgical procedures. N Engl J Med. 1977;297:845-50.
33. Charlson ME, MacKenzie CR, Gold JP, Ales KL, Topkins M, Shires GT. Risk for postoperative congestive heart failure. Surg Gynecol Obstet. 1991;172:95-104.
34. Mangano DT, Browner WS, Hollenberg M, London MJ, Tubau JF, Tateo IM. Association of perioperative myocardial ischemia with cardiac morbidity and mortality in men undergoing noncardiac surgery. The Study of Perioperative Ischemia Research Group. N Engl J Med. 1990;323:1781-8.
35. McConkey PP. Postobstructive pulmonary oedema--a case series and review. Anaesth Intensive Care. 2000;28:72-6.
36. Fleisher LA, Beckman JA, Brown KA, Calkins H, Chaikof EL, Fleischmann KE, et al. 2009 ACCF/AHA focused update on perioperative beta blockade incorporated into the ACC/AHA 2007 guidelines on perioperative cardiovascular evaluation and care for noncardiac surgery: a report of the American college of cardiology foundation/American heart association task force on practice guidelines. Circulation. 2009;120:e169-276.
37. The American Society of Anesthesiologists Task Force on Perioperative Management of Patients with Cardiac Implantable Electronic Devices presents a Practice Advisory for the Perioperative Management of Patients with Cardiac Implantable Electronic Devices: Pacemakers and Implantable Cardioverter-Defibrillators. Anesthesiology. 2011;114:247-61.
38. Rooke GA, Bowdie TA. Perioperative management of pacemakers and implantable cardioverter defibrillators: it's is not just about the magnet. Anasth Analg. 2013;117:292-4.
39. Rooke GA, Natrajan K, Lombaard S, Dziersk J, Van Norman G, Poole J. Initial experience of an anesthesia-based service for perioperative management of CIEDs. Anesthesiology 2012;117: A835.
40. Poirier P, Alpert MA, Fleisher LA, Thompson PD, Sugerman HJ, Burke LE, et al. Cardiovascular evaluation and management of severely obese patients undergoing surgery: a science advisory from the American Heart Association. Circulation. 2009;120:86-95.
41. Priebe HJ. Preoperative cardiac management of the patient for non-cardiac surgery: an individualized and evidence-based approach. British Journal of Anaesthesia. 2011;107: 83-96.
42. Moonesinghe SR. Risk stratification tools for major noncardiac surgery. Anesthesiology. 2013;119:959-8.
43. Goldman L, Caldera DL, Nussbaum SR, Southwick FS, Krogstad D, Murray B, et al. Multifactorial index of cardiac risk in noncardiac surgical procedures. N Engl J Med. 1977;297:845-50.
44. Detsky AS, Abrams HB, McLaughlin JR, Drucker DJ, Sasson Z, Johnston N, et al. Predicting cardiac complications in patients undergoing noncardiac surgery. J Gen Intern Med. 1986;1:211-9.
45. Younis LT, Miller DD, Chaitman BR. Preoperative strategies to assess cardiac risk before noncardiac surgery. Clin Cardiol. 1995;18:447-54.
46. Lee TH, Marcantoni, ER, Mangion, CM, et al. Derivation and prospective validation of a simple index for prediction of cardiac risk of major noncardiac surgery. Circulation. 1999; 100:1043-9.
47. Ford MK, Beattie WS, Wijeysundera DN. Systematic review: prediction of perioperative cardiac complications and mortality by the revised cardiac risk index. Ann Intern Med. 2010;152:26-35.
48. Eagle KA, Coley CM, Newell JB, Brewster DC, Darling RC, Strauss HW, et al. Combining clinical and thallium data

optimizes preoperative assessment of cardiac risk before major vascular surgery. Ann Intern Med. 1989;110:859-66.
49. Fleisher LA, Eagle KA. Clinical practice: Lowering cardiac risk in noncardiac surgery. N Engl J Med. 2001;345:1677-82.
50. Gupta PK, Gupta H, Sundaram A, Kaushik M, Fang X, Miller WJ et al. Development and validation of a risk calculator for prediction of cardiac risk after surgery. Circulation. 2011;124:381-7.
51. Johansson T, Fritsch G, Flamm M, Hansbauer B, Bock NM, Sonnichsen AC. Effectiveness of non-cardiac preoperative testing innon-cardiac elective surgery: a systematic review. BJA. 2013;110:926-39.
52. Auerbach A, Goldman L. Assessing and reducing the cardiac risk of noncardiac surgery. Circulation. 2006;113:1361-7.
53. Kertai MD, Boersma E, Bax JJ, Heijenbrok-Kal MH, Hunink MG, L'talien GJ, et al. A meta-analysis comparing the prognostic accuracy of six diagnostic tests for predicting perioperative cardiac risk in patients undergoing major vascular surgery. Heart. 2003;89:1327-34.
54. Young EL, Karthikesalingam A, Huddart S, Pearse RM, Hinchliffe RJ, Loftus IM, et al. A systematic review of the role of cardiopulmonary exercise testing in vascular surgery. Eur J Vasc Endovasc Surg. 2012;44:64-71.
55. Poldermans D, Arnese M, Fioretti PM, Salustri A, Boersma E, Thomson IR, et al. Improved cardiac risk stratification in major vascular surgery with dobutamine-atropine stress echocardiography. J Am Coll Cardiol. 1995;26:648-53.
56. Boersma E, Poldermans D, Bax JJ, Steyerberg EW, Thomson IR, Banga JD, et al. Predictors of cardiac events after major vascular surgery: Role of clinical characteristics, dobutamine echocardiography, and beta-blocker therapy. JAMA. 2001; 285:1865-73.
57. Day SM, Younger JG, Karavite D, Bach DS, Armstrong WF, Eagle KA. Usefulness of hypotension during dobutamine echocardiography in predicting perioperative cardiac events. Am J Cardiol. 2000;85:478-83.
58. Poldermans D, Schouten O, Vidakovic R, Bax JJ, Thomson IR, Hoeks SE, et al. A clinical randomized trial to evaluate the safety of a noninvasive approach in high-risk patients undergoing major vascular surgery: the DECREASE-V Pilot Study. J Am Coll Cardiol. 2007;49:1763-9.
59. POISE Study Group. Effects of extended-release metoprolol succinatein patients undergoing non-cardiac surgery (POISE trial): arandomised controlled trial. Lancet. 2008;371:1839-47.
60. Fleisher LA, Beckman JA, Brown KA, Calkins H, Chaikof EL, Fleischmann KE, et al. 2009 ACCF/AHA focused update on perioperative beta blockade incorporated into the ACC/AHA 2007 guidelines on perioperative cardiovascular evaluation and care for noncardiac surgery: a report of the American college of cardiology foundation/American heart association task force on practice guidelines. Circulation. 2009;120:e169.
61. Poldermans D, Bax J, Boersma E, De Hert S, Eeckhout E, Fowkes G, et al. Guidelines for pre-operative cardiac risk assessment and peri-operative cardiac management in non-cardiac surgery: the Task Force for Preoperative Cardiac Risk Assessment and Peri-operative Cardiac Management in Non-cardiac Surgery of the European Society of Cardiology (ESC) and endorsed by the European Society of Anaesthesiology (ESA). Eur Heart J. 2009; 30:2769-812.
62. Libby P, Aikawa M. Mechanisms of plaque stabilization with statins. Am J Cardiol. 2003;91:4B-8B;
63. Ito MK, Talbert RL, Tsimikas S. Statin-associated pleiotropy: possiblebeneficial effects beyond cholesterol reduction. Pharmacotherapy. 2006;26:85S-97S.
64. Ray KK, Cannon CP. The potential relevance of the multiplelipid-independent (pleiotropic) effects of statins in the management of acute coronary syndromes. J Am Coll Cardiol. 2005;46: 1425-33.
65. Klingenberg R, Hansson GK. Treating inflammation in atherosclerotic cardiovascular disease: emerging therapies. Eur Heart J. 2009;30:2838-44.
66. Hindler K, Shaw A, Samuels J, Fulton S, Collard C, Riedel B. Improved postoperative outcomes associated with preoperative statin therapy. Anesthesiology. 2006;105:1260-72.
67. Le Manach Y, Godet G, Coriat P, et al. The impact of postoperative discontinuation or continuation of chronic statin therapyon cardiac outcome after major vascular surgery. Anesth Analg. 2007;104:1326-33.
68. Schouten O, Hoeks SE, Welten GMJM, et al. Effect of statin withdrawalon frequency of cardiac events after vascular surgery. Am J Cardiol. 2007;100:316-20.
69. McFalls EO, Ward HB, Moritz TE, Goldman S, Krupski WC, Littooy F, et al. Coronary-artery revascularizationbefore elective major vascular surgery. N Engl J Med. 2004;351:2795-804.
70. Garcia S, Moritz TE, Goldman S , Littooy F, Pierpont G, Larsen GC, et al. Perioperative complications after vascular surgery are predicted by the revised cardiac risk index but are not reduced in high-risk subsets with preoperative revascularization. Circ Cardiovasc Qual Outcomes. 2009;2:73-7.
71. Monaco M, Stassano P, Di Tommaso L, Pepino P, Giordano A, Pinna GB, et al. Systematic strategy of prophylactic coronary angiography improves long-term outcome after major vascular surgery in medium- to high-risk patients: a prospective, randomized study. J Am Coll Cardiol. 2009;54:989-96.
72. Bartels C, Bechtel JF, Hossmann V, Horsch S. Cardiac risk stratification for high-risk vascular surgery. Circulation. 1997;95: 2473-5.
73. Froehlich JB, Karavite D, Russman PL, Erdem N, Wise C, Zelenock G, et al. American College of Cardiology/American Heart Association preoperative assessment guidelines reduce resource utilization before aortic surgery. J Vasc Surg. 2002; 36:758-63.
74. Almanaseer Y, Mukherjee D, Kline-Rogers EM, Kesterson SK, Sonnad SS, Rogers B, et al. Implementation of the ACC/AHA guidelines for preoperative cardiac risk assessment in a general medicine preoperative clinic: improving efficiency and preserving outcomes. Cardiology. 2005;103:24-29.
75. Mangano DT, Goldman L. Preoperative assessment of patients with known or suspected coronary disease. N Engl J Med. 1995; 333:1750-6.
76. Girish M, Trayner E Jr, Dammann O, Pinto-Plata V, Celli B. Symptom-limited stair climbing as a predictor of postoperative cardiopulmonary complications after high-risk surgery. Chest. 2001;120:1147-51.
77. Reilly DF, McNeely MJ, Doerner D, Greenberg DL, Staiger TO, Geist MJ, et al. Self-reported exercise tolerance and the risk of serious perioperative complications. Arch Intern Med. 1999; 159:2185-92.
78. Rade JJ, Hogue CW. Noncardiac surgery for patients with coronary artery stents, timing is everything. Anesthesiology. 2008;109:573-5.

28

Minimally Invasive Cardiac Surgery: Has it Delivered its Promise?

Yugal K Mishra, Syed Asrar Ahmed Qadri

INTRODUCTION

Endoscopic procedures have been introduced in nearly all surgical disciplines during the last few decades and have become the standard of care. Patients are increasingly requesting less invasive procedures. In an attempt to achieve this and also maintain or improve on results of full median sternotomy many minimally invasive and endoscopic approaches have been tried in the cardiac surgery. In the 1990s when minimally invasive cardiac surgery (MICS) was introduced, concern centered on longer operations, greater risk, and more complications for the perceived benefit of better cosmetic results, better respiratory function, and less pain and bleeding. The adoption of minimally invasive techniques in cardiac surgery and especially for coronary artery bypass grafting (CABG) is challenging due to following reasons. First, cardiac surgery is not straightforward and adding endoscopic approaches further increases the complexity; second, until recently the cardiac surgery community had no endoscopic surgical tradition; and third, the use of conventional thoracoscopic instrumentation in early attempts to perform cardiac surgery failed completely.[1]

Open operations for acquired heart disease have been standardized, but cardiac surgery results are heavily scrutinized despite low mortality and excellent results, so the bar has been raised for any new technique that will cause a paradigm shift in the scenario of cardiac surgery, which has slowed its adoption.

Surgical outcomes are better with minimal access (Fig. 28.1) as compared to full sternotomy in terms of cosmesis, postoperative pain, bleeding and transfusion, respiratory function and length of ICU and hospital stay.[2-4] However, there is also a concern about longer operation times, greater risk, and more complications.

Less bleeding and fewer transfusions are likely due to the less extensive mediastinal dissection required for the minimally invasive approach. Less pain is likely due to less surgical dissection, and less spreading of the sternum and no stretch on the posterior rib head and costovertebral ligaments as chest is not widely opened as a trap door. The better pulmonary function can be explained by no interference with the diaphragm or dissection along it.

Also with less chest wall pain, patients might have less splinting of the chest and thus can breathe easy.

Robotic cardiac surgery was developed in order to overcome the limitations and difficulties associated with minimally invasive surgery and to improve the abilities of cardiac surgeon. A surgical robot allows the surgeon to perform surgery by instruments on robotic arms that are controlled by him from a console situated away from the operating table. A wide array of procedures is possible through small 1–2 cm incisions using robotic control, visualization, dexterity, and precision.

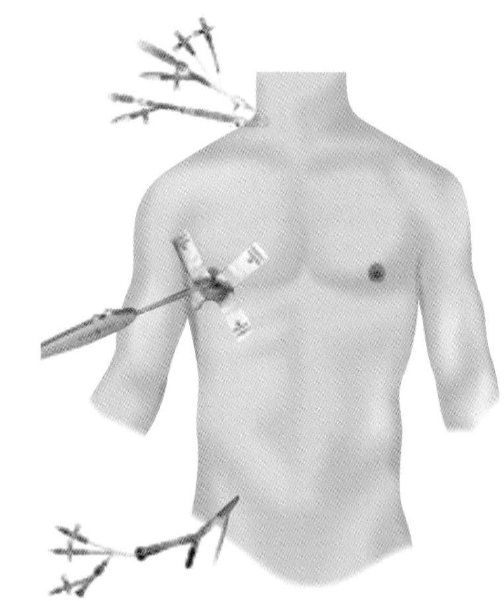

Fig. 28.1 Minimal access cardiac surgery

The aim of advanced cardiac surgery is to ameliorate two potentially invasive components of conventional cardiac surgery: (1) cardiopulmonary bypass (CPB) machine and (2) sternotomy. In order to reduce the morbidity of conventional cardiac surgery and to maintain same safety and efficiency, surgeons were mandated to develop and adopt lesser invasive approaches.

INVASIVENESS OF CONVENTIONAL CARDIAC SURGERY

There are four major invasive aspects of conventional cardiac surgery, which have demerits of their own:

1. *CPB machine*: Use of pump has been the backbone of all cardiac surgeries till recently when off-pump techniques were developed for CABG. Use of pump causes a multitude of derangements in many homeostatic mechanisms like coagulation and compliments. In short, it causes systemic inflammatory response syndrome. Normal body organs have lot of reserve capability to overcome this trauma, but CPB can have a major influence in case of a patient with borderline organ dysfunction like chronic renal failure, liver dysfunction, and chronic obstructive pulmonary disease (COPD). CPB is also associated with neurocognitive changes either short-term or long-term.
2. *Sternotomy*: The trauma of access is much more than trauma of surgery. It is a cause of major morbidity especially in old patients with osteoporotic sternum, diabetes, immunocompromised status, obesity and also in redo cases.
3. *Aortic manipulation*: Cannulation, partial or complete clamping of aorta is not tolerated well especially in patients with aortic atherosclerosis and can be a cause of major or minor stroke.
4. *Conduits harvest*: Harvest of conduits like long saphenous vein, radial artery requires pretty long incision that can be much more morbid than main operation, especially in patients with obesity, diabetes, and old age.

The various minimally invasive cardiac procedures are listed below:

1. Coronary artery surgery
   a. MIDCAB—minimally invasive direct coronary artery bypass
      i. Anterior
      ii. Lateral
      iii. Anterolateral
      iv. Transabdominal
   b. MICS CABG—minimally invasive cardiac surgery coronary artery bypass grafting
2. Endoscopic conduit harvest
3. Minimally invasive valve surgery
4. Minimally invasive atrial septal defect (ASD) surgery
5. Other minimally invasive cardiac procedures
6. Robotic cardiac surgery
   a. Robot-assisted CABG (RACABG)
   b. Totally endoscopic coronary artery bypass (TECAB)
   c. Robotic ASD closure
   d. Robotic valve surgery.

MINIMALLY INVASIVE CORONARY ARTERY BYPASS GRAFTING

Early attempts at sternal sparing techniques for coronary bypass surgery began in mid-1990s.[5] These mostly involved a left anterior thoracotomy, direct harvest of left internal mammary artery (LIMA), and beating heart anastomosis to the left anterior descending (LAD) coronary artery. This procedure was called MIDCAB for minimally invasive direct coronary artery bypass.

However, the relatively anterior thoracotomy led to cartilage disruption, which was frequently more painful than a sternotomy. Access to LIMA was limited by medial incision; only the LAD artery could be approached easily, the ascending aorta remained out of reach and instruments for this approach were not well developed.

In 2005, Mc Ginn at Staten Island University introduced MICS CABG. This is a sternal sparing technique that is versatile and easier to perform. A more lateral incision avoids cartilage disruption and gives a good view of the LIMA allowing complete harvest from first rib to the bifurcation. With easier access to the lateral wall of left ventricle, all the coronary arteries can be approached. Lower profile single shafted instruments enhance visibility. It allows safe access to the aorta. Aortic proximal anastomosis can now be performed using any technique that the surgeon prefers.

MICS CABG offers the ability to perform multivessel bypass with access to aorta and thus preserves the proven configuration of grafts performed with sternotomy techniques. This is done in a less invasive way without violating the bony integrity of the thorax. Preserving the structural integrity of the chest helps in a faster recovery and an earlier return to work. Elderly, deconditioned patients can resume upper body weight bearing sooner without the burden of sternal precautions.

MINIMALLY INVASIVE DIRECT CORONARY ARTERY BYPASS

The major advantages of MIDCAB are avoidance of CPB and avoidance of sternotomy. Avoidance of sternotomy decreases risk of infection and shortens hospital stay compared to conventional CABG. The various types of MIDCAB approaches used are described below:

1. *Anterior MIDCAB*: The LAD or the diagonal braches on the front of the heart are often the only arteries that

have significant blockages requiring surgical bypass. The conduit used most often is LIMA. MIDCAB is done without the support of CPB.[6] Surgery is accomplished through a 5 cm skin incision.
2. *Anterolateral MIDCAB*: This approach is used for grafting of ramus intermedius that is not accessible through the anterior or lateral approach. This graft is brought up to its new blood supply in the neck with a small incision under the left clavicle and then directed into the chest. A separate small incision high on the anterolateral aspect of the chest allows the graft to be anastomosed to the ramus intermedius artery.
3. *Lateral MIDCAB*: The circumflex coronary artery and its obtuse marginal branch run along the left side of the heart. They can be reached and grafted through a small lateral incision on the left side of chest below the armpit. This approach is particularly important when prior cardiac surgery has resulted in grafts on the anterior aspect of heart that are patent and should be left undisturbed during surgery.
4. *Transabdominal MIDCAB*: This approach is used to revascularize the right coronary artery and its posterior descending branch that travel along the base of the heart. A small subcostal incision in the upper abdomen provides access to the right coronary artery and the posterior descending artery. The right gastroepiploic artery can be harvested without compromising the blood supply to the stomach and it easily reaches through base of heart.

MINIMALLY INVASIVE CARDIAC SURGERY/CORONARY ARTERY BYPASS GRAFTING

The differences between MICS CABG operation and MIDCAB operation that are restricted to the performance of a single graft[7,8] are following:

1. MICS CABG is not restricted to single vessel grafting but allows complete revascularization in the presence of triple vessel or diffuse coronary artery disease.
2. Approach in the MICS CABG is smaller and more lateral on the chest wall that allows for maximal rib spreading without the risk of costochondral or rib injury, and also the space occupied by the left lung is used to work inside the chest as lung deflated during the surgery.
3. As the pericardium is widely opened, all the three coronary arteries and their branches are visualized, which allows proper selection of the anastomotic site.
4. The internal mammary arteries can be easily harvested either along with the pedicle or skeletonized, right from the origin up to the bifurcation avoiding the possibility of steal phenomenon from the side branches of internal mammary artery.[9,10]
5. Proximal anastomoses are routinely performed onto the ascending aorta.

It is wise to begin with single vessel bypass (LIMA to LAD) and gain experience with exposure of aorta and other coronary targets. One may then progress to diagonal and lateral wall targets. Surgical team must constantly assess its abilities and stay within its limitations. Absolute contraindications to MICS CABG include severe chest wall deformity, severe COPD, emergency surgery, morbid obesity, aortoiliac disease, left subclavian stenosis; diffuse coronary artery disease, and severe left ventricular (LV) dysfunction.

MICS CABG requires experience in off-pump surgery. It is done under direct vision, using single lung ventilation. Defibrillation pads are placed before starting surgery. The patient is placed supine with a longitudinal roll under the left chest. A 6–10 cm incision is given just below and medial to the nipple in males and extended laterally. An inframammary incision is given in Figure 28.2. The thoracic cavity is entered through fourth or fifth intercostal space. Some surgeons use additional ports in subxiphoid area and seventh intercostal space to pass coronary stabilizers.

LIMA is harvested by elevating the anterior chest wall with the help of Rultract attached to anterior blade of Thoratrak retractor. The ascending aorta should be brought as close access to the right coronary artery and the posterior as possible to the incision and the proximal anastomosis may be performed using a partial occlusion clamp, a clampless anastomotic device (heartstring, Macquet Inc.) or a fully automated anastomotic connector (passport, Cardica Inc.).

The apical suction device (starfish) can be placed through the subxiphoid port and the tissue stabilizer (Octo Nova) is placed through the sixth or seventh intercostal port. It is possible to access virtually any coronary artery with the help of pericardial traction sutures and patient positioning. One should not hesitate to assist the circulation with peripheral cannulation in the event of hemodynamic instability.

ENDOSCOPIC HARVEST OF CONDUITS

Having added surgical endoscope in the armamentarium has allowed us to reduce the morbidity associated with conduit harvest for CABG, especially in elderly patients, patients with diabetes, obesity, and immunocompromised status. It is a technique that has made a great impact on patients undergoing CABG. Endoscope is inserted and advanced over the anterior portion of the conduit in a cephalad direction. With continuous CO_2 insufflation a space is created in the subcutaneous tissue within which the dissection is carried out. Branches are then clipped and cut with vascular clips and endoscopic scissors. Once the conduit is freed, the proximal portion is first ligated with a large clip and then cut with endoscopic scissors. Two to four transverse incisions of 2 cm are employed for the whole procedure.

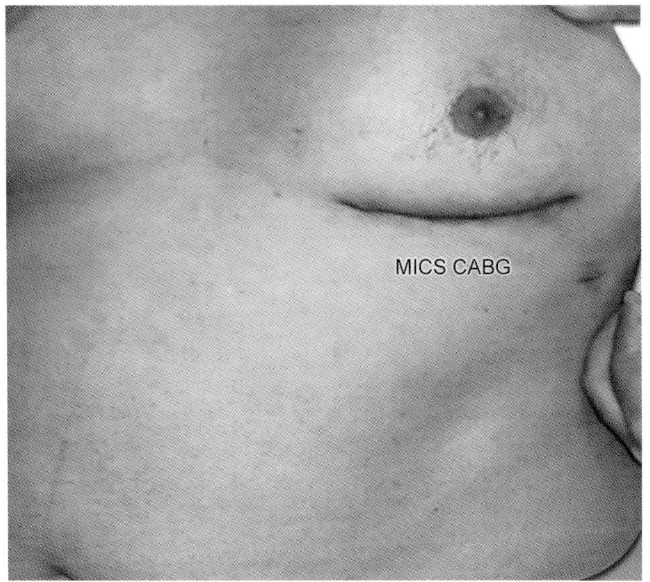

Fig. 28.2 Minimally invasive cardiac surgery (MICS)/ Coronary artery bypass grafting (CABG)

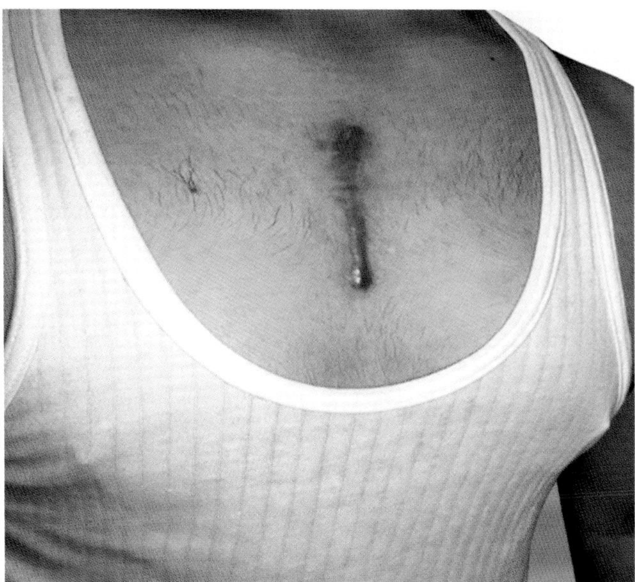

Fig. 28.3 Upper partial sternotomy

MINIMALLY INVASIVE VALVE SURGERY

Majority of valve surgeries are performed through a conventional median sternotomy. There have been many attempts, however, to make the procedure less invasive by reducing incision size and keeping apportion of sternum intact. Since the detailed vascular anastomosis is not needed, less invasive approach to valve surgery has been proved to be more interesting and promising than less invasive approaches for CABG. Many surgeons have shown excellent results with low surgical morbidity and mortality[11-15] by using ministernotomy and parasternal incisions.

Minimally invasive mitral valve surgery started in the early 1996. The Stanford group used intra-aortic balloon occlusion with cardioplegia to perform the surgery. Video assistance through tiny incisions offers better visualization than through direct vision. Carpentier repaired mitral valve successfully through minithoracotomy with video assistance using cold ventricular fibrillation in February, 1996. Chitwood performed the minimally invasive mitral valve surgery with the use of a percutaneous clamp and cardioplegia in March, 1996.

Minimally invasive options should be explored for all patients who present for an isolated valve disease. The integrity, completeness, and safety of an operation must not be compromised in favor of a desire to be minimally invasive. The various types of minimal access approaches for valvular surgery performed frequently are described further.

Upper Partial Sternotomy

The sternum is divided in midline down through the third or fourth intercostals space and then incised in a shape of T into that space. A variation in this is J shape into the third or fourth intercostal space, leaving the left table of sternum intact. Central cannulation is straightforward and venous cannulation can either be peripheral or through the robot-assisted appendage. Using pericardial stay stitches will provide excellent exposure of the aorta and after aortotomy the aortic valve. Traditional aortic valve replacement (AVR), mitral valve (MVR), Ross procedures, aortic aneurysmorrhaphy, and some limited bypass procedures can be performed through this exposure. The mitral valve is accessed through the roof of left atrium under the aorta and superior vena cava. This approach has several advantages, including a lack of internal mammary ligation or injury, direct and conventional access, and cannulation and avoiding dividing the lower portion of sternum that bears the majority of stress from chest wall (Fig. 28.3).

Lower Partial Sternotomy

The incision is made from the level of third intercostals space to the xiphoid and the sternum is incised in the shape of T at the third space. A J modification can also be done; however, the exposure of aorta for cannulation may be more difficult. Central aortic cannulation is done by retracting the upper

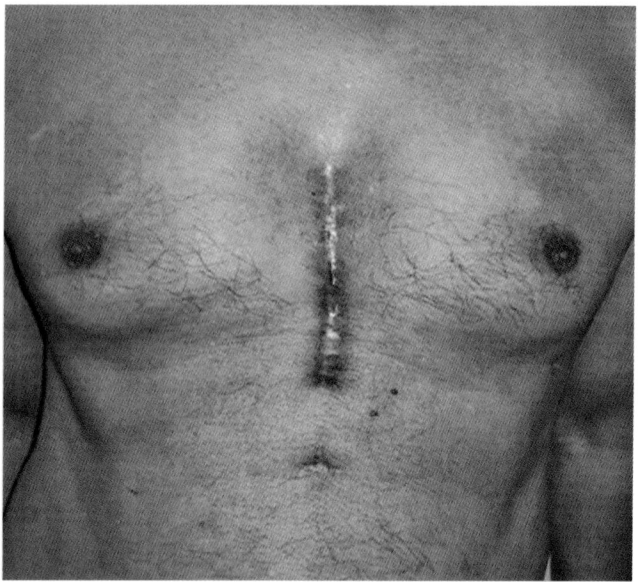

Fig. 28.4 Lower partial sternotomy

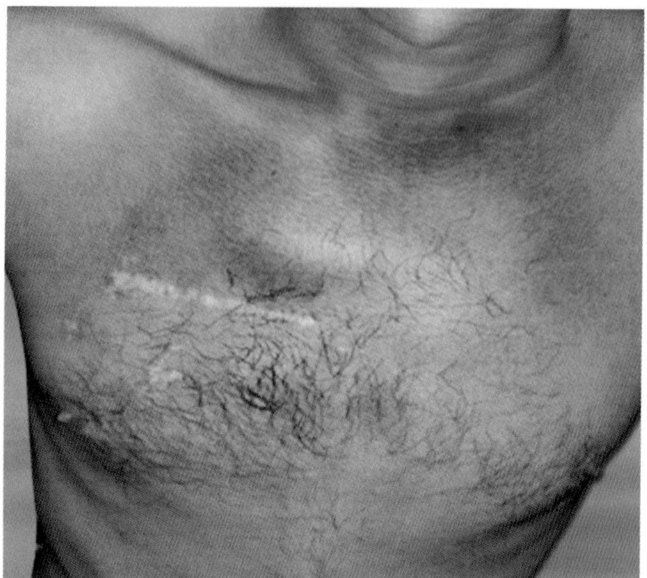

Fig. 28.5 Right anterior thoracotomy

sternal segment. Bicaval cannulation is accomplished using a stab incision in the right thorax and going through the right thorax into the upper right atrium. The inferior vena cava (IVC) can be drained through stab incision in right costal margin and right atrial cannulation or through femoral vein. The mitral valve is accessed in the standard fashion through the Waterston's groove or through the right atrium and interatrial septum. Exposure for the aortic valve and tricuspid valve is excellent and the incision provides access to the entire heart so double and triple valve operations are possible. This also is the best minimally invasive incision if a coronary artery bypass is necessary in addition to aortic valve replacement (Fig. 28.4).

Right Anterior Thoracotomy for Aortic Valve Replacement

This approach is typically performed through the second or third intercostal space and cannulation can be central or peripheral. Well-placed pericardial stay sutures will bring the right side of the aorta into the field well and them the operation in as usual. If further exposure is needed, a transverse sternotomy can be performed (Fig. 28.5).

Right Thoracotomy (Heart Port)

Platform was developed at Stanford University and New York University Hospital in 1994. It is based on a small right anterolateral 5–7 cm thoracotomy incision through the third or fourth interspace with peripheral cannulation and balloon occlusion of ascending aorta (Fig. 28.6). Several specialized

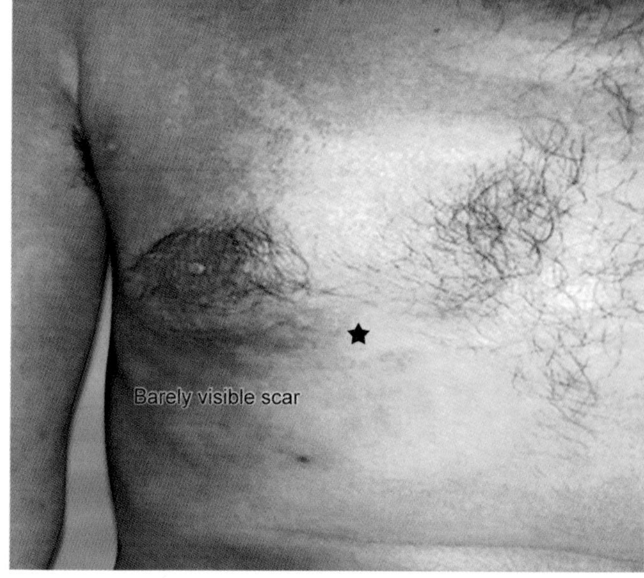

Fig. 28.6 Right thoracotomy (heart port) for MVR. Asterisk shows scar site

cannulae are used to put the patient on CPB. Arterial cannulation is done through the femoral artery. Direct aortic cross clamping is done with a long vascular clamp inserted through a stab incision in the second intercostal space. Cardioplegia is given directly into the aortic root or via the coronary sinus. Mitral valve, tricuspid valve, and ASDs are accessed comfortably through this approach. Initially the procedure was done under direct vision. Visual assistance has been added using a 10 mm port in the anterior axillary line at second or third intercostal space.[16] Advantages of this approach include a very small incision with minimal distraction of ribs resulting in rapid healing and rehabilitation with excellent cosmesis.[17]

MINIMALLY INVASIVE ATRIAL SEPTAL DEFECT CLOSURE

A small anterior thoracotomy through third or fourth intercostal space is performed.[13] Cannulation is done through femoral artery and vein. Right internal jugular vein is cannulated to drain the blood from upper body. Cross clamp is passed through the second intercostal space. Antegrade cardioplegia cannula is inserted under direct vision into the ascending aorta. Visual assistance has now been added using a 10 mm port through the second IC space in the anterior axillary line (Fig. 28.7).

OTHER MINIMALLY INVASIVE CARDIAC PROCEDURES

Besides above-mentioned cardiac procedures, there are a wide variety of cardiac procedures that are performed through minimal access approach, such as:

- Left atrial clot removal
- Right/left atrial myxoma excision
- Maze procedure
- Epicardial lead implantation
- Ruptured sinus of valsalva repair
- Radiofrequency ablation.

ROBOTIC CARDIAC SURGERY

Robotic cardiac surgery was developed in order to overcome the limitations of minimally invasive surgery and to improve the abilities of cardiac surgeon performing the conventional cardiac surgery. In robot-assisted cardiac surgery, the surgeon performs the normal movements associated with the surgery on a telemanipulator, which are translated through the robotic arms to carry out the movements using end effectors and manipulators to perform the surgery inside the body of patient.

Robotic cardiac surgery started in 1997 when Falk et al. used the AESOP 3000 to perform port access mitral surgery using endoaortic clamping.[18] In 1998, Chitwood's group performed a mitral operation using AESOP 3000 robotic arm and a vista three-dimensional camera.[19] Carpentier in 1998 performed the first totally robotic, endoscopic ASD closure.[20] Mohr and Falk in 1998 harvested LIMA by using da Vinci system and through a small left anterior thoracotomy performed the coronary anastomosis.[21] Loulmet et al. performed the world's first TECAB using robotic assistance in 1998 (Fig. 28.8).[22]

During subsequent years, development has been significant but at a low pace. In the early stages, only single vessel grafting was done using robotic assistance, then gradually as the surgeons became well acquainted with the system now multiple and complex coronary revascularization is performed. Further development of robotic systems was carried out with the introduction of the third generation of surgical telemanipulators, which provide improvement in the areas of three-dimensional video, range of motion of robotic arm, instrument reach, surgeon comfort, and have the capability of intraoperative training with a dual-console system (Fig. 28.9).[23]

Robotic cardiac surgery is performed through multiple, small 1–2 cm incision for passage of instruments and camera (Fig. 28.10). A wide array of procedures is possible by using robotic visualization, dexterity, precision, and control. During the operation, surgeon sits on a console in the surgical suite and directs the robotic arm through the telemanipulator.

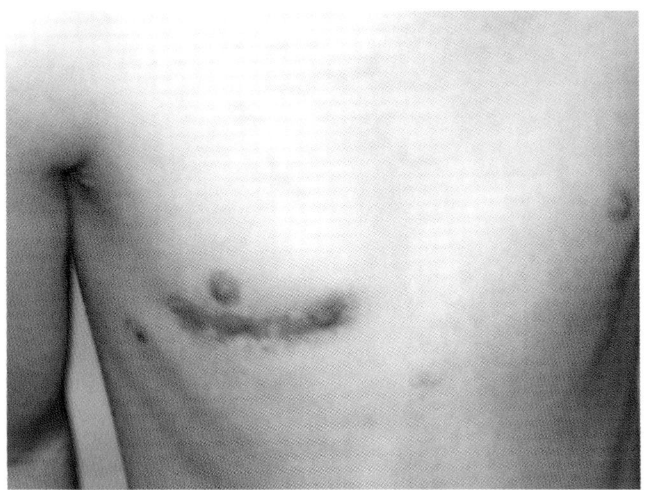

Fig. 28.7 Anterior thoracotomy for ASD

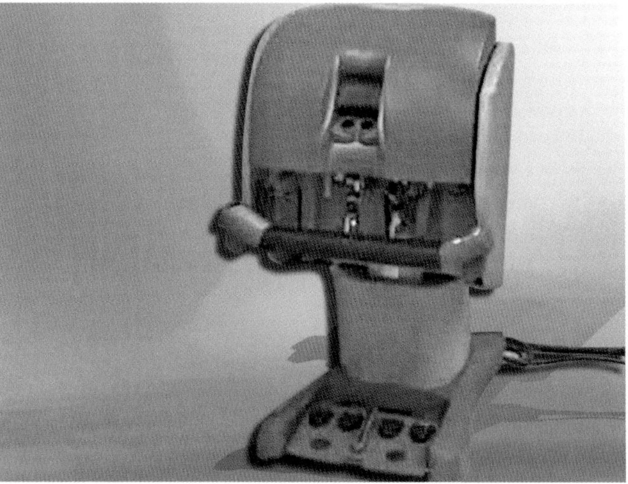

Fig. 28.8 Surgical robot

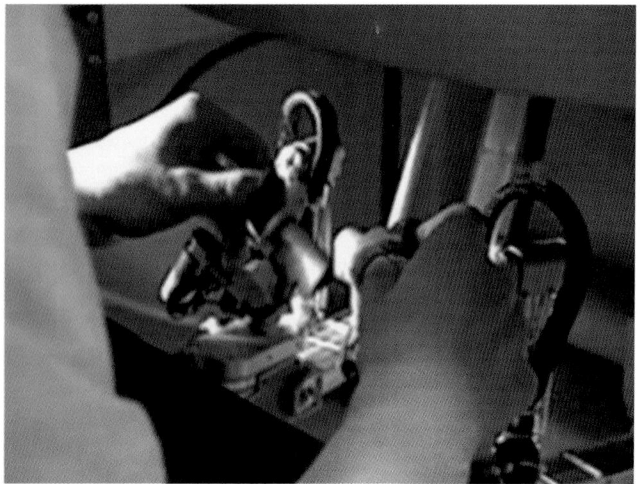

Fig. 28.9 Surgeon working at console

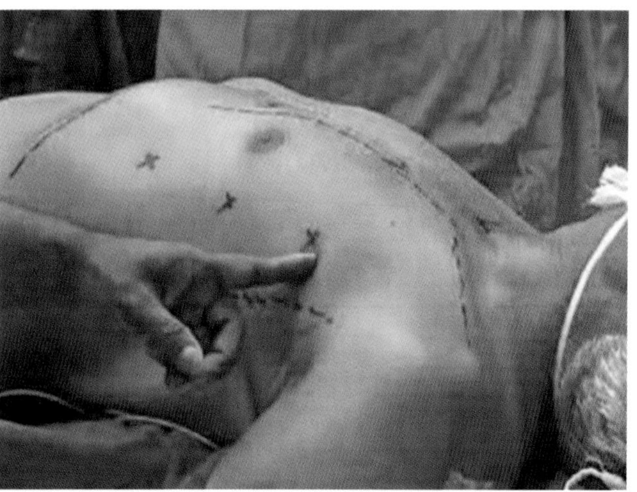

Fig. 28.10 Marking for surgical ports

The robotic arms seamlessly and directly translate the moments of surgeon's wrist, hand, and fingers from control at the consol to the instruments inside the patient.

Advantages of robotic assistance to a cardiac surgeon are the following:

1. It provides the surgeon with a greater range of motion and precision.
2. It provides a magnified, high-definition, three-dimensional view.
3. It enables the surgeon with instruments that resemble the extension of his own hands and fingers to move the small instruments in a precise and delicate manner.

Advantages of robotic cardiac surgery for the patient are the following:

1. Sternotomy is avoided
2. Less postoperative pain

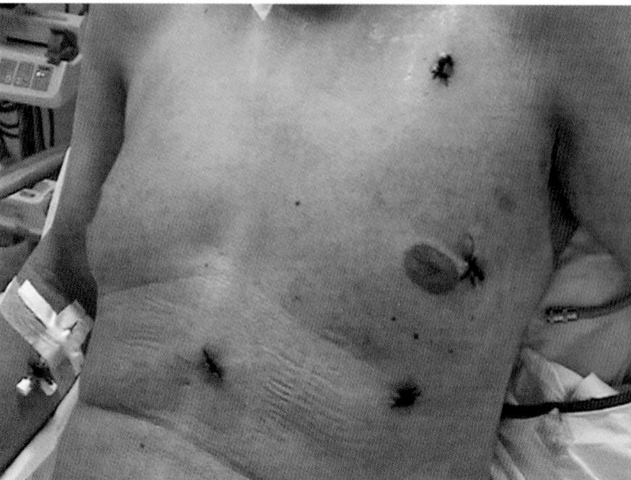

Fig. 28.11 Post-robotic surgery appearance

3. Shorter hospital stay
4. Reduced blood loss and need for transmission
5. Quick recovery and return to normal activity and
6. Better cosmesis (Fig. 28.11).

ROBOT-ASSISTED CORONARY ARTERY BYPASS GRAFTING

The learning curve for any robotic procedure is steep and so is true for robot-assisted CABG. So a stepwise approach should be adopted for learning RACABG.

ROBOTIC INTERNAL MAMMARY HARVEST

Single lung ventilation is used. After isolating from ventilation, the lung gets collapsed, a camera is inserted through left fifth intercostal space is the mild axillary line. Instruments are inserted through ports made in the left third and seventh intercostal space, for instrument arms. LIMA as well as right internal mammary artery (RIMA) can be harvested after proper port placement. Retrosternal tissue is dissected and right pleura opened for harvesting RIMA.

ROBOT-ASSISTED MINIMALLY INVASIVE DIRECT CORONARY ARTERY BYPASS

After LIMA harvest, small thoracotomy is done through left fourth intercostal space and anastomosis of target vessel usually LAD is accomplished by direst hand suturing. Apical suction positing devices (starfish) and stabilizers area placed through the thoracotomy or through same small ports so as to expose the circumflex and right coronary target vessels.

OPEN CHEST ROBOTIC ANASTOMOSIS

After mastering the robotic internal mammary harvesting techniques, one should start doing robotic anastomosis via midline sternotomy as part of standard CABG. It is a reasonable step to enable a safe subsequent totally endoscopic approach.

TOTALLY ENDOSCOPIC CORONARY ARTERY BYPASS ON ARRESTED HEART

Robotic totally endoscopic coronary artery bypass is performed very safely on an arrested heart. CPB is initiated through bifemoral cannulation and endoaortic balloon is used for occlusion of the ascending aorta and for cardioplegia. Coronary anastomosis is performed very precisely on an arrested heart as the heart is not moving robotic instruments act as natural extension of surgeon's hand and fingers. Arrested heart can be easily rotated for access to the circumflex and right coronary artery and also as the lung can be collapsed, the intrathoracic space is significantly enhanced.

Coronary anastomosis is performed with the use of double armed 7.0 Prolene sutures, U-clip, or other anastomotic device. Single, multiple, sequential, and even Y-grafts can be constructed robotically.[24,25] Rate of revision of anastomosis for bleeding is higher as compared to conventional CABG; however, with increased experience and management of port hole bleeding, these complications have been greatly reduced.

TOTALLY ENDOSCOPIC CORONARY ARTERY BYPASS ON BEATING HEART

This is often regarded as the ultimate goal in TECAB. The familiarity with beating heart TECAB is mandatory especially for managing patients with contradiction to remote access perfusion and balloon endo-occlusion of ascending aorta (e.g. severe peripheral vascular disease and ascending aorta dilation); with the availability of endoscopic stabilizers this procedure has been made easy. Latest generation of robots includes a suction stabilizer that is inserted as a robotic instrument and controlled from the telemanipulator. The target coronary artery is stabilized and opened. Coronary anastomosis is performed after putting an endoluminal stent. Doing a TECAB on beating heart is taxing and technically difficult and one should always have a low threshold for conversion to open technique, which should not be regarded as failure but as a second option.

Grafting of lateral and posterior wall of the heart is particularly difficult without CPB, but this situation can be overcome by putting the patient on CPB while allowing the heart to beat (pump supported). This dramatically reduces the technical difficulty of beating heart TECAB by emptying the heart and permitting bilateral lung deflation that provides greater space to work within the closed chest. Technical difficulties like myocardial ischemia, arrhythmia during coronary occlusion, hemodynamic instability, bleeding from target vessels, and organ injuries due to robotic instruments can be managed with prophylactic cannulation and standby CPB.

ROBOTIC CORONARY ARTERY BYPASS GRAFTING AS PART OF HYBRID CORONARY INTERVENTION

The concept of hybrid coronary interventions has come as viable alternative to open CABG and multivessel percutaneous coronary intervention so that advantages of both types of coronary revascularization procedures are brought together. Long-term therapeutic concept with potentially enhanced survival with internal mammary artery conduits is an established fact. Hence, it is a valuable element of hybrid coronary revascularization procedures. TECAB involving placement of LIMA to LAD artery or placement of both internal mammary artery grafts to the left ventricle can be followed by percutaneous intervention of other coronary vessels in the same hybrid suite. An increasing number of complex and advanced hybrid coronary interventions are performed these days including multivessel TECAB and/or multivessel percutaneous coronary intervention.[26,27]

ROBOTIC ATRIAL SEPTAL DEFECT SURGERY

The patient is intubated with a double lumen endotracheal tube so that right lung can be isolated. After heparinization, an appropriate size arterial cannula is inserted in the superior vena cava through the right internal jugular vein. Transesophageal echocardiographic probe is inserted and left in place throughout the procedure in order to confirm the position of cannulae and endoaortic balloon. A transthoracic clamp can also be used for clamping ascending aorta. External defibrillation pads are placed on the chest wall. The patient is positioned with the right side of chest inclined by 30° and the right arm slightly beneath the posterior axillary line. The right lung is deflated, and the camera is introduced through a port in the right fourth intercostal space midway between the nipple and the anterior axillary line. In the third and fifth intercostal spaces on the anterior axillary line, two additional ports are made for the introduction of the robotic instruments. An accessory port is made in the fourth intercostal space on the posterior axillary line. The pericardium is opened and both venae cavae are dissected and encircled by umbilical tapes. After putting the patient on CPB through cannulation of right femoral artery and vein in connection with cannula in the superior vena cava, ASD is closed in the usual manner (Fig. 28.12).

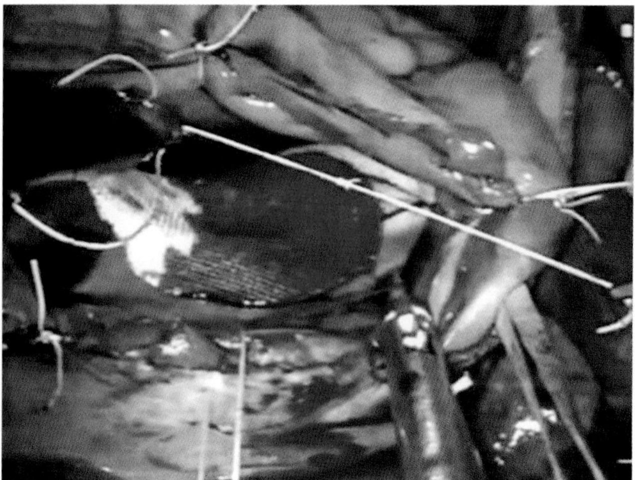

Fig. 28.12 Robotic ASD closure with Dacron patch

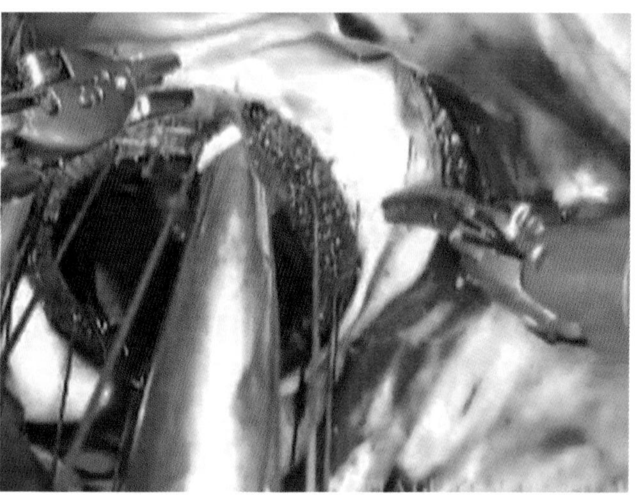

Fig. 28.13 Robotic mitral valve replacement

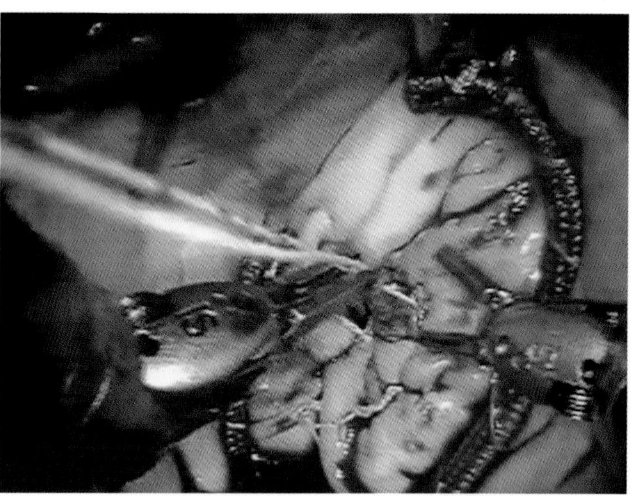

Fig. 28.14 Robotic mitral valve repair

ROBOTIC MITRAL VALVE SURGERY

It is usually performed with the use of robotic instruments through a minithoracotomy or endoscopic ports. CPB is established through cannulation of femoral artery and vein. Occasionally, superior vena cava can be cannulated through the right internal jugular vein proper venous drainage. The ascending aorta can be occluded with a transthoracic clamp or occasionally with an endoballoon. One arm of the robot is inserted through the third intercostal space in the anterior-axillary line and the other arm is inserted through the fifth intercostal space in the midaxillary line. Through the fourth intercostal space a small thoracotomy or working port is created in the mid-axillary line, and an left atrial retractor is placed in the midclavicular line. Replacement or repair of the valve can be accomplished (Figs 28.13 and 28.14). Acceptance for robotic mitral valve surgery has been limited, despite initial favorable reports, because of the complexity associated with the procedure, high cost of the procedure, as well as its quality and safety.[28]

REFERENCES

1. Stevens J, Burdon T, Siegel L, et al. Port-access coronary artery bypass with cardioplegic arrest: acute and chronic canine studies. Ann Thorac Surg. 1996;62:435-40.
2. Mihaljevic T, Cohn LH, Unic D, et al. One thousand minimally invasive valve operations. Early and late results. Ann Surg. 2004;240:529-34.
3. Bonacchi M, Prifti E, Giunti G, et al. Does ministernotomy improve postoperative outcome in aortic valve operation? A prospective randomized study. Ann Thorac Surg. 2002;73:460-6.
4. Sharony R, Gross EA, Saunders PC, et al. Minimally invasive aortic valve surgery in the elderly: a case-control study. Circulation. 2003;108(Suppl. 1):II43-7.
5. Subramanian VA, McCabe JC, Geller CM. Minimally invasive direct coronary artery bypass grafting: two-year clinical experience. Ann Thorac Surg. 1997;64:1648-55.
6. Mishra Y, Mairal M, Maheshwari P, et al. Mammary coronary anastomosis through minithoracotomy without extracorporeal circulation. Indian Heart J. 1996;48(5) (abst).
7. Boodhwani M, Ruel M, Mesana TG, et al. Minimally invasive direct coronary artery bypass for the treatment of isolated disease of the left anterior descending coronary artery. Can J Surg. 2005;48:307-10.
8. Holzhey DM, Jacobs S, Mochalski M, et al. Seven-year follow-up after minimally invasive direct coronary artery bypass: experience with more than 1300 patients. Ann Thorac Surg. 2007;83:108-14.
9. Tsakiridis K, Mikroulis D, Didilis V, et al. Internal thoracic artery side branch ligation for post coronary surgery ischemia. Asian Cardiovasc Thorac Ann. 2007;15:339-41.
10. Pagni S, Bousamra M II, Shirley MW, et al. Successful VATS ligation of a large anomalous branch producing IMA steal syndrome after MIDCAB. Ann Thorac Surg. 2001;71:1681-2.
11. Cosgrove DM 3rd, Sabik JF. Minimally invasive approach for aortic valve operations. Ann Thorac Surg. 1996;62:596-7.
12. Cosgrove DM 3rd, Sabik JF, Navia JL. Minimally invasive valve operations. Ann Thorac Surg. 1988;65:1535-9.

13. Konertz W, Waldenberger F, Schmutzler M, et al. Minimal access valve surgery through superior partial sternotomy: a preliminary study. J Heart Valve Dis. 1996;5:638-40.
14. Arom KM, Emery RW. Minimally invasive mitral operations [Letter]. Ann Thorac Surg. 1996;62:1542-4.
15. Navia JL, Cosgrove DM 3rd. Minimally invasive mitral valve operations. Ann Thorac Surg. 1996;62:1542-4.
16. Trehan N, Mishra YK, Sharma M, et al. Robotically controlled video-assisted port-access mitral valve surgery. Asian Cardiovasc Thorac Ann. 2002;10(2):133-6.
17. Mishra YK, Khanna SN, Wasir H, et al. Port-access approach for cardiac surgical procedures: our experience in 776 patients. Indian Heart J. 2005;57(6):688-93.
18. Falk V, Walther T, Autschbach R, et al. Robot-assisted minimally invasive solo mitral valve operation. J Thorac Cardiovasc Surg. 1998;115(2):470-1.
19. Chitwood WR Jr1, Wixon CL, Elbeery JR, et al. Video-assisted minimally invasive mitral valve surgery. J Thorac Cardiovasc Surg. 1997;114(5):773-80; discussion 780-2.
20. Carpentier A1, Loulmet D, Aupècle B, et al. Computer assisted open heart surgery. First case operated on with success C R Acad Sci III. 1998;321(5):437-42.
21. Mohr FW, Falk V, Diegeler A,et al. Computer-enhanced coronary artery bypass surgery. J Thorac Cardiovasc Surg. 1999;117(6): 1212-4.
22. Loulmet D, Carpentier A, d'Attellis N, et al. Endoscopic coronary artery bypass grafting with the aid of robotic assisted instruments. J Thorac Cardiovasc Surg. 1999;118:4-10.
23. Lehr EJ, Grigore A, Reicher B, et al. Dual console robotic system to teach beating heart total endoscopic coronary artery bypass grafting: a video presentation. Interact Cardiovasc Thorac Surg. 2010;8:S113-S114.
24. Bonatti J, Schachner T, Bonaros N, et al. Robotic totally endoscopic double-vessel bypass grafting: a further step toward closed-chest surgical treatment of multivessel coronary artery disease. Heart Surg Forum. 2007;10:E239-E242.
25. Dogan S, Aybek T, Andressen E, et al. Totally endoscopic coronary artery bypass grafting on cardiopulmonary bypass with robotically enhanced telemanipulation: report of forty-five cases. J Thorac Cardiovasc Surg. 2002;123:1125-31.
26. Jansens J, De Croly P, De Cannie`re D. Robotic hybrid procedure and triple-vessel disease. J Cardiac Surg. 2009;24:449-50.
27. Argenziano M, Katz M, Bonatti J, et al. Results of the prospective multicenter trial of robotically assisted totally endoscopic coronary artery bypass grafting. Ann Thorac Surg. 2006;81: 1666-74.
28. Chitwood WR, Rodriguez E, Chu MWA, et al. Robotic mitral valve repairs in 300 patients: a single center experience. J Thorac Cardiovasc Surg. 2008;136:436-41.

29

Management of Advanced Heart Failure

Vishal Rastogi, Bhumika S Anand

INTRODUCTION

Last few years have seen decrease in coronary artery disease-related mortality. At the same time, morbidity and mortality due to acute and chronic heart failure have been increasing relentlessly despite tremendous development in the diagnosis and management of this condition. The principle of management of patients with systolic heart failure is "remodel, repair, or replace" the damaged ventricle, depending on the clinical status of the patient (NYHA class) and the stage of heart failure (ACC/AHA stage of heart failure). Remodeling therapies include drugs, heart failure surgeries, and valve procedures including MitraClip and transcatheter aortic valve implantation (TAVI). The ventricle can be repaired by revascularization and stem cell therapy. However, patients with end-stage heart failure and selected cases of acute decompensated heart failure will require temporary or permanent cardiac replacement treatment. The gold standard treatment of these end-stage heart failure patients remains cardiac transplantation, but the shortage of available organs makes it necessary to use mechanical circulatory support devices in some of these patients.

The idea of a replacement with mechanical assistance first appeared in the 1950s and evolved over more than half a century, yet the first device that is the intra-aortic balloon pump (IABP) appeared only in the late 1960s. It remains, even today, the most common, economical, and easily available cardiac mechanical support device. It is effective in selected case scenarios, but as it does not provide full cardiac support and is dependent on the intrinsic cardiac function as well as stable rhythm of the patient, improvement in clinical outcome has not been demonstrated in clinical studies. In light of these facts, efforts were invested in the development of mechanical devices to support the failing heart, which are classified as acute short-term mechanical assistance devices or surgically implantable ventricular assist devices for a wide range of indications: from long-term replacement of failing hearts as bridge-to-transplantation or as destination therapy or in the temporary support of cardiogenic shock (*bridge-to recovery*) or even its prophylactic use in certain invasive coronary or valvular procedures.[1]

Over the past several years, there has been a progressive development from large pulsatile devices to the smaller continuous-flow left ventricular assist devices (LVADs) for the provision of mechanical circulatory support. An LVAD receives oxygenated blood from the left ventricle or left atrium and delivers it to the aorta. A right ventricular assist device (RVAD) receives blood from either the right atrium or right ventricle and delivers it to the pulmonary artery. Some VADs can function either as LVAD or an RVAD, or both (BiVAD). VADs have improved appreciably in the last few years in terms of providing survival and quality of life among recipients.[2]

SURGICALLY IMPLANTED VENTRICULAR ASSIST DEVICE

Ventricular assist devices (VADs) are of various types and sizes and their components too differ according to their versions. The device in general has a pump unit, a control system, and an energy supply. Figure 29.1 shows HeartMate II VAD with its components.

PREPROCEDURAL PLANNING

As a general note, the success of a LVAD implantation procedure depends on more than just implantation technique. Judicious preoperative evaluation and preparation must be combined with vigilant postoperative management of both the usual issues encountered in the intensive care unit (ICU) and the issues arising in the outpatient setting. Only through the efforts of an active and engaged multidisciplinary team, this can be accomplished.

Issues that must be taken into account in planning the care of an LVAD patient include underlying cardiovascular disease and anticoagulation. Normally functioning right ventricle is

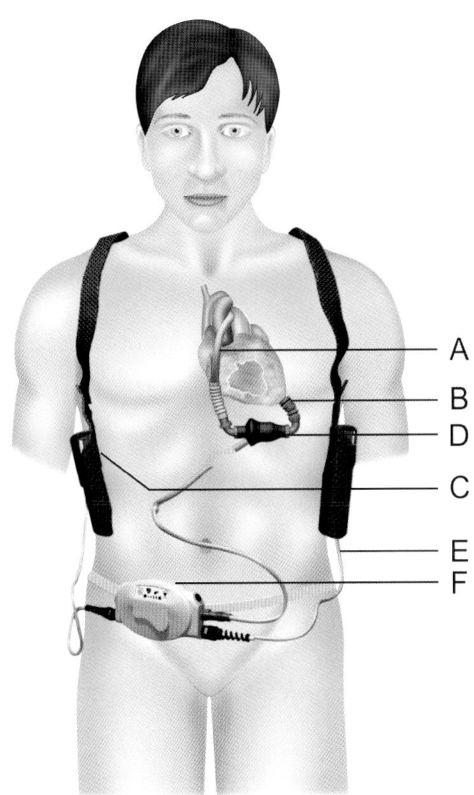

Fig. 29.1 Diagram of HeartMate II VAD with its components. (A) Outflow graft/tube: connected to the aorta (the main artery that carries oxygenated blood away from the heart). (B) Inflow graft/tube: attached to the left ventricular (LV) apex—the lowest and bottom portion of the LV. (C) Power source: electrical power or battery power is necessary to run the pump. The diagram shown above is operating on battery supply. (D) Pump unit: the device with the inflow and outflow grafts. (E) Driveline: it is an electrical cable from the internal device that exits the patient's skin and connects the pump to an external controller outside the body. (F) External controller: The controller is powered by either lithium ion batteries or an electricity outlet. The controller monitors the pump's function and displays the operations of the pump, alarms, and the battery status in a LED screen. The controller and batteries are carried in a case, designed to be worn around the waist or over the shoulder

of paramount importance in these patients receiving LVADs. To the extent possible, all patent grafts must be protected at the time of surgery.

General guidelines for associated valve disease are as follows[3]:

- Aortic stenosis—This is generally not a problem and can be left alone.
- Aortic insufficiency—This must be fixed if it is more than mild as it causes closed loop circulation; options include bioprosthetic aortic valve replacement (AVR), collagen-impregnated Dacron patch to oversew the valve (e.g. Hemashield; Maquet, Rastatt, Germany), and approximation of the nodes of Arantius; oversewing the valve makes the patient completely dependent on the LVAD for LV ejection and hence many surgeons do not prefer.
- Prosthetic AVR—A bioprosthetic AVR is not a trouble, but there are no data till date suggesting what to do with a mechanical AVR; some surgeons recommend oversewing or replacement with a bioprosthetic AVR (especially in destination therapy patients), whereas others might consider leaving the prosthesis in place; this scenario was an exclusion criteria for patients in current trials.
- Mitral stenosis—This must be repaired to allow LV inflow; options include tissue valve replacement and, if the situation is compliant, valvuloplasty.
- Mitral regurgitation—This can be left alone unless myocardial recovery and explantation are being considered. In many of these patients, mitral regurgitation is secondary to LV dilatation that may decrease on its own once LV is unloaded with LVAD.
- Tricuspid regurgitation—Although the practice is controversial, most operators perform annuloplasty in the face of severe tricuspid regurgitation.

Warfarin is usually administered when the patient is extubated and taking oral medications; the ultimate goal is to achieve an international normalized ratio (INR) of 1.7–2.5.

PERCUTANEOUS LEFT VENTRICULAR ASSIST DEVICES

Currently, percutaneous insertable devices are mainly used for additional treatment of hemodynamically unstable patients in cardiogenic shock, as well as for selected patients undergoing high-risk percutaneous coronary interventions (PCI). These devices are also approved as bridge to bridge and as bridge to decision. Mainly due to the lack of sufficient scientific evidence, there are wide variations in the use of the different available devices (Fig. 29.2).

TANDEMHEART

The *TandemHeart* creates a percutaneous left atrial to aortic shunt. Blood is collected from the left atrium through trans-septal puncture and directed to abdominal aorta through extracorporeal pump. Using a two-stage [14–21 French (Fr)] dilator, the interatrial septum is dilated to harbor a 21-Fr left atrial drainage cannula. While a 15-Fr cannula allows a maximal estimated flow of 3.5 L/min, the 17-Fr allows 4–5 L/min, depending on systemic vascular resistance. The pump's efficacy is determined by proper suction of blood from the left atrium, which could be hampered by inadequate filling of the atrium or a deeply positioned cannula thrust against the atrial wall. Proper positioning of the cannula

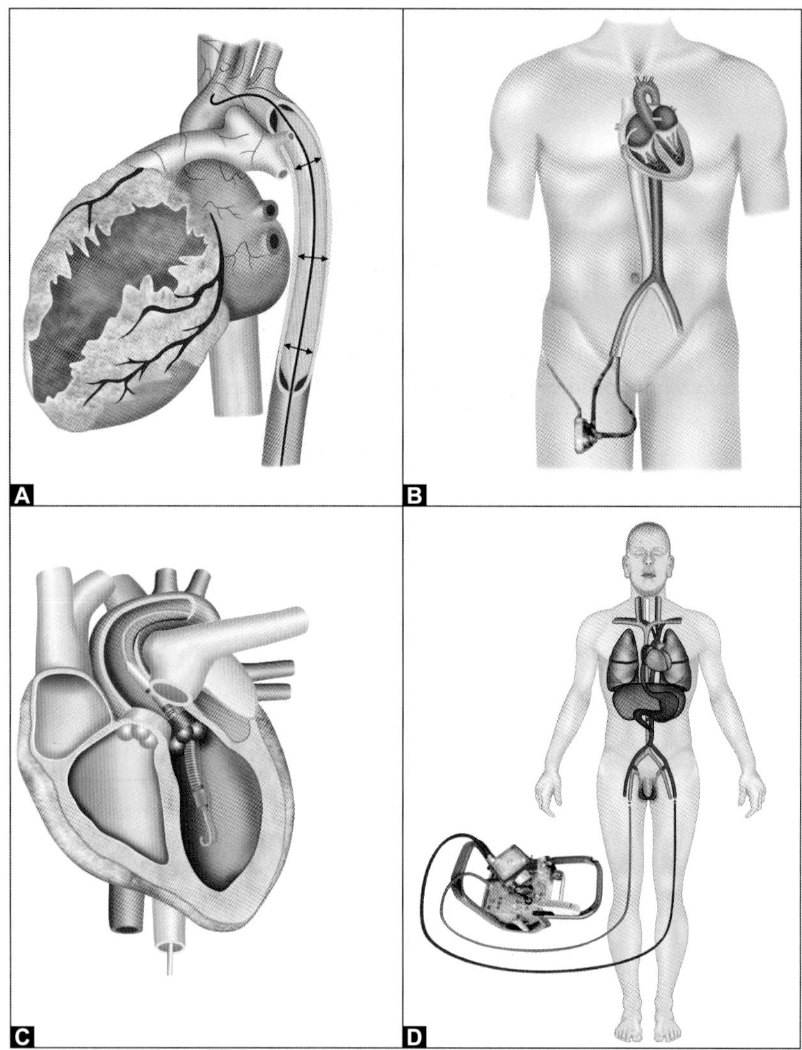

Figs 29.2A to D Overview of the different devices for percutaneous hemodynamic support. (A) Intra-aortic balloon pump (IABP); (B) TandemHeart; (C) Impella Recover LP 2.5; and (D) Extracorporeal membrane oxygenation (ECMO)

is also important to avoid displacement or kinking of the inflow cannula, as dislodgement of the cannula into the right atrium would result in a functional right-to-left shunt as a consequence to loss of oxygenation. The *TandemHeart* allows support from hours to up to 4 weeks and a gradual weaning process (about 500 mL/min every hour) is initiated appropriately. Surgical closure is often required to achieve hemostasis, owing to the large cannula size. However, care should be taken in patients with significant right ventricular failure as the trans-septal puncture site remains patent.

IMPELLA

The Impella Recover LP 2.5 L/min works on the principle of an Archimedes screw. The impeller is a 12-Fr axial flow pump that is inserted via a 13-Fr peel-away sheath using the standard catheterization procedure through the femoral artery. A 5-Fr JR is introduced across the aortic valve into the left ventricle and the 12-Fr device is then inserted to draw blood out of the left ventricle into the ascending aorta. An output of 2.5 L/min is achieved at a maximum speed of 50,000 rpm. Nine intensities can be adjusted, allowing subtle support. The pump, at minimum speed, compensates for the aortic regurgitation induced by the catheter. Hemostasis is achieved by manual compression. The conventional catheterization technique with single arterial puncture and no trans-septal puncture or extracorporeal blood flow makes the implantation process of impeller faster than TandemHeart. However, the pump support is feeble than the TandemHeart and usually is of shorter duration too (from hours up to 5 days). Although arterial occlusion is uncommon, hemolysis typically occurs within the first 48 hours of support and has been reported in one-fifth patients. A similar version, the Impella LP 5.0, requires a surgical procedure and gives an output of 5 L/min. The aorta-iliac and femoral vessel angiography is necessary to assess vessel diameter, presence of obstruction, or tortuosity prior to implantation of either of the device. The use of Impella Recover 2.5 has been studied by the Euroshock registry in 120 patients with cardiogenic shock after acute myocardial infarction.[4] The significant predictors of 30-day mortality (64.2%) were age above 65 and plasma lactate of >3.8 mmol/L at the time of admission and 15% of patients reported major cardiac and cerebral events. When compared to other studies, the initial hemodynamic profile of patients was poor reflecting the last-resort use of percutaneous VAD (pVAD). Anticoagulation with heparin is necessary for both pVADs with recommended activated clotting time of 250 seconds during the procedure and an activated clotting time of 200 seconds during the support phase.

EXTRACORPOREAL LIFE SUPPORT

Extracorporeal membrane oxygenation (ECMO) or extracorporeal life support (ECLS) is a form of cardiopulmonary bypass providing support for either lung, or both lung and heart. The basic circuit is composed of a 4000 rpm centrifugal pump with flow up to 7 L/min, a membrane oxygenator, a heat exchanger, a venous cannula carrying deoxygenated blood, and a returning cannula with oxygenated blood. The two most common modalities of ECMO are the venovenous (VV) cannulation that bypasses the lungs and supports in respiratory failure and the venoarterial (VA) cannulation where the oxygenated blood is pumped back to the arterial system bypassing lungs and heart providing both respiratory and hemodynamic support. In V-A ECLS, 22–30-Fr venous cannula is placed in inferior vena cava or right atrium via the femoral or subclavian vein and a 15–23-Fr arterial cannula is placed in the iliac artery through the common femoral artery. To prevent lower limb ischemia, an extra-arterial cannula may be inserted distal to the femoral artery. In situations where the lower limb vessels are not accessible, the right common carotid or axillary artery cannulation can be done. Anticoagulation using continuous unfractionated heparin infusion with recommended activated clotting time between 210 and 230 seconds is recommended. Sheer forces and exposure to foreign body continuously abuse the platelets and hence care should be taken to maintain platelet count >100,000/μL. The duration for femoral access is from 15 to 21 days and up to 2 months for central thoracic access. Local hemorrhage, thromboembolism, lower limb ischemia, ischemic and hemorrhagic stroke, hemolysis, infections, and systemic inflammatory response syndrome are some of the complications encountered. Special attention must be taken when cardiac function recovers with flow competing against the ECLS returning blood into the aorta. A switch from VA to VV ECLS may be required in case of persistent respiratory failure, the *Harlequin syndrome* with classical blue-headed (deoxygenated blood directed to the upper body) and red-legged patient (deoxygenated blood directed to the upper body). There have been no randomized trials to evaluate the efficacy of ECLS in hemodynamic support till date, but observational studies reveal promising results. Two studies showed a benefit of ECLS performed in cardiac arrest.[5,6] When compared with conventional cardiopulmonary resuscitation (CPR), short-term and 6-month survival rate was significantly high in 59 and 85 patients under ECLS-CPR. Another study reported a long-term survival rate of 36% in 81 patients who benefitted from ECLS in severe refractory cardiogenic shock. ECLS was constructive in recovery of fulminant myocarditis with faster renal and hepatic recuperation when compared to biventricular assist devices (Table 29.1).[7]

Table 29.1 Technical details of percutaneous mechanical circulatory support devices

	IABP	ECLS (ECMO)	Impella LP2.5	Impella LP 5.0	TandemHeart
Cannula size (Fr)	–	17–21 (venous) 16–18 (arterial)	12	21	21 (venous) 12–19 (arterial)
Catheter size (Fr)	7–8	–	9	9	–
Insertion site	Femoral artery	Femoral artery Femoral vein	Femoral artery	Femoral artery cut down	Femoral artery Femoral vein
Pump speed (maximum rpm)	As per heart rate	5000	51,000	33,000	7500
Flow rate L/min		7.0	2.5	5.0	4.0
Maximum recommended duration	30 days	7 days	10 days	10 days	14 days
FDA/CE	+/+	+/+	+/+	+/+	+/+
Cost in comparison to IABP	–	++	+++	++++	++++++

Abbreviations: IABP, intra-aortic balloon pump; ECLS, extracorporeal life support; ECMO, extracorporeal membrane oxygenation; rpm, rate per minute.

CONCLUSION

End-stage heart failure requires innovative management strategies. Today in our armamentarium we have large number of effective devices that can improve morbidity and mortality in patients suffering from heart failure. However, these devices are not yet approved by DGCI and are sparingly available on case-to-case basis. Moreover, the cost of these devices can be prohibitive for large number of patients in this country. Yet it is necessary for the cardiologists taking care of these patients to be aware of all the options so that these therapies can be offered to them as a rescue or salvage option when significant progress is not achieved by the conventional modalities of treatment.

REFERENCES

1. Birks E, Tansley PD, Hardey J, et al. Left ventricular assist device and drug therapy for the reversal of heart failure. N Eng J Med. 2006;355(18):1873-84.
2. Osaki S, Edwards NM, Velez M, et al. Improved survival in patients with ventricular assist device therapy: the University of Wisconsin experience. Eur J Cardiothorac Surg. 2008;34(2):281-8.
3. Rao V, Slater JP, Edwards NM, et al. Surgical management of valvular disease in patients requiring left ventricular assist device support. Ann Thorac Surg. 2001;71(5):1448-53.
4. Lauten A, Engström AE, Jung C, Empen K, Erne P, Cook S, et al. Percutaneous left-ventricular support with the Impella-2.5-assist Device in acute cardiogenic shock: results of the Impella-EUROSHOCK-Registry. Circ Heart Fail. 2013;6:23-30.
5. Shin TG, Choi J-H, Jo IJ, et al. Extracorporeal cardiopulmonary resuscitation in patients with in-hospital cardiac arrest: a comparison with conventional cardiopulmonary resuscitation. Crit Care Med. 2011;39(1):1-7.
6. Chen YS, Lin JW, Yu HY, et al. Cardiopulmonary resuscitation with assisted extracorporeal life-support versus conventional cardiopulmonary resuscitation in adults with in hospital cardiac arrest: an observational study and propensity analysis. The Lancet. 2008;372(9638):554-61.
7. Pages ON, Aubert S, Combes A, et al. Paracorporeal pulsatile biventricular assist device versus extracorporeal membrane oxygenation-extracorporeal life support in adult fulminant myocarditis. J Thorac Cardiovasc Surg. 2009;137(1):194-7.

30

Diastolic Heart Failure

Sameer Srivastava, Avinash Verma

"The greatest trick the devil ever pulled was convincing the world he didn't exist."
—*Charles Baudelaire*

Such is the case with diastolic heart failure (DHF). As a term, DHF was first introduced by Kessler[1] in as late as 1988. The obliviousness about this entity is apparent in lack of any consensus on its definition or even its relevance as a separate disease. Diastolic heart failure is a part pathophysiology of systolic heart failure (SHF). The relative contribution of DHF in the symptomatology and prognosis of SHF is a subject of consideration. Existing clinical studies suggest that the frequency of DHF among patients with heart failure (HF) ranges from 13% to 74%.[2] However, in isolation it is as distinct a syndrome from SHF as there could be. None of the advances made in the field of management of SHF, viz., mortality benefits with angiotensin-converting-enzyme (ACE) inhibitors, beta-blocker, mineralocorticoids receptors antagonists, and cardiac devices demonstrate benefit in isolated DHF.[3]

Heart failure is defined as "a pathophysiological state in which an abnormality of cardiac function is responsible for failure of the heart to pump blood at a rate commensurate with metabolic requirements or to do so only from an elevated filling pressure."[3,4] Although conveying the message and having stood test of time, this definition is generalized and unquantifiable and cannot be incorporated into trials or day-to-day clinical practice. In 1980s, when large-scale trials began for what is now current standard of therapy in HF, left ventricular ejection fraction (LVEF) was taken as diagnostic indicator for HF.[5] Even though the symptom complex of DHF and SHF is indistinguishable from each other, this reliance on LVEF as indicator of HF led to exclusion of patients with isolated DHF [heart failure with preserved ejection fraction (HFpEF)] from the evidence base. It has led to arbitrary generalization of cardiac dysfunction as systolic cardiac dysfunction and thus leaving diastolic cardiac dysfunction out of favor and understudied. Hence, a working definition of DHF was need of the hour (Table 30.1).

Table 30.1 Prevalence of specific symptoms and signs in systolic and diastolic heart failure (HF)[6]

Symptoms	*Systolic HF*	*Diastolic HF*
Dyspnea on exertion	96	85
Paroxysmal nocturnal dyspnea	50	55
Orthopnea	73	60
Physical examination		
Jugular venous distension	46	35
Rales	70	72
Displaced apical impulse	60	50
S3	65	45
S4	66	45
Hepatomegaly	16	15
Edema	40	30
Chest radiograph		
Cardiomegaly	96	90
Pulmonary venous hypertension	80	85

Source: Adapted from Zile MR, Brutsaert DL. New concepts in diastolic dysfunction and diastolic heart failure. Part I: Diagnosis, prognosis, and measurements of diastolic function. Circulation. 2002;105(11):1387-93.

DEFINITION OF DIASTOLIC HEART FAILURE

Isolated DHF is a subset of more widely used HF with preserved or normal EF. Heart failure with preserved ejection fraction includes various types of left ventricular (LV) diastolic dysfunction, including delayed myocardial relaxation and myocardial restriction, as well as mild or long-axis LV systolic dysfunction, valve disease such as mitral stenosis (MS) and acute mitral regurgitation (MR), arrhythmias [predominantly atrial fibrillation (AF)], right ventricular dysfunction, and pericardial diseases. Diastolic heart failure as a term is used to describe a group of chronic heart failure (CHF) patients characterized by concentric remodeling, normal LV diastolic volume, and predominant abnormalities in LV diastolic properties including slow and delayed active relaxation and increased passive stiffness (Table 30.2).[7]

To fill this diagnostic void, the European Study Group of Diastolic Heart Failure[8] came out with a primary DHF criteria in 1998 (Table 30.3). It utilized noninvasive Doppler assessment for diagnosing DHF.[8] It was a consensus document and was not validated in trials.[9]

In 2000, Vasan and Levy[10] attempted to give a standardized definition to diagnose DHF (Table 30.4). However, their definition required invasive LV diastolic properties measurements by cardiac catheterization for making a diagnosis of definite DHF. Though a step forward it was impractical. Both these definitions used EF cutoff of 50% and 45%, respectively for DHF. Because LVEF > 45–50% appears to be normal, DHF was now termed as HFNEF or more accurately HFpEF. Systolic heart failure was termed as HFrEF.

In another approach, ACC/AHA in their 2013 HF guideline has used a cutoff of LVEF > 50% for differentiating HFpEF from HFrEF.[11] The definition also defines HFrEF cutoff as <40% keeping LVEF 40–50% as borderline. This definition is purely from treatment perspective and demarcates patients who are going to benefit from current HF management measures (that are mostly for LVEF < 40%) from those who are not (LVEF >50%). It is not a pathophysiological definition and does not take into account any diastolic function assessment.

Table 30.2 Causes of heart failure with preserved or normal ejection fraction[7]

DHF
Pressure-overload hypertrophy
Ischemic heart disease
Hypertrophic cardiomyopathy
Diabetes/metabolic syndrome
Valvular heart disease
Acute aortic
Mitral regurgitation
Mitral stenosis
Aortic stenosis
Pericardial disease
Constriction
Tamponade
Circulatory congestive states
Rapid fluid administration
Arteriovenous fistula
Severe anemia
Thyrotoxicosis

40% OR 50%—WHAT SHOULD BE THE CUT-OFF?

The LVEF cutoff value for diagnosis of DHF, however, is somewhat arbitrary. It is apparent that EF can remain preserved or normal (>50%) with drastically reduced stroke volume (SV) and cardiac output accompanied with raised filling pressures if the end-diastolic volume (EDV) is small thus giving rise to syndrome of DHF. The corollary is that LVEF at higher EDV has to be low to give a small SV required for low cardiac output in pathophysiology of SHF. So in effect an EF below or above 40% or 50% distinguishes between increased or normal/reduced left ventricular end-diastolic volumes (LVEDV) in HF patients. Thereby, it distinguishes between two different pathophysiologies of HF; both having reduced SV and increased filling pressures, but in one (SHF) LV dilates associated with reduced EF and in another (DHF) LV size remains normal or gets reduced with normal EF. The cutoff of 40% for HFrEF has arisen largely because in the past most patients of HF admitted to hospitals for investigation or entered into clinical trials have had dilated hearts with a reduced EF <35 or 40%.

At present there appears to be a consensus between American and European societies concerning the cutoffs for HFrEF, i.e. LVEF <40% (SHF) and HFpEF, i.e. LVEF > 50% (DHF).[3,11] Range between 40% and 50% is still a gray zone as European Society of Cardiology's 2012 Heart Failure guidelines mentions "patients with an EF in the range 35–50% therefore represent a 'gray area' and most probably have primarily mild systolic dysfunction".[3] ACC/AHA also defines LVEF range between 40% and 50% as borderline.

Epidemiology

Heart failure is a modern-day epidemic. It has reached epidemic proportions due to even widespread prevalence of its harbingers, viz., hypertension, diabetes mellitus (DM), and coronary artery disease (CAD). Aging population has furthered its scope.

Many studies have shown that approximately half of patients with HF have a normal EF. Senni et al. in Olmsted County, Minnesota, HF study in 1991 reported that in patients receiving first diagnosis of HF 43% had a normal EF (≥0.50) and 57% had a reduced EF (<0.50).[12] An echocardiographic study of 73 Framingham Heart Study subjects with HF found

Table 30.3 ASE/ESE recommendations for the evaluation of left ventricular diastolic function by echocardiography[46]

- Morphologic and functional correlates of diastolic dysfunction
  - Left ventricular hypertrophy
  - Left atrial (LA) volume
  - LA function
  - Pulmonary artery systolic and diastolic pressures
- Mitral inflow
- Valsalva maneuver
- Pulmonary venous flow
- Color M-mode flow propagation velocity
- Tissue Doppler annular early and late diastolic velocities
- Deformation measurements
- Left ventricular untwisting
- Estimation of left ventricular relaxation
  - Direct estimation
    - Isovolumic relaxation time
    - Aortic regurgitation CW signal
    - MR CW signal
  - Surrogate measurements
    - Mitral inflow velocities
    - Tissue Doppler annular signals
    - Color M-mode Vp
- Estimation of left ventricular stiffness
  - Direct estimation
  - Surrogate measurements
    - Declaration time of mitral E velocity.
    - A-wave transit time
- Diastolic stress test
- Other reasons for heart failure symptoms in patients with normal ejection fractions.
  - Pericardial diseases
  - Mitral stenosis
  - MR
- Estimation of left ventricular filling pressures in special populations
  - Atrial fibrillation
  - Sinus tachycardia
  - Restrictive cardiomyopathy
  - Hypertrophic cardiomyopathy
  - Pulmonary hypertension

Abbreviation: MR CW, mitral regurgitation continuous wave.

Table 30.4 Assessment of LV filling pressures in special populations[46]

Diseases	*Echocardiographic measurements and cutoff values*
Atrial fibrillation	Peak acceleration rate of mitral E velocity (≥1,900 cm/s^2), IVRT (≤65 ms), DT of pulmonary venous diastolic velocity (≤220 ms), E/Vp ratio (≥1.4), and septal E/e' = ratio (≥11)
Sinus tachycardia	Mitral inflow pattern with predominant early LV filling in patients with EFs < 50%, IVRT ≤ 70 ms is specific (79%), systolic filling fraction ≤ 40% is specific (88%), lateral E/e' > 10 (a ratio >12 has highest the specificity of 96%)
Hypertrophic cardiomyopathy	Lateral E/e' (≥10), Ar – A (≥30 ms), PA pressure (>35 mm Hg), and LA volume (≥34 mL/m^2)
Restrictive cardiomyopathy	DT (<140 ms), mitral E/A (>2.5), IVRT (<50 ms has high specificity), and septal E/e' (>15)
Non-cardiac pulmonary hypertension	Lateral E/e' can be applied to determine whether a cardiac etiology is the underlying reason for the increased PA pressures (cardiac etiology: E/e' > 10; non-cardiac etiology: E/e' < 8)
Mitral stenosis	IVRT (<60 ms has high specificity), IVRT/$T_{E\text{-}e'}$ (<4.2), mitral A velocity (>1.5 m/s)
MR	Ar – A (≥30 ms), IVRT (<60 ms has high specificity), and IVRT/$T_{E\text{-}e'}$ (<3) may be applied for the prediction of LV filling pressures in patients with MR and normal EFs, whereas average E/e' (>15) is applicable only in the presence of a depressed EF

Abbreviations: MR, mitral regurgitation continuous wave; IVRT, isovolumic relaxation time; LV, left ventricular; EF, ejection fraction; DT, deceleration time.

that 51% had a normal EF (≥0.50) and 49% had a reduced EF (<0.50).[13]

Similarly in Redfield et al study, the population prevalence of HF was 2.2% and among the HF patients, 44% had an EF ≥ 0.50,[14] whereas Cortina et al reported a population prevalence of HF as 5% and that among the HF patients, 59% had an EF ≥ 0.50.[15] Owan et al in 2005[2] reviewed epidemiology of DHF and reviewed nine cross-sectional epidemiological studies. In these studies, the prevalence of DHF within the population varies from 1.14% to 5.5%.

Risk Factors

In the general population, patients with HFpEF are usually older women with a history of hypertension. Obesity, CAD, DM, AF, and hyperlipidemia are also highly prevalent in HFpEF in population-based studies and registries.[16,17] Despite these associated cardiovascular risk factors, hypertension remains the most important cause of HFpEF, with a prevalence of 60–89% from large controlled trials, epidemiological studies, and HF registries.[18]

Prognosis

Studies have shown that both patients with a normal EF and those with a reduced EF have poor prognosis. Senni et al reported that the prognosis of patients with a new diagnosis of HF was worse than age- and gender-matched controls. Survival of HF patients was 86% at 3 months, 76% at 1 year, and 35% at 5 years.[12] There was no significant difference in adjusted survival between HF patients with an EF ³ 0.50 and those with an EF < 0.50 (Fig. 30.1). On the contrary, Vasan et al reported that HF patients with a reduced EF (<0.50) had significantly higher annual mortality than age- and gender-matched cases

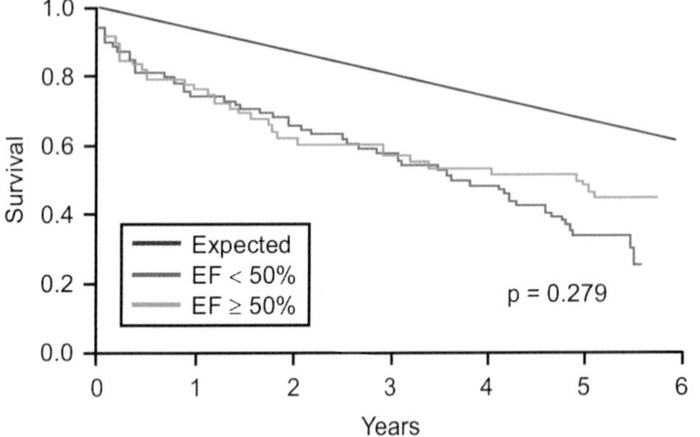

Fig. 30.1 Survival of heart failure patients with an ejection fraction of ≥50% and <50%

Source: Adapted from Senni M, Tribouilloy CM, Rodeheffer RJ, et al. Congestive heart failure in the community: a study of all incident cases in Olmsted County, Minnesota, in 1991. Circulation. 1998;98(21):2282-9.

[18.9% vs. 4.1%; adjusted HR (95% CI), 4.31 (1.98–9.36)].[13] Similarly, HF patients with a normal EF (≥0.50) had significantly higher annual mortality than age- and gender-matched cases [8.7% vs. 3.0%; adjusted HR (95% CI), 4.06 (1.61–10.3)].[13]

An echocardiographic substudy from the Irbesartan in HFpEF (I-PRESERVE) trial showed that increased LV mass, mass/volume ratio, and left atrial (LA) size were independently associated with (p < 0.05) an increased risk of both primary endpoint (death or cardiovascular hospitalization) of HF events.[19]

Pathophysiology of DHF

Diastolic Relaxation

Relaxation of the contracted myocardium begins at the onset of diastole. This is a dynamic process that takes place during isovolumic relaxation [the period between aortic valve closure and mitral valve opening (MVO) during which LV pressure declines with no change in volume] and then continues during the three phases of diastole (Fig. 30.3). The remaining three phases encompass the auxotonic phase, which begins with opening of the MV and early rapid passive filling of the LV (seen as the E wave on Doppler echocardiography).[20] The rapid pressure decay and the concomitant "untwisting" and elastic recoil of the left ventricle produce a suction effect that augments the left atrial (LA) to LV pressure gradient and pulls blood into the ventricle, thereby promoting diastolic filling.[21] The E-wave velocity reflects the high LA to LV pressure gradient and the elastic recoil of LV, creating a suction effect and pulling in blood from the left atrium. During the later phases of diastole, the normal left ventricle is composed of completely relaxed cardiomyocytes and is very compliant and easily distensible, offering minimal resistance to LV filling over a normal volume range. This phase is known as diastasis, when there is slow filling of the LV. Toward the end of diastole, atrial contraction results in an additional 20–30% filling of the LV (seen as the A wave on Doppler echocardiography) with increase of diastolic pressures by <5 mm Hg.[21]

During exercise in normal patients, relaxation rate is increased and early diastolic pressures decrease, augmenting elastic recoil and diastolic suction and resulting in more rapid filling during a shortened diastolic filling period at increasing heart rates (Fig. 30.2).[22,23]

Pathophysiology—Organ Level

- *Left ventricular myocardial*
  - Near normal or reduced LVEDV, increased LV mass, concentric left ventricular hypertrophy (LVH), increased relative wall thickness (RWT = 2 × Posterior wall thickness in diastole/LVIDd), i.e. RWT ≥ 0.42 suggestive of concentric hypertrophy (Fig. 30.3).[24]

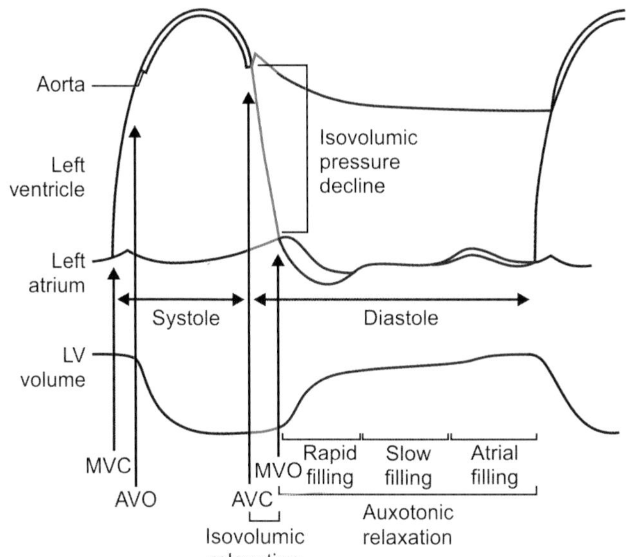

Fig. 30.2 Changes in left ventricular pressure and volume throughout the cardiac cycle. The cardiac cycle is divided into systole, the time period from mitral valve closure (MVC) to aortic valve closure (AVC), and diastole. Diastole is further divided into isovolumic relaxation [the time period from AVC to MVO during which left ventricular (LV) pressure declines with no change in volume] and auxotonic relaxation (the time period from MVO to MVC during which LV volume increases at variable pressure). AVO, atrial valve opening

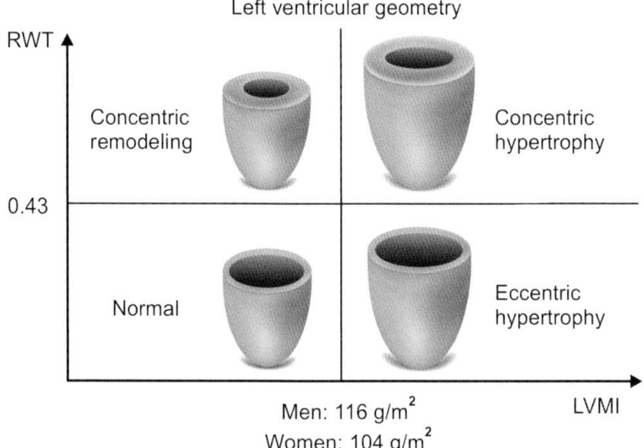

Fig. 30.3 Relationship of relative wall thickness (RWT) to left ventricular mass index (LVMI)

- *Reduced LV isovolumic relaxation*: Isovolumic relaxation can be measured by peak instantaneous rate of LV pressure decline (peak dP/dt) and the time constant of LV isovolumic pressure decline (Tau).[6] When the natural log of LV diastolic pressure is plotted versus time, Tau equals the slope of this linear relationship. Conceptually, Tau is the "time required for LV pressure to fall by approximately two-thirds of its initial value."[21] When isovolumic pressure decline is slowed, Tau is prolonged and its numerical value increases. Isovolumic relaxation time (IVRT) can also be noninvasively assessed using echocardiography.
- Reduced LV elastic recoil/suction.
- *Increased LV chamber stiffness and reduced distensibility*: Left ventricular diastolic stiffness and distensibility are quantified by the position and shape of the LV diastolic pressure–volume (P–V) relationship, which plots LV diastolic pressure as a function of LV diastolic volume throughout diastole (Fig. 30.4). A relatively stiff, nondistensible ventricle will require higher pressures to achieve filling of a given volume. Thus, an increase in LV diastolic chamber stiffness or a decrease in distensibility shifts the LV diastolic P–V curve upward and often increases its slope.

- Pericardial restraint.
- Right ventricular pressure/volume overload.

The major abnormalities in LV diastolic function that contribute to or occur during the development of DHF include:

- Slowed, delayed, and incomplete myocardial relaxation
- Impaired rate and extent of LV filling (Fig. 30.4)
- Shift of filling from early to late diastole (Fig. 30.4)
- Decreased early diastolic suction/recoil contributing to decrease dP/dt
- Augmented LA pressure during the early filling
- Altered passive elastic properties of the ventricle, resulting in increased passive stiffness and decreased diastolic distensibility
- Inability to sufficiently augment cardiac output during exercise
- Inability to sufficiently augment relaxation during exercise
- Inability to utilize the Frank–Starling mechanism during exercise
- Increased diastolic LV, LA, and pulmonary venous pressures at rest or during exercise.

Pathophysiology—Tissue Level

- Decreased myocardial relaxation
- Increased myocardial stiffness
- Abnormal force-frequency relationship
  - Increased HR results in decreased contractility
  - Increased HR results in decreased relaxation.

Pathophysiology—Cellular and Protein Level

- Increased myocyte diameter without an increase in length
- Reduced myocyte relaxation
- Post-translational modification of myofilaments
- Extracellular matrix, e.g. increased collagen, fibrosis

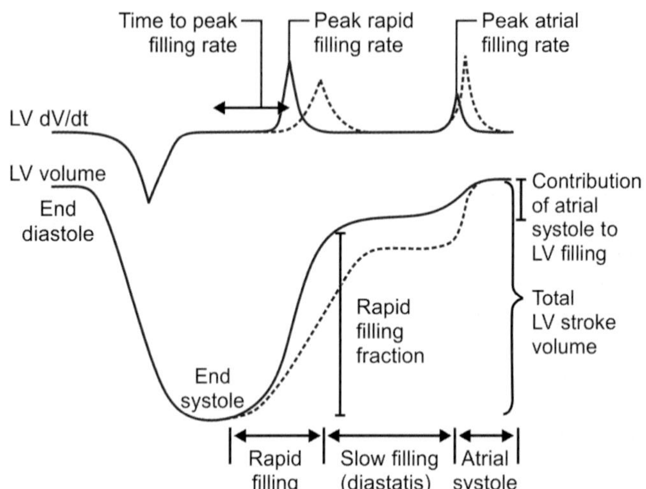

Fig. 30.4 In diastolic heart failure, peak dV/dt is reduced during early filling phase of diastole due to fall in dP/dt value. Simultaneously, the peak atrial filling rate (dV/dt during atrial systole) and relative contribution of atrial systole in ventricular filling rises

Source: Adapted from Bonnema DD, Baicu CF, Zile MR. Pathophysiology of diastolic heart failure: relaxation and stiffness. In: Klein AL, Garcia MJ (Eds). Diastology: Clinical Approach to Diastolic Heart Failure, 1st edition. Philadelphia: Saunders/Elsevier; 2008. p. 12.

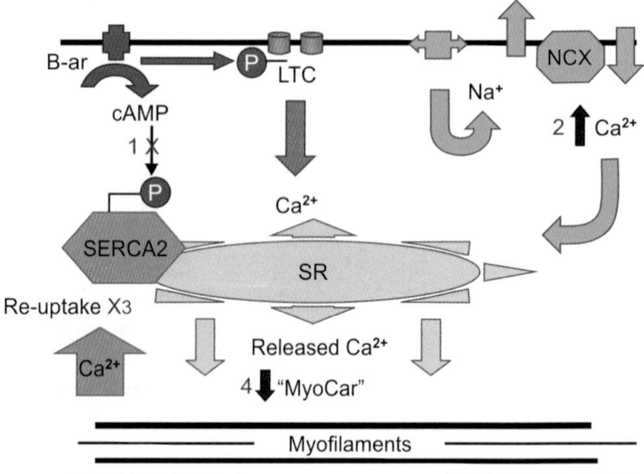

Fig. 30.5 Major cellular mechanisms of diastolic dysfunction. (1) Inhibition of cyclic adenosine monophosphate (cAMP) formation via adenylate cyclase due to β-receptor down-regulation. cAMP mediates phosphorylation of SERCA2 and the myofilaments, which reduces Ca^{2+} uptake and increases myofilament Ca^{2+}responsiveness, respectively. Ca^{2+} entry via the L-type Ca^{2+} channels is also increased. (2) Enhancement of Na^+/Ca^{2+} exchange. (3) Blockade of reuptake of Ca^{2+} by SERCA2 by non-cAMP-dependent mechanisms. (4) Decreased myofilament Ca^{2+} responsiveness by non-cAMP-dependent mechanisms. (B-ar, β-adrenergic receptor; p, phosphorylation site; SR, sarcoplasmic reticulum.)

Source: Adapted from Quraishi A, Morgan JP. Molecular, gene, and cellular mechanisms. In: Klein AL, Garcia MJ (Eds). Diastology: Clinical Approach to Diastolic Heart Failure, 1st edition. Philadelphia: Saunders/Elsevier; 2008. p. 5.

- Down regulation and uncoupling of β-receptors[25,26]
- Titin isoform changes
- *Decreased SERCA2a activity (Fig. 30.5)*[27]
  - Inhibition of cyclic adenosine monophosphate (cAMP) formation via adenylate cyclase. cAMP mediates phosphorylation of SERCA2 and the myofilaments, inhibition of which reduces Ca^{2+} uptake and increases myofilament Ca^{2+} responsiveness (MyoCAr), respectively. Ca^{2+} entry via the L-type Ca^{2+} channels is also increased[28]
  - Blockade of reuptake of Ca^{2+} by SERCA2 by non-cAMP-dependent mechanisms
  - Decreased myofilament Ca^{2+} responsiveness by non-cAMP-dependent mechanisms
- Reduced phospholamban m-RNA but increased SERCA2a to phospholamban ratio[29,30]
- Increased Ca^{2+} leak through RyR[31]
- Decreased sarcoplasmic reticulum (SR) Ca^{2+} transport leading to increased intracellular Ca^{2+} concentration leading to enhancement of Na^+/Ca^{2+} exchange (NCX). In humans, only 25% of the calcium is extruded by the NCX, and the other 75% is removed by SERCA2a pumps (Fig. 30.5).[32]

Pathophysiology—Gene Level

- Re-expression of fetal genes for myocyte hypertrophy
- Decreased SERCA2a expression[33,34]
- Increased NCX exchange expression.[35,36]

Role of Ischemia in LVH Causing DHF

Left ventricular hypertrophy and ischemia have important interactions. For a given degree of ischemia, a greater decline in diastolic function is seen in hypertrophied hearts.[37,38] Hearts with concentric LVH are highly susceptible to subendocardial ischemia for several reasons:[39]

1. Inadequate coronary growth relative to muscle mass, with a resultant decrease in capillary density.[40]
2. The increase in ventricular wall thickness raises the epicardial–endocardial distance. Thus, coronary perfusion pressure is dissipated in proportion to LV wall thickness, leaving the subendocardium as the region most vulnerable to ischemia.[39]
3. Increased LV diastolic pressures can cause vascular compression, thereby reducing coronary flow and perfusion of the subendocardial layer.[39]
4. Coronary flow reserve is diminished: Vascular tone at rest is often abnormally reduced, and coronary flow at rest is increased in the hypertrophied heart.[41,42] Thus, when metabolic demand and the need for oxygen increase,

coronary reserve is often inadequate to meet the increased oxygen requirements, and ischemia ensues.[42]

5. The incidence and severity of coronary atherosclerosis is increased in the presence of systemic arterial hypertension, a frequent cause of concentric LVH.

Clinical Features

Patients with either HFrEF or HFpEF often present with dyspnea, impaired exercise tolerance, orthopnea, and paroxysmal nocturnal dyspnea. Each may have signs suggestive of HF, including tachycardia, elevated neck veins, gallop, inspiratory crackles, displaced apical impulse, hepatomegaly, and dyspnea (Table 30.1). The frequency of these various signs and symptoms is not statistically different between patients with HFpEF versus those with HFrEF.[6] Also the biventricular filling pressures and pulmonary artery pressures are similarly elevated in HFpEF and HFrEF, although cardiac output is somewhat lower in HFrEF. In addition, exercise capacity is impaired in both HFpEF and HFrEF.

A history of hypertension and AF is slightly more prevalent in patients with HFpEF than in those with HFrEF, whereas CAD is more prevalent in HFrEF.[17,37] Rapid onset of dyspnea in patients who are markedly hypertensive (often termed "flash" pulmonary edema), particularly in elderly women, is more common in HFpEF. Slower-onset HF with a history of coronary disease, particularly in middle-aged men, is more likely to be related to HFrEF.[17,37] Atrial fibrillation or LVH on the electrocardiogram (ECG) is more suggestive of HFpEF. Left bundle branch block (LBBB) or evidence of prior ischemic injury is more suggestive of HFrEF.[37,43]

ASSESSMENT OF DIASTOLIC HEART FAILURE

Electrocardiography

An ECG should be performed in all patients with suspected HF. Although an abnormal ECG has little predictive power for the presence of HF, common abnormal findings in patients with HFpEF include evidence of ventricular hypertrophy, presence of LV strain, LA abnormality, and AF.[44,45]

Chest X-ray

A chest X-ray is routinely ordered to detect pulmonary vascular congestion and cardiomegaly.[44,45] Radiographic signs of pulmonary congestion, including increased interstitial markings, Kerley "B" lines, and pleural effusion, frequently indicate pulmonary venous hypertension and elevated LA pressure in a patient with HFpEF. Cardiomegaly in a patient with HFpEF generally reflects ventricular hypertrophy due to long-standing pressure overload as well as atrial and right heart enlargement. These findings may be considered indicative, if not diagnostic, of the HF syndrome.

Echocardiographic Assessment of DHF

Echocardiography is the mainstay of cardiac diastolic function assessment. It is immense in possibility, and a detailed discussion of its role and techniques is beyond the scope of this chapter. Readers are advised to read "ASE/ESE Recommendations for the Evaluation of Left Ventricular Diastolic Function by Echocardiography" and references provided in this chapter.

ASE/ESE recommends following parameters for study of diastolic functions of the heart (Table 30.3). Some of the variables are mainstream but others like deformation measurements and LV untwisting are still mainly used as research tools.

1. *Morphologic and functional correlates of diastolic dysfunction*
   A. *Left ventricular hypertrophy*: The ASE-recommended formula for estimation of LV mass is:[24]
      $$\text{LV mass} = 0.8 \times \{1.04[(\text{LVIDd} + \text{PWTd} + \text{SWTd})^3 - (\text{LVIDd})^3]\} + 0.6 \text{ g}$$
      where PWTd and SWTd are posterior wall thickness and septal wall thickness at end diastole, respectively.
      Relative wall thickness calculated by the formula (2 × PWTd)/LVIDd categorizes an increase in LV mass as either concentric (RWT $\geq$ 0.42) or eccentric (RWT < 0.42) hypertrophy and allows identification of concentric remodeling (normal LV mass with increased RWT.[24]
   B. *Left atrial volume*: Increased filling pressure will result in remodeling of left atrium that is reflected in the measure of LA volume. Left atrial volume is regarded as a "barometer" of the chronicity of diastolic dysfunction and "to analogize, LA volume is to diastolic function and to all forms of heart disease as the HbA1c is to diabetes."[47] Left atrial volume index $\geq$ 34 mL/m^2 is an independent predictor of death, HF, AF, and ischemic stroke.[48]
   C. *Left atrial function*: The atrium modulates ventricular filling through its reservoir, conduit, and pump functions.
      i. *Reservoir function*: When the atrioventricular (AV) valves are closed (i.e. during ventricular systole and isovolumic relaxation) atrial chambers work as distensible reservoirs accommodating blood flow from the venous circulation [reservoir volume is defined as LA maximum volume – LA minimum volume; atrial expansion index = [(LAmax – LAmin)/LAmin] × 100].[49]
      ii. *Pump function*: The atrium is a pumping chamber, which adds to adequate LVEDV by actively emptying at end-diastole [LA stroke volume is LA volume at the onset of the electrocardiographic P wave minus LA minimum volume; active atrial

emptying fraction = [(LApreA – LAmin)/LApreA] × 100], as an index of LA active function.[49]

iii. *Conduit function*: The atrium behaves as a conduit that starts with AV valve opening and terminates before atrial contraction and can be defined as LV stroke volume minus the sum of LA passive and active emptying volumes [Passive atrial emptying fraction (LA passive) = [(LAmax – LApreA)/ LAmax] × 100, as an index].[49]

LA functional assessment is not routinely recommended.

D. *Pulmonary artery systolic and diastolic pressures (PASP and PADP)*: With normal pulmonary resistance and no pulmonary vein obstruction normal PASP and PADP denotes normal LA pressure. Pulmonary artery pressures is not reflective of LA pressures in patients with pulmonary vascular resistance > 200 dynes × s × cm^{-5} or mean PA pressures > 40 mm Hg in which PA diastolic pressure is higher (>5 mm Hg) than mean wedge pressure.

2. *Mitral inflow velocities*: PW Doppler is performed to record peak E and A velocities, E/A ratio, deceleration time (DT), and IVRT. Mitral inflow patterns comprise normal, impaired LV relaxation, pseudonormal flow, and restrictive LV filling.

A. *Isovolumic relaxation time*: Left ventricular IVRT is the interval from aortic valve closure to MVO and the start of mitral inflow. In patients with impaired relaxation filling and normal pressures, a prolonged IVRT (>110 ms) is an early indicator of LV diastolic dysfunction. A short IVRT of 40–60 ms can be seen in young, healthy, normal individuals or in patients with very high mean LA pressure and restrictive filling.

B. *Peak mitral inflow velocity*: The mitral/LVOT velocity ratio is about 80% in younger individuals, decreasing to 70% in middle aged and 60% in the elderly as LV relaxation slows slightly and E-wave velocity decreases. An *E wave/LVOT velocity ratio* lower than expected indicates impaired LV relaxation and normal mean LA pressure. A normal ratio with increased or decreased E- and A-wave velocities is seen with reduced or increased cardiac output. Higher than expected ratios indicate that peak E-wave velocity is elevated, which may occur in MS, MR, or increased mean LA pressure.

C. *Mitral deceleration time*: Mitral DT is the most important mitral variable for prognosis when heart disease is present, regardless of LVEF. In cardiac patients, mitral DT relates to LV chamber stiffness; the shorter the mitral DT and the more "restrictive" the LV filling pattern, the higher the mortality.

i. With impaired LV relaxation and normal mean LA pressure, early diastolic filling is reduced (E/A wave ratio < 1) and mitral DT is prolonged roughly in proportion to the slowing in the rate of LV relaxation.

ii. With pseudonormal mitral filling, the elevated mean LA pressure increases filling in early diastole into the noncompliant ventricle, and the rapid filling wave shortens the DT, with values that appear more normal for age.

iii. More advanced disease and further decreases in LV compliance cause such high a pressure that blood is forced rapidly into a stiff ventricle in early diastole, which causes a very rapid, abnormal rise in LV pressure. A short mitral DT (<140 ms) characterizes this restrictive filling, which is most commonly seen in advanced dilated or restrictive cardiomyopathies.

D. *Mitral flow velocity at the start of atrial contraction*: If mitral flow velocity does not have sufficient time to fall below 20 cm/s before atrial contraction, early and late diastolic filling (E and A waves) begin to merge. The fusion of early and late diastolic filling most often occurs when the heart rate is too fast for a diastolic filling period that is shortened by impaired LV relaxation (very long IVRT) from LVH, an LBBB, or CAD.

E. *Peak mitral A-wave velocity*: The mitral A-wave velocity is determined by the late diastolic transmitral pressure gradient and varies from 50 cm/s in younger individuals to 75 cm/s in normal individuals over 60 years of age. In patients with impaired relaxation filling and reduced E-wave velocity, an increased A-wave velocity and TVI are expected and necessary to maintain a normal LVEDV and cardiac output. An A-wave velocity below 1 m/s or atrial DT that is unusually short (<110 ms) may indicate a decrease in late diastolic LV chamber compliance and an increase in LV A-wave and end diastolic pressures.

F. *Mitral A-wave duration*: In pseudonormal or restricted LV filling patterns, the mitral A-wave duration is shortened because excessive rise in LV pressure with atrial contraction abruptly terminates transmitral flow. The reduced time of a positive transmitral pressure gradient is indicated by a shorter mitral A-wave duration whose DT is shorter than its acceleration time.

G. *Mitral peak E/A wave velocity ratio*: The E/A ratio is most helpful when the mitral DT is linear and preA velocity is below 20 cm/s. If there is partial fusion of E and A-wave velocities, then the LV filling pattern needs a careful assessment in relation to the other echo-Doppler findings.

i. *Mitral E/A ratio < 1 (Grade I)*: The "true" impaired relaxation filling pattern is due to slow LV relaxation with "normal mean LA pressure." Criteria include normal LA volume, with "hypercontractile"-appearing LA systolic function due to ejection into a ventricle with a lower than normal preA pressure. Left atrial pressures can be elevated despite with "impaired relaxation" pattern in following circumstances. *First*, it occurs when the mitral velocity at atrial contraction is above 20 cm/s and there is fusion of early and late diastolic LV filling. *Second*, an E/A ratio of <1 with increased filling pressures can also be seen in patients with marked LVH and severely impaired LV relaxation. The presence of *moderate or severe LVH, increased LA volume, E-wave velocity that approaches or exceeds LVOT velocity, and increased E/E' ratio* are all clues that despite the E/A wave ratio of below 1, mean LA pressure is elevated.

ii. *Pseudonormalization (Grade II)*: The MIP can be altered or pseudonormalized by changes in LA pressure. When diastolic dysfunction occurs, relaxation is slowed and incomplete, early LV diastolic pressures rise, early diastolic suction falls, and LV filling becomes increasingly dependent on an increase in LA pressure to push blood into the left ventricle during diastole. As LA pressures rise, the value of the E wave increases and the E/A ratio increases to a "normal" (or pseudonormal) value (Fig. 30.6). As a result, the E velocity and E/A ratio will now increase, and the mitral inflow velocity profile may appear normal (E/A = 0.9–1.5 and DT = 160–240, grade II diastolic dysfunction).

iii. *Mitral E/A ratio > 1 (Grades III and IV)*: When LA pressures are severely increased, a "restrictive" pattern may develop in which the IVRT may be decreased and the E/A ratio further increased. Similarly, individuals with grade III diastolic dysfunction, E/A > 2, and DT < 140 ms who are able to favorably influence their mitral inflow velocity profile with hemodynamic manipulation, often the Valsalva maneuver, declare themselves of less severe diastolic dysfunction than those with grade IV diastolic dysfunction who have an irreversible restrictive pattern and a very poor prognosis (Fig. 30.6).

3. *Valsalva maneuver*: During the Valsalva maneuver, LV preload is reduced during the strain phase (phase II), and changes in mitral inflow are used to distinguish normal from pseudo normal flow pattern (PNF pattern) (Fig. 30.6). A decrease of 20 cm/s in mitral peak E velocity is usually considered an adequate effort in patients without restrictive filling. In cardiac patients, a decrease of >50% in the E/A ratio is highly specific for increased LV filling pressures.

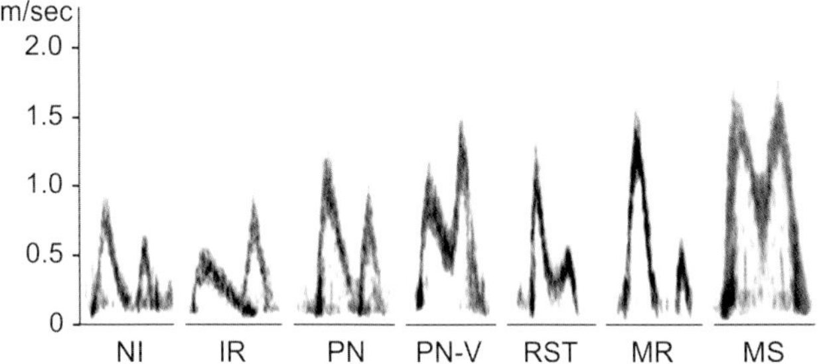

Fig. 30.6 Mitral E/A velocity ratios and their interpretation. (NI, normal; IR, impaired relaxation; PN, pseudonormal; PN-V, pseudonormal Valsalva; RST, restrictive; MR, mitral regurgitation; MS, mitral stenosis.)

4. *Pulmonary venous flow*: With increased LVEDP, atrial reversal (Ar) velocity and duration increase, as well as the Ar–A duration. D velocity is related to changes in LV filling and compliance and changes together with mitral E velocity. Pulmonary venous Ar velocity and duration are influenced by LV late diastolic pressures, atrial preload, and LA contractility. A reduction in LA compliance and a rise in LA pressure decrease the S velocity and increase the D velocity, resulting in an S/D ratio > 1, a systolic filling fraction < 40%, 63 and a shortening of the DT of D velocity, usually <150 ms.
5. *Color M-mode flow propagation velocity*: Vp > 50 cm/s is considered normal. In patients with reduced EFs, Vp is reduced, and should other Doppler indices appear inconclusive, an E/Vp ratio ≥ 2.5 predicts PCWP ≥ 15 mm Hg with reasonable accuracy. Patients with HFpEF with normal LV volume can have falsely normal Vp.
6. *Tissue Doppler annular early and late diastolic velocities*: PW DTI is performed in the apical views to acquire mitral annular velocities.
   A. Systolic and early (e´) and late (a´) diastolic velocities. The ratios include annular e'/a' and the mitral inflow E velocity to tissue Doppler e' (E/e') ratio.
      i. Septal e' is usually lower than lateral e' velocity. Therefore, the Septal E/e' ratio is higher than the lateral E/e' ratio. The average (septal and lateral) e' velocity should be used in the presence of regional dysfunction.
      ii. With age, e' velocity decreases, whereas a' velocity and the E/e' ratio increase.
      iii. By the septal E/e' ratio, a ratio <8 is usually associated with normal LV filling pressures, whereas a ratio >15 is associated with increased filling pressures.[50] When the value is between 8 and 15, other echocardiographic indices should be used.
      iv. The E/e' ratio is not accurate in patients with heavy annular calcification, MV disease, and constrictive pericarditis.
   B. $T_{E\text{-}e'}$: It is derived by subtracting the time interval between the QRS complex and the onset of mitral E velocity from the time interval between the QRS complex and e' onset.
      i. $T_{E\text{-}e'}$ is dependent on the time constant of LV relaxation (τ) and LV minimal pressure.
      ii. It is useful in subjects with normal cardiac function[51] or those with MV disease[52] and when the E/e' ratio is 8–15.[53] An IVRT/$T_{E\text{-}e'}$ ratio < 2 has reasonable accuracy in identifying patients with increased LV filling pressures.

7. *Deformation [strain/strain rate (StR)] measurements*: Hypertensive patients have a lower mean relaxation based on StR E and StR E/A at the basal, mid, and apical regions, with the basal parts appearing more compromised and with higher segmental diastolic dysfunction compared with controls.[46] Researchers have shown a significant relation between segmental[54] and global[55] early diastolic strain rate and the time constant of LV relaxation (τ).
8. *Estimation of LV relaxation*:
   A. *Direct estimation*:
      i. IVRT. When myocardial relaxation is impaired, IVRT is prolonged. Time constant of LV relaxation τ using noninvasive estimates of LV end-systolic pressure and LA pressure can be derived as τ. This approach can be used to provide a quantitative estimate of τ in place of a qualitative assessment of LV relaxation.[56]
   B. *Surrogate measurements*:
      i. *Mitral inflow velocities*: E/A ratio <1 is suggestive of markedly delayed myocardial relaxation with DT > 220 ms. In the presence of bradycardia, a characteristic low mid-diastolic (after early filling) mitral inflow velocity may be seen, due to a progressive fall in LV diastolic pressure related to slow LV relaxation (Fig. 30.7).
      ii. *Tissue Doppler annular signals*: Most patients with e' (lateral) < 8.5 cm/s or e' (septal) < 8 cm/s have impaired myocardial relaxation.
9. *Special circumstances*: Table 30.4.

Blood Test

Essential blood tests include plasma levels of the natriuretic peptides BNP and N-terminal pro-BNP (NT-proBNP). Other essential studies include complete blood counts to evaluate anemia, serum electrolytes, creatinine, glucose, liver function, and urinalysis.[44,45] Levels of both BNP and NT-proBNP though elevated are usually lower in patients with HFpEF than in those with HFrEF.[57] Accuracy of

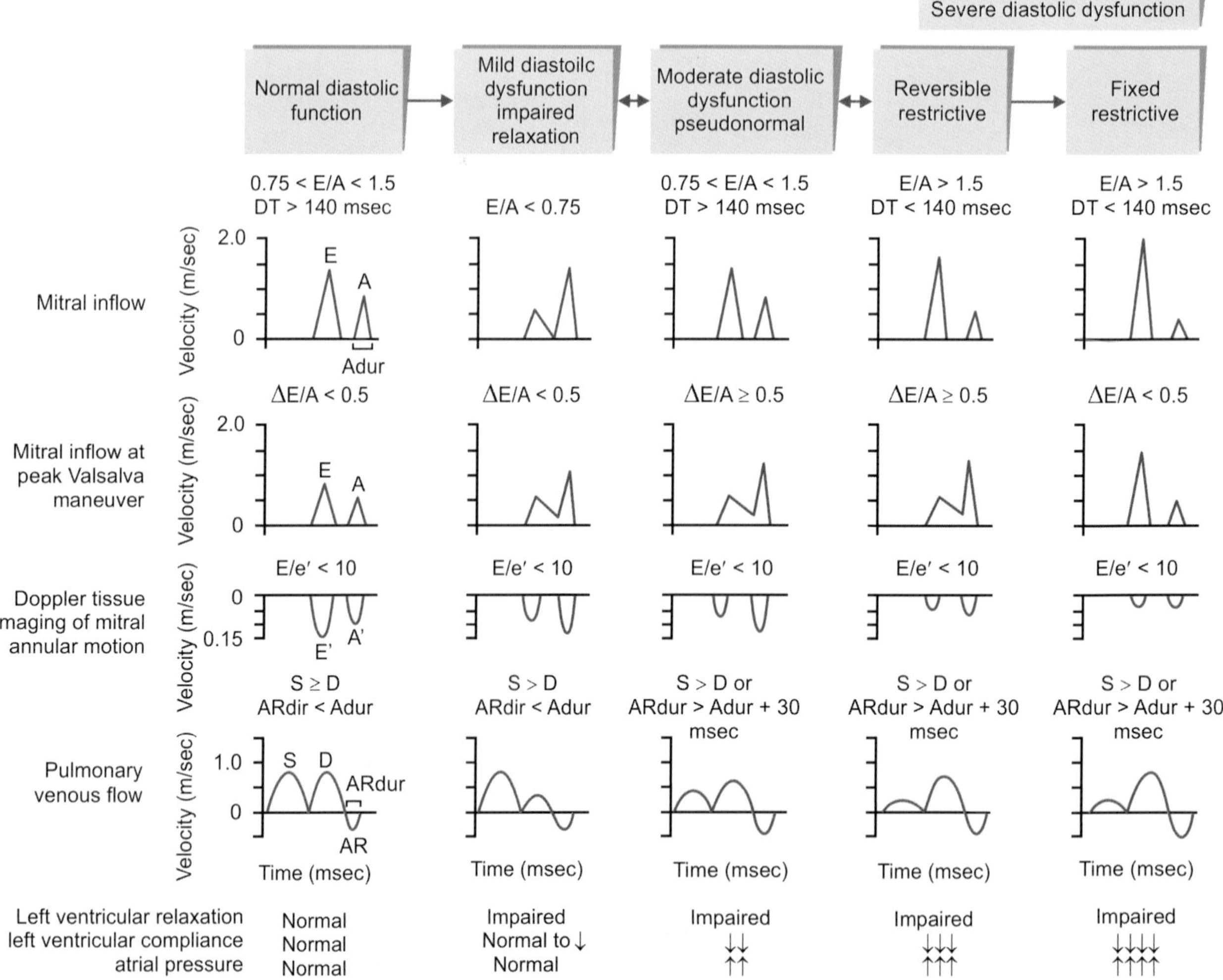

Fig. 30.7 Assessment and grading of diastolic dysfunction

NT-proBNP is generally superior than BNP levels due to higher sensitivity.[58]

On average, HFpEF patients presenting with acute decompensated heart failure have a BNP value of 100–500 pg/mL versus HFrEF patients with 500–1,500 pg/mL.[59] N-terminal proBNP at cutpoints > 450 pg/mL for patients <50 years of age and >900 pg/mL for patients ≥50 years of age are highly sensitive and specific for the diagnosis of acute HF in the emergency department.[58,60]

BNP and NT-proBNP are now essential elements of the diagnostic criteria for HFpEF proposed in HF guidelines.[3] Furthermore, BNP and NT-proBNP have become essential inclusion criteria in randomized controlled trails in HFpEF. The criterion diagnostic values of BNP = 100 pg/mL and NT-proBNP = 800 pg/mL have been suggested to support the diagnosis of HFpEF.[3] Both elevated NT-proBNP and BNP are strong independent predictors of clinical events in patients with HFpEF (Flow chart 30.1).

MANAGEMENT

Acute Heart Failure

Patients with HFpEF presenting with acute decompensation should be treated immediately with diuretics for pulmonary vascular congestion.[61] Nitrates, oxygen, and in some cases morphine sulfate are commonly used. Ventilatory support in form of noninvasive positive pressure ventilation or intubation may be required. In HFpEF, the diastolic P–V curve is steep, hence even small changes in volume result in large changes in pressure, and therefore an unmonitored drop in cardiac volume can produce hypotension and reduced cardiac output. Intravenous furosemide and nitrates should be employed judiciously.[61] Beta-adrenoceptor blockers or nondihydropyridine calcium channel blockers are useful for ventricular rate control during rapid AF or flutter.[61] Accelerated hypertensive episodes should be controlled with nitroglycerin or other antihypertensive agents as they are often the major cause of exacerbations (Flow chart 30.2).

Chronic Heart Failure

General measures such as daily monitoring of weight, attention to diet and lifestyle, patient education, and close medical follow-up are as helpful in HFpEF as in HFrEF. In patients with HFpEF, rigid control of hypertension, tachycardia, and other potential precipitants of HF decompensation should be addressed. Systolic and diastolic blood pressure should be controlled in patients with HFpEF in accordance with published clinical practice guidelines to prevent morbidity.[62,63] Diuretics should be used for relief of symptoms due to volume overload in patients with HFpEF.[61]

Renin Angiotensin System Inhibition in Diastolic Heart Failure

In the perindopril in elderly people with chronic heart failure (PEP-CHF) study, 850 elderly patients with LVEF between 40% and 50% and a history of HF and abnormal diastolic dysfunction were randomized either to perindopril or to placebo.[64] The primary endpoint was a composite of all-cause mortality and HF hospitalizations and was achieved in 25.1% of patients randomized to placebo versus 23.6% of patients randomized to perindopril ($p = 0.545$). However, in the interim analysis conducted at 1-year follow-up, patients randomized to perindopril had significantly fewer HF hospitalizations, improvement in New York Heart Association (NYHA) class, and an increase in 6 minutes walking distance. Explanation given for lack of significant benefit at the end of mean study duration of 29 months was that by end of 1 year, a large proportion of the patients were unblinded, and about one-third were taking ACE inhibitors by the end of the study.[65]

The first large randomized clinical trial in patients with HF and preserved EF conducted is the CHARM-Preserved trial.[66] CHARM-Preserved enrolled 3,023 patients, randomizing them to either candesartan or placebo with a mean follow-up of 36.6 months. There was a slight relative risk reduction of 11% in the combined primary outcome of cardiovascular death and hospitalizations related to HF among LV preserved patients treated with candesartan; however, this improvement was marginal (unadjusted $p = 0.118$, covariate adjusted $p = 0.051$). Although cardiovascular death did not differ between the two groups, there did appear to be a significant reduction in HF hospitalizations with use of candesartan ($p = 0.017$).

ARBs have consistently demonstrated an improvement in LVH regression; in fact, the greatest reduction (13%) of LV mass index in a meta-analysis on antihypertensive therapy was observed with ARBs.[67] A study of hypertensive patients using losartan for 12 months, with endomyocardial biopsies at follow-up demonstrated losartan causing significant regression of myocardial fibrosis and that this was associated with reduction of echocardiographically assessed LV chamber stiffness.[68]

So far the largest study in HFpEF I-PRESERVE enrolled 4,128 patients ≥ 60 years of age and had NYHA class II, III, or IV HF and an LVEF ≥ 45% and randomly assigned them to receive 300 mg of irbesartan or placebo per day.[69] During a mean follow-up of 49.5 months, the primary outcome (death from any cause or hospitalization for a cardiovascular cause) occurred in 742 patients (100.4 per 1,000 patient-years) in the irbesartan group and 763 (105.4 per 1,000 patient-years) in the placebo group [hazard ratio, 0.95; 95% confidence interval (CI), 0.86–1.05; $p = 0.35$]. Overall rates of death ($p = 0.98$) and rates of hospitalization for cardiovascular ($p = 0.44$) were similar. Irbesartan did not improve the outcomes of

Flow chart 30.1 Heart Failure and Echocardiography Associations of the European Society of Cardiology algorithm for diagnosing diastolic heart failure

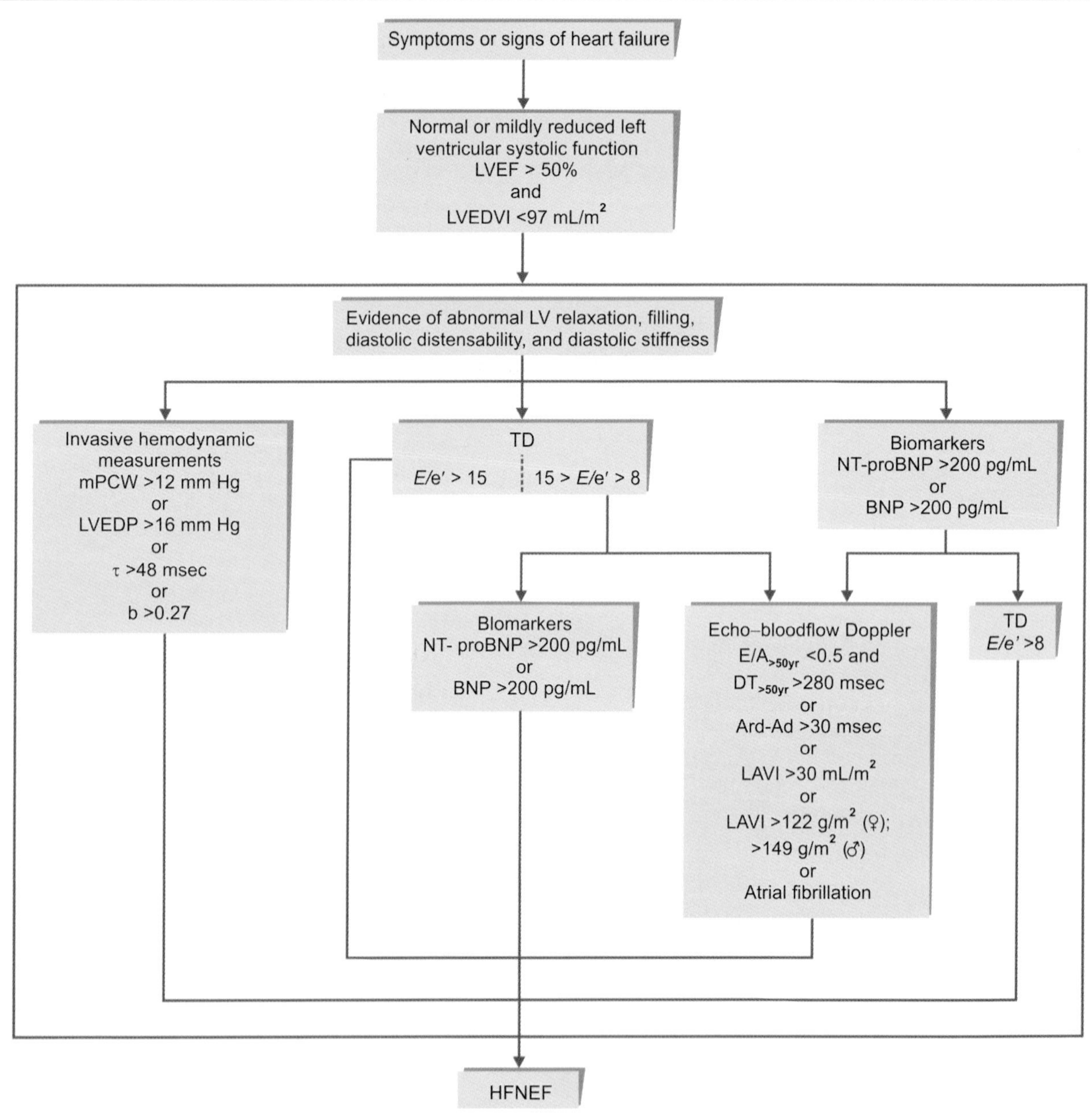

Source: Adapted from Paulus WJ, Tschope C, Sanderson JE, et al. Eur Heart J. 2007;28(21):2686.

patients with HFpEF.[69] The I-PRESERVE trial as compared to the older CHARM-Preserved study enrolled patients with greater incidence of HF due to hypertension (63 vs. 23%), as compared to an ischemic etiology (24 vs. 63%).[70] Still it failed to show any benefit in this favorable subset of HF patients.

Recently in 2013 a systematic review of RAS inhibition in HFpEF patients was done by Agarwal et al in which a total of 12 studies with 11,259 participants were included in the analysis. The authors reported that among the randomized clinical trials, with the use of RAS inhibitors over standard treatment, there was no improvement in all-cause mortality ($p = 0.88$), while there was a trend toward lowered rates of hospitalization ($p = 0.08$). As per the 2013 ACCF/AHA Heart Failure Guidelines the use of ARBs might be considered to decrease hospitalizations for patients with HFpEF (class IIb, Level of Evidence B).[61]

Flow chart 30.2 Management: treatment of heart failure with preserved ejection fraction

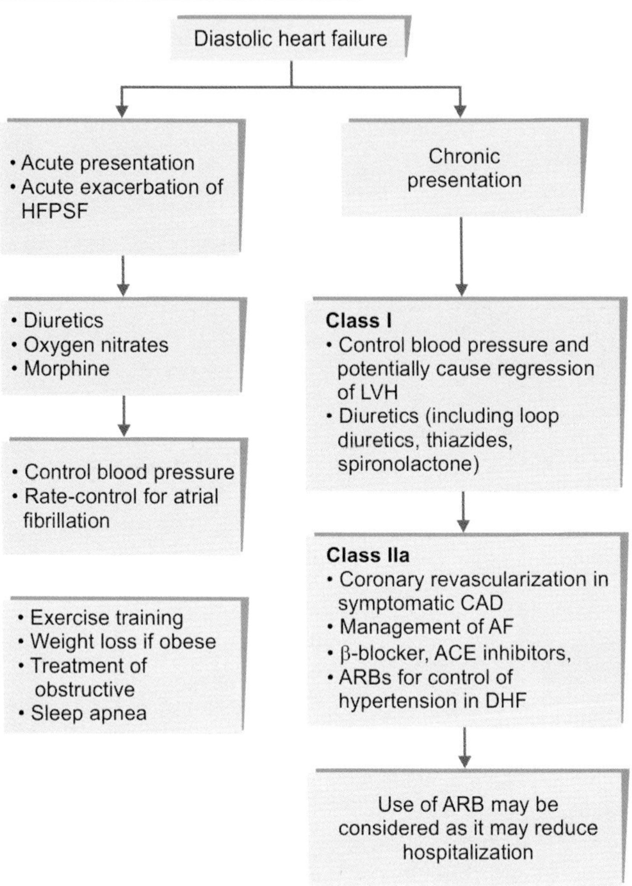

Beta-Blockers

The SENIORS trial randomized 2,128 elderly patients with HF to nebivolol versus placebo.[71] Nebivolol is a β-1-selective blocker that modulates nitric oxide and serves as a vasodilator. Only 35% of patients had an EF > 35%. The primary outcome consisted of a composite of all-cause mortality or cardiovascular hospitalizations. Subgroup analyses were performed in patients with EFs <35% and >35%. The hazard ratios for the primary outcome were 0.87 and 0.82, respectively, indicating no differential effect on preserved or low EF. However, beta-blockers could not offer same magnitude of benefit that they did in SHF, such as was established with carvedilol in the COPERNICUS[72] and bisoprolol in the CIBIS II studies.[73]

The Swedish Doppler echocardiographic study (SWEDIC) was comprised solely of patients with HF and preserved systolic function.[74] In this study, 113 patients were randomized to carvedilol or placebo for 6 months. A statistically significant improvement in E/A ratio was found in patients treated with carvedilol ($p = 0.046$). On subgroup analysis, the benefit of carvedilol on E/A ratio was exclusive to patients with baseline heart rates > 71 bpm ($p = 0.002$). In those with low heart rates (<71 bpm), there was no effect.

In the Organized Program to Initiate Lifesaving Treatment in Hospitalized Patients with Heart Failure Registry (OPTIMIZE-HF), the cohort with HFPSF treated with a beta-blocker showed no mortality benefit at 1 year.[75] After treatment with carvedilol in Carvedilol Heart Failure Registry (COHERE), patients with an LVEF of >40% had improved functional status and lower rates of hospitalization, though it did not amount to the improvements seen in patients with systolic dysfunction.[76]

Beta-blockers may also be beneficial in patients with AF to control heart rate, lower blood pressure, and alleviate myocardial ischemia. As per the recent 2013 ACCF/AHA Heart Failure Guideline, the use of beta-blocking agents was not recommended for mortality of repeat hospitalization prevention owing to lack of data. However, beta-blocking agents along with ACE inhibitors, and ARBs in patients with hypertension can reasonably be used to control blood pressure in patients with HFpEF (class IIa, Level of Evidence C).[61]

Other Drugs

Aldosterone Antagonists

A recent trial Aldo-DHF randomized 422 patients with DHF to spironolactone 25 mg per day or placebo.[77] Inclusion criteria was age ≥ 50 years, NYHA II/III, preserved LVEF > 50%, and diastolic dysfunction evaluated by echo. After 12 months spironolactone significantly improved diastolic function (E/é, echocardiography) ($p < 0.001$) but did not significantly enhance maximal exercise capacity ($p = 0.81$). Spironolactone was found to be safe and effective. However, spironolactone also modestly increased serum potassium levels (+0.2 mmol/L; 95% CI, +0.1 to +0.3; $p < .001$) and decreased estimated glomerular filtration rate (–5 mL/min/1.73 m^2; 95% CI, –8 to –3 mL/min/1.73 m^2; $p < .001$) without affecting hospitalizations.[77] As of now, aldosterone antagonists are not recommended for HFpEF patients routinely.[61]

TOPCAT trial randomized 3,445 patients with symptomatic HFpEF from 270 sites in six countries in double-blind fashion to treatment with spironolactone (target dose 30 mg daily) or matching placebo.[78] The mean age was 68.6 ± 9.6 years with a slight female predominance (52%). History of hypertension (91% prevalence in TOPCAT) exceeded all other major HFpEF clinical trials and CAD was present in 57%.[79] The result is eagerly awaited.

PDE-5 Inhibitors

The RELAX study is double-blinded, placebo-controlled, randomized trial in patients with DHF assessing the use of chronic sildenafil therapy.[80] Patients with NYHA class II–IV symptoms, EF ≥ 50%, elevated (>400 pg/mL) NT-proBNP or elevated rest or exercise filling pressures (catheterization) and peak VO_2 ≤60% predicted with respiratory exchange ratio ≥ 1 on screening cardiopulmonary exercise test were enrolled. Two hundred and sixteen participants were randomized 1:1 to either sildenafil or placebo. It was a negative trial and it demonstrated that there was a 91% and 80% ($p = 0.90$) change in peak VO_2 for the sildenafil group (n = 91) and placebo group (n = 94), respectively.[80]

FUTURE

Use of BNP as a therapeutic agent by using neutral endopeptidases (neprilysin) inhibitor to increase in vivo levels of BNP is being tested in a phase 2 study. PARAMOUNT is a randomized, double-blind multicenter trial in patients with NYHA class II-III HFpEF (EF > 45%), and NT-proBNP >400 pg/mL.[81] One hundred and forty-nine patients were assigned to LCZ696 (an angiotensin receptor and neprilysin inhibitor, 200 mg BID) or 152 patients to valsartan (160 mg BID) for 36 weeks. At 12 weeks, LCZ696 significantly reduced NT-proBNP by approximately 15% compared with valsartan (p = 0.005). At 36 weeks, LCZ696 significantly reduced LA volume by approximately 5% compared with valsartan (p = 0.003). LCZ improved NHYA class versus valsartan (p = 0.05). LCZ696 was well tolerated with adverse effects similar to those of valsartan. LCZ696 effect on clinical outcomes will be tested in a large randomized trial (PARAGON-HF).[59]

Zile et al[82] reported that treatment with the selective endothelin type A [ETA] receptor antagonist sitaxentan appears safe and significantly increased exercise tolerance in patients with DHF, as measured by time on the treadmill. In a phase 2, multicenter, double-blind, placebo-controlled study, they enrolled 148 patients aged 18 years and older (mean age ~64 years) with signs and symptoms of CHF NYHA functional class (FC) 2 or 3 and LVEF[3] 50%. Patients were randomized in a 2:1 ratio to placebo (n = 52) or to a target dose of 100 mg of sitaxsentan once daily (n = 96). Sitaxsentan significantly increased median treadmill time compared with placebo (90 second increase vs. 37 second increase; p = .03). There were no changes in E/E' ratio, LV mass, quality of life (QoL), NYHA FC, deaths, or HF hospitalization. The incidence of adverse events (all causalities and treatment-related) was reported similar for both groups.[82]

Advanced glycation end-product (AGEs) crosslink breakers alagebrium directly targets the biochemical pathway leading to myocardial and vascular stiffness. Advanced glycation end-products irreversibly crosslink the collagen molecule and make it less susceptible to degradation by MMPs and therefore leads to increased stiff ness. In a phase 2 trial (DIAMOND study) patients who received alagebrium had a statistically significant reduction in LV mass, as well as a marked improvement in the early LV diastolic filling and better QoL in the absence of blood pressure reduction.[83] The results from another study investigating alagebrium (PEDESTAL study) showed trends consistent with the DIAMOND study results.[84] However, in spite of proof of concept there were recent safety concerns regarding liver toxicity and further studies on this molecule have been given up.[84]

MCC-135 (calderet) is an agent that demonstrates improving effects for cardiac diastolic dysfunction and protective effects for cardiac necrosis by enhancing Ca^{2+} uptake by the SR and inhibiting the sarcolemmal Na^+/Ca^{2+} exchange.[85] It is under study in a phase 2 trial in patients symptomatic of DHF.[86]

Devices for HF monitoring are also going to be helpful in the management of HFpEF. The Champion trial (CardioMEMS Heart Sensor Allows Monitoring of Pressure to Improve Outcomes in NYHA Class III Heart Failure Patients) management of HFpEF based on knowledge of LVDP resulted in a 152% decrease in pressures and a 52% decrease in HF events (both $p < 0.001$ vs. control).[87]

Role of existing neurohormonal antagonists will be better defined in future and they will show their presence in the DHF treatment. In future drugs, working on calcium homeostasis will become more prominent. New targets will emerge, like AGE crosslink breakers, MMP modulators, and gene therapy will be tested. Intracardiac hemodynamic monitoring devices will play an important role in directing management of HFpEF.

CONCLUSION

Diastolic heart failure is the problem child of modern medicine. Of late, success has been achieved in defining the entity and formulating diagnostic criteria. Echocardiography has promoted our understanding of cardiac diastole and has made important contribution in formulating a noninvasive and relevant diagnostic criterion of DHF. Though quite simplistic in nature and easily amenable to understand, DHF has constantly defined any attempt of altering its prognosis by intervention. Till date, all the evidence guides us to treat the causal factors of DHF such as CAD and hypertension for prevention of DHF. Stages B, C, and D of DHF have very little evidence for even a class II recommendation. There are newer trials in the pipeline and hopefully we shall have some answers. More research in this field is need of the hour.

REFERENCES

1. Kessler KM. Diastolic heart failure. Diagnosis and management. Hosp Pract (Off Ed). 1989;24(7):137-41, 46-8, 58-60 passim.
2. Owan TE, Redfield MM. Epidemiology of diastolic heart failure. Prog Cardiovasc Dis. 2005;47(5):320-32.
3. McMurray JJ, Adamopoulos S, Anker SD, et al. ESC Guidelines for the diagnosis and treatment of acute and chronic heart failure 2012: The Task Force for the Diagnosis and Treatment of

Acute and Chronic Heart Failure 2012 of the European Society of Cardiology. Developed in collaboration with the Heart Failure Association (HFA) of the ESC. Eur Heart J. 2012;33(14):1787-847.
4. Braunwald E. Pathophysiology of heart failure. In: Braunwald E (Ed). Heart Disease : A Textbook of Cardiovascular Medicine, 4th edn. Philadelphia: WB Saunders; 1992. p. 393.
5. Marantz PR, Alderman MH, Tobin JN. Diagnostic heterogeneity in clinical trials for congestive heart failure. Ann Intern Med. 1988;109(1):55-61.
6. Zile MR, Brutsaert DL. New concepts in diastolic dysfunction and diastolic heart failure: Part I: Diagnosis, prognosis, and measurements of diastolic function. Circulation. 2002;105(11): 1387-93.
7. Zile MR, Baicu CF, Bonnema DD. Diastolic heart failure: definitions and terminology. Prog Cardiovasc Dis. 2005;47(5):307-13.
8. How to diagnose diastolic heart failure. European Study Group on Diastolic Heart Failure. Eur Heart J. 1998;19(7):990-1003.
9. Yturralde RF, Gaasch WH. Diagnostic criteria for diastolic heart failure. Prog Cardiovasc Dis. 2005;47(5):314-9.
10. Vasan RS, Levy D. Defining diastolic heart failure: a call for standardized diagnostic criteria. Circulation. 2000;101(17):2118-21.
11. Yancy CW, Jessup M, Bozkurt B, et al. 2013 ACCF/AHA Guideline for the Management of Heart Failure: A Report of the American College of Cardiology Foundation/American Heart Association Task Force on Practice Guidelines. J Am Coll Cardiol. 2013;62(16):e147-e239. doi:10.1016/j.jacc.2013.05.019
12. Senni M, Tribouilloy CM, Rodeheffer RJ, et al. Congestive heart failure in the community: a study of all incident cases in Olmsted County, Minnesota, in 1991. Circulation. 1998;98(21):2282-9.
13. Vasan RS, Larson MG, Benjamin EJ, et al. Congestive heart failure in subjects with normal versus reduced left ventricular ejection fraction: prevalence and mortality in a population-based cohort. J Am Coll Cardiol. 1999;33(7):1948-55.
14. Redfield MM, Jacobsen SJ, Burnett JC Jr., et al. Burden of systolic and diastolic ventricular dysfunction in the community: appreciating the scope of the heart failure epidemic. JAMA. 2003;289(2):194-202.
15. Cortina A, Reguero J, Segovia E, et al. Prevalence of heart failure in Asturias (a region in the north of Spain). Am J Cardiol. 2001;87(12):1417-9.
16. Owan TE, Hodge DO, Herges RM, et al. Trends in prevalence and outcome of heart failure with preserved ejection fraction. N Engl J Med. 2006;355(3):251-9.
17. Lee DS, Gona P, Vasan RS, et al. Relation of disease pathogenesis and risk factors to heart failure with preserved or reduced ejection fraction: insights from the framingham heart study of the national heart, lung, and blood institute. Circulation. 2009;119(24):3070-7.
18. Bhuiyan T, Maurer MS. Heart failure with preserved ejection fraction: persistent diagnosis, therapeutic enigma. Curr Cardiovasc Risk Rep. 2011;5(5):440-9.
19. Zile MR, Gottdiener JS, Hetzel SJ, et al. Prevalence and significance of alterations in cardiac structure and function in patients with heart failure and a preserved ejection fraction. Circulation. 2011;124(23):2491-501.
20. Lanier GM, Vaishnava P, Kosmas CE, et al. An update on diastolic dysfunction. Cardiol Rev. 2012;20(5):230-6.
21. Bonnema DD, Baicu CF, Zile MR. Pathophysiology of diastolic heart failure: relaxation and stiffness. In: Klein AL, Garcia MJ (Eds) . Diastology: Clinical Approach to Diastolic Heart Failure, 1st edition. Philadelphia: Saunders/Elsevier; 2008. p. 12.
22. Brutsaert DL, Sys SU, Gillebert TC. Diastolic failure: pathophysiology and therapeutic implications. J Am Coll Cardiol. 1993;22(1):318-25.
23. Leite-Moreira AF. Current perspectives in diastolic dysfunction and diastolic heart failure. Heart. 2006;92(5):712-8.
24. Lang RM, Bierig M, Devereux RB, et al. Recommendations for chamber quantification: a report from the American Society of Echocardiography's Guidelines and Standards Committee and the Chamber Quantification Writing Group, developed in conjunction with the European Association of Echocardiography, a branch of the European Society of Cardiology. Journal of the American Society of Echocardiography: official publication of the American Society of Echocardiography. 2005;18(12):1440-63.
25. Brodde OE. Beta-adrenoceptors in cardiac disease. Pharmacol Ther. 1993;60(3):405-30.
26. Ungerer M, Bohm M, Elce JS, et al. Altered expression of beta-adrenergic receptor kinase and beta 1-adrenergic receptors in the failing human heart. Circulation. 1993;87(2):454-63.
27. Pieske B, Maier LS, Bers DM, et al. Ca^{2+} handling and sarcoplasmic reticulum Ca^{2+} content in isolated failing and nonfailing human myocardium. Circ Res. 1999;85(1):38-46.
28. Quraishi A, Morgan JP. Molecular, gene, and cellular mechanisms. In: Klein AL, Garcia MJ (Eds). Diastology: Clinical Approach to Diastolic Heart Failure, 1st edn. Philadelphia: Saunders/Elsevier; 2008. p. 5.
29. Meyer M, Schillinger W, Pieske B, et al. Alterations of sarcoplasmic reticulum proteins in failing human dilated cardiomyopathy. Circulation. 1995;92(4):778-84.
30. Schwinger RH, Bohm M, Schmidt U, et al. Unchanged protein levels of SERCA II and phospholamban but reduced Ca^{2+} uptake and Ca(2+)-ATPase activity of cardiac sarcoplasmic reticulum from dilated cardiomyopathy patients compared with patients with nonfailing hearts. Circulation. 1995;92(11):3220-8.
31. Scoote M, Poole-Wilson PA, Williams AJ. The therapeutic potential of new insights into myocardial excitation-contraction coupling. Heart. 2003;89(4):371-6.
32. Hasenfuss G. Calcium pump overexpression and myocardial function. Implications for gene therapy of myocardial failure. Circ Res. 1998;83(9):966-8.
33. Cain BS, Meldrum DR, Joo KS, et al. Human SERCA2a levels correlate inversely with age in senescent human myocardium. J Am Coll Cardiol. 1998;32(2):458-67.
34. Hasenfuss G, Reinecke H, Studer R, et al. Relation between myocardial function and expression of sarcoplasmic reticulum Ca(2+)-ATPase in failing and nonfailing human myocardium. Circ Res. 1994;75(3):434-42.
35. Flesch M, Schwinger RH, Schiffer F, et al. Evidence for functional relevance of an enhanced expression of the Na(+)-Ca^{2+} exchanger in failing human myocardium. Circulation. 1996;94(5):992-1002.
36. Golden KL, Ren J, O'Connor J, et al. In vivo regulation of Na/Ca exchanger expression by adrenergic effectors. Am J Physiol Heart Circ Physiol. 2001;280(3):H1376-82.
37. Aurigemma GP, Gaasch WH. Clinical practice. Diastolic heart failure. N Engl J Med. 2004;351(11):1097-105.
38. Eberli FR, Apstein CS, Ngoy S, et al. Exacerbation of left ventricular ischemic diastolic dysfunction by pressure-overload hypertrophy. Modification by specific inhibition of cardiac angiotensin converting enzyme. Circulation research. 1992;70(5):931-43.
39. Isayama S. Interplay of hypertrophy and myocardial ischemia. In: Lorell BH, Grossman W (Eds). Diastolic Relaxation of

the Heart: The Biology of Diastole in Health and Disease, 2nd edn. Boston: Kluwer Academic; 1994. p. 203-12.
40. Tomanek RJ, Wessel TJ, Harrison DG. Capillary growth and geometry during long-term hypertension and myocardial hypertrophy in dogs. Am J Physiol. 1991;261(4 Pt 2):H1011-8.
41. Eberli FR, Ritter M, Schwitter J, et al. Coronary reserve in patients with aortic valve disease before and after successful aortic valve replacement. Eur Heart J. 1991;12(2):127-38.
42. Marcus ML, Koyanagi S, Harrison DG, et al. Abnormalities in the coronary circulation that occur as a consequence of cardiac hypertrophy. Am J Med. 1983;75(3A):62-6.
43. Udelson JE. Heart failure with preserved ejection fraction. Circulation. 2011;124(21):e540-3.
44. Jessup M, Abraham WT, Casey DE, et al. 2009 focused update: ACCF/AHA Guidelines for the Diagnosis and Management of Heart Failure in Adults: a report of the American College of Cardiology Foundation/American Heart Association Task Force on Practice Guidelines: developed in collaboration with the International Society for Heart and Lung Transplantation. Circulation. 2009;119(14):1977-2016.
45. Paulus WJ, Tschope C, Sanderson JE, et al. How to diagnose diastolic heart failure: a consensus statement on the diagnosis of heart failure with normal left ventricular ejection fraction by the Heart Failure and Echocardiography Associations of the European Society of Cardiology. Eur Heart J. 2007;28(20): 2539-50.
46. Nagueh SF, Appleton CP, Gillebert TC, et al. Recommendations for the evaluation of left ventricular diastolic function by echocardiography. J Am Soc Echocardiogr. 2009;22(2):107-33.
47. Lester SJ, Tajik AJ, Nishimura RA, et al. Unlocking the mysteries of diastolic function: deciphering the Rosetta Stone 10 years later. J Am Coll Cardiol. 2008;51(7):679-89.
48. Abhayaratna WP, Seward JB, Appleton CP, et al. Left atrial size: physiologic determinants and clinical applications. J Am Coll Cardiol. 2006;47(12):2357-63.
49. Marsan NA, Tops LF, Nihoyannopoulos P, et al. Real-time three dimensional echocardiography: current and future clinical applications. Heart. 2009;95(22):1881-90.
50. Ommen SR, Nishimura RA, Appleton CP, et al. Clinical utility of Doppler echocardiography and tissue Doppler imaging in the estimation of left ventricular filling pressures: a comparative simultaneous Doppler-catheterization study. Circulation. 2000;102(15):1788-94.
51. Rivas-Gotz C, Khoury DS, Manolios M, et al. Time interval between onset of mitral inflow and onset of early diastolic velocity by tissue Doppler: a novel index of left ventricular relaxation: experimental studies and clinical application. J Am Coll Cardiol. 2003;42(8):1463-70.
52. Diwan A, McCulloch M, Lawrie GM, et al. Doppler estimation of left ventricular filling pressures in patients with mitral valve disease. Circulation. 2005;111(24):3281-9.
53. Min PK, Ha JW, Jung JH, et al. Incremental value of measuring the time difference between onset of mitral inflow and onset of early diastolic mitral annulus velocity for the evaluation of left ventricular diastolic pressures in patients with normal systolic function and an indeterminate E/E'. Am J Cardiol. 2007;100(2):326-30.
54. Kato T, Noda A, Izawa H, et al. Myocardial velocity gradient as a noninvasively determined index of left ventricular diastolic dysfunction in patients with hypertrophic cardiomyopathy. J Am Coll Cardiol. 2003;42(2):278-85.
55. Wang J, Khoury DS, Thohan V, et al. Global diastolic strain rate for the assessment of left ventricular relaxation and filling pressures. Circulation. 2007;115(11):1376-83.
56. Scalia GM, Greenberg NL, McCarthy PM, et al. Noninvasive assessment of the ventricular relaxation time constant (tau) in humans by Doppler echocardiography. Circulation. 1997;95(1): 151-5.
57. Iwanaga Y, Nishi I, Furuichi S, et al. B-type natriuretic peptide strongly reflects diastolic wall stress in patients with chronic heart failure: comparison between systolic and diastolic heart failure. J Am Coll Cardiol. 2006;47(4):742-8.
58. Grewal J, McKelvie RS, Persson H, et al. Usefulness of N-terminal pro-brain natriuretic Peptide and brain natriuretic peptide to predict cardiovascular outcomes in patients with heart failure and preserved left ventricular ejection fraction. Am J Cardiol. 2008;102(6):733-7.
59. Zile MR, Baicu CF. Biomarkers of diastolic dysfunction and myocardial fibrosis: application to heart failure with a preserved ejection fraction. J Cardiovasc Transl Res. 2013;6(4):501-15.
60. Januzzi JL, Jr, Camargo CA, Anwaruddin S, et al. The N-terminal Pro-BNP investigation of dyspnea in the emergency department (PRIDE) study. Am J Cardiol. 2005;95(8):948-54.
61. Yancy CW, Jessup M, Bozkurt B, et al. 2013 ACCF/AHA Guideline for the Management of Heart Failure: A Report of the American College of Cardiology Foundation/American Heart Association Task Force on Practice Guidelines. J Am Coll Cardiol. 2013; 62(16):e147-e239.
62. Chobanian AV, Bakris GL, Black HR, et al. Seventh report of the Joint National Committee on Prevention, Detection, Evaluation, and Treatment of High Blood Pressure. Hypertension. 2003;42(6): 1206-52.
63. Levy D, Larson MG, Vasan RS, et al. The progression from hypertension to congestive heart failure. JAMA. 1996;275(20): 1557-62.
64. Cleland JG, Tendera M, Adamus J, et al. Perindopril for elderly people with chronic heart failure: the PEP-CHF study. The PEP investigators. Eur J Heart Fail. 1999;1(3):211-7.
65. Kanderian AS, Bhargava A, Francis GS. General treatment of diastolic heart failure. In: Klein AL, Garcia MJ (Eds). Diastology: Clinical Approach to Diastolic Heart Failure, 1st edn. Philadelphia: Saunders/Elsevier; 2008. p. 415.
66. Yusuf S, Pfeffer MA, Swedberg K, et al. Effects of candesartan in patients with chronic heart failure and preserved left-ventricular ejection fraction: the CHARM-Preserved Trial. Lancet. 2003;362(9386):777-81.
67. Klingbeil AU, Schneider M, Martus P, et al. A meta-analysis of the effects of treatment on left ventricular mass in essential hypertension. Am J Med. 2003;115(1):41-6.
68. Diez J, Querejeta R, Lopez B, et al. Losartan-dependent regression of myocardial fibrosis is associated with reduction of left ventricular chamber stiffness in hypertensive patients. Circulation. 2002;105(21):2512-7.
69. Massie BM, Carson PE, McMurray JJ, et al. Irbesartan in patients with heart failure and preserved ejection fraction. N Engl J Med. 2008;359(23):2456-67.
70. Agarwal V, Briasoulis A, Messerli FH. Effects of renin-angiotensin system blockade on mortality and hospitalization in heart failure with preserved ejection fraction. Heart Fail Rev. 2013;18(4):429-37.
71. Flather MD, Shibata MC, Coats AJ, et al. Randomized trial to determine the effect of nebivolol on mortality and cardiovascular hospital admission in elderly patients with heart failure (SENIORS). Eur Heart J. 2005;26(3):215-25.

72. Packer M, Fowler MB, Roecker EB, et al. Effect of carvedilol on the morbidity of patients with severe chronic heart failure: results of the carvedilol prospective randomized cumulative survival (COPERNICUS) study. Circulation. 2002;106(17):2194-9.
73. The Cardiac Insufficiency Bisoprolol Study II (CIBIS-II): a randomised trial. Lancet. 1999;353(9146):9-13.
74. Bergstrom A, Andersson B, Edner M, et al. Effect of carvedilol on diastolic function in patients with diastolic heart failure and preserved systolic function. Results of the Swedish Doppler-echocardiographic study (SWEDIC). Eur J Heart Fail. 2004;6(4): 453-61.
75. Hernandez AF, Hammill BG, O'Connor CM, et al. Clinical effectiveness of beta-blockers in heart failure: findings from the OPTIMIZE-HF (Organized Program to Initiate Lifesaving Treatment in Hospitalized Patients with Heart Failure) Registry. J Am Coll Cardiol. 2009;53(2):184-92.
76. Massie BM, Nelson JJ, Lukas MA, et al. Comparison of outcomes and usefulness of carvedilol across a spectrum of left ventricular ejection fractions in patients with heart failure in clinical practice. Am J Cardiol. 2007;99(9):1263-8.
77. Edelmann F, Wachter R, Schmidt AG, et al. Effect of spironolactone on diastolic function and exercise capacity in patients with heart failure with preserved ejection fraction: the Aldo-DHF randomized controlled trial. JAMA. 2013;309(8):781-91.
78. Desai AS, Lewis EF, Li R, et al. Rationale and design of the treatment of preserved cardiac function heart failure with an aldosterone antagonist trial: a randomized, controlled study of spironolactone in patients with symptomatic heart failure and preserved ejection fraction. Am Heart J. 2011;162(6):966-72 e10.
79. Shah SJ, Heitner JF, Sweitzer NK, et al. Baseline characteristics of patients in the treatment of preserved cardiac function heart failure with an aldosterone antagonist trial. Circ Heart Fail. 2013; 6(2):184-92.
80. Redfield MM, Chen HH, Borlaug BA, et al. Effect of phosphodiesterase-5 inhibition on exercise capacity and clinical status in heart failure with preserved ejection fraction: a randomized clinical trial. JAMA. 2013;309(12):1268-77.
81. Solomon SD, Zile M, Pieske B, et al. The angiotensin receptor neprilysin inhibitor LCZ696 in heart failure with preserved ejection fraction: a phase 2 double-blind randomised controlled trial. Lancet. 2012;380(9851):1387-95.
82. Zile MR, Barst RJ, Bourge R, et al. A phase 2 randomized, double-blind, placebo-controlled exploratory efficacy study of sitaxsentan sodium to improve impaired exercise tolerance in subjects with diastolic heart failure. J Card Fail. 2009;15(6):S63.
83. Little WC, Zile MR, Kitzman DW, et al. The effect of alagebrium chloride (ALT-711), a novel glucose cross-link breaker, in the treatment of elderly patients with diastolic heart failure. J Card Fail. 2005;11(3):191-5.
84. Tang WHW. Future therapies in diastolic heart failure. In: Klein AL, Garcia MJ (Eds). Diastology: Clinical Approach to Diastolic Heart Failure, 1st edn. Philadelphia: Saunders/Elsevier; 2008. p. 435.
85. Satoh N, Kitada Y. Effects of MCC-135 on Ca^{2+} uptake by sarcoplasmic reticulum and myofilament sensitivity to Ca^{2+} in isolated ventricular muscles of rats with diabetic cardiomyopathy. Mol Cell Biochem. 2003;249(1-2):45-51.
86. Zile M, Gaasch W, Little W, et al. A phase II, double-blind, randomized, placebo-controlled, dose comparative study of the efficacy, tolerability, and safety of MCC-135 in subjects with chronic heart failure, NYHA class II/III (MCC-135-GO1 study): rationale and design. J Card Fail. 2004;10(3):193-9.
87. Abraham WT, Adamson PB, Bourge RC, et al. Wireless pulmonary artery haemodynamic monitoring in chronic heart failure: a randomised controlled trial. Lancet. 2011;377(9766):658-66.

31

Stem Cells: A New Horizon toward Cardiac Regenerative Medicine

Vinay Sanghi, Khushboo Choudhury, Kenneth Lee Harris, Venkatesh Ponemone

INTRODUCTION

Coronary artery disease (CAD) and MI causes significant mortality, morbidity, and economic burden in our society in the present times. Coronary atherosclerosis plays a pivotal part as the underlying substrate in many patients. In addition, a new definition of MI has recently been introduced that has major implications from the epidemiological, societal, and patient points of view. The most common cause of heart failure is CAD, a narrowing of the small blood vessels that supply blood and oxygen to the heart. Symptoms of heart failure often begin slowly. At first, they may only occur when a person is very active. Over time, they may notice breathing problems and other symptoms even when in a resting position. Heart failure symptoms may also begin suddenly; for example, after a heart attack or sudden decompensation associated with high blood pressure or blood volume changes.

Most myocardial infarctions (MIs) are caused by a disruption in the vascular endothelium associated with an unstable atherosclerotic plaque that stimulates the formation of an intracoronary thrombus, which results in epicardial coronary artery blood flow occlusion. The development of chronic atherosclerotic plaque occurs over a period of years to decades. When a life-threatening sudden occlusion of the arterial lumen occurs due to the thrombus, and if it subsequently persists for more than 20 minutes, irreversible myocardial cell damage and cell death occurs resulting in a congestive heart failure (CHF). The degree of loss of viable myocardium in patients with MI serves as a main predictor of contractile ventricular dysfunction, the occurrence of acute complications and subsequent development of CHF. Therefore, the timely intervention for treating coronary occlusion is of particular importance for improving both survival and quality of life after CHF. The death of myocardial cells first occurs in the area of myocardium most distal to the epicardial arterial blood supply—the endocardium. As the duration of the occlusion increases, the area of myocardial cell death enlarges, extending from the endocardium to the myocardium and ultimately to the epicardium. The area of myocardial cell death then spreads laterally to areas of water shed or collateral perfusion. Generally, following a 6–8-hours period of coronary occlusion, most of the distal myocardium will be dead. The extent of myocardial cell death defines the magnitude of the MI. However, if blood flow can be restored to at-risk myocardium as soon as a symptomatic CHF appears, more heart muscle can be saved from the irreversible damage or death.

Congestive heart failure, commonly known as a heart failure is the inability of the heart to supply sufficient blood flow to meet the needs of the body. Cardiovascular disease remains the leading cause of death in industrialized nations despite major advances over the past 60 years in medical and surgical therapy. Largely, this relates to the growing worldwide epidemic of CHF currently affecting ~15 million patients and which carries a 5-year mortality of 50%. After MI, chronically ischemic (hibernating) myocardium may persist in association with variable degrees of scar tissue. In most circumstances, native angiogenesis is insufficient to prevent the resultant remodeling when significant injury occurs. As a consequence, infarct-related heart failure remains a major cause of morbidity and mortality. Heart failure—severe ventricular dysfunction—has numerous etiologies but is most often seen as a result of ischemic cardiomyopathy. Early rapid revascularization—be it with pharmacotherapy, stenting, or surgery—may potentially improve myocardial blood flow with resultant improvement in the function of remaining viable myocardium. However, current therapeutics cannot regenerate myocytes which have been lost to necrosis. As a result, complete cardiovascular functional restoration remains unattainable with the currently available conventional therapies. Despite application of pharmacotherapeutics and mechanical interventions, the cardiomyocytes lost during cardiac failure cannot be regenerated. The recent finding that a small population of cardiac muscle cells is able to replicate itself is encouraging but is still consistent with the concept that such regeneration is restricted to viable myocardium.

Despite the recent advances in percutaneous intervention, drug and device therapy, patients with acute myocardial infarction (AMI) and resulting left ventricular (LV) impairment have almost 13% mortality in 1 year. AMI as a consequence of CAD has significant detrimental effects. The affected left ventricle of patients who survived AMI may undergo negative remodeling (characterized by the replacement of necrotic myocardium with scar tissue which is made of fibroblasts and collagen) in about 6 months despite successful revascularization of the infarct artery. Eventually, it deteriorates into heart failure as the left ventricle function is compromised. After the loss of over one billion cardiomyocytes in a functionally significant MI, the surviving cardiomyocytes undergo abnormal remodeling, which eventually leads to cardiac failure. This has become one of the leading causes of death and disability in the developed world. It has also been associated with a 5-year mortality rate of up to 70% in symptomatic patients.[1] The advent of coronary-care units in all major hospitals plus the results of randomized clinical trials based on reperfusion therapy, percutaneous coronary intervention (PCI), and chronic medical treatment with various pharmacological agents have substantially changed the therapeutic approach, in-hospital mortality showing a decrease, and improved the long-term outlook in survivors of the acute phase of MI. In the present times, new treatments will continue to emerge, but the greatest challenge we face will be to implement preventive actions effectively in all high-risk individuals and also to expand the timely delivery of treatment of eligible patients in the acute phase. Ischemic heart failure occurs when cardiac tissue becomes seriously deprived of oxygen. If and when the ischemic abuse is severe enough to lead to a loss of critical amounts of cardiac muscle cells (cardiomyocytes), this initiates a cascade of detrimental events, including the formation of a noncontractile scar, ventricular wall thinning, an overload of blood flow and pressure, ventricular remodeling (the overstretching of viable cardiac cells to sustain cardiac output), heart failure, and subsequent death. Restoring this damaged heart muscle tissue, through repair, regeneration or remodeling, therefore represents a fundamental strategy to treat heart failure. Current pharmacologic interventions for heart disease, that includes beta-blockers, diuretics, and angiotensin-converting enzyme inhibitors, and surgical treatment options, such as changing the shape of the left ventricle and implanting assistive devices such as pacemakers or defibrillators, do not necessarily restore function to damaged tissue. Moreover, while the implantation of mechanical ventricular assist devices can provide long-term improvement in heart function, complications such as infections and blood clots remain an issue. There are certain factors that certainly necessitate exploration of new therapeutic modalities for long-term management of heart disease. One of these is the inability of all the available treatment options to repair and replace infarcted segment and prevent progressive left ventricle remodeling and systolic dysfunction. The other is a socioeconomic burden that is present on both the individual and society as a result of time and economic loss due to postinfarction failure. Stem cell transplantation can result in myocardial regeneration by halting the detrimental hemodynamic and neurohormonal effects that result in postinfarction heart failure. It has been postulated that the mechanism of action of BMSC therapy is via the release of paracrine factors. More importantly, implanted cells have not been shown to survive in myocardium for long periods. It is not known whether they can survive long enough to synthesize the paracrine factors necessary to affect cardiac repair and regeneration, or whether they release preformed cellular content, perhaps even in the act of dying, is not known.

The only therapeutic option that currently addresses cardiomyocyte loss is heart transplantation. But also due to stringent selection criteria and a chronic shortage of donor hearts, a vast majority of patients are deemed unsuitable or never able to receive a transplant. Therefore, preventing this progression post-MI is a major challenge requiring novel therapeutic strategies such as stem cell transplantation to improve prognosis and the quality of life for these patients. It has been a traditional view that the heart is a terminally differentiated organ that has been challenged by the discovery of stem cells transforming into cardiomyocytes in animal and human hearts. This in turn has led to the exciting possibility for regenerative therapy for cardiomyocyte loss after an MI. The demonstration of functional recovery of myocardium through cardiomyogenesis and neoangiogenesis in AMI in murine models has generated a tremendous interest in the potential of BMSCs.[2]

Progenitor cells are primitive bone marrow (BM) cells that have the capacity to proliferate, migrate, and differentiate into various mature cell types. Currently, one of the major sources of adult cells that have been used for basic research as well as in clinical trials originates from the BM. The bone marrow mononuclear subset is a heterogeneous population and comprises of hematopoietic progenitor cells, mesenchymal stem cells (MSCs) and endothelial progenitor cells (EPCs). The differentiation capacity of different populations of BMSCs into cardiomyocytes has been studied intensively. Since different isolation and identification methods have been used to determine the cell population studied, the results are rather confusing and sometimes difficult to compare. Till date, only MSCs have shown evidence to form cardiomyocytes, and only a small percentage of this population do so in vitro or in vivo. Pragmatically, the translation of the basic science into clinical research has followed a common trail: the injection of bone marrow-derived mononuclear cells (BMMNCs) as a source of stem cells into the heart. Autologous BMSC therapy has emerged as a novel approach to treat patients with LV dysfunction following AMI despite successful revascularization by PCI and patients with chronic ischemia and heart failure who have received surgical revascularization.[3] Since heart disease is reaching pandemic proportions in developed and developing countries and the heart, being an organ of limited regenerative capacity; most of the research using stem cell therapy is focused on the regeneration of the myocardium. Therefore, a major chunk of the studies focusing on stem cell differentiation and cell fusion are often looking at the heart. The implanted cells retain their contractile phenotype and express necessary elements for intercellular electrical communications.[2] It has been demonstrated that BM could be a source of extracardiac source of progenitor cells with the ability to differentiate into cardiomyocytes and restore cardiac function. Cell fusion of transplanted stem cells with the presence of resident cardiomyocytes has been proven as a feasible mechanism for differentiation. Fusion of BM-derived cells with Purkinje neurons, hepatocytes and cardiomyocytes was reported for the first time.[4]

Despite hopeful results with experiments looking at fusion and differentiation, the mechanism by which BMSCs work to repair damaged tissue remains unclear even in the light of seemingly successful studies. Furthermore, inconsistent results when researching stem cell regenerative capacity have been linked to improper labeling of donor cells and an inability to consistently track them in vivo, making it very difficult to distinguish them from background tissue leading to misinterpretation. One major limitation of cell therapy is the low therapeutic efficacy of transdifferentiated cells at the site of injury. This low rate of sustained transplanted engrafted stem cells has been attributed to insufficient blood supply, cell stress, hostile environment due to inflammation and hypoxia, and an elaboration of inflammatory cytokines resulting from ischemia and cell death. Research has shown that stem cell differentiation and fusion alone cannot account for enhanced cardiac function, evidence of the presence of a non-myogenic pathway of cardiac repair is being explored increasingly. The debate surrounding fusion and differentiation is of little importance now because the number of reported cardiomyocytes derived from exogenous stem cells is too low to account for the impressive enhancement of physiological function. Thus, it has been proposed that stem cell transplantation possesses therapeutic effect because of the endogenous repair mechanisms secreted by the BMSCs that account for functional benefits of cell therapy in cases such as cardiac repair. Indications for stem cell therapy in cardiac regenerative medicine include ischemic heart disease (IHD), CHF and AMI. These diseases can be managed by cell therapy that replaces the damaged heart tissue with new tissue that can be regenerated through stem cells and factors that activate endogenous cardiac myocytes. Under normal circumstances, dead myocardial tissue forms scar tissue as the capillary network does not meet the demands of the hypertrophied cells. This inevitable lack of oxygen and nutrients leads to apoptosis and necrosis. Moreover, inducing angiogenesis requires coordinated interactions between monocytes/macrophages, endothelial cells (EC), smooth muscle cells, and pericytes. Human BM-derived multipotent stem cells allow for angiogenesis by paracrine factors and are believed to influence adjacent cells via mechanisms including myocardial protection, neovascularization, and most the activation of resident cardiac stem cells (CSC) and/or stimulation of endogenous cardiomyocyte replication. Also, cytokines can be isolated from the media of cultured cells and have shown to have positive effects on experimental blood flow recovery.

Encouraged by pioneer preclinical studies, a number of early phase clinical trials have been conducted. It is generally accepted that stem cell therapy for post-MI cardiac repair should ideally be conducted within 2 weeks post-AMI before scar formation, and autologous cells are most suitable for transplantation because they obviate the need for immunosuppression. Most of the clinical trials were conducted to evaluate a safety index for administration of stem cells on the MI site. For trials that involve invasive procedures, it is important to establish correct risk-benefit associations. Due to the positive results obtained from early phase trials and several preclinical studies, it has been established that stem cell therapy for AMI is a feasible procedure for cardiac patients. The marginal and sometimes transient clinical benefits appear to be significant statistically rather than clinically. Such effects have been considered as secondary effects not associated with the direct cardiogenesis of implanted cells. There is so far little evidence suggesting transdifferentiation of implanted BM-derived cells into any cardiac cell lineages in vivo. Accumulating evidences have attributed the clinical benefits to several effects, including paracrine effects, angiogenic effects, cell fusion, passive mechanical effects, and endogenous responses of CSC.

Although heart transplantation offers a viable option to replace the damaged myocardium in affected individuals, organ availability and transplant rejection complications limit the practicality of this approach. A number of stem cell types, including embryonic stem (ES) cells, CSC that are endogenous to the heart reside within, myoblasts (muscle stem cells), adult BM-derived cells, mesenchymal cells (BM-derived cells that give rise to tissues such as muscle, bone, tendons, ligaments, and adipose tissue), EPCs (cells that give rise to the endothelium, the interior lining of blood vessels), and umbilical cord blood cells, have been investigated to varying extents as possible sources for regenerating damaged myocardium. All of these cell types have been tested in mouse or rat models, and some have also been tested in large animal models such as pigs. Preliminary clinical data for many of these cell types have been gathered in selected patient populations.

SOURCES OF PROGENITOR STEM CELLS

Embryonic Stem Cells

Since ES cells are pluripotent, they can potentially give rise to the variety of cell types that are instrumental in regenerating damaged myocardium, including cardiomyocytes, EC, and smooth muscle cells. To this end, mouse and human ES cells have been shown to differentiate spontaneously to form endothelial and smooth muscle cells in vitro and *in vivo*[5] and human ES cells differentiate into myocytes with the structural and functional properties of cardiomyocytes. Moreover, ES cells that were transplanted into ischemically-injured myocardium in rats differentiated into normal myocardial cells that remained viable for up to 4 months suggesting that these cells may be candidates for regenerative therapy in humans.[6]

However, several key hurdles must be overcome before human ES cells can be used for clinical applications. Foremost, ethical issues related to embryo access currently limit the avenues of investigation. In addition, human ES cells must go through rigorous testing and purification procedures before the cells can be used as sources to regenerate tissue.

Skeletal Myoblasts

While skeletal myoblasts (SMs) are committed progenitors of skeletal muscle cells, their autologous origin, high proliferative potential, commitment to a myogenic lineage, and resistance to ischemia promoted their use as the first stem cell type to be explored extensively for cardiac application. Studies in rats and humans have demonstrated that these cells can repopulate scar tissue and improve LV function following transplantation.[7]

Human Adult Bone Marrow-Derived Cells

Scientists have demonstrated that cardiomyocytes and EC could be regenerated in a mouse heart attack model through the introduction of adult mouse BMSCs.[8] Researchers have investigated the potential of human adult BM as a source of stem cells for cardiac repair. Adult bone marrow contains several stem cell populations, including hematopoietic stem cells, EPCs, and MSCs; successful application of these cells usually necessitates isolating a particular cell type on the basis of its unique cell-surface receptors. Several studies, including the Bone Marrow Transfer to Enhance ST-Elevation Infarct Regeneration (BOOST) and the Transplantation of Progenitor Cells and Regeneration Enhancement in Acute Myocardial Infarction (TOPCARE-AMI) trials, have shown that intracoronary infusion of BMMNCs following a heart attack significantly improves the LV ejection fraction (LVEF), or the volume of blood pumped out of the left ventricle with each heartbeat.[9]

Mesenchymal (Bone Marrow Stromal) Cells

Mesenchymal stem cells are precursors of nonhematopoietic tissues (e.g. muscle, bone, tendons, ligaments, adipose tissue, and fibroblasts) that are obtained easily from autologous BM. Characteristically, they remain multipotent following expansion *in vitro*, exhibit relatively low immunogenicity, and can be frozen easily. While these properties make the cells amenable to preparation and delivery protocols in vivo, scientists can also culture them under special conditions to differentiate them into cells that resemble cardiomyocytes. This property enables their application for cardiac regeneration. MSCs differentiate into EC when cultured with vascular endothelial growth factor (VEGF) and cardiomyogenic cells when treated with the DNA-demethylating agent, 5-azacytidine.[10] More important, however, is the observation that MSCs can differentiate into cardiomyocytes and EC in vivo when transplanted into the heart following MI or noninjury in pig, mouse, or rat models. Additionally, the ability of MSCs to restore functionality may also be enhanced by the simultaneous transplantation of other stem cell types.

Resident Cardiac Stem Cells

Recent evidence suggests that the heart contains a small population of endogenous stem cells that most likely facilitate minor repair and turnover-mediated cell replacement. These cells have been isolated and characterized in mouse, rat, and human tissues.[11] They can be harvested in very limited quantities from human endomyocardial biopsy specimens and can directly be injected into the site of infarction to promote cardiomyocyte formation and improvements in systolic function. Separation and expansion ex vivo over a period of weeks is necessary to obtain sufficient quantities of these cells for experimental purposes.

Endothelial Progenitor Cells

The endothelium is a layer of specialized cells that lines the interior surface of all blood vessels in the body (including the heart). It provides an interface between circulating blood and the vessel wall. EPCs are cells that have been derived from the BM that are recruited into the peripheral blood in response to tissue ischemia. EPCs are precursor cells that express a few cell-surface markers characteristic of mature endothelium and some of hematopoietic cells. EPCs home in on ischemic areas, where they differentiate into new blood vessels; following a heart attack, intravenously injected EPCs home to the damaged region within 48 hours. The new vascularization induced by these cells prevents cardiomyocyte apoptosis (programmed cell death) and LV remodeling, thereby preserving ventricular function.

ROUTES OF PROGENITOR STEM CELL ADMINISTRATION

Progenitor stem cells are administered via various routes into cardiac tissue:

- *Intracoronary injection*: This is the most common approach used and involves the injection of the stem cells directly into the arteries of the heart using a stent or balloon catheter. The main concern with this approach is the possibility of embolism and plugging of the small vessels by the injected cells that may reduce the blood flow to the heart. However, it has shown an excellent safety profile in the clinical studies.
- *Intravenous injection*: This method involves the injection of stem cells via a vein and is considered the least invasive.
- *Transepicardial injection*: This is the most invasive route but also the most dependable and it delivers cells directly to the infarcted or scarred myocardium during a planned open heart procedure. It can thus be used with routine bypass surgery to inject stem cells into the areas that cannot be grafted.
- *Transendocardial injection*: This delivery method involves injection of the stem cells through the inner wall of the heart using a catheter. It employs a sophisticated imaging and guidance system to ensure delivery to the correct areas. This is comparatively less invasive than the transepicardial injection.

The goal of any cell delivery strategy is to transplant enough cells into the area of interest to achieve maximum retention in that area. Moreover, the local environment determines the success of cell delivery since it is the milieu that will influence short-term cell survival, cell properties in regard to adhesion, transmigration through vasculature, and tissue invasion. Therefore, the targeted administration of cells is preferred.[12] In context to various cardiac trials which make use of stem cells, intracoronary infusion of stem cells has been deemed best for the treatment of MI and chronic heart failure. This is attributed to the fact that intracoronary infusion offers a target directed local delivery, thus increasing the number of cells that reach the target tissue comparative to the number that will home in cardiac tissue once they have been placed in the circulation. However, these strategies may be of limited benefit to those who have poor circulation, and stem cells are often injected directly into the ventricular wall of these patients. This endomyocardial injection may be carried out either via a catheter or during open-heart surgery. To determine the ideal site for administration of stem cells, few studies used mapping or direct visualization techniques to identify the locations of scars and viable cardiac tissue. Despite improvements in delivery efficiency, however, the success of these methods remains limited by the death of the transplanted cells as a result of physical stress, inflammation and hypoxia. Timing of delivery may slow the rate of deterioration of tissue function and this issue could remain a hurdle for therapeutic approach.

CELL MIGRATION AND HOMING

Cell homing, transmigration, adhesion, and tissue invasion are a result of many complex processes. Stromal cell-derived factor-1 (SDF-1) is a chemotactic cytokine that enhances the homing of mobilized progenitor cells to areas of SDF-1 production. SDF-1 acts as a potent chemoattractant for lymphocytes and monocytes, and also enhances B-cell proliferation. The mechanism of action of SDF-1 involves promotion of cell migration and proliferation.[13] SDF-1 delivered locally, either as free protein or via plasmid-mediated gene expression, enhances EPC recruitment into ischemic tissue resulting in augmented angiogenesis.[14-16] SDF-1 is highly expressed in ischemic tissues.[17,18] SDF-1 mobilizes BM progenitor cells by binding to the cell surface receptor CXCR4, and which ultimately enter the peripheral circulation and migrate to the ischemic site following the SDF-1 gradient. On arrival, bone marrow mononuclear cells (BMCs) promote angiogenesis by providing cellular elements such as EC and perivascular cells and also by secreting signaling proteins that mature the angiogenesis process. BMC surface CXCR4 expression and the SDF-1/CXCR4 interaction are essential for BMC homing at the injured site. However, the strategies to augment cell function via better localization/homing of these cells is crucial if there is to be any therapeutic benefit using BMSCs for targeted regenerative therapy. To augment cell function via localization/homing is crucial if there has to be any therapeutic benefit using BMSCs for targeted regenerative therapy. Additional strategies for better homing of BMSCs include inducing hypoxia for the upregulation of CXCR-4 protein receptor expression at the BMSC cell surface. CXCR-4 are chemokine protein receptors that are expressed in cells that are going to be dead, which can be complexed with SDF-1 protein ligands.[19] The CXCR 4/SDF-1 complex allows for stem cell migration and homing via chemotaxis where expression of the CXCR-4 receptor and the presence of SDF-1 receptor are required to regulate and make cell migration possible. It has been found that CXCR-4 expression can be induced by exposure to a pool of cytokines such as stem cell factor (SCF), IL-6, Flt-ligand, hepatocyte growth factor (HGF), and IL-3. Administering homologous cytokines directly is one way to encourage the proliferation of injected stem cells. Furthermore, increasing affinity of the stem cells can also be done by increasing the concentration of the chemoattractant SDF-1.

HUMAN CLINICAL TRIALS

Strauer et al. 2001, 2002 conducted and published the results of intracoronary BM mononuclear cell infusion in patients with chronic MI which showed that autologous intracoronary mononuclear BM cell-derived stem cells regenerate infarcted myocardium. The BOOST trial included 60 patients, of which 30 received intracoronary injections of unfractionated mononuclear cells as an average of 6 days after occlusion, whereas 30 patients formed the control group.[20] MRI showed that the cell therapy group had a significant increase in ejection fraction compared with controls (50.0–56.7% in treated versus 51.3–52% in controls), associated with nonsignificant trends for improved end-diastolic and end-systolic volumes. Chen et al., 2004[21] performed intracoronary delivery of autologous BM-derived mesenchymal cells in 34 patients, an average of 18 days after the revascularization procedure. Although derived from BM, MSCs differ significantly from hematopoietic stem cells in that they can form bone, fat, and cartilage, with some evidence for forming occasional cardiomyocytes after intracoronary infusion. Furthermore, there is evidence that MSCs can induce local immune tolerance and hence may be tolerated after allogeneic transplantation. By year 2006, several important BMSC trials had been conducted, the most important one was the Reinfusion of Enriched Progenitor Cell and Infarct Remodeling in Acute Myocardial Infarction (REPAIR-AMI) trial,[22] the BOOST,[23] and the Autologous Bone Marrow-Derived Stem-Cell Transfer in Patients with ST-Segment Elevation Myocardial Infarction (STEMI) double-blind, randomized control trial.[24] Together, these studies reported an increase in LVEF of 3.3–5.9% in patients treated with intracoronary BMSCs. This modest magnitude of LVEF increase was corroborated in two meta-analyses, which evaluated 13 clinical trials with a total of 811 patients[25] and 18 studies with a total of 999 patients[26] and found significant improvements in LVEF of 2.99% and 3.66% in the cell-treated groups, respectively. Furthermore, a recent meta-analysis of 7 RCTs, which included a total of 237 patients, reported a similarly modest increase in LVEF of 3.7% in patients who received intracoronary circulating progenitor cells or intracoronary/intramyocardial peripheral blood stem cells.[27] Most clinical trials have used autologous whole BM as a cell therapeutic.[12,23-25] Other clinical indications for catheter-based BM cell injections have included refractory ischemia and heart failure.[28] In these settings, cells were delivered through an endoventricular catheter guided by electromechanical mapping (NOGA). The authors of these pilot experiments have reported striking improvements in outcomes (Table 31.1), but this enthusiasm must be tempered by the small size of the investigated patient populations and the lack of control groups.

Recent studies have indicated to the fact that bone marrow-derived MSCs (BMMSCs) may significantly improve LVEF in patients with AMI. Lee et al, 2014,[29] conducted a randomized pilot study to assess the safety and efficacy of administering MSCs in AMI patients. After randomly assigning 80 patients for receiving autologous BMMSCs into infarct artery at 1 month of successful reperfusion therapy, 58 patients completed the trial. Upon follow-ups after 6 months, changes in the LVEF was assessed using single-photon emission computer-aided tomography, where it was found that the BM-derived group had a higher LVEF than the control patients. No significant adverse event was noted during the duration of the trial which established the safety of the procedure.

One of the pioneering trials conducted to establish the safety and efficacy of using autologous stem cells for MI was the BOOST trial.[22] In the trial, 60 patients with STEMI and successful PCI were randomized to a control and a cell therapy group. As previously reported, BMC transfer led to an improvement of LVEF by 6.0% at 6 months ($P = 0.003$) and 2.8% at 18 months ($P = 0.27$). In conclusion, it was found that a single intracoronary application of BMCs does not promote a sustained improvement of LVEF in STEMI patients with relatively preserved systolic function. It is conceivable that a subgroup of patients with more infarcts may derive a sustained benefit from BMC therapy. Another clinical trial was conducted[30] to determine the effect of intracoronary autologous BMC delivery following STEMI on recovery of global and regional LV function and if timing of BMC delivery (3 versus 7 days following reperfusion) influences this effect. Between July 2008 and November 2011, 120 patients were enrolled in a randomized, 2 × 2 factorial, double-blind, placebo-controlled trial of the patients with LV dysfunction (LVEF ≤ 45%) following successful primary PCI of anterior STEMI. Intracoronary infusions were administered on day 3 and day 7. LVEF increased similarly in both BMC (45.2 +/- 10.6 to 48.3 +/- 13.3%) and placebo groups (44.5 +/- 10.8 to 47.8 +/- 13.6 %). No detectable treatment effect on regional LV function was observed in either infarct or border zones. Differences between therapy groups in the change in global LV function over time when treated at day 3 or day 7 were not significant, nor were they different from each other. Also, timing of treatment had no detectable effect on recovery of regional LV function. Major adverse events were rare with no difference between groups. Overall, the improvement in LV function observed 6 months after reperfusion of STEMI did not appear to be influenced by BMCs, regardless of the timing of delivery, within the initial week following reperfusion.

Assmus et al, 2014[31] conducted a randomized placebo-controlled, multicenter, double-blind REPAIR-AMI trial (extension of the REPAIR-AMI trial, 2010), 204 patients received either intracoronary infusion of BMCs or placebo into the infarct vessel 3–7 days following successful PCI. Mortality was reported in 15 patients in control group compared to 7 patients in the BMC-treated group. Nine patients in

Table 31.1 Summary of cardiac stem cell clinical trials during the year 2009–2012

Trial	*Cell type and delivery mode*	*Time of delivery*	*Results*	*F/U (months)*	*Patients (age)*
Van Ramshorst et al., 2009[32]	Autologous BMMNC, 1 $\times$ 10^8 cells, IM	CMI	Modest improvements of summed stress score, increase of QoL at 6 months	3, 6	Placebo 25(62), cell 25(64), RCT
Tendera et al. REGENT trial, 2009[33]	Autologous BMC 24.6 $\times$ 10^8, IC	5 days	EF decrease by 3.3 +/– 9.5% in control, 2.5 +/– 11.9% in BMC	61	Control 30(59.2), BMC 30(53.4), RCT
Beitnes et al., ASTAMI trial, 2009[34]	BMC, 7 $\times$ 10^8 , IC	PCI after 12-hour MI onset	EF: 39 to 39 in control, 37–40 in MNC, 35–38 in CD34 + grp.	6	Control 40 (59), nonselected MNC 80(55), selected MNC 80(58), RCT
Hare et al., Prochymal, 2009[35]	Allogeneic BMMNC, 0.5, 1.6, 5 $\times$ 10^8 cells/kg, IV	1–10 days	LVEF increase	12	Placebo 21 (55.1) hMSC 39(59.0), RCT
Assmus et al., REPAIR-AMI, 2010[31]	Auto-BMC, 236 +/– 174 $\times$ 10^8, IC	3–7 days after reperfusion	Still safe	24	Placebo 103(57), BMC 101(55)
Strauer et al., STAR-heart study, 2010[36]	BMC, 6.6 +/– 3.3 $\times$ 10^7, IC	Chronic HF EF < 35% (mean post-MI interval: 8.5 years)	Hemodynamics, exercise capacity, oxygen uptake, LV contractility, long-term mortality increase in BMC group	3, 12, 60	Control 200 (60) Stem cell 191 (59), RCT
Mansour et al.,[37] COMPARE-AMI, 2011	CD_{133} + HSC, 1 $\times$ 10^7, IC	3–7 days after PCI	Safe, EF 41.2 +/– 1 at base, 51.1 +/– 2.5 at 4 months, 52.3 +/– at 12 months	12	Placebo 20, cell 20 (52.2)
Bolli et al.,[38] SCIPIO, 2011	CSCs, IC, I million (*n* = 15), 0.5 million (*n* = 1)	EF < 40%, CABG, ischemic cardiomyopathy	EF 35.9–39.2% (4 months), to 42.5% (12 months), infarct size 32.6 to 24.8 (4 months) to 22.8 (12 months)	12	Control 7(57.3), treatment 16 (56.0), RCT
Roncalli et al.,[39] BONAMI trial, 2011	Auto-BMC, IC	9.3 days after STEMI	Myocardial viability 16% (control), 34% (BMC), active significant adverse role of smoking	3	Control 49 (55), BMC 52(56), RCT
Ahmadi et al., 2012[40]	BM-CD_{133}^{+} BMC 1.77 $\times$ 10^6 +/– 1.14 $\times$ 10^6 CD_{133}^{+}cells, IM	Candidate of CABG, after MI	Safe, no benefit	60	Control 5, BMC 13, RCT

Abbreviations: BMMNCs, bone marrow-derived mononuclear cells; BMC, bone marrow mononuclear cells; IC, intracoronary; IM, intramuscular; HSC, hematopoietic stem cell; CSC, cardiac stem cells; CMI, chronic myocardial ischemia; PCI, percutaneous coronary intervention; CABG, coronary artery bypass grafting; EF, ejection fraction; LVEF, LV ejection fraction; STEMI, ST-segment elevation myocardial infarction; REGENT, myocardial regeneration by intracoronary infusion of selected population of stem cells in acute myocardial infarction; REPAIR-AMI, reinfusion of enriched progenitor cell and infarct remodeling in acute myocardial infarction; COMPARE-AMI, comparison of intracoronary injection of CD133 bone marrow stem cells to placebo in patients after acute myocardial infarction and left ventricular dysfunction; SCIPIO, cardiac stem cells in patients with ischemic cardiomyopathy; BONAMI, bone marrow in acute myocardial infarction; ASTAMI, autologous stem cell transplantation in acute myocardial infarction.

the control arm and five in BMC-treated arm required rehospitalization for chronic heart failure. Cardiac-related adverse event (death or rehospitalization) was observed more in the control arm than the BMC treatment arm.

Meta-analyses review carried out by the scientists of various medium and small trials proves that feasibility and short-term safety of the use of stem cells for cardiac repair has been proved through the studies. All the trials that have been taken into consideration have substantial confirmation of improvement of cardiac function. Autologous BMSC therapy has emerged as a novel approach to treat patients with AMI or chronic ischemia and heart failure following percutaneous or surgical revascularization, respectively. Fischer et al, 2006 carried out meta-analyses from various databases and found that cell therapy for patients with IHD with no hope for revascularization showed significantly improved quality of life, exercise and performance and LVEF. Nine trials were eligible for inclusion. BMSC treatment significantly reduced the risk of mortality ($P = 0.001$).

The therapeutic effects of MSC transplantation after AMI have been investigated in two clinical trials. Infusion of autologous MSCs by intracoronary route and it was demonstrated that no arrhythmias or other side effects were noticed.[41] After 6 months of MSC transfer, regional wall motion and global LVEF were improved, and left ventricular end-diastolic volume (LVEDV) was decreased compared with a randomized control group that had received an intracoronary infusion of saline. Unfortunately, it was not reported whether intracoronary MSC delivery promoted ischemic damage to the myocardium, a complication that had occurred after intracoronary MSC infusions in dogs. An extensive meta-analysis done on eighteen eligible studies ($N =$ 999 patients) involving adult BMSCs such as BMMNC, MSCs, and EPCs measuring the same outcomes demonstrated that, as compared to controls, BM transplantation improved LVEF (pooled difference of 3.66%; $P < 0.001$), reduced infarct scar size (–5.49%; $P = 0.003$), and reduced left ventricular end-systolic volume (LVESV) (–4.8%mL; $P = 0.006$). The available evidence suggests that BMC transplantation is associated with modest improvements in physiologic and anatomic parameters in patients with both acute MI and chronic IHD, above and beyond conventional therapy (Table 31.1). Poole and Quyyumi, 2013,[42] pooled in data from major cardiac trials that have made use of cell therapy as a first line of treatment. Through meta-analyses and thorough study of these trials, they mention that the intracoronary injection of BMMNCs after AMI was proven to be safe and is associated with modest improvement in LVEF. Meta-analyses suggest that intracoronary cell therapy procedures performed right after AMI holds a greater chance at cell fusion since it is in the repair phase. This further suggests carrying out multicentric randomized large trials targeted to address the impact of intracoronary cell therapy on important outcomes and long-term event-free survival as compared to the conventional therapy.

MECHANISM OF ACTION

The ability of an injured myocardium to recruit extracardiac stem cells following cardiac injury is critical in myocardial repair and regeneration. Little has been known with regard to the regulatory mechanisms that control the homing and localization of progenitor stem cells to injured tissues. The precise time course and factors that have shown to stimulate BM mobilization remain the subject of intense investigation. Several crucial factors show a promotion of the mobilization of BMSCs into peripheral circulation, including granulocyte colony-stimulating factor (G-CSF), granulocyte/macrophage colony-stimulating factor (GM-CSF), SCF, VEGF, HGF, and erythropoietin (EPO).[43] Myocardial ischemia is known to induce several "mobilizing cytokines", including, but not limited to, G-CSF, SCF, VEGF, SDF-1, and EPO.[44] These cytokines may be responsible for the observed homing of BMSCs following MI. Mobilization of BMSCs through cytokine stimulants increases their concentration in the peripheral circulation substantially. In addition to well-recognized HSCs mobilizing agents such as G-CSF and SCF, VEGF, and EPO and statins have been shown to promote EPC recruitment. EPCs, in particular, possess the ability to mature into the cells that line the lumen of blood vessels.[45] The first evidence indicating the presence of EPCs in the adult circulation emerged when mononuclear blood cells from healthy human volunteers were shown to acquire an endothelial cell-like phenotype in vitro and to incorporate into capillaries in vivo.

Since these cytokines are known to promote angiogenesis and vascularization, the conclusion that was reached was that it was not direct cell incorporation but rather the paracrine signaling that may be responsible for the effects of BM cell therapy in a setting of acute ischemic injury. It may also be likely that the paracrine mediators are expressed in a specific temporal and spatial manner that can enhance cell survival and activate endogenous mechanisms of endogenous repair and regeneration. Angiogenesis consists of several distinct processes which include sprouting and proliferation of pre-existing capillaries to form new networks. This process is tightly and highly regulated by hypoxia through a number of proangiogenic factors that include VEGF, fibroblast growth factors (FGFs), placental growth factor (PIGF), and HGF. The rapid proliferation of already existing collateral arteries is characterized by the arteriogenesis that involves the basic remodeling of smaller vessels into the larger ones. This is triggered in part by a steady increase in the stress in arterioles that run parallel to the occluded artery. Recruitment of monocytes that differentiate into macrophages and produce abundant angiogenic growth factors such as VEGF, nitrous oxide (NO), monocyte chemoattractant protein-1 (MCP-1), and other cytokines, is also essential and ultimately leads to endothelial and smooth muscle proliferation, migration, vessel remodeling, and extracellular matrix synthesis.[46] Recent studies like Cardiopoietic Stem Cell Therapy in

Heart Failure (C-CURE) which is a prospective, randomized, multicenter trial where patients with cardiac failure of ischemic origin either received standard of care or standard of care plus lineage specified stem cells. For this trial, in the therapy arm, the bone marrow was harvested and cells were exposed to a cardiogenic cocktail. At follow-up, it was noticed that there was no evidence of increased cardiac or systemic toxicity and LVEF improved by significant fractions. Another study is the JUVENTAS SDF-1 trial where the trial is hoping to prove that the SDF1:CXCR4 pathway is critical in stem cell-based cardiac repair. Moreover, this study also suggests critical mechanisms that, if ignored by scientists, would lead to poorly designed studies eventually yielding negative results.

Stem cell potency is a double-aged sword, and therefore, although the initial experimental studies confirmed that the infusion of BMSCs does not cause major side effects; several issues were raised such as, increased restenosis, or progression of atherosclerotic disease in the future. However, none of the clinical studies with BMSCs so far have reported an increased incidence of arrhythmias, bleeding complications, additional ischemic injury, or promoted inflammatory reaction as no further increase in C-reactive protein. Available state-of-the-art imaging techniques and end-point evaluation by external core laboratories are required to unmistakably demonstrate the moderate functional effects of cell therapy.

CONCLUSION

Cardiovascular ischemic disease is the leading cause of morbidity and mortality worldwide and constitutes a major health burden. The realization that endogenous and transplanted adult stem and progenitor cells promote functional and repair after ischemic injury, has led to a new understanding of the pathobiology of cardiovascular disease. Translation of these concepts from disease models into the clinic could lead to the development of completely new therapeutic approaches for patients with AMI and chronic heart disease. Early clinical trials provide a signal that cell therapy can enhance tissue perfusion and contractile performance of the infarcted human heart. While the initially perceived rapid chance for a complete cardiac repair by stem/progenitor cell therapy after MI has generated high expectations, now the potential of this therapy needs to be carefully developed by addressing important remaining questions, including the optimal cell types and preconditioning, the timing and dosing of cells to be used, how to augment the functional repair capacity of transplanted cells, how to optimize their homing and engraftment in the heart, and how to select the patients that may benefit most from this therapy. An important focus of present basic and clinical studies is therefore directed toward optimizing the outcome and effect of stem/progenitor cell-based therapies, such as by improving stem/progenitor cell repair capacity and the process of cardiac cell homing. Notably, the vascular and proangiogenic repair capacity of autologous stem/progenitor cells is reduced by cardiovascular risk factors, such as diabetes.

Bone marrow-derived stem cells and their paracrine factors have shown all the necessary attributes for tissue regeneration, namely, homing, immunosuppression, differentiation, angiogenesis, stimulation of endogenous cells, and possible regulation of specific metabolic pathways, only to name a few. Thus, research into paracrine factors and mechanisms has shown that stem cell therapy is much more complicated and greatly enhances the potential and variety of therapeutic applications. Mediating angiogenic factors, cell proliferation, and all of the above-mentioned characteristics are crucial to stem cell therapy and provide many new approaches for therapy. The initial studies of cell-based human clinical trials for cardiac repair using autologous adult BM have demonstrated safety. With clinical trials of cell-based cardiac repair just getting under way, there is a great deal of excitement, and expectations are high. We need to take a long-term view, however, and if these initial trials are not optimally successful, we must return to the laboratory to refine scientific proof of concept hypotheses. It may require close interaction between clinical investigators and basic scientists over a decade before we have optimized techniques for rebuilding the heart. But, if we succeed, cell-based cardiac repair will offer hope for millions of patients worldwide each year who would otherwise suffer from inexorable progression of heart failure.

REFERENCES

1. Arnous S, Mozid A, Martin J, Mathur A. Bone marrow mono nuclear cells and acute myocardial infarction. Stem Cell Res Ther. 2012;3(1):2.
2. Orlic D, Kajstura J, Chimenti S, et al. Mobilized bone marrow cells repair the infarcted heart, improving function and survival. Proc Natl Acad Sci U S A. 2001;98(18):10344-9.
3. Clifford DM, Fisher SA, Brunskill SJ, et al. Long-term effects of autologous bone marrow stem cell treatment in acute myocardial infarction: factors that may influence outcomes. PLoS One. 2012;7:e37373.
4. Alvarez-Dolado M, Pardal R, Garcia-Verdugo JM, et al. Fusion of bone-marrow-derived cells with Purkinje neurons, cardio myocytes and hepatocytes. Nature. 2003;425(6961):968-73.
5. Marchetti S, Gimond C, Iljin K, et al. Endothelial cells genetically selected from differentiating mouse embryonic stem cells incorporate at sites of neovascularization in vivo. J Cell Sci. 2002; 115:2075-85.
6. Min JY, Yang Y, Converso KL, et al. Transplantation of embryonic stem cells improves cardiac function in postinfarcted rats. J Appl Physiol. 2002;92:288-96.
7. Dowell JD, Rubart M, Pasumarthi KB, Soonpaa MH, Field LJ. Myocyte and myogenic stem cell transplantation in the heart. Cardiovasc Res. 2003;58:336-50

8. Jackson KA, Majka SM, Wang H, et al. Regeneration of ischemic cardiac muscle and vascular endothelium by adult stem cells. J Clin Invest. 2001;107:1395-402.
9. Schächinger V, Assmus B, Britten MB, et al. Transplantation of progenitor cells and regeneration enhancement in acute myocardial infarction: final one-year results of the TOPCARE-AMI Trial. J Am Coll Cardiol. 2004; 44:1690.
10. Davani S, Marandin A, Mersin N, et al. Mesenchymal progenitor cells differentiate into an endothelial phenotype, enhance vascular density, and improve heart function in a rat cellular cardiomyoplasty model. Circulation. 2003;108:253-8.
11. Boyle AJ, Schulman SP, Hare JM. Is stem cell therapy ready for patients? Stem cell therapy for cardiac repair. Circulation. 2006; 114:339-52.
12. Strauer BE, Kornowski R. Stem cell therapy in perspective. Circulation. 2003;107(7):929-34.
13. Grunewald M, Avraham I, Dor Y, et al. VEGF-induced adult neo vascularization: recruitment, retention, and role of accessory cells. Cell. 2006;124:175-89.
14. Yamaguchi J, Kusano KF, Masuo O, et al. Stromal cell-derived factor-1 effects on ex vivo expanded endothelial progenitor cell recruitment for ischemic neovascularization. Circulation. 2003; 107:1322-8.
15. Hiasa K, Ishibashi M, Ohtani K, et al. Gene transfer of stromal cell derived factor-1alpha enhances ischemic vasculo genesis and angiogenesis via vascular endothelial growth factor/endothelial nitric oxide synthase-related pathway: next-generation chemokine therapy for therapeutic neovascularization. Circulation. 2004; 109:2454-61.
16. Carr AN, Howard BW, Yang HT, et al. Efficacy of systemic administration of SDF-1 in a model of vascular insufficiency: support for an endothelium-dependent mechanism. Cardiovasc Res. 2006;69:925-35.
17. Askari AT, Unzek S, Popovic ZB, et al. Effect of stromal-cell-derived factor 1 on stem-cell homing and tissue regeneration in ischaemic cardiomyopathy. Lancet. 2003;362:697-703.
18. Ceradini DJ, Kulkarni AR, Callaghan MJ, et al. Progenitor cell trafficking is regulated by hypoxic gradients through HIF-1 induction of SDF-1. 2004; 10: 858-64.
19. Hung SC, Pochampally RR, Hsu SC, et al. Short term exposure of multipotent stromal cells to low oxygen increases their expression of CX3CR1 and CXCR4 and their engraftment in vivo. PLoS One. 2007;2(5):416.
20. Wollert KC, Meyer GP, Lotz J, et al. Intracoronary autologous bone marrow cell transfer after myocardial infarction: the BOOST randomized controlled clinical trial. Lancet. 2004;364:141-8.
21. Chen SL, Fang WW, Ye F, et al. Effect on left ventricular function of intracoronary transplantation of autologous bone marrow mesenchymal stem cell in patients with acute myocardial infarction. Am J Cardiol. 2004;94:92-5
22. Meyer GP, Wollert KC, Lotz J, et al. Intracoronary bone marrow cell transfer after myocardial infarction: eighteen months' follow-up data from the randomized, controlled BOOST (BOne marrOw transfer to enhance ST-elevation infarct regeneration) trial. Circulation. 2006;113:1287-94.
23. Janssens S, Dubois C, Bogaert J, et al. Autologous bone marrow-derived stem-cell transfer in patients with ST-segment elevation myocardial infarction: double-blind, randomized controlled trial. Lancet. 2006;367:113-21.
24. Martin-Rendon E, Brunskill SJ, Hyde CJ, et al. Autologous bone marrow stem cells to treat acute myocardial infarction: a systematic review. Eur Heart J. 2008;29:1807-18.
25. Abdel-Latif A, Bolli R, Tleyjeh IM, et al. Adult bone marrow-derived cells for cardiac repair: a systematic review and meta-analysis. Arch Intern Med. 2007;167:989-97.
26. Wen Y, Meng L, Ding Y, Ouyang J. Autologous transplantation of blood-derived stem/progenitor cells for ischaemic heart disease. Int J Clin Pract. 2011;65:858-65.
27. Tse HF, Kwong YL, Chan JK, et al. Angiogenesis in ischaemic myocardium by intramyocardial autologous bone marrow mononuclear cell implantation. Lancet. 2003;361:47-9.
28. Perin EC, Dohmann HF, Borojevic R, et al. Transendocardial, autologous bone marrow cell transplantation for severe, chronic ischemic heart failure. Circulation. 2003;107:2294-302.
29. Lee JW, Lee SH, Youn YJ, et al. A randomized, open-label, multi center trial for the safety and efficacy of adult mesenchymal stem cells after acute myocardial infarction. J Korean Med Sci. 2014; 29:23-31.
30. Traverse JH, Henry TD, Pepine CJ, et al. Effect of the use and timing of bone marrow mononuclear cell delivery on left ventri cular function after acute myocardial infarction: The TIME randomized trial. JAMA. 2012;308(22):2380-9.
31. Assmus B, Rolf A, Erbs S, et al. Clinical outcome 2 years after intracoronary administration of bone marrow-derived pro genitor cells in acute myocardial infarction. Circ Heart Fail. 2010;3:89-96.
32. van Ramshorst J, Bax JJ, Beeres SL, et al. Intramyocardial bone marrow cell injection for chronic myocardial ischemia: a rando mized controlled trial. JAMA. 2009;301:1997-2004.
33. Tendera M, Wojakowski W, Ruzyłło W, et al. Intracoronary infusion of bone marrow-derived selected CD34+CXCR4+ cells and non-selected mononuclear cells in patients with acute STEMI and reduced left ventricular ejection fraction: results of randomized, multicentre Myocardial Regeneration by Intracoronary Infusion of Selected Population of Stem Cells in Acute Myocardial Infarction (REGENT) trial. Eur Heart J. 2009;30:1313-21.
34. Beitnes JO, Hopp E, Lunde K, et al. Long-term results after intra coronary injection of autologous mononuclear bone marrow cells in acute myocardial infarction: the ASTAMI randomised, controlled study. Heart. 2009;95:1983-9.
35. Hare JM, Traverse JH, Henry TD, et al. A randomized, double-blind, placebo-controlled, dose-escalation study of intravenous adult human mesenchymal stem cells (prochymal) after acute myocardial infarction. J Am Coll Cardiol. 2009; 54:2277-86
36. Strauer BE, Yousef M, Schannwell CM. The acute and long-term effects of intracoronary Stem cell Transplantation in 191 patients with chronic heARt failure: the STAR-heart study. Eur J Heart Fail. 2010; 12:721-9.
37. Mansour S, Roy DC, Bouchard V, et al. One-year safety analysis of the COMPARE-AMI trial: comparison of intracoronary injec tion of CD133 bone marrow stem cells to Placebo in patients after acute myocardial infarction and left ventricular dysfunction. Bone Marrow Res. 2011; 2011:385124.
38. Bolli R, Chugh AR, D'Amario D, et al. Cardiac stem cells in patients with ischaemic cardiomyopathy (SCIPIO): initial results of a randomised phase 1 trial. Lancet. 2011; 378:1847-57.

39. Roncalli J, Mouquet F, Piot C, et al. Intracoronary autologous mononucleated bone marrow cell infusion for acute myocardial infarction: results of the randomized multicenter BONAMI trial. Eur Heart J. 2011; 32:1748-57.
40. Ahmadi H, Farahani MM, Kouhkan A, et al. Five-year follow-up of the local autologous transplantation of CD133+ enriched bone marrow cells in patients with myocardial infarction. Arch Iran Med. 2012;15:32-5.
41. Chen SL, Fang WW, Ye F, et al. Effect on left ventricular function of intracoronary transplantation of autologous bone marrow mesenchymal stem cell in patients with acute myocardial infarction. Am J Cardiol. 2004;94:92-5.
42. Poole JC, Quyyumi AA. Progenitor cell therapy to treat acute myocardial infarction: The promise of high-dose autologous CD34 bone marrow mononuclear cells. Stem Cells Int. 2013; 2013:658480.
43. Dewald O, Ren G, Duerr GD, et al. Of mice and dogs: species-specific differences in the inflammatory response following myocardial infarction. Am J Pathol. 2004; 164(2):665-77.
44. Heeschen C, Aicher A, Lehmann R, et al. Erythropoietin is a potent physiologic stimulus for endothelial progenitor cell mobilization. Blood. 2003;102(4): 1340-6.
45. Asahara T, Murohara T, Sullivan A, et al. Isolation of putative progenitor endothelial cells for angiogenesis. Science. 1997;275:964-7.
46. Forrester JS, White AJ, Matsushita S, Chakravarty T, Makkar RR. New paradigms of myocardial regeneration post-infarction tissue preservation, cell environment, and pluripotent cell. JACC Cardiovasc Interv. 2009;2(1):1-8.

32

Left Main Stenting: Appropriate in Current Era

Pramod Joshi, S Yadav, Dheeraj Gandotra, Suman Bhandari

INTRODUCTION

Significant unprotected left main coronary artery (ULMCA) disease occurs in 5–7% of patients undergoing coronary angiography [1,2] and patients with ULMCA disease treated medically have a 3-year mortality rate of 50%.[3,4] Various studies have shown a significant benefit following the treatment of left main (LM) stenosis with coronary bypass grafting (CABG) compared with medical treatment.[5-8] Left main coronary artery (LMCA) stenosis is considered an appropriate target for the percutaneous coronary intervention (PCI) because of its large vessel size, no tortuosity, and shorter lesion size, but bifurcation lesion require some important techniques and skills. This small group of patients with unique anatomy whose importance has been magnified because of the jeopardized myocardium requires bypass surgery, and thereby drawing special attention from surgeons and skilled interventionists. Clinical outcome is variable according to the disease complexity and atherosclerotic plaque location. Now the evidence-based treatment modality needs to be used for this group of patients.

IMPORTANCE OF LEFT MAIN CORONARY ARTERY STENOSIS

The LMCA supplies 75% of the left ventricular (LV) cardiac mass in patients with right dominant type and 100% in the case of left dominant type. As a result, severe LMCA disease would reduce flow to large portion of the myocardium, placing the patient at high risk for life-threatening LV dysfunction and arrhythmias.[9] The LMCA is anatomically divided into three regions: the ostium, the mid-shaft, and the distal portion.[10] The distal LMCA, by definition, always ends in a bifurcation, or even trifurcation, giving rise to the left anterior descending (LAD) and left circumflex (LCx) arteries, and probably an intermedius artery. Greater elastic content of this artery explains elastic recoil and high restenosis following balloon angioplasty.[11] Seventy percent of significant LMCA lesions involve the distal bifurcation. Intimal atherosclerosis in the LMCA bifurcation is accelerated primarily in area of low shear stress in the lateral wall close to the LAD and LCx bifurcation (Figs 32.1A and B). Why single-stent strategy can be successfully performed in patients with no or moderate disease by angiography, because carina is usually free of disease.

SURGICAL OUTCOME IN LEFT MAIN DISEASE

Coronary artery bypass surgery is a well-established technique, with excellent proven results for the treatment of coronary artery disease, dating back to the early 1970s.[3]

A recent review by Taggart et al.[12] published in 2008 reported on a series of studies, all of which had an in-hospital mortality of between 2% and 3% after CABG for LM stenosis, and although long-term follow-up data are very less, studies with report on long-term outcomes had results showing 5–6% mortality at 5 years (Table 32.1).

The Cleveland Clinic experience of CABG for patients with LM stenosis, Sabik et al.[13] report a 20-year follow-up of all patients operated on between 1971 and 1998. They have shown that for the 3,803 patients with LM stenosis, 30-day survival is 97.6%, with 93.6% at 1 year and 83% at 5 years. Ten-year survival rate is 64%. Importantly, rates of freedom from coronary reintervention are 99.7% at 30 days, 98.9% at 1 year, and 89% at 5 years. At 10 years, 76% of surviving patients remain free from reintervention and 61% at 20 years.

RESULTS OF PERCUTANEOUS CORONARY INTERVENTION WITH BARE-METAL STENTS IN LEFT MAIN STENOSIS

The balloon angioplasty of the LMCA was performed first in 1979 by Gruntzig as one of five angioplasties that he performed.[14] After the first series of 129 patients, reports of Hartzler and O'Keefe in 1989[15] showed a 10% in-hospital mortality and 64% 3-year mortality; this was quickly abandoned due to poor outcomes and better surgical results.

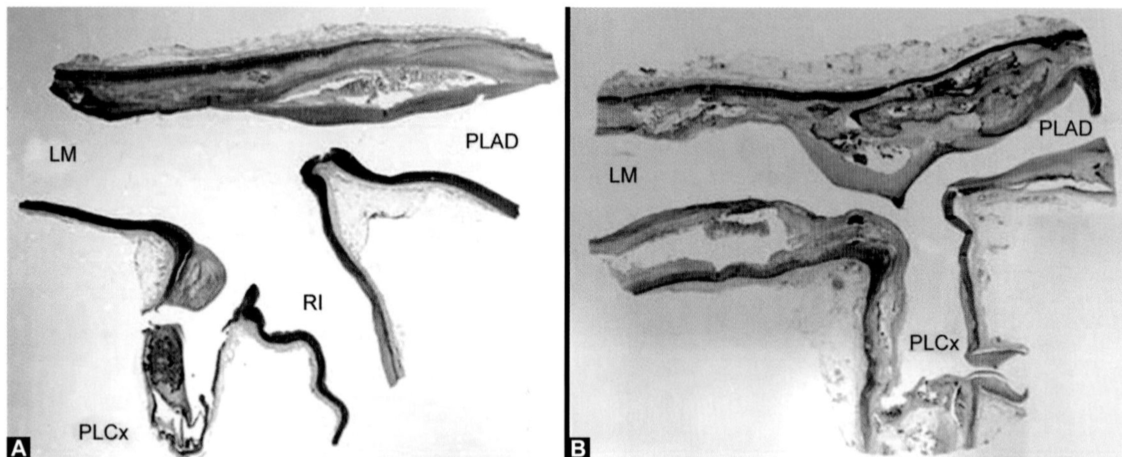

Figs 32.1A and B Longitudinal section of bifurcation of the left main coronary artery showing distribution of the atherosclerotic plaque. Note plaque is located in the lateral wall (area of low shear stress) while sparing the flow divider region (high shear)

Abbreviations: PLAD, proximal left anterior descending artery; PLCx, proximal left circumflex artery; RI, ramus intermedius; LM, left main

Table 32.1 In-hospital and long-term mortality after coronary bypass grafting for left main coronary artery disease (adapted from Taggart et al.)

Author (year)	*Year of surgery*	*n*	*Mortality (%)*			
			Hospital	*30 days*	*1 year*	*2 years*
Jonsson et al. (2006)	1970–99	1888	27	–	–	–
Lu et al. (2006) (2005)	1997–2003	1197	28	3	5	6
Keogh and Kinsman (2003)	2003	5003	3	–	–	–
Dewey et al. (2006) (2001)	1998–99	728	–	4.2	–	–
Yeatman et al. (2006) (2001)	1996–2000	387	24	–	–	5
Eilis et al. (2006) (1998)	1990–95	1585	23	–	–	–
Weighted average	–	10788	28	–	–	–

However, the development of newer stenting techniques and dual antiplatelet regimes allowed LM stenting to be again considered as a treatment by the mid-1990s, and no looking backward since then.

Stenting of the LM with bare-metal stents (BMS) was characterized by high procedural success rates, a 17–20% target lesion revascularization (TLR), and a 10–20% mortality rate at 1 year.[16-21]

EVIDENCE OF PERCUTANEOUS CORONARY INTERVENTION WITH DRUG-ELUTING STENT IN LEFT MAIN CORONARY ARTERY STENOSIS

The evolution of drug-eluting stent (DES) has been a major revolution in PCI of LMCA stenosis that has led to significant reduction in restenosis and target lesion revascularization when compared with initial experiences with BMS limited by poor mid-term results, higher rates of restenosis, and in some series sudden deaths.[22-41] Three single-center studies[23-25] showed high procedural success rates, low procedural complication rates, and encouraging long-term outcome. It was again confirmed by the French multicenter Registry for stenting uNprotecteD LMCA stenosis (FRIEND) registry.[26] Several single-center and multicenter registries show good safety and efficacy profile for DES in LMCA PCI.[22-24,28,31-41]

A meta-analysis of 17 trials involving PCI for ULMCA identified a distal lesion as the most significant predictor of repeated revascularization and overall major adverse cardiac event (MACE).[27] In LMCA bifurcation, however, different outcomes have been described depending on lesion complexity (simple vs. complex distal lesions with extensive involvement of both branches) and consequent stenting strategies (one- vs. two-stent approach). Current evidence suggests that the results in cases of simple bifurcation lesions treated with a one-stent approach are more favorable compared with complex bifurcation lesions treated with a two-stent approach.[31,42] The TLR rate is relatively low (<5%) with a one-stent approach, reaching nearly equivalent results to those obtained with DES for ostial or mid-ULMCA lesions.[24,43] Distal ULMCA approached with two-stent strategy show TLR rate as high as 255 with restenosis confined mainly to LCx ostium.[62] Since stent thrombosis can have clinically disastrous consequences following PCI for ULMCA bifurcation, distal LMCA bifurcation stenting should be performed only by skilled interventionist.

Comparison between CABG and PCI with DES

Several observational studies revealed that the clinical events of LMCA stenting were similar or superior to those of coronary artery bypass graft (CABG) because of significant increase in periprocedural myocardial infarction (MI) or stroke in CABG patients and that mortality between 30 days and 3 years was similar in both the groups.[40,44–46] The risk of target vessel revascularization was higher with PCI than CABG. Recently, the 5-year results from the MAIN-COMPARE (Revascularization for Unprotected Left Main Coronary Artery Stenosis: Comparison of Percutaneous Coronary Angioplasty vs. Surgical Revascularization) showed similar findings.[40] Recent data from ASAN-MAIN (ASAN Medical Centre-Left MAIN Revascularization) registry demonstrated that stenting showed similar long-term mortality and rates of death, Q wave MI, or stroke.[47]

The randomized trials comparing CABG and PCI in LMCA disease is limited. The Study of Unprotected Left Main Stenting versus Bypass Surgery (LEMANS) trial showed a significant benefit of ejection fraction improvement and favorable clinical outcomes after PCI than after CABG.[48] In the LMCA subgroup analysis from the SYNTAX (Synergy between PCI with TAXUS and Cardiac Surgery) trial,[49] PCI demonstrated the 12 months rate of major adverse cardiac or cerebrovascular events, death, MI or stroke, similar to those seen after CABG, but target vessel revascularization rate was found higher in DES arm. Drug-eluting stent (DES) in LMCA PCI has been evaluated in several observational single- and multicenter registries showing a good efficacy and safety profile.[22–24,28,33–41]

Moreover, other nonrandomized registries have shown no difference in the occurrence of MACCE between patients treated with DES compared with CABG in this subset of patients up to 5 years of clinical follow-up (Table 32.2).[47,50–58]

Table 32.2 Clinical outcome after left main stenting with drug-eluting stents

Treatment	DES/BMS/CABG	DES/BMS/CABG	DES/CABG	DES vs. CABG	DES/CABG	DES/CABG
Patients. n	1102/1138	52/53	107/147	157/154	50/123	96 vs. 245
Study design	Registry	Randomized	Registry	Registry	Registry	Registry
Age (mean, years)	62/64	61/61	64/68	73/69	72/70	66/66
Diabetes (%)	29.7/34.7	19/17	18.7/23.2	26.1/25.3	36/31	19/32
Distal lesion (%)	49.5/53.8	56/60	81.3/NA	80.3/82.5	60/NA	62/NA
EuroSCORE (mean)	NA	3.3/3.5	4.4/4.3	6/5	NA	27/25.3[b]
SYNTAX score (mean)	NA	25/24	28/29	NA	NA	NA
Follow-up time (years)	5	1	5	1	1	1
Cardiac death (%)	9.9[a]	NA	7.5/11.9		2/1.6	NA
MI (%)	1[a]	1.9/5.6	0.9/7.7	8/5	NA	0/1.3
TLR (%)	NA	NA	18.7/8.4****	25.5/2.6****	NA	NA
TVR (%)	9.7***	28.8/9.4*	28/8.4	NA	7/1	5.2/0.8**
CVA (%)	1.8[a]	0/3.7	0.9/4.2	NA	NA	0/0.8
ST/symptomatic graft occlusion	NA	NA	0.93/2.8	NA	NA	NA
MACCE (%)	NA	30.7/24.5	32.4/38.3	NA	17/25	10.4/11.4

Abbreviations: MI, myocardial infarction; TLR, target lesion revascularization; CVA, cerebrovascular accidents; ST, ARC definite/probable stent thrombosis; MACCE, major adverse cerebrovascular events; NA, not available; TVR, target vessel revascularization.

[a]Cumulative for overall study population

[b]Euroscore >6

**P* = 0.01, ***P* = 0.02, ****P* = 0.001, *****P* = 0.0001.

SYNTAX Trial Results

The SYNTAX trial compared PCI with paclitaxel-eluting stent (PES) implantation versus CABG for left main/multivessel CAD.[41] Recently, the 3-year results of the ULMCA subgroup from the SYNTAX trial (PCI arm 348 patients vs. CABG arm 357 patients) were presented by Serruys at Transcatheter Cardiovascular Therapeutics 2010. Percutaneous coronary intervention with PES implantation (348 patients) resulted in equivalent 3-year overall MACCE to CABG (22.3% CABG vs. 26.8% PCI; $P = 0.20$). Notably, the MACCE rate was similar between the groups for patients with low (23% CABG vs. 18% PCI; $P = 0.33$) and intermediate (23.4% CABG vs. 23.4% PCI; $P = 0.90$) SYNTAX score, but was significantly higher in the PCI arm in the high SYNTAX score group (21.2% CABG vs. 37.3% PCI; $P = 0.003$). Even the overall safety outcomes (death/cerebrovascular event [CVE]/MI) were similar between the two groups (14.3% CABG vs. 13% PCI; P = NS).

As reported at 1-year follow-up,[49] there was a higher revascularization rate in the PCI group (11.7% CABG vs. 20% PCI, $P = 0.004$) and a higher rate of CVE in the CABG group (4% CABG vs. 1.2% PCI, $P = 0.2$) even at 3-year follow-up (Table 32.3). Moreover, favorable results of PCI for ULMCA disease treatment were also reported in a gender subanalysis.[43]

Table 32.4 lists the variables influencing revascularization strategy in clinical practice.

Table 32.3 SYNTAX trial: results from the left main subgroup analysis

	PCI n = 358	CABG n = 357	P
One-year clinical outcomes			
Death (%)	4.2	4.4	0.88
Stroke (%)	0.3	2.7	0.0009
MI (%)	4.3	4.1	0.97
Revascularization (%)	12	6.7	0.02
ST or graft occlusion (%)	2.7	3.7	0.49
Overall MACCE (%)	15.8	13.6	0.44
MACCE, low SYNTAX score (0–17)	7.7	1.3	0.19
MACCE intermediate SYNTAX score (23–32)	12.6	15.5	0.54
MACCE high SYNTAX score (≥33)	25.3	12.9	0.008
Three-year clinical outcomes			
Death	7.3	8.4	0.64
Stroke (%)	1.2	4	0.02
MI (%)	6.9	4.1	0.14
Revascularization (%)	20	11.7	0.004
ST or graft occlusion (%)	4.1	3.7	0.80
Overall MACCE (%)	26.8	22.3	0.20
MACCE low SYNTAX score (0–17)	18	23	0.33
MACCE intermediate SYNTAX score (23–32)	23.4	23.4	0.90
MACCE high SYNTAX score (≥33)	37.3	21.2	0.003

Abbreviations: CABG, coronary artery bypass graft; MACCE, major adverse cerebrovascular events; MI, myocardial infarction; PCI, percutaneous coronary intervention; ST, definite/probable stent thrombosis.

Risk Stratification for Procedural and Long-term Outcomes

The SYNTAX score[49] could be an effective tool for stratification of patients with complex LMCA disease for appropriateness of revascularization strategy. In the LMCA subgroup of SYNTAX trial, the patients with a low SYNTAX score have a higher rate of nondistal LMCA lesions with mainly isolated LMCA disease or LMCA disease associated with single-vessel disease where PCI could be favored over CABG. In contrast, high SYNTAX score patients have a higher rate of distal LMCA lesions and are associated with two or three vessels disease, where CABG stand better than PCI. Combining the SYNTAX and the EuroSCORE into a common risk model [global risk classification [GRC]) was correlated with a significant improvement in predicting cardiac mortality in patients for LMCA PCI.[59]

GRC System

The additive EuroSCORE was calculated according to the original methodology.[60] The GRC is a combination of both EuroSCORE and SYNTAX score. The EuroSCORE was stratified into three groups for identification of different risks (low risk: 0–3; intermediate risk: 4–5; high risk: 6). Whereas SYNTAX score was stratified into three groups according to tertiles (lowest tertile: <28, intermediate tertile: 28–38, highest tertile: >38). The GRC system was classified into three risk groups. The low-risk group was composed of patients with both low/intermediate EuroSCORE and low/intermediate SYNTAX score. The intermediate-risk group was composed of patients with high EuroSCORE or high SYNTAX score. The high-risk group was composed of patients with both high EuroSCORE and high SYNTAX score.

The vessel distribution is LM population according to SYNTAX score tertiles shown in Figure 32.2. The definition of GRC is presented in Figure 32.3.[59]

Table 32.4 Clinical and lesion characteristics influencing the choice of stenting versus coronary artery bypass grafting in unprotected left main coronary artery disease in everyday clinical practice

Pro-stenting

- Isolated (ostial or mid-shaft) lesion or ULMCA plus 1 vessel disease (SYNTAX score <32)
- Isolated (distal) lesion or ULMCA (distal) plus 1 vessel disease anatomically suitable for stenting (SYNTAX score <32)
- No contraindications for prolonged dual antiplatelet therapy
- High-surgical risk comorbidities: advanced age; chronic lung disease; limited life expectancy, etc.
- Patient refusal of surgery

Pro-bypass surgery

- Complex coronary anatomy (SYNTAX score ≥33 due to ULMCA lesion associated with severe multivessel coronary disease, total occlusions of ≥2 major coronary epicardial vessels, severe calcifications, or tortuosity)
- Diabetes
- Renal dysfunction
- Severe compromised left ventricular systolic function
- Severe peripheral vascular disease unsuitable for catheterization
- Contraindication to antiplatelet therapy (allergy or intolerance to aspirin, clopidogrel, ticlopidine, high bleeding risk)

Abbreviations: ULMCA, unprotected left main coronary artery; SYNTAX, Synergy between PCI with TAXUS and Cardiac Surgery.

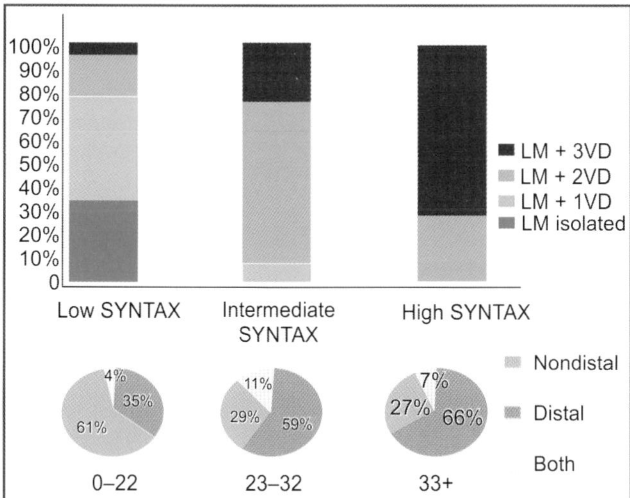

Fig. 32.2 Vessel distribution in left main population according to SYNTAX score tertiles

		SYNTAX score		
		<28	28–38	>38
EuroSCORE	0–3	L	L	I
	4–5	L	L	I
	≥6	I	I	H

Fig. 32.3 Global risk classification (GRC) are classified as follows. Patients classified as high-risk group are those who have both EuroSCORE _ 6 and SYNTAX score >38; patients classified as low-risk group (L) are those who have none of EuroSCORE _ 6 or SYNTAX score >38; otherwise, patients are classified as intermediate-risk group (I)

DES Choice in Treating LMCA

Several small observational studies have compared outcomes following "first-generation" DES implantation.[24,61] In the "Intracoronary Stenting and Angiographic Results: Drug-Eluting Stents for Unprotected LM Lesions" (ISAR-LM) randomized trial,[62] 607 patients were assigned to ULMCA PCI with SES or PES to compare the 1-year composite of death, MI, TLR. At 12-month follow-up, no significant differences were reported in the composite outcome of death, MI, and TLR [13.6% PES vs. 15.8% SES; relative risk: 0.85; 95% confidence interval (CI): 0.56–1.29] at 12-month follow-up. Angiographic restenosis (6–9 months of follow-up 16% PES vs. 19.4% SES; P = 0.30) and 2-year LM-specific revascularization (9.2% PES vs. 10.7% SES, P = 0.47). The incidence of definite Stent thrombosis (ST) (0.7% PES vs. 0.3% SES) and probable ST (0.3% PES vs. 0% SES) was also similar at 2-year follow-up.

In the Left Main Taxus and LEft MAin Xience (LEMAX) nonrandomized registry, 173 patients with ULMCA disease treated with everolimus-eluting stent (EES) were compared with a historical cohort of 291 patients treated with PES for ULMCA stenosis. At 12-month clinical follow-up, EES was associated with lower target lesion failure (a composite of cardiac death, target vessel MI, and TLR) and ST when compared with PES.[49] The ongoing ISAR-LM2 randomized trial, which evaluating the safety and efficacy of EES versus zotarolimus-eluting stent, will provide some newer information about the efficacy of new-generation DES platforms in this complex lesions.

WHO IS THE GOOD CANDIDATE FOR LMCA STENTING?

- The first step in safety in performing PCI is careful patient selection.
- The PCI or CABG for treatment of unprotected LMCA stenosis depends on several clinical and anatomical features.
- LMCA disease is mostly associated with lesions in the other coronary arteries also. The treatment strategy of this subset and the feasibility of a complete revascularization approach are very essential.
- The group of patients with ULMCA disease who are likely to have favorable clinical outcomes with PCI as that of CABG:
  - Ostial and/or mid-shaft LMCA disease
  - Isolated LMCA disease
  - LMCA disease plus single-vessel disease
  - LMCA bifurcational disease treatable by single-stent approach
  - Low or intermediate SYNTAX score (SYNTAX score <33).

IMPACT OF DIABETES ON THE CLINICAL OUTCOME

SYNTAX trial subgroup analysis at 1 year suggests the following key findings[63]:

1. In patients with LM and/or 3VDs, MACCE rates were significantly higher in the PES arm compared with the CABG arm in diabetic patients and directionally higher (but nonsignificant) in nondiabetic patients. Although there was no statistically powered prespecified primary endpoint of this subgroup analysis, this result suggests that MACCE after PES treatment might be inferior to CABG treatment for diabetic patients with LM and/or three-vessel disease.
2. There were no significant differences in composite death/cerebrovascular accident/MI or in the individual components of death or MI between the CABG and PES groups, regardless of diabetic status or lesion complexity. Compared with nondiabetic patients, patients with diabetes had increased mortality in both the CABG and PES groups.
3. In both diabetic and nondiabetic patients with the greatest anatomical complexity (SYNTAX scores ≥33), mortality was significantly increased with PES treatment compared with CABG.
4. Repeat revascularization was higher with PES compared with CABG in both diabetic and nondiabetic patients.
5. Patients with diabetes had significantly increased repeat revascularization rates compared with nondiabetic patients when treated with PES, but not when treated with CABG.
6. Repeat revascularization rates after PES treatment (and hence the relative difference between the PES and CABG groups) tended to increase with increasing lesion complexity (i.e. higher SYNTAX score), particularly in patients with diabetes; in nondiabetic patients with low lesion complexity, repeat revascularization rates were similar between treatment arms.

Acute ULMCA Occlusion in the Setting of ST-elevation MI—Is Percutaneous Coronary Intervention the Preferred Revascularization Approach?

Acute occlusion involving the ULMCA accounts for 0.8% of patients who undergo primary PCI.[64] This event is often associated with catastrophic events such as cardiogenic shock, lethal arrhythmias, and sudden death. Uncertainty surrounds the optimal revascularization strategy for ST-elevation MI (STEMI) patients due to acute ULMCA occlusion. The revised 2004 American College of Cardiology (ACC)/ American Heart Association (AHA) STEMI guidelines[65] indicate that PCI and CABG have a class Ia indication in patients with cardiogenic shock, but do not provide specific treatment recommendations for ULMCA disease.

Regardless of the revascularization strategy chosen, the in-hospital mortality rate of STEMI patients with ULMCA occlusion treated with primary PCI is very high and it ranges between 35% and 44%, 65–67 while a rate of 46% was reported after emergency CABG in the same clinical setting. Considering the high clinical risk profile of this subset of patients, a treatment bias favoring PCI over CABG prohibits direct comparison between the two revascularization modalities.

In the AMIS (acute myocardial infarction in Switzerland) plus registry experience, Pedrazzini et al.[66] reported results of 348 patients who underwent LM primary PCI, either isolated (n = 208) or concomitant to PCI for other vessel segments (n = 140). They were compared with 6,318 patients undergoing PCI of non-LM vessel segments only. The LM patients with higher rates of cardiogenic shock (12.2% vs. 3.5%; P = 0.001) had a remarkably high (89%) in-hospital survival and concurrent LM, and non-LM PCI had worse outcomes than isolated LM PCI.

Percutaneous coronary intervention may be performed more expeditiously than CABG to promptly reperfuse the infarcted artery, potentially reversing arrhythmic, and hemodynamic instability in STEMI substrate. Delays to reperfusion with CABG, which may take 1 hour or more during off-peak hours to establish cardiopulmonary bypass, can be catastrophic in this situation. Hence, emergency PCI performed in a timely by experienced operators should be considered as a better alternative to CABG in such situations.[67]

Primary aim should be made to decrease the time from the first medical contact to balloon inflation. Intra-aortic balloon pump should be implemented before or immediately after urgent coronary angiography prior to PCI. This strategy may reduce the incidence of ventricular tachycardia/fibrillation and need for cardiopulmonary resuscitation during the intervention. Thrombus aspiration instead of standard balloon predilatation has been shown to improve microvascular reperfusion. One must avoid stent oversizing and high-pressure postdilatation to avoid "slow" or "no-reflow" phenomenon, which may be catastrophic especially when patient in a cardiogenic shock with LM occlusion (Table 32.5).

Table 32.5 European Society of Cardiology/European Association for Cardiothoracic Surgery Recommendations for coronary artery bypass grafting versus percutaneous coronary intervention in patients with unprotected left main stenosis

Favors CABG Favors PCI		
• Left main (isolated or 1-VD ostium/shaft)	IA	IIa B
• Left main (isolated or 1-VD, distal bifurcation)	IA	IIb B
• Left main +2-VD or 3-VD and SYNTAX score <32	IA	IIb B
• Left main +2-VD or3-VD and SYNTAX score >33	IA	III B

Abbreviations: CABG, coronary bypass grafting; PCI, percutaneous coronary intervention.

Different Strategies and Techniques for Percutaneous Coronary

Intervention of Left Main Lesions

Although once ULMCA considered a relative contraindication and widely discouraged, PCI for ULMCA is now rapidly emerging as safe option to CABG. Left main disease is usually associated with lesions in the other coronary vessels, giving a complex multivessel disease. The treatment of complex lesions needs to be considered when deciding on the treatment strategy of the LM and the possibility of a complete revascularization.

Ostial and Midvessel Lesions

These lesions can be stented as in any other artery and good result achieved with single-stent strategy. Good angiographic views must be performed to ensure adequate visualization of the ostium and adjacent aorta. Usually, anterior-posterior cranial and/or slightly left anterior oblique cranial projections give the best visualization. The guide catheter may be occlusive with severe stenosis. The Amplatz guides should be avoided in ostial lesions. Ostial lesions are often predilated. The stent needs to be placed carefully with 1–2 mm protruding into the aorta. After deployment, the balloon should be withdrawn slightly into the aorta and the proximal part of the stent postdilated to flare it that ensures good stent apposition at the ostium. Intravascular ultrasound (IVUS) may be used to ensure a satisfactory result (Figs 32.4A and B).

LMCA Bifurcation Lesion

In LMCA bifurcation stenosis, intervention may result in occlusion of the ostium of LAD or LCx with clinical catastrophe. Various interventional techniques have been tested or eliminated the side branch occlusion risk in bifurcation lesions.

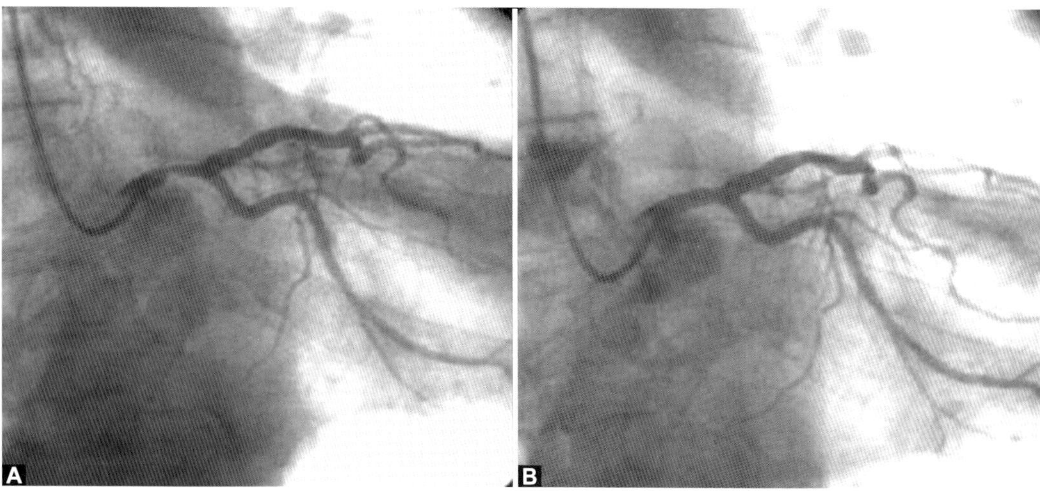

Figs 32.4A and B Direct stenting of isolated mid-shaft left main stenosis. (A) Baseline angiography: short, noncalcified lesion of mid-left main treated by direct stenting; (B) Final angiographic result

Distal LMCA lesions are mostly treated as true bifurcation. The exception to this is when one branch is small (usually the LCx), when one branch is chronically occluded or if protected by a patent graft. In these circumstances, the distal lesion may be addressed with a single-stent technique across the ostium of the other vessel. True bifurcation lesions may be treated either by single-stent or by a two-stent strategy. Choice of strategy depends on vessel and lesion characteristics (plaque distribution, the diameter of the branches, the angle between them and anatomy of side branch). The provisional stenting is a single-stent strategy, although it allows the placement of a second stent if required [T stenting, T and protrusion (TAP), culotte technique]. More complex lesions may require double-stent strategy (T stenting, TAP, mini-crush, culotte, V stenting). No single interventional technique has been found to guarantee preserved patency of the parent vessel and side branch; it is technically demanding, requiring expertise.

Strategy for Bifurcation Stenting

The size of the LCx and the anatomy of the ostium are two important features. If the LCx is either occluded, its diameter <2.5 mm, it can be ignored and a stent can be placed between the LMCA and the LAD.[68] Better to put a wire placed in a small LCx may help to maintain flow after a single stent is placed across the ostium. For a healthy LCx ostium, if the bifurcation angle is of T shape, it is the operator's choice to place a protective wire but it is often not necessary.

If the bifurcation angle is of Y shape, a protective wire is definitely recommended. For a significant and diseased LCx ostium, there are several techniques depending on the angle of bifurcation, if the angle is of T shape, the T-stent or mini-crush kissing stent technique is recommended. If the angle is of Y shape, the culotte, mini-crush or double kiss (DK) crush technique is recommended, while T stenting is not.[69]

When double stents are used, a final simultaneous inflation of both stents (kissing balloon inflation) at medium pressure (8-10 atm) with noncompliant balloons is considered critical to optimize outcomes. Finally, IVUS should be performed to ensure adequate stent expansion, complete stent strut apposition to the vessel wall, and absence of persistent dissection.

Single-stent Strategy

The Provisional T Stenting

This is a single-stent strategy but allows the positioning of a second stent if required (Figs 32.5A to D). The LAD and LCx are wired. A stent is positioned from LMCA to the LAD to fully cover the lesion and then deployed at 12–14 atm. The wires are then exchanged, the LAD wire can be withdrawn and passed through the stent struts to the LCx, and the "jailed" wire in the LCx can be withdrawn and advanced to the LAD. High pressure postdilatation may be applied if it is required. If LCx ostium is compromised, a kissing balloon technique can be performed. If the ostium of the LCx is severely compromised, the provisional T stenting, TAP, or culotte technique may be applied. Final kissing inflation (FKI) is performed if two stents have been used (Table 32.6).

Table 32.6 Favorable or unfavorable anatomical features for single-stent crossover stenting in treatment of unprotected left main coronary artery stenosis[80]

	Anatomical features
Favorable	Insignificant stenosis at the ostial LCX with Medina classification 1,1,0 or 1,0,0,
	Diminutive LCx with <2.5 mm in diameter, right dominant coronary system
	Wide angle with LAD
	No concomitant disease in LCx
	Focal disease in LCx
Unfavorable	Insignificant stenosis at the ostial LCx with Medina classification 1,1,1; 1,0,1; or 0,1,1
	Large size of LCx with ≥2.5 mm in diameter; left dominant coronary system
	Narrow angle with LAD
	Concomitant disease in LCx
	Diffuse disease in LCx

Abbreviations: LCx artery, left circumflex artery; LAD, left anterior descending artery.

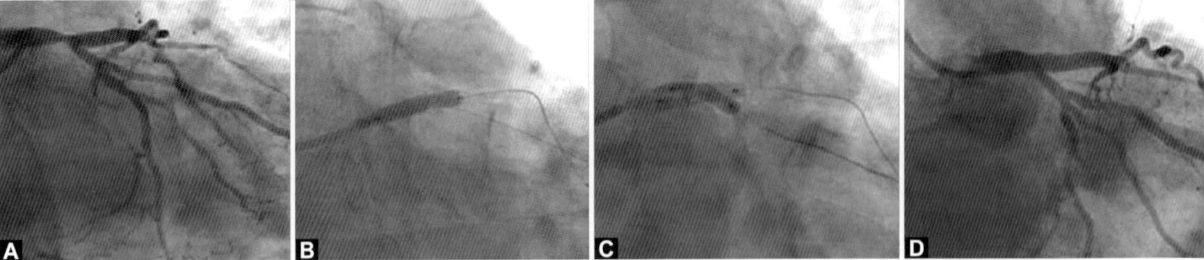

Figs 32.5A to D Provisional stenting. (A) Initial appearance; (B) Stent to left main-left anterior descending; (C) Kissing balloon poststent deployment; (D) Final result

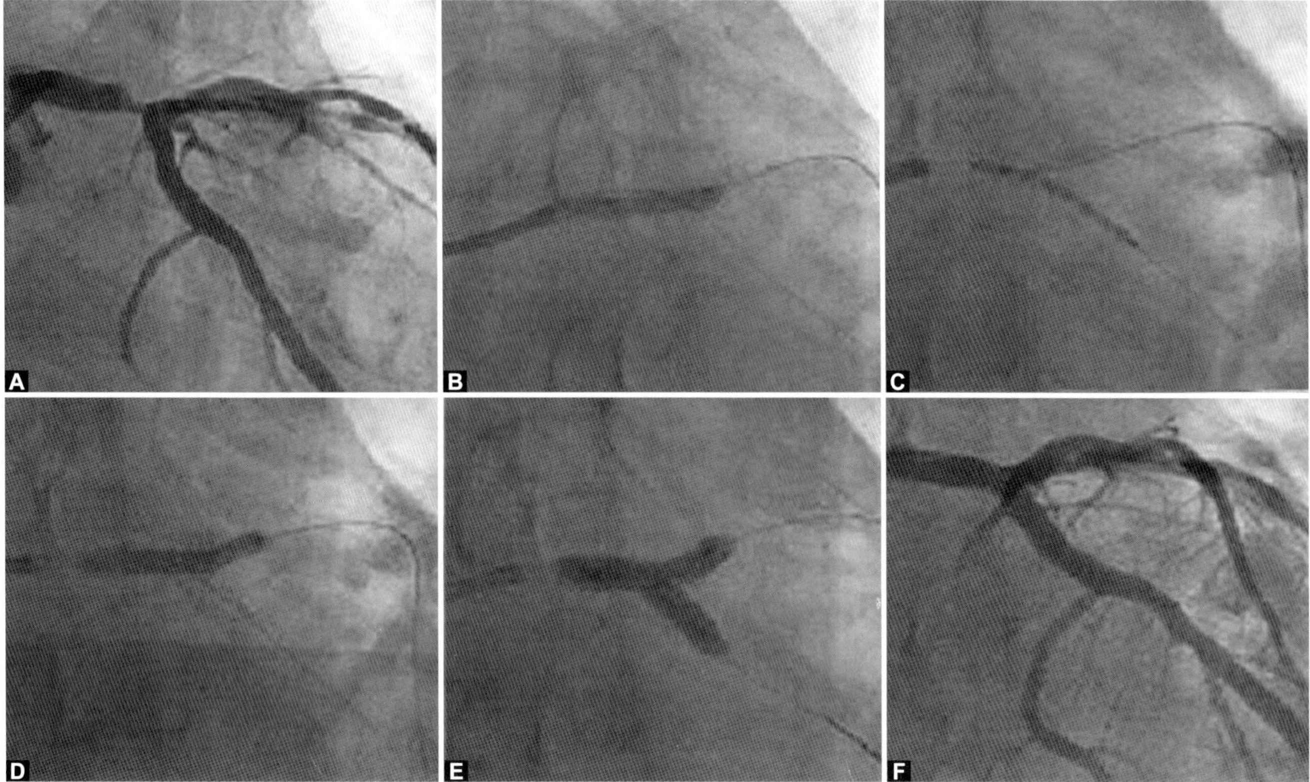

Figs 32.6A to F Culotte stenting. (A) Initial appearance; (B) Predilatation of the left anterior descending; (C) First stent deployed in the left circumflex; (D) Second stent deployed in the left anterior descending after recrossing with wire and predilatation; (E) Kissing balloon postdilatation; (F) Final result

Double-Stent Strategy

The Culotte Stenting

Double stent strategy is useful when the ostium of LCx is diseased, the angulation between LAD and LCx is <60° and when two vessels are of similar diameter. The main branch (MB) usually the LMCA-LAD is stented. The LCx is rewired through the stent struts and dilated. A second stent is advanced through the struts of the first into the side vessel. The LMCA-LCx stent is deployed. Each limb of the culotte is dilated at high pressure (16 atm) using noncompliant balloon followed by FKI at 8–12 atm (Figs 32.6A to F). This technique gives near-perfect coverage of the carina and SB ostium. The main disadvantage of the technique is that rewiring both branches through stent struts can be technically demanding and time-consuming. Open-cell stents are preferred for this technique.

The Classical T Stenting

This technique is suited when the angle between the two vessels is close to 90°. A stent is deployed in LCx, making sure to cover the ostium with minimal protrusion into the LAD. The LMCALAD lesion is then stented. LCx is rewired and dilated followed by FKI. This technique provides good reconstruction of distal LMCA bifurcation, but is associated with the risk of leaving a small gap between the branches, hence restenosis at the ostium of LCx. For this reason, this technique has largely been replaced by the modified T-stenting technique (Figs 32.7A to F).

The Modified T Stenting

It is performed by simultaneously positioning stents at LCx and LAD with LCx stent minimally protruding into the LAD, when the angulations between the branches approach 90°. The LCx stent is deployed first, and then after removal of the wire and balloon from LCx, the LAD stent is deployed. The procedure is completed with FKI.

The TAP Stenting

In majority of the bifurcation lesions, this TAP technique is used. It can provide good reconstruction of distal LMCA bifurcation with minimal stent overlap.

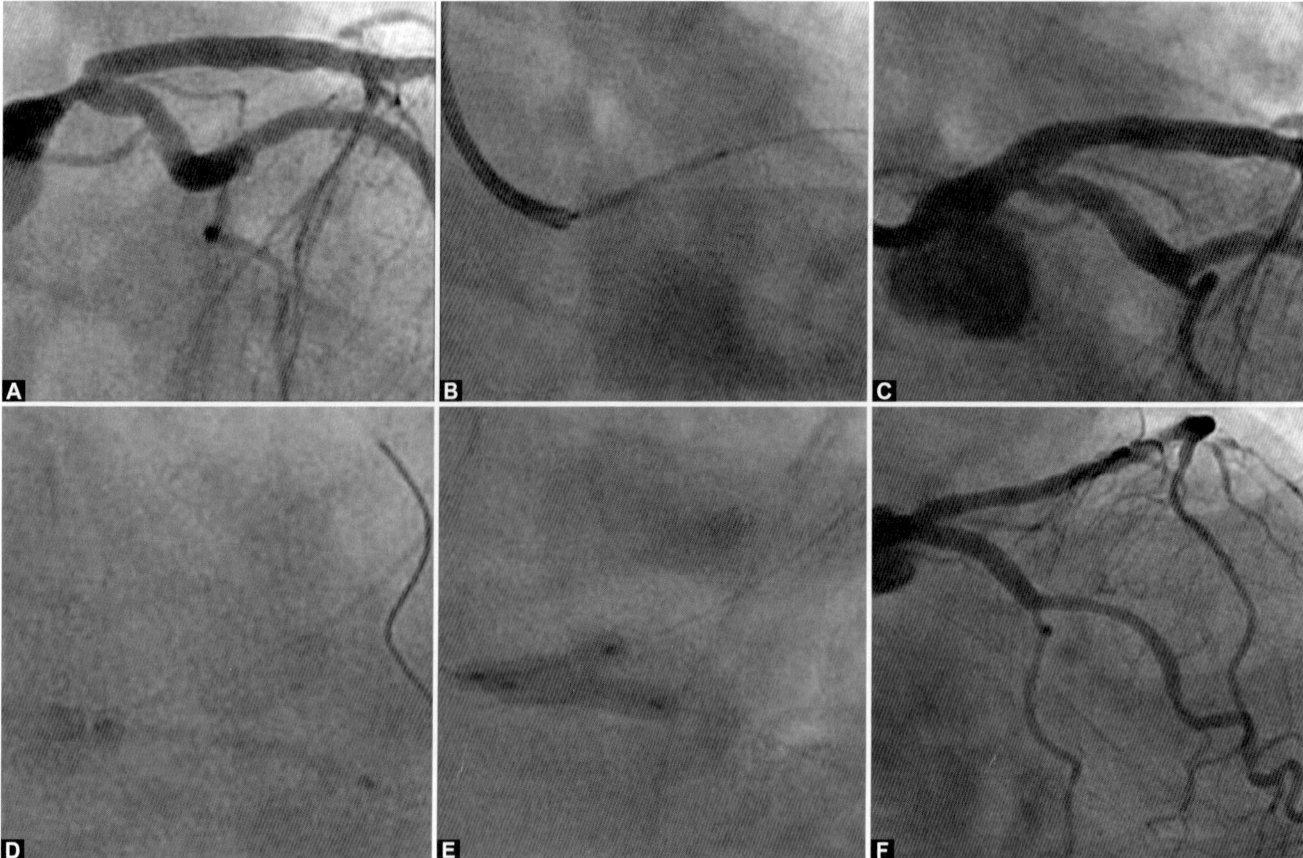

Figs 32.7A to F T stenting. (A) Initial appearance; (B) Stent to left main-left anterior descending; (C) Dissection of ostial left circumflex; (D) Advancement of the stent into left circumflex; (E) Kissing balloons; (F) Final result

The MB (LMCA-LAD) is stented jailing the SB (LCx) wire. Kissing balloon inflation is performed after rewiring the SB. After positioning the proximal edge of the SB stent 1–2 mm inside the MB stent, the SB stent is deployed at high pressure with deflated balloon kept in the MB stent. Then, SB balloon is slightly retrieved and aligned to the MB balloon. An FKI is performed to reshape the carina (Figs 32.8A to F).

The Mini-crush Stenting

This technique is mainly for LM bifurcation patient with ostial and proximal stenosis of the MB (LAD) and SB (LCx), in which the diameter of LAD is greater than LCx and the angle between LAD and LCx is <60°. The immediate patency of both branches is assured and it should be used in conditions of instability or complex anatomy. This technique is used for excellent coverage of the SB ostium. In almost all true bifurcation lesions, this technique is used but must be avoided in wide angle bifurcations. The disadvantage to perform FKI is that there is need to recross multiple struts with wire and a balloon. The SB stent is positioned in the SB followed by advancement of MB stent. The SB stent is pulled back into the MB about 1–2 mm and is deployed at least at 12 atm. The MB is stented at high pressure, usually above 12 atm that crushes the proximal SB stent against the LMCA wall. LCx is rewired through the stent struts of LAD and crushed LCx stent to perform FKI (Figs 32.9A to G).

The DK-Crush Stenting

A stent is placed into LCx and a balloon placed in LMCA-LAD. The stent and balloon are positioned as in the standard crush technique. The LCx stent is deployed and then the wire and balloon from the LCx are removed. The prepositioned balloon in LMCA-LAD is inflated to crush the protruding segment of LCx stent against the vessel wall of the LM. The balloon is removed and a stent is deployed in the LMCA-LAD. The wire is then recrossed into the LCx, and FKI is applied to finish the procedure (Figs 32.10A to H).

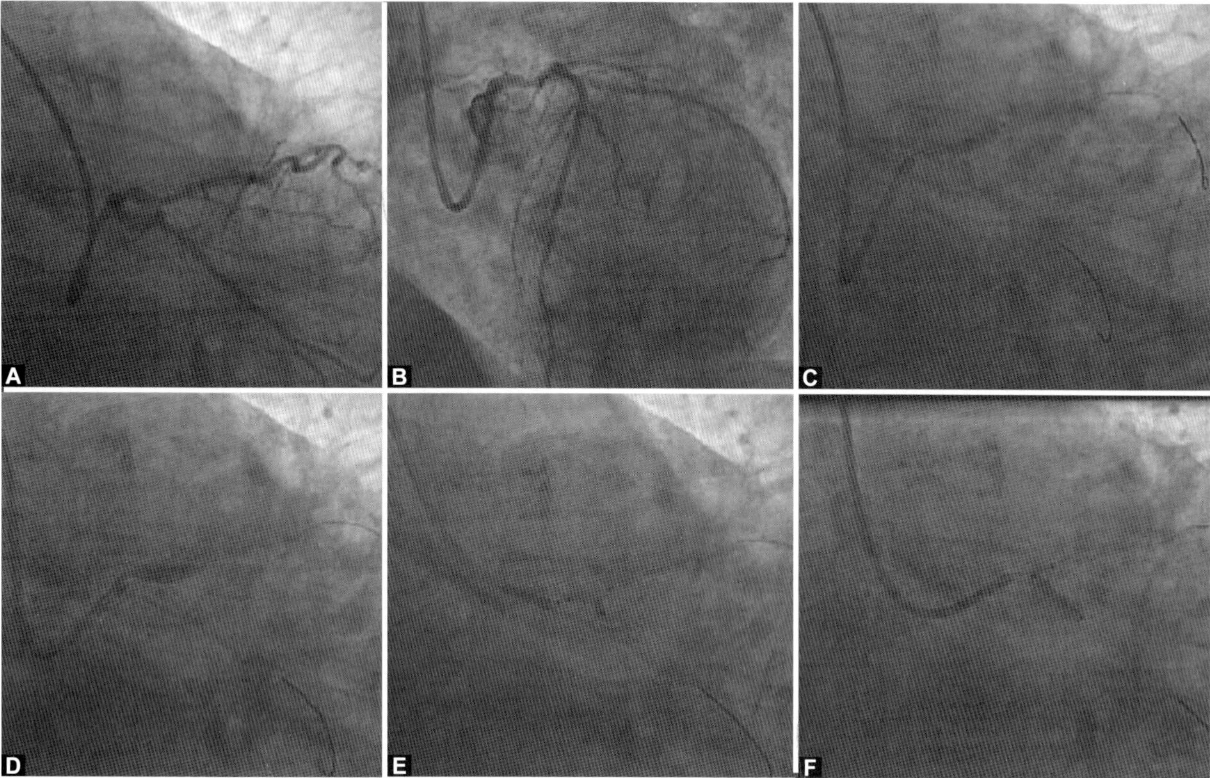

Figs 32.8A to F T stenting and protrusion technique. (A and B) Baseline angiography: severe eccentric distal left main stenosis; (C and D) 3.5 × 18 mm DES implanted in left main-left anterior descending. Postdilatation with a 4.0 mm balloon; (E) 2.5 mm balloon inflated in left main-left circumflex through the stent struts; (F) 3.5 × 18 mm drug-eluting stents placed in left circumflex with proximal edge inside the left main and a deflated 3.5 mm balloon in the left main

DK-Crush II is the only randomized trial to suggest that double stenting may be superior to provisional stenting and associated with a lower rate of restenosis and repeat revascularization.[70]

The V and the Simultaneous Kissing Stent

When the two stents are deployed together then V and simultaneous kissing stent (SKS) techniques are performed.[71,72] Wires are placed in LAD and LCx, with or without predilatation. The two stents are placed into the LMCA and the respective branches and deployed by simultaneous inflation. Some operators allow a variable amount of protrusion creating a rather long double barrel; the technique is called SKS. The main advantage of this technique is that access to both branches is always preserved with no need for rewiring. V stenting is relatively easy and fast and thus ideal in emergencies. It is indicated in patients with a short LMCA-free disease and critical disease of the LAD and LCx ostia.

The SKS can also be performed when the LMCA is very large resulting in a significant diameter mismatch with the LAD and LCx, as this technique will ensure apposition and full coverage of the large LMCA with drug (Figs 32.11A to F).

ADJUNCTIVE MANAGEMENT

IVUS and Optical Coherence Tomography

Intravascular ultrasound (IVUS) guidance is helpful in assessing vessel size, adequate stent expansion, and absence of stent malapposition. Intravascular ultrasound criteria for the significant LMCA disease are stenosis of >50% of the vessel diameter, stenosis of >60% of the area, an absolute cross-sectional area, 7 mm^2 in symptomatic patients, or <6 mm^2 in asymptomatic patients.

A subgroup analysis from the MAIN-COMPARE registry reported that IVUS guidance was associated with improved 3-year mortality compared with a conventional angiography-guided procedure after adjustment with propensity-score matching [6.3% IVUS vs. 13.6% angiography, log-rank $p = 0.063$, hazard ratio (HR): 0.54; 95% CI, 0.28–1.03].[73] In particular, for

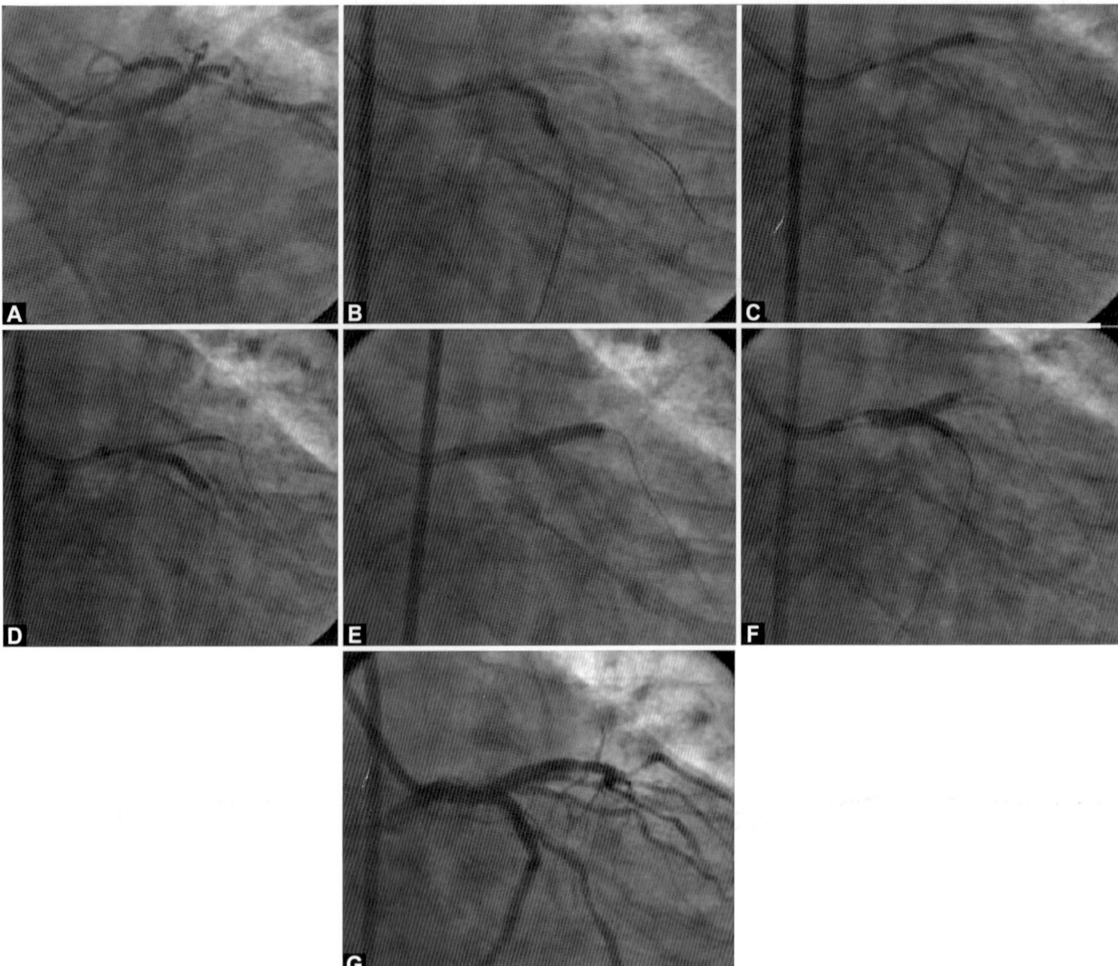

Figs 32.9A to G Mini-crush technique. (A) Baseline angiogram revealing significant stenosis of left-main (LM) bifurcation involving proximal left anterior descending (LAD) and left circumflex (LCx) artery; (B) Predilatation of LCx artery; (C) Predilatation of LAD artery; (D) Stent to LCx with protrusion into LAD artery; (E) Crushing of LCx stent with left main coronary artery (LMCA) to LAD stent; (F) Rewiring of LCx followed by final kissing balloon inflation; (G) Final angiographic result

patients receiving DES, IVUS-guided PCI was associated with a significantly lower 3-year incidence of mortality compared with angioguided PCI (4.7% IVUS vs. 16% angiography; log rank $p = 0.048$; HR: 0.39; 95% CI: 0.15–1.02).[73,74]

Optimal coherence tomography has been recently reported to assess vascular response to LMCA stenting.[75,76]

Fractional Flow Reserve

Fractional flow reserve (FFR) has been used to distinguish that LM patients require revascularization. It may be reasonable to defer LM revascularization in patients with a FFR >0.80. The FFR drawbacks for LMCA assessment, in the presence of concomitant lesions in the LAD and LCx without repairing the downstream lesions, the FFR usually underestimate the true significance of the LM lesion. In ostial LM lesions with catheter-induced damping upon engagement, uncomfortable maneuvers are sometimes repetitively required to engage, inject intracoronary adenosine, and disengage the guide. The administration of intravenous adenosine should be considered under these circumstances. There may be a discrepancy between angiographic percent diameter stenosis and FFR in jailed LCx lesions after LMCA-LAD stenting. A study by Nam et al. reports that the need for revascularization of the ostial LCx after LMCA-LAD crossover stenting may be reduced, if the procedure is guided by FFR.

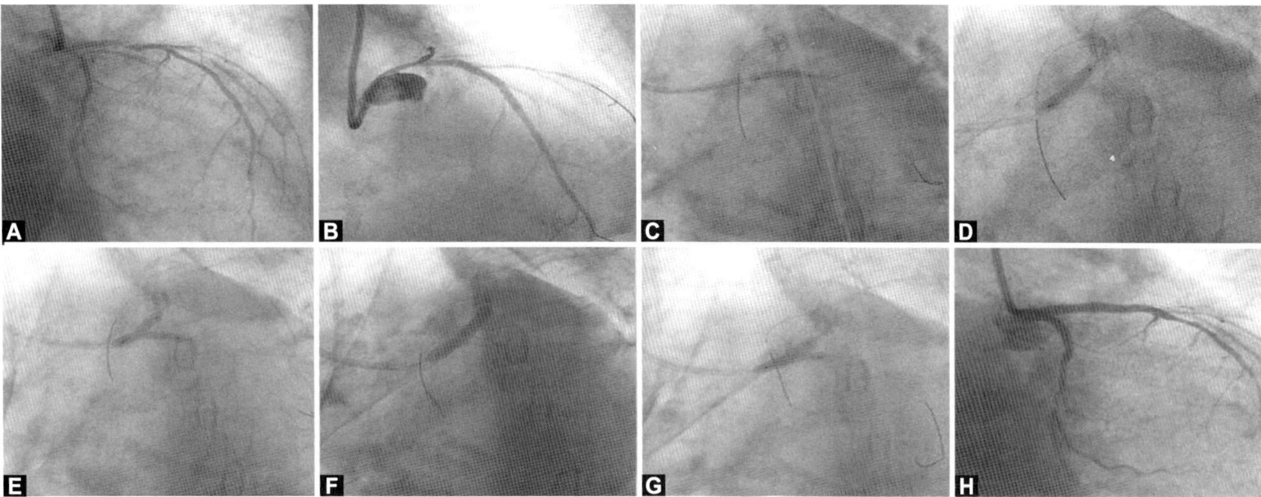

Figs 32.10A to H Double kiss crush technique. (A) Baseline angiography showing critical distal left main (LM), proximal left anterior descending (LAD) and ostioproximal left circumflex (LCx) artery; (B) Predilatation followed by stenting of proximal LAD; (C) Predilatation followed by subsequent stenting of LM-LCx; (D) Crushing of LCx stent with noncompliant balloon placed in LM-LAD artery; (E) First kissing balloon inflation; (F) Deployment of stent from LM-LAD with second crushing of LCx stent; (G) Second kissing balloon inflation; (H) Final result

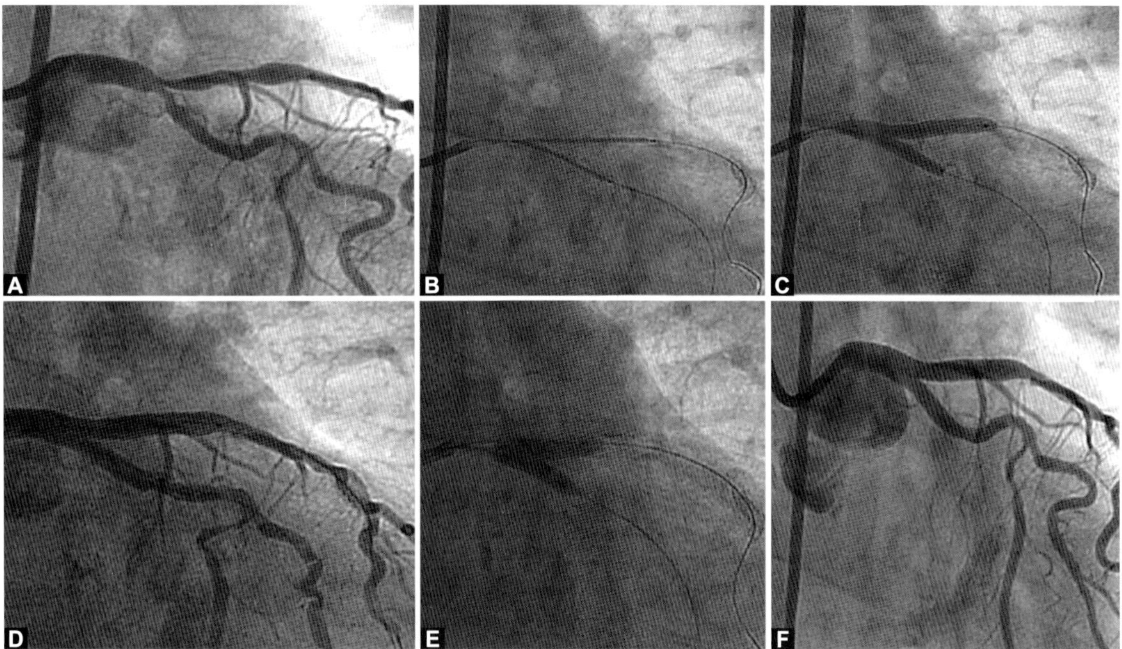

Figs 32.11A to F V stenting. (A) Initial appearance (medina 0, 1, 1); (B and C) Two drug-eluting stents implanted in left anterior descending and left circumflex; (D) Intermediate result; (E) Postdilatation (kissing); (F) Final angiographic result

Dual Antiplatelet Therapy

The optimal duration of DAPT in patients with ULMCA disease to be defined. The current guidelines suggest long-term aspirin administration and at least 6- to 12-month dual antiplatelet therapy (DAT) in patients receiving a DES (class: I, level of evidence: B); however, this is not specific for ULMCA stenting.[77,78] Although the risk-benefit ratio of long-term DAT is not well defined, many clinicians prolong DAT long term after ULMCA stenting with DES. Migliorini et al.[79] reported the outcomes of 215 patients treated with DES for ULMCA who had prospective platelet reactivity assessment by light transmittance aggregometry after a loading dose of 600 mg of clopidogrel. The incidence of high residual platelet reactivity (HRPR) after clopidogrel loading was 18.6%. The 3-year cardiac mortality and ST rate were significantly reduced in the low residual platelet reactivity group compared with the HRPR group. High residual platelet reactivity after clopidogrel loading was the only independent predictor of cardiac death and ST. Additional studies are strongly required in order to resolve these issues and to determine the optimal duration of DAT administration after DES placement in ULMCA disease. The new antiplatelet agents (Prasugrel and Ticagrelor) have been evaluated in acute coronary syndromes but not yet in LMPCI.

THE FUTURE

New generation of DES, dedicated bifurcation stents, and improvement of procedural techniques will probably improve the clinical outcome. The new antiplatelet agents (Prasugrel and Ticagrelor) could improve the safety of PCI in complex LM lesions, but they need to be evaluated in this particular setting. The future EXCEL trial (evaluation of Xience Prime or Xience V-eluting stent vs. CABG for effectiveness of LM revascularization) will evaluate the safety and efficacy of PCI with Xience Prime or Xience V EES vs. CABG in patients with ULMCA disease with a low or intermediate SYNTAX score (<33). The composite measure of all-cause mortality, MI, or stroke at an anticipated median follow-up duration of 3 years will be the primary endpoint.

CONCLUSION

Current guidelines indicate CABG as the optimal treatment for LMCA lesions. However, data from worldwide registries and LM subset of SYNTAX are encouraging toward a noninferiority of PCI with DES versus CABG with regard to MI, death and cardiovascular events at medium-term follow-up. The LMCA stenting is feasible and is generally technically safe, although there are some special considerations during the stenting process. Stenting of ostial and shaft of LMCA can be achieved without major technical difficulties and with good immediate and long-term results. Distal LMCA bifurcational lesions continue to pose a considerable challenge and require expertise and performance of unique approaches for optimal results. An integrated approach that combines advanced devices, specialized techniques, adjunctive imaging support, as well as adjunctive pharmacological agents would continue to improve PCI success rate and long-term outcomes for these complex subsets. The EXCEL trial will demonstrate whether PCI with new generation of DES will compete with CABG as regards safety endpoint.

REFERENCES

1. Stone P, Goldschlager N. Left main coronary artery disease: review and appraisal. Cardiovasc Med. 1979;4:165-77.
2. DeMots H, Rosch J, McAnulty J. Left main coronary artery disease. Cardiovasc Clin. 1977;8:201-11.
3. Taylor H, Deumite N, Chaitman B, et al. Asymptomatic left main coronary artery disease in the Coronary Artery Surgery Study (CASS) registry. Circulation. 1989;79:1171-9.
4. Cohen M, Gorlin R. Main left coronary artery disease: clinical experience from 1964–1974. Circulation. 1975;52:275-85.
5. Yusuf S, Zucker D, Peduzzi P, et al. Effect of coronary artery bypass graft surgery on survival: overview of 10-year results from randomised trials by the Coronary Artery Bypass Graft Surgery Trialists Collaboration. Lancet. 1994;344:1446.
6. Chaitman BR, Fisher LD, Bourassa MG, et al. Effect of coronary bypass surgery on survival patterns in subsets of patients with left main coronary artery disease: report of the Collaborative Study in Coronary Artery Surgery (CASS). Am J Cardiol. 1981;48:765-77.
7. Takaro T, Peduzzi P, Detre KM, et al. Survival in subgroups of patients with left main coronary artery disease: Veterans Administration Cooperative Study of Surgery for Coronary Arterial Occlusive Disease. Circulation. 1982;66:14-22.
8. Caracciolo EA, Davis KB, Sopko G, et al. Comparison of surgical and medical group survival in patients with left main equivalent coronary artery disease: long-term CASS experience. Circulation. 1995;91:2335-44.
9. Kalbfleisch H, Hort W. Quantitative study on the size of coronary artery supplying areas postmortem. Am Heart J. 1977;94:183-8.
10. Farinha JB, Kaplan MA, Harris CN, et al. Disease of the left main coronary artery. Surgical treatment and long-term follow up in 267 patients. Am J Cardiol. 1978;42:124-8.
11. Macaya C, Alfonso F, Iniguez A, et al. Stenting for elastic recoil during coronary angioplasty of the left main coronary artery. Am J Cardiol. 1992;70:105-7.
12. Taggart D, Kaul S, Boden WE, et al. Revascularisation for unprotected left main stem coronary artery stenosis: stenting or surgery. J Am Coll Cardiol. 2008;51:885-92.
13. Sabik JF, Blackstone EH, Firstenberg M, et al. A benchmark for evaluating innovative treatment of left main coronary disease. Circulation. 2007;116(Suppl. I):I-232-9.
14. Gruntzig AR, Senning A, Siegenthaler WE. Nonoperative dilatation of coronary-artery stenosis: percutaneous transluminal coronary angioplasty. N Engl J Med. 1979;301:61-8.
15. O'Keefe JH Jr, Hartzler GO, Rutherford BD, et al. Left main coronary angioplasty: early and late results of 127 acute and elective procedures. Am J Cardiol. 1989;64:144-7.

16. Park SJ, Park SW, Hong MK, et al. Long-term (three-year) outcomes after stenting of unprotected left main coronary artery stenosis in patients with normal left ventricular function. Am J Cardiol. 2003;91:12-6.
17. Silvestri M, Barragan P, Sainsous J, et al. Unprotected left main coronary artery stenting: immediate and medium-term outcomes of 140 elective procedures. J Am Coll Cardiol. 2000;35:1543-50.
18. Park SJ, Park SW, Hong MK, et al. Stenting of unprotected left main coronary artery stenoses: immediate and late outcomes. J Am Coll Cardiol. 1998;31:37-42.
19. Takagi T, Stankovic G, Finci L, et al. Results and long-term predictors of adverse clinical events after elective percutaneous interventions on unprotected left main coronary artery. Circulation. 2002;106:698-702.
20. Black A, Cortina R, Bossi I, et al. Unprotected left main coronary artery stenting: correlates of midterm survival and impact of patient selection. J Am Coll Cardiol. 2001;37:832-8.
21. Tan WA, Tamai H, Park SJ, et al. Long-term clinical outcomes after unprotected left main trunk percutaneous revascularization in 279 patients. Circulation. 2001;104:1609-14.
22. de Lezo JS, Medina A, Pan M, et al. Rapamycin-eluting stents for the treatment of unprotected left main coronary disease. Am Heart J. 2004;148:481-5.
23. Park SJ, Kim YH, Lee BK, et al. Sirolimus-eluting stent implantation for unprotected left main coronary artery stenosis: comparison with bare metal stent implantation. J Am Coll Cardiol. 2005;45:351-6.
24. Valgimigli M, van Mieghem CA, Ong AT, et al. Short- and long-term clinical outcome after drug-eluting stent implantation for the percutaneous treatment of left main coronary artery disease: insights from the Rapamycin-Eluting and Taxus Stent Evaluated at Rotterdam Cardiology Hospital registries (RESEARCH and T-SEARCH). Circulation. 2005;111:1383-9.
25. Pavei A, Oreglia J, Martin G, et al. Long-term follow-up of percutaneous coronary intervention of unprotected left main lesions with drug eluting stents. Predictors of clinical outcome. EuroIntervention. 2009;4:457-63.
26. Carrie D, Eltchaninoff H, Lefevre T, et al. Twelve month clinical and angiographic outcome after stenting of unprotected left main coronary artery stenosis with paclitaxel-eluting stents-results of the multicentre FRIEND registry. EuroIntervention. 2009;4:449-56.
27. Biondi-Zoccai GG, Lotrionte M, Moretti C, et al. A collaborative systematic review and meta-analysis on 1278 patients undergoing percutaneous drug-eluting stenting for unprotected left main coronary artery disease. Am Heart J. 2008;155:274-83.
28. Price MJ, Cristea E, Sawhney M, et al. Serial angiographic follow-up of sirolimus-eluting stents for unprotected left main coronary revascularization. J Am Coll Cardiol. 2006;47:871-7.
29. Tamburino C, Di Salvo ME, Capodanno D, et al. Comparison of drug-eluting stents and bare-metal stents for the treatment of unprotected left main coronary artery disease in acute coronary syndrome. Am J Cardiol. 2009;103:187-93.
30. Kim YH, Park DW, Lee SW, et al. Long-term safety and effectiveness of unprotected left main coronary stenting with drug-eluting stents compared with bare-metal stents. Circulation. 2009;120:400-7.
31. Kim YH, Park SW, Hong MK, et al. Comparison of simple and complex stenting techniques in the treatment of unprotected left main coronary artery bifurcation stenosis. Am J Cardiol. 2006;97:1397-601.
32. Kim YH, Dangas GD, Solinas E, et al. Effectiveness of drug-eluting stent implantation for patients with unprotected left main coronary artery stenosis. Am J Cardiol. 2008;101:801-6.
33. Tamburino C, Di Salvo ME, Capodanno D, et al. Are drug-eluting stents superior to bare-metal stents in patients with unprotected non-bifurcational left main disease? Insights from a multicentre registry. Eur Heart J. 2009;30:1171-9.
34. Christiansen EH, Lassen JF, Andersen HR, et al. Outcome of unprotected left main percutaneous coronary intervention in surgical low-risk, surgical high-risk, and myocardial infarction patients. EuroIntervention. 2006;1:403-8.
35. Gao RL, Xu B, Chen JL, et al. Immediate and long-term outcomes of drug-eluting stent implantation for unprotected left main coronary artery disease: comparison with bare-metal stent implantation. Am Heart J. 2008;155:553-61.
36. Palmerini T, Marzocchi A, Tamburino C, et al. Two year clinical outcome with drug-eluting stents versus bare-metal stents in a real-world registry of unprotected left main coronary artery stenosis from the Italian Society of Invasive Cardiology. Am J Cardiol. 2008;102:1463-8.
37. Carrie D, Lhermusier T, Hmem M, et al. Clinical and angiographic outcome of paclitaxel-eluting stent implantation for unprotected left main coronary artery bifurcation narrowing. EuroIntervention. 2006;1:396-402.
38. Chieffo A, Park SJ, Meliga E, et al. Late and very late stent thrombosis following drug-eluting stent implantation in unprotected left main coronary artery: a multicentre registry. Eur Heart J. 2008;29:2108-15.
39. Sanmartin M, Baz JA, Claro A, et al. Comparison of drug-eluting stents versus surgery for unprotected left main coronary artery disease. Am J Cardiol. 2007;100:970-3.
40. Seung KB, Park DW, Kim YH, et al. Stents versus coronary artery bypass grafting for left main coronary artery disease. N Engl J Med. 2008;358:1781-92.
41. Meliga E, Garcia-Garcia HM, Valgimigli M, et al. Longest available clinical outcomes after drug-eluting stent implantation for unprotected left main coronary artery disease the DELFT (Drug Eluting stent for LeFT main) registry. J Am Coll Cardiol. 2008;51(23):2212-9.
42. Valgimigli M, Malagutti P, Rodriguez Granillo GA, et al. Single-vessel versus bifurcation stenting for the treatment of distal left main coronary artery disease in the drug-eluting stenting era. Clinical and angiographic insights into the Rapamycin-Eluting Stent Evaluated at Rotterdam Cardiology Hospital (RESEARCH) and Taxus-Stent Evaluated at Rotterdam Cardiology Hospital (T-SEARCH) registries. Am Heart J. 2006;152:896-902.
43. Chieffo A, Stankovic G, Bonizzoni E, et al. Early and mid-term results of drug-eluting stent implantation in unprotected left main. Circulation. 2005;111:791-5
44. Chieffo A, Morici N, Maisano F, et al. Percutaneous treatment with drug-eluting stent implantation versus bypass surgery for unprotected left main stenosis: a single-centre experience. Circulation. 2006;113:2542-7.
45. Lee MS, Kapoor N, Jamal F, et al. Comparison of coronary artery bypass surgery with percutaneous coronary intervention with drug-eluting stents for unprotected left main coronary disease. J Am Coll Cardiol. 2006;47:864-70.

46. Park DW, Seung KB, Kim YH, et al. Long-term safety and efficacy of stenting versus coronary artery bypass grafting for unprotected left main coronary artery disease: 5-year results from the MAIN-COMPARE (Revascularization for Unprotected Left Main Coronary Artery Stenosis; Comparison of Percutaneous Coronary Angioplasty versus Surgical Revascularization) registry. J Am Coll Cardiol. 2010;56:117-27.
47. Park DW, Kim YH, Yun SC, et al. Long-term outcomes after stenting versus coronary artery bypass grafting for unprotected left main coronary artery disease: 10-year results of bare-metal disease and 5-year results of drug-eluting stents from the ASAN-MAIN (ASAN Medical Center-Left Main Revascularization) registry. J Am Coll Cardiol. 2010;56:1366-75.
48. Buszman PE, Kiesz SR, Bochenek A, et al. Acute and late outcomes of unprotected left main stenting in comparison with surgical revascularization. J Am Coll Cardiol. 2008;51:538-45.
49. Morice MC, Serruys PW, Kappetein AP, et al. Outcomes in patients with de novo left main disease treated with either percutaneous coronary intervention using paclitaxel-eluting stents or coronary artery bypass graft treatment in the Synergy between Percutaneous Coronary Intervention with TAXUS and Cardiac Surgery (SYNTAX) trial. Circulation. 2010;121:2645-53.
50. Lee MS, Kapoor N, Jamal F, et al. Comparison of coronary artery bypass surgery with percutaneous coronary intervention with drug-eluting stents for unprotected left main coronary artery disease. J Am Coll Cardiol. 2006;47:864-70.
51. Brener SJ, Galla JM, Bryant R 3rd, et al. Comparison of percutaneous versus surgical revascularization of severe unprotected left main coronary stenosis in matched patients. Am J Cardiol. 2008;101:169-72.
52. Chieffo A, Morici N, Maisano F, et al. Percutaneous treatment with drug-eluting stent implantation versus bypass surgery for unprotected left main stenosis: a single-center experience. Circulation. 2006;113:2542-7.
53. Palmerini T, Marzocchi A, Marrozzini C, et al. Comparison between coronary angioplasty and coronary artery bypass surgery for the treatment of unprotected left main coronary artery stenosis (the Bologna Registry). Am J Cardiol. 2006;98: 54-9.
54. Rodes-Cabau J, Deblois J, Bertrand OF, et al. Nonrandomized comparison of coronary artery bypass surgery and percutaneous coronary intervention for the treatment of unprotected left main coronary artery disease in octogenarians. Circulation. 2008;118:2374-81.
55. Wu C, Hannan EL, Walford G, et al. Utilization and outcomes of unprotected left main coronary artery stenting and coronary artery bypass graft surgery. Ann Thorac Surg. 2008;86:1153-9.
56. Buszman PE, Kiesz SR, Bochenek A, et al. Acute and late outcomes of unprotected left main stenting in comparison with surgical revascularization. J Am Coll Cardiol. 2008;51:538-45.
57. Park DW, Seung KB, Kim YH, et al. Long-term safety and efficacy of stenting versus coronary artery bypass grafting for unprotected left main coronary artery disease: 5-year results from the MAIN-COMPARE (Revascularization for Unprotected Left Main Coronary Artery Stenosis: Comparison of Percutaneous Coronary Angioplasty versus Surgical Revascularization) registry. J Am Coll Cardiol. 2010;56:117-24.
58. Chieffo A, Magni V, Latib A, et al. 5-year outcomes following percutaneous coronary intervention with drug-eluting stent implantation versus coronary artery bypass graft for unprotected left main coronary artery lesions the Milan experience. JACC Cardiovasc Interv. 2010;3:595-601.
59. Capodanno D, Miano M, Cincotta G, et al. EuroSCORE refines the predictive ability of SYNTAX scoring patients undergoing left main percutaneous coronary intervention. Am Heart J. 2010;159:103-9.
60. Roques F, Nashef SA, Michel P, et al. Risk factors and outcome in European cardiac surgery: analysis of the EuroSCORE multinational database of 19030 patients. Eur J Cardiothorac Surg. 1999;15:816-22.
61. Lee SH, Ko YG, Jang Y, et al. Sirolimus-versus paclitaxel-eluting stent implantation for unprotected left main coronary artery stenosis. Cardiology. 2005;104:181-5.
62. Mehilli J, Katrati A, Byrne RA, et al. Paclitaxel-versus sirolimus-eluting stents for unprotected left main coronary artery disease. J Am Coll Cardiol. 2009;53:1760-8.
63. Banning A, Westaby S, Morice MC, et al. Diabetic and nondiabetic patients with left main and/or 3-vessel coronary artery disease: comparison of outcomes with cardiac surgery and paclitaxel-eluting stents. J Am Coll Cardiol. 2010;55:1067-75.
64. De Luca G, Suryapranata H, Thomas K, et al. Outcome in patients treated with primary angioplasty for acute myocardial infarction due to left main coronary artery occlusion. Am J Cardiol. 2003;91:235-8.
65. Antman EM, Anbe DT, Armstrong PW, et al., ACC/AHA guidelines for the management of patients with ST-elevation myocardial infarction—executive summary: a report of the American College of Cardiology/American Heart Association Task Force on Practice Guidelines (Writing Committee to Revise the 1999 Guidelines for the Management of Patients With Acute Myocardial Infarction). Circulation. 2004;110:588-636.
66. Pedrazzini GB, Radovanovic D, Vassilli G, et al. On behalf of the AMIS plus Investigators. Primary percutaneous coronary intervention for unprotected left main disease in patients with acute ST-segment elevation myocardial infarction. J Am Coll Cardiol Interv. 2011;4:627-33.
67. Lee MS, Bokhoor P, Park SJ, et al., Unprotected left main coronary disease and ST-segment elevation myocardial infarction: a contemporary review and argument for percutaneous coronary intervention. JACC Cardiovasc Interv. 2010;3:791-5.
68. Fajadet J, Chieffo A. Current management of left main coronary artery disease. Eur Heart J. 2012;33:36-50.
69. Teirstein PS. Unprotected left main intervention: patient selection, operator technique and clinical outcomes. J Am Coll Cardiol Interv. 2008;1:5-13.
70. Chen SL, Santoso T, Zhang J, et al. A randomized clinical study comparing double kissing crush with provisional stenting for treatment of coronary bifurcation lesions: results from the DKCRUSH-II (double kissing crush versus provisional stenting technique for treatment of coronary bifurcation lesions) trial. J Am Coll Cardio. 2011;57:914-20.
71. Schampaert E, Fort S, Adelman AG, et al. The V-stent: a novel technique for coronary bifurcation stenting. Cathet Cardiovasc Diagn. 1996;39:320-6.
72. Sharma SK. Simultaneous kissing drug-eluting stent for percutaneous treatment of bifurcation lesions in large-size vessels. Catheter Cardiovasc Interv. 2005;65:10-6.
73. Park SJ, Kim YH, Park DW, et al. Impact of intravascular ultrasound guidance on long-term mortality in stenting for

unprotected left main coronary artery stenosis. Circ Cardiovasc Interv. 2009;2:167-77.
74. Tyczynski P, Pregowski J, Mintz GS, et al. Intravascular ultrasound assessment of ruptured atherosclerotic plaques in left main coronary arteries. Am J Cardiol. 2005;96:794-8.
75. Parodi G, Maehara A, Giuliani G, et al. Optical coherence tomography in unprotected left main coronary artery stenting. EuroIntervention. 2010;6:94-9.
76. Nam CW, Hur SH, Koo BK, et al. Fractional flow reserve versus angiography in left circumflex ostial intervention after left main crossover stenting. Korean Circ J. 2011;41:304-7.
77. Smith SC Jr, Allen J, Blair SN, et al. AHA/ACC guidelines for secondary prevention for patients with coronary and other atherosclerotic vascular disease: 2006 update endorsed by the National Heart, Lung, and Blood Institute. J Am Coll Cardiol. 2006;47:2130-9.
78. The Task Force on Myocardial Revascularization of the European Society of Cardiology (ESC) and the European Association for Cardio-Thoracic Surgery (EACTS); European Association for Percutaneous Cardiovascular Interventions (EAPCI); Wijns W, Kolh P, Danchin N, et al. Guidelines on myocardial revascularization. Eur Heart J. 2010;31:2501-55.
79. Migliorini A, Valenti R, Marcucci R, et al. High residual platelet reactivity after clopidogrel loading and long-term clinical outcome after drug-eluting stenting for unprotected left main coronary disease. Circulation. 2009;120:2214-21.
80. Moussa ID, Colombo A. Tips and Tricks in Interventional Therapy of Coronary Bifurcation Lesions, 1st edition. London: Informa Healthcare; 2010. p. 135.

33

Cardiomyopathies: Revisit Beyond 2013

Nishith Chandra, Nishant Kumar

INTRODUCTION

Heart muscle disease have a notable and evolving history, by mid-18th century the only recognized form of heart muscle disease was chronic myocarditis and in early 19th century the term primary myocardial disease was used introduced. The term "cardiomyopathy" was introduced first in 1957. Cardiomyopathies represent a heterogeneous group of diseases that cause mechanical and/or electrical dysfunction that are due to ventricular hypertropohy or dilation, the cause of this are frequently genetic. They are either confined to the heart or a part of systemic disorder. It can be divided into two major groups based on predominant organ involvement:

1. Primary (genetic, nongenetic, acquired) are those solely or predominantly confined to heart muscle and are relatively few in number (Flow chart 33.1).
2. Secondary show pathological myocardial involvement as part of a large number and variety of generalized systemic (multiorgan) disorders.

HYPERTROPHIC CARDIOMYOPATHY

Hypertrophic cardiomyopathy (HCM) is defined by the presence of myocardial hypertrophy unexplained by loading conditions, primary due to genetic disorder caused by mutation in sarcomere protein gene.[1]

Conventional diagnostic tools [electrocardiogram (ECG), two-dimensional echocardiogram (2D echo)] have undergone substantial refinement over the last decade but overall sensitivity remained low, newer imaging techniques such as 3D echo deformation, cardiac magnetic resonance imaging (CMR) have changed the scenario. The ability of CMR (Figs 33.1A to F) to detect the "invisible" myocardial segment to 2D echo (posterior septum and apex) and the ability to image scar by late gadolinium enhancement (LGE).

Premature sudden cardiac death and/or decades of poor health due to worsening heart failure symptoms have afflicted many with HCM for decade, the current state of art management focuses on:

- Individuals who are at high risk for sudden cardiac death
- Left ventricular outflow tract (LVOT) obstruction reduction
- Providing better management for systolic and diastolic dysfunction.

Despite advancement in few area the treatment however remains suboptimal, role of septal myectomy and septal alcohol ablation for reduction of LVOT obstruction reduction have been studied by various meta-analysis,[2-5] which have shown alcohol septal ablation is associated with broadly similar mortality rates and improvement in functional status compared to surgical treatment but with higher risk for permanent pacemaker implantation, higher post-intervention gradient and few showing higher death rates, raising safety concerns for the procedure.[3] Radiofrequency ablation and dual chamber atrioventricular (RV) sequential pacing for reduction of outflow tract reduction is been looked as alternative method.[6-8] Invasive treatment of LV outflow obstruction is recommended only in patients with drug-refractory symptoms.

The role of Perhexiline, an inhibitor of mitochondrial fatty acid uptake is begin studied as it has been hypothesized and the excessive sarcomeric energy consumption is the important pathophysiology of HCM and other heart muscle disease.[9] The drug has shown improved exercise capacity and diastolic functions in symptomatic patients with nonobstructive HCM.[10]

Arrhythmogenic Right Ventricular Cardiomyopathy

Arrhythmogenic right ventricular cardiomyopathy (ARVC) is an autosomal dominant trait with incomplete penetrance characterized histologically by cardiomyocyte loss and replacement by fibrous or fibrofatty tissue, causing fatal

Flow chart 33.1 Classification of cardiomyopathies

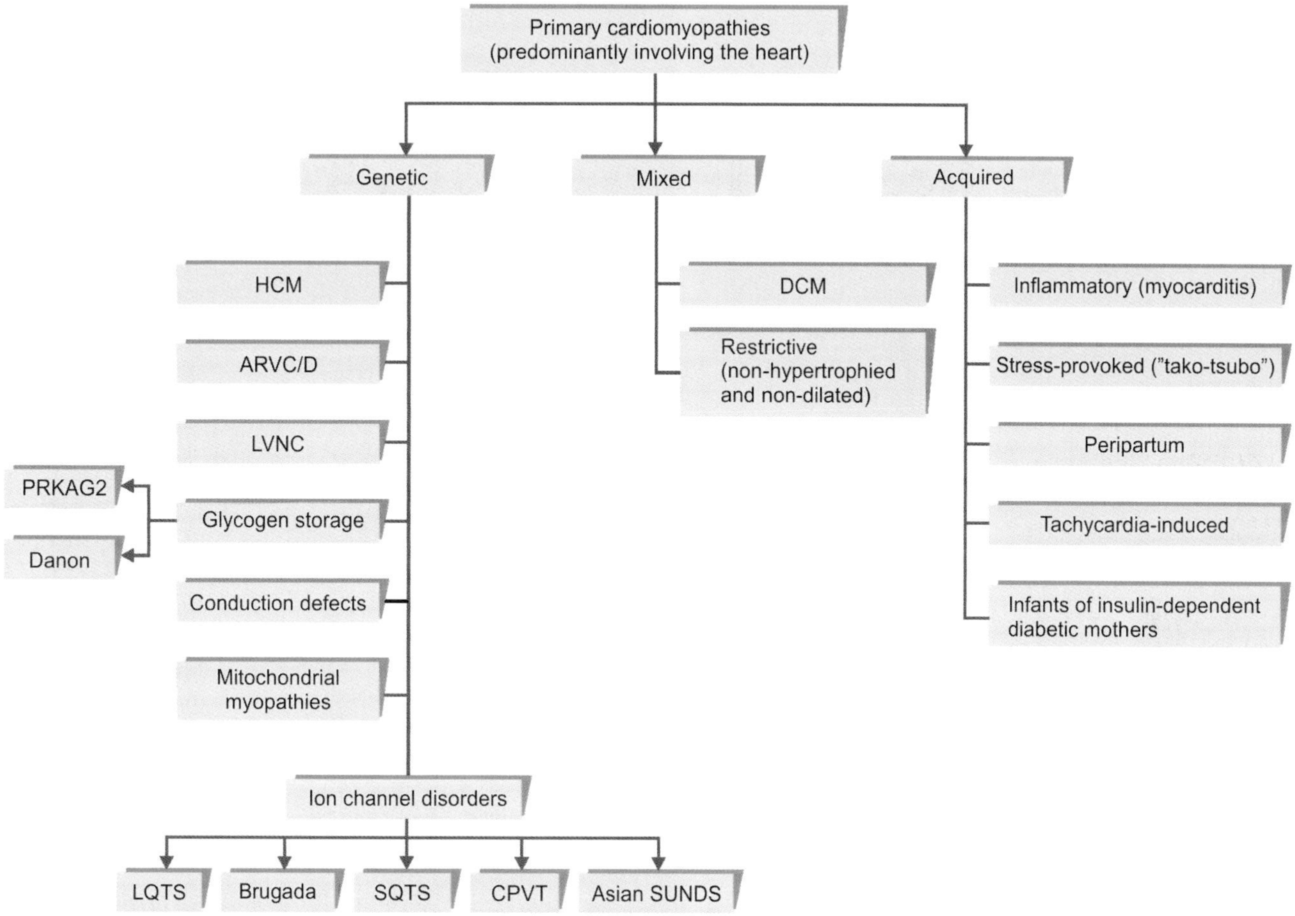

- Primary cardiomyopathies (predominantly involving the heart)
  - Genetic
    - HCM
    - ARVC/D
    - LVNC
    - Glycogen storage
      - PRKAG2
      - Danon
    - Conduction defects
    - Mitochondrial myopathies
    - Ion channel disorders
      - LQTS
      - Brugada
      - SQTS
      - CPVT
      - Asian SUNDS
  - Mixed
    - DCM
    - Restrictive (non-hypertrophied and non-dilated)
  - Acquired
    - Inflammatory (myocarditis)
    - Stress-provoked ("tako-tsubo")
    - Peripartum
    - Tachycardia-induced
    - Infants of insulin-dependent diabetic mothers

Abbreviations: HCM, hypertrophic cardiomyopathy; ARVC, arrhythmogenic right ventricular cardiomyopathy; LVNC, left ventricular non-compaction cardiomyopathy; DCM, dilated cardiomyopathy; SUNDS, sudden unexplained nocturnal death syndrome; LQTS, long QT syndrome; SQTS, short QT syndrome; CPVT, catecholaminergic polymorphic ventricular tachycardia.

arrhythmia, sudden cardiac death, and symptoms of heart failure caused by mutation in the gene encoding for components of intercalated disk of cardiomyocytes.[11] Familial cases are caused by heterozygous mutations in genes encoding desmosomal proteins, in majority of cases but other genes have been implicated, transforming growth factor β3 and transmembrane protein 43 (TMEM43), a cytoplasmic membrane protein.[11-13]

Recent evidence of gene heterogeneity has been demonstrated by the discovery of pathogenic mutations in desmin, an intermediate filament protein, and titin.[14-16]

Studies continue to report complex genetic status in many patients with multiple variants in different desmosomal genes.[17] The presence of multiple mutations appears to increase the severity of the clinical phenotype, and possessing a challenge for the interpretation of genetic testing, particularly with regard to variant in normal populations which do not cause disease, but might alter disease susceptibility in the presence of other genetic or environmental factors. Diagnosis is often difficult and requiring data of sudden cardiac death among family members, genetic testing, ECG and imaging techniques, have been used to study the various manifestation of the histological phenotype.[18-20]

It is recommend that (ICD) implantation to be done in patients with ARVC who have documented ventricular tachycardia or ventricular fibrillation, on optimal medical therapy and with life expectancy with good functional status more than 1 year. Recommendations in patients without these features are necessarily more speculative. The study by Corrado and colleagues published a study on 106 consecutive patients with ARVC who received an ICD based on one or more arrhythmic risk factors, such as syncope, nonsustained VT, familial sudden death and inducibility at programmed ventricular stimulation. During follow-up, 24% of patients had appropriate ICD interventions, 17 of which (16%) were for ventricular flutter (VF). All patients survived to 48 months. Syncope was the most important predictor of ICD

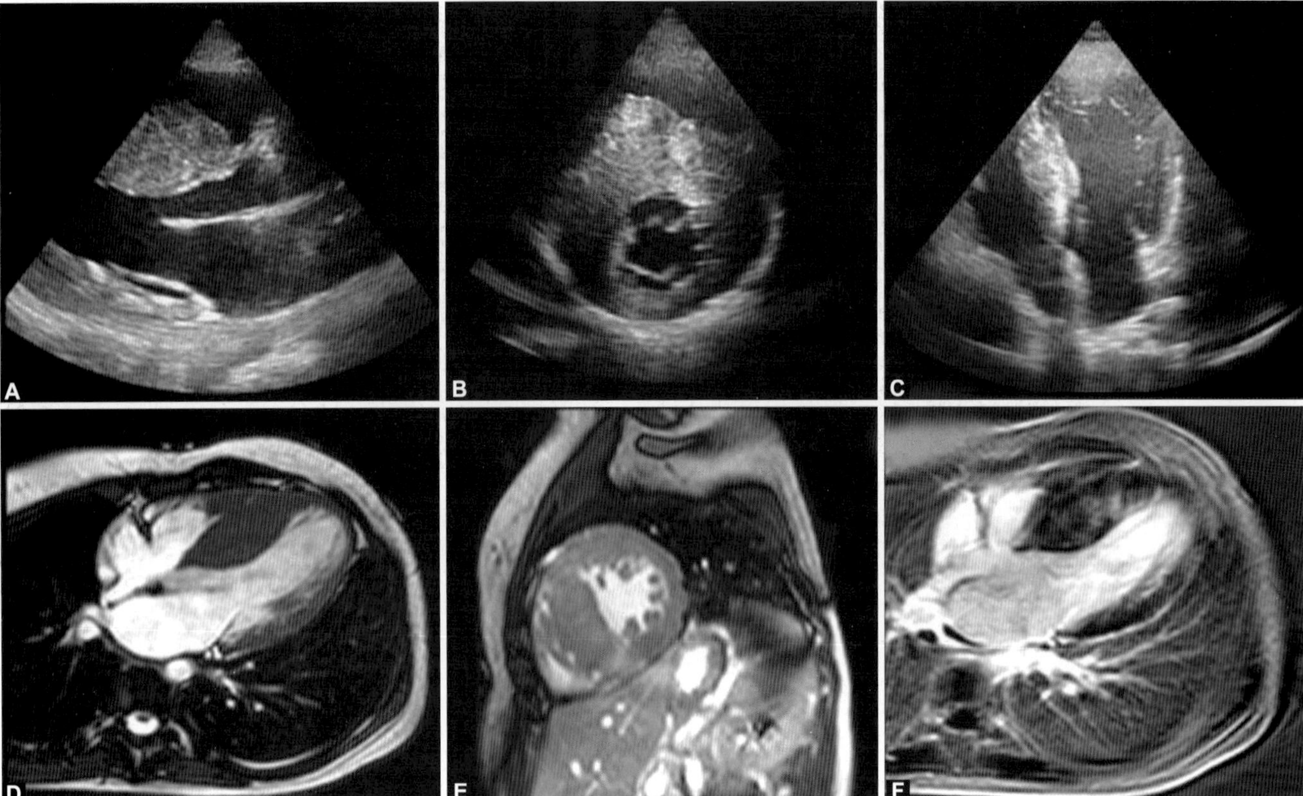

Figs 33.1A to F Echocardiographic and cardiac magnetic resonance images from a patient with hypertrophic cardiomyopathy (HCM). Parasternal long and short axis views show severe left ventricular (LV) thickness values (maximum LV wall thickness—31 mm), with redundant mitral leaflets (A, B and D) and small cavity size. Apical 4 chambers view shows massive hypertrophy of the septum and the anterolateral wall (C and E). Image of late gadolinium enhancement showing limited and non-transmural area of fibrosis of the interventricular septum (IVS) (F)

intervention but programmed ventricular stimulation had a low accuracy for predicting ICD treatment. These data add to current advice for ICD implantation in symptomatic patients, but the issue of primary prevention in asymptomatic patients remains a question for the future.

DILATED CARDIOMYOPATHY

Dilated cardiomyopathy (DCM) is characterized by LV dilatation and systolic impairment in the absence of previous myocardial infarction. It may be genetics in the etiology or acquired. The identification of etiology is of paramount importance in sporadic cases (absence of affected family member) causative agent could be circumstantial (inflammatory, infective, toxins, heart rate induced or metabolic abnormalities). However, recent evidence genetic studies have challenged the accepted concept.[21]

Cardiac magnetic resonance (CMR) helps in tissue characterization and provides additional diagnostic, prognostic information and can easily differentiate between normal myocardium from edematous, fibrotic and infiltrated myocardium and can detect fatty change. In certain clinical situations, the profile, spatial distribution and temporal characteristics of tissue abnormalities, can distinguished between causes of cardiac damage.[22] Myocardial LGE though not specific are detected in one-third [23]of cases of DCM and are typically in mid-wall or subepicardial. Few recent studies suggest LGE may be a marker of diseases severity and has prognostic implication.[23,24] CMR play an important role in diagnosis in acute and chronic myocarditis and it progression to DCM and to development of heart failure[25,26] but its role as a prognostic tool need to be verified by larger studies.

The standard management is in line of symptomatic heart failure and device implantation for prevention of sudden cardiac death.

The indications for device therapy (both ICD and cardiac resynchronization therapy), major guidelines suggest slightly different criteria for non-ischemic than for ischemic heart failure that recognize on average, non-ischemic DCM may have a better prognosis.[27,28] Recent work

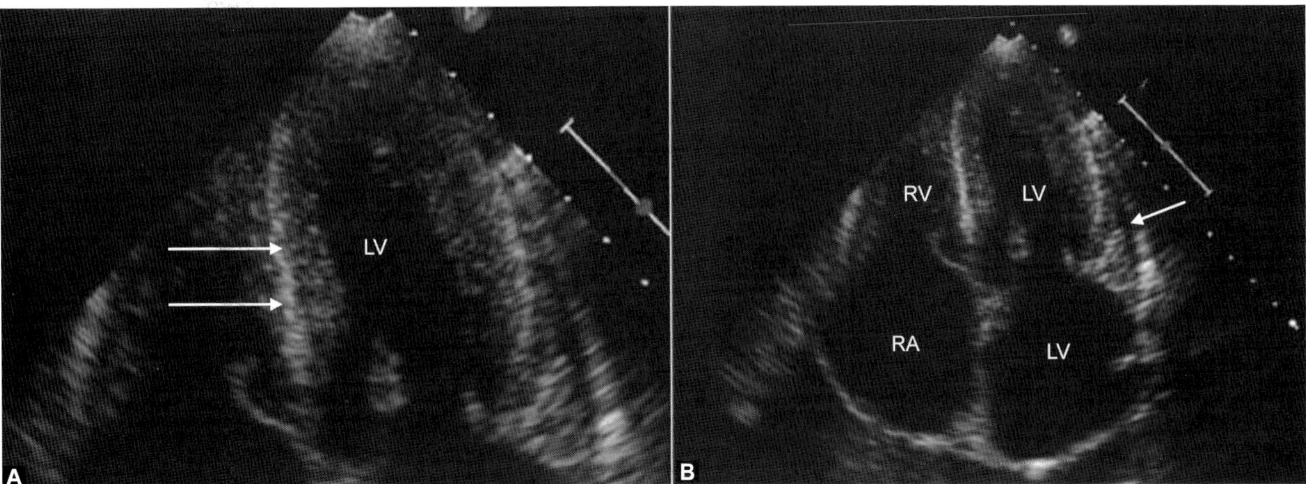

Figs 33.2A and B (A) Apical four chamber 2D echocardiogram in a patient with cardiac amyloid, showing thickened left ventricular walls with increased echogenicity (arrows); (B) Apical four chamber 2D echocardiogram in the same patient, showing left ventricular hypertrophy with enlarged atria and small pericardial effusion (arrow)

Abbreviations: LA, left atrium; LV, left ventricle; RA, right atrium; RV, right ventricle

by Millat et al.[29]demonstrated that nearly 10% of unrelated patients with DCM had mutations in LAMIN A/C, a cause of DCM associated with particularly high risks of ventricular arrhythmias and progressive conduction disease.[30] Recent publications describe the prognostic importance of functional mitral regurgitation, a feature of DCM related to LV geometry, contractility and dyssynchrony. Rossi et al. demonstrated, in nonischemic DCM, that functional mitral regurgitation is associated with doubling of a combined end point of all-cause mortality hospitalization and worsening heart failure.

INFILTRATIVE CARDIOMYOPATHY

It represents a wide spectrum of both inherited and acquired condition with varying systemic manifestation, with adverse prognosis. Cardiac amyloidosis remains the archetypal infiltrative cardiomyopathy.

Cardiac Amyloidosis

It is clinical disorder caused by extracellular deposition of insoluble abnormal fibrils derived from aggregation of misfolded, normally soluble protein.[31-33] There are about 20 different forms of amyloid fibril in vivo which share a pathognomonic ultrastructure. Various forms of amyloidosis in which the deposits are confined to specific organ or tissue. Cardiac amyloidosis involves the heart and echocardiography shows a wide spectrum of finding, the most common benign feature of increased thickness of LV wall particularly in absence of hypertension (Figs 33.2A and B). This is referred incorrectly as hypertrophy as the pathological process is infiltration not myocyte hypertrophy. This is very nonspecific feature and occurs commonly in various other diseases. However, the combination of increased LV mass in absence of high ECG voltage is more specific for infiltrative disease of which amyloid is more common (72% sensitivity and 91% specificity). 2D echo of the myocardium shows increased echogenicity of myocardium, particularly with a granular or a sparkling appearance .

The CMR using LGE has the ability to profile various forms of cardiomyopathy with high spatial resolution. In amyloidosis there is qualitative global and subendocardial gadolinium enhancement of myocardium (Figs 33.3A and B), subendocardial longitudinal relaxation time is shorter .The CMR hyperenchantment represents the interstitial expansion from amyloid infiltration.

The CMR in patients with no echocardiography, morphological changes of amyloid can be detected with high sensitivity if LGE proves to be a sensitive marker. Perugini et al. studied an Italian population with histologically proven systemic amyloidosis and echodiagnosis of cardiac involvement gadolinium enhancement was detected in 76% of patients, however the pattern of LGE was much variable, i.e. localized or diffuse, and subendocardial or transmural.

SARCOIDOSIS

It is a systemic disorder causing granulomatous infiltration of various organs. The involvement of heart produces a variety of echocardiographic abnormalities from regional motion wall abnormalities, regional thinning, aneurysms, systolic, diastolic dysfunction pulmonary hypertension and

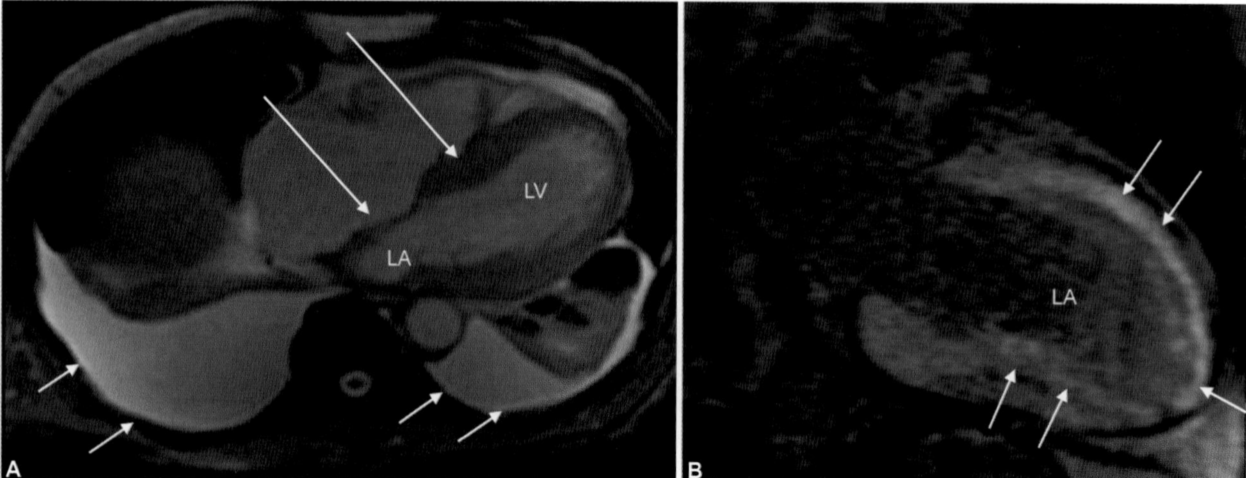

Figs 33.3A and B (A) Cardiovascular magnetic resonance (CMR) steady state free precession image in a horizontal long axis view demonstrating increased left ventricle (LV), atrial wall thickness (long arrows) and bilateral pleural effusions (small arrows), in a patient with cardiac amyloid (CA); (B) CMR late gadolinium imaging in vertical long axis view. There is global subendocardial hyperenhancement (arrows) in the LV and right ventricle, typical of CA

Abbreviation: LA, left atrium

pericardial effusion. Case reports have sarcoidosis mimicking coronary artery disease, takotsubo cardiomyopathy, right ventricular cardiomyopathy, HCM, and valvular dysfunction. Newer modalities of tissue Doppler and ultrasonic tissue characterization by myocardial integrated backscatter have demonstrated in absence abnormalities in absence of 2D echo feature. The use of thallium 201, which shows characteristic pattern of reverse redistribution in which resting perfusion defect improve on stress is helpful in differentiating from ischemic causes.

Its role as screening tool is of suspect as these findings are nonspecific. Gallium-67 scintigraphy has also been used to diagnose cardiac sarcoid as it accumulates in the presence of active inflammation. Hence, the absence of uptake may not exclude sarcoid involvement but suggests lack of active disease and has been shown to predict response to corticosteroid therapy.[34] (18)-F-fluoro-2-deoxyglucose positron emission tomography (FDG PET) has high diagnostic accuracy in the assessment of cardiac sarcoidosis. Langah et al., using FDG PET in 30 patients with systemic sarcoidosis and suspected cardiac sarcoidosis, showed a specificity of 90% and sensitivity of 85%.[35]

The CMR is useful in identifying even small areas of myocardial edema and fibrosis leading to postinflammatory scarring. Global, regional function and, LGE technique has been most widely evaluated in clinical studies using CMR. A study by Smedma and colleagues evaluated the utility of LGE in 58 patients with biopsy proven pulmonary sarcoidosis, 25% of whom also had symptoms suggestive of cardiac involvement. All patients underwent clinical assessment, 12-lead ECG, ambulatory ECG monitoring, transthoracic echocardiography, 201-thallium single photon emission CT (SPECT), and CMR (cine and LGE). The modified Japanese Ministry of Health and Welfare (JMHW) criteria were used as the gold standard. CMR revealed LGE, mostly involving the epicardium of the basal and lateral segments, in 73% of patients diagnosed with cardiac involvement by the Japanese criteria (Flow chart 33.2). In about half of these patients scintigraphy was normal, while patchy LGE was present, underlining the differences in spatial resolution. This study is limited in that only a minority of patients had correlation between LGE-CMR results and endomyocardial biopsy. Other studies have confirmed the predilection of LGE for the basal-lateral segments, although subendocardial or transmural hyperenhancement has been also observed, mimicking the ischemic pattern. Apart from LGE, both functional and anatomical ("white blood" and "black blood") CMR sequences can help in detecting cardiac sarcoid by demonstrating some of its characteristic features—septal thinning, LV/RV dilatation and systolic dysfunction, and pericardial effusion. T2 weighted sequences may also help in identifying myocardial edema.[36] CMR also identifies pulmonary features of sarcoid, such as enlarged hilar lymph nodes and lung fibrosis.

FABRY'S DISEASE[37-39]

X-linked occurs due to deficiency of alpha glactosidase deficiency leading to accumulation of glycosphingolipids in lysosomes of various cells and organ including the heart. It results in myocyte vacuolations, hypertrophy, and regional

Flow chart 33.2 Organization of family screening

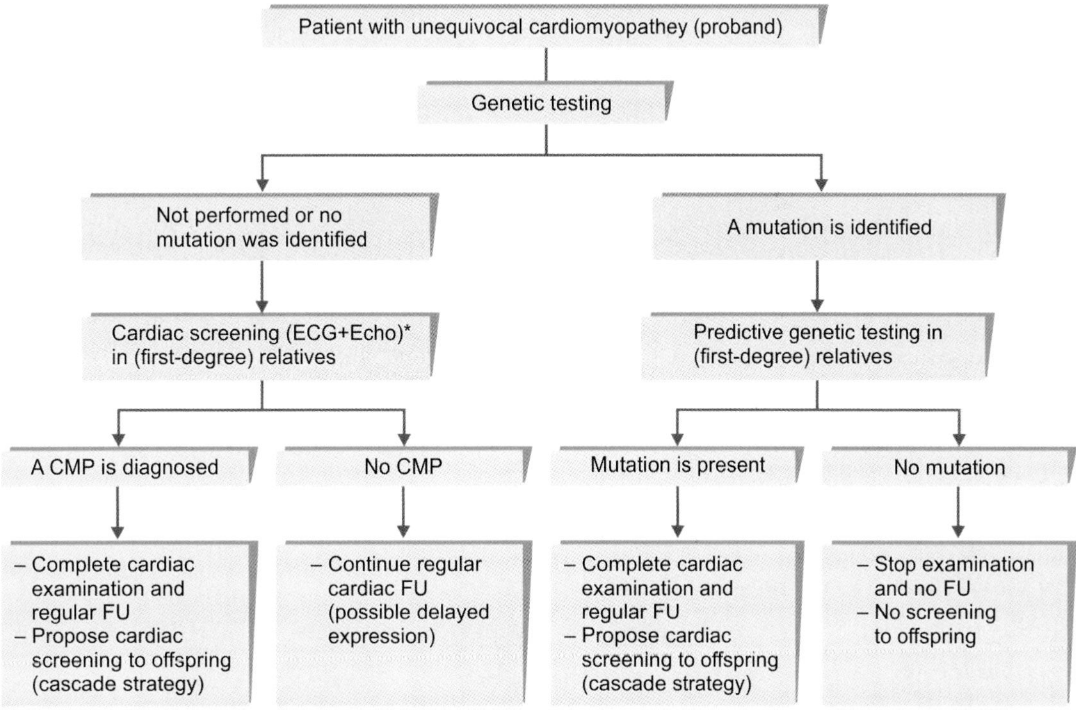

Asterisk (*) indicates additional cardiac examination in selected cardiomyopathies (i.e. Holter-ECG, SAECG, MRI, etc.)

Abbreviations: FU, follow-up; CMP, cardiomyopathy

fibrosis, which can leads to heart failure and conduction abnormality causing death. Fabry's disease is not rare as it was earlier thought a study revealed 6% of male patients diagnosed as HCM in fact had Fabry's disease on biochemical and genetic testing. 2D echo findings are typically concentric LVH with persevered systolic function and abnormal diastology without cavity dilatation.

Cardiac magnetic resonance (CMR) feature of the disease is sparse, however, Moon et al. reported LGE patterns in a unique distribution involving the basal inferolateral wall, sparing endocardium in 50% of the cases.[40]

Late gadolinium enhancement (LGE) in this respect represent interstitial expansion secondary to replacement fibrosis, although why this reason is favored is unclear.

The extent of fibrosis on LGE CMR determines the response to enzyme replacement therapy (ERT). A study by Weisemann and colleagues studied 41 patients over 3 years and found that patient without myocardial fibrosis ERT resulted in significant reduction in LV mass, and improvement in myocardial function or exercise capacity, than compared with patients with mild-to-severe fibrosis.[41,42]

Pronounced deposition of glycolipid in the myocardium leads to prolongation of myocardial T2 relaxation time. This has been suggested as useful marker of the disease in some patients, however, there is a wide overlap in myocardial T2 values of Fabry's disease patients when compared with patients with LVH from other causes.

ROLE OF GENETIC TEST

Background

The heterogeneous group of inherited cardiovascular disorder caused by genetic mutation has variable expression they include:

1. Hypertrophic, dilated, restrictive, arrhythmogenic and LV noncompaction cardiomyopathies.
2. *Ion channel diseases:* Long QT syndrome, short QT syndrome, Brugada syndrome, catecholaminergic polymorphic ventricular tachycardia, familial atrial fibrillation, and inherited conduction disorders.
3. *Aortopathies:* Marfan syndrome, Ehler Danlos syndrome type 4, Loeys-Dietz syndrome, and familial thoracic aortic aneurysms as well as familial pulmonary hypertension.

The concept of one gene one disease have been challenged by fact that a proportion of affected patients carry more than one mutation in the same or different and this effect the clinical expression or the severity of the disease.[43-46]

Determination of the pathogenicity of individual sequence variants can be challenging.[47] It is important to differentiate between the polymorphism and mutation the arbitrary cut off point begin 1% (the least common allele has the frequency in general population more than 1% to be polymorphic and less than 1% then it is a mutation).[48] Once the mutation is identified the aim is establish absence in healthy controls its cosegregation in affected families.[47]

The next step is identify type of mutation (frame-shift, nonsense, missense mutations, or ones that affect coding or noncoding regions—exons and introns) and the relevance of the protein affected domain and its conservation in different species and isoform (phylogenetic conservation).

The role of genetic testing is however limited to selected patients with certain type of cardiomyopathies, after detailed clinical and family assessment such as:[43,44]

- In ARVC for identification of genetic mutation.
- In atypical phenotypic feature (example enzyme replacement therapy in Anderson-Fabry disease, liver transplantation in transthyretin-related amyloidosis or early prophylactic defibrillator implantation in dilated cardiomyopathy caused by a lamin A/C gene mutation) where specific therapy is required.
- For patients and families with cardiomyopathy where an acquired cause cannot be demonstrated.

Genetic testing is not indicated in:

- To gain prognostic information
- Confirm the diagnosis
- Diagnose borderline or doubtful cardiomyopathy.

The reason for this being very few correlation between specific genotypes and outcome have been described, data are based on very small and usually retrospective cohorts with selected mutation.

Newer researches have proven:

- Association between mutations in the *TNNT2* gene and sudden death in patients with hypertrophic cardiomyopathy.[49]
- Risk of sudden cardiac death in patients with dilated cardiomyopathy is much higher in individuals carrying mutations in the lamin A/C gene.
- Patients with multiple mutations (especially in hypertrophic cardiomyopathy and arrhythmogenic cardiomyopathy) present with a more severe phenotype.

Role of Genetic Counseling and Testing

The Heart Failure Society of America, the European Society of Cardiology (ESC) and the Canadian Cardiovascular Society have suggested guidelines for genetic counseling and testing.[43-46] The ESC guidelines make recommendations to clinicians involved in genetic testing on many levels:

1. Information to give during genetic counseling in families with cardiomyopathies.
2. Protocol for clinical family screening when genetics is not available.
3. Protocol for clinical screening in asymptomatic relatives who carry a disease-causing mutation.

They also have recommendations regarding:

1. Positive diagnosis (as a complete analysis of potential genes of interest in the proband of a family).
2. Prognostic diagnosis.
3. Predictive testing.
4. Prenatal diagnosis, interpretation, and organization of genetic counseling.

Cardiologists should be proactive in referring patients to specialized inherited cardiovascular conditions or cardiomyopathy clinics for genetic testing, where a multidisciplinary team of physicians, geneticists, genetic counselors, and laboratory scientists will collaborate in the delivery of the clinical service. By this genotyping method, it is possible to analyze a very large number of genes simultaneously and even the entire genome quickly and at a reasonable cost.

REFERENCES

1. Hagege AA, Caudron E, Damy T, Roudaut R, Millaire A, Etchecopar-Chevreuil C, et al. Screening patients with hypertrophic cardiomyopathy for fabry disease using a filter-paper test: the focus study. Heart. 2011;97:131-6.
2. Agarwal S, Tuzcu EM, Desai MY, Smedira N, Lever HM, Lytle BW, et al. Updated meta-analysis of septal alcohol ablation versus myectomy for hypertrophic cardiomyopathy. J Am Coll Cardiol. 2010;55:823-34.
3. Ten Cate FJ, Soliman OI, Michels M, Theuns DA, de Jong PL, Geleijnse ML, et al. Long-term outcome of alcohol septal ablation in patients with obstructive hypertrophic cardiomyopathy: a word of caution. Circ Heart Fail. 2010;3:362-9.
4. Nishimura RA, Ommen SR. Septal reduction therapy for obstructive hypertrophic cardiomyopathy and sudden death: what statistics cannot tell you. Circ Cardiovasc Interv. 2010;3:91-3.
5. Leonardi RA, Kransdorf EP, Simel DL, Wang A. Meta-analyses of septal reduction therapies for obstructive hypertrophic cardiomyopathy: comparative rates of overall mortality and sudden cardiac death after treatment. Circ Cardiovasc Interv. 2010;3:97-104.
6. Lawrenz T, Borchert B, Leuner C, Bartelsmeier M, Reinhardt J, Strunk-Mueller C, et al. Endocardial radiofrequency ablation for hypertrophic obstructive cardiomyopathy: acute results and 6 months' follow-up in 19 patients. J Am Coll Cardiol. 2011;57:572-6.
7. Galve E, Sambola A, Saldana G, Quispe I, Nieto E, Diaz A, et al. Late benefits of dual-chamber pacing in obstructive hypertrophic cardiomyopathy: a 10-year follow-up study. Heart. 2010;96:352-6.
8. Mohiddin SA, Page SP. Long-term benefits of pacing in obstructive hypertrophic cardiomyopathy. Heart. 2010;96:328-30.
9. Gao D, Ning N, Niu X, Hao G, Meng Z. Trimetazidine: a meta-analysis of randomised controlled trials in heart failure. Heart. 2011;97:278-86.

10. Abozguia K, Elliott P, McKenna W, Phan TT, Nallur-Shivu G, Ahmed I, et al. Metabolic modulator perhexiline corrects energy deficiency and improves exercise capacity in symptomatic hypertrophic cardiomyopathy. Circulation. 2010;122:1562-9.
11. Corrado D, Basso C, Pilichou K, Thiene G, et al. Molecular biology and clinical management of arrhythmogenic right ventricular cardiomyopathy/dysplasia. Heart. 2011;97:530-9.
12. Marcus FI, McKenna WJ, Sherrill D, Basso C, Bauce B, Bluemke DA, et al. Diagnosis of arrhythmogenic right ventricular cardiomyopathy/dysplasia: proposed modification of the task force criteria. Eur Heart J. 2010;31:806-14.
13. Fressart V, Duthoit G, Donal E, Probst V, Deharo JC, Chevalier P, et al. Desmosomal gene analysis in arrhythmogenic right ventricular dysplasia/cardiomyopathy: spectrum of mutations and clinical impact in practice. Europace. 2010;12:861-8.
14. Otten E, Asimaki A, Maass A, van Langen IM, van der Wal A, de Jonge N, et al. Desmin mutations as a cause of right ventricular heart failure affect the intercalated disks. Heart Rhythm. 2010;7:1058-64.
15. Klauke B, Kossmann S, Gaertner A, Brand K, Stork I, Brodehl A, et al. De novo desmin-mutation n116s is associated with arrhythmogenic right ventricular cardiomyopathy. Hum Mol Genet. 2010;19:4595-607.
16. Taylor M, Graw S, Sinagra G, Barnes C, Slavov D, Brun F, et al. Genetic variation in titin in arrhythmogenic right ventricular cardiomyopathy-overlap syndromes. Circulation. 2011;124: 876-85.
17. Kapplinger JD, Landstrom AP, Salisbury BA, Callis TE, Pollevick GD, Tester DJ, et al. Distinguishing arrhythmogenic right ventricular cardiomyopathy/dysplasia-associated mutations from background genetic noise. J Am Coll Cardiol. 2011;57:2317-27.
18. Cox MG, van der Zwaag PA, van der Werf C, van der Smagt JJ, Noorman M, Bhuiyan ZA, et al. Arrhythmogenic right ventricular dysplasia/cardiomyopathy: pathogenic desmosome mutations in index-patients predict outcome of family screening: Dutch arrhythmogenic right ventricular dysplasia/cardiomyopathy genotype-phenotype follow-up study. Circulation. 2011;123: 2690-700.
19. La Gerche A, Robberecht C, Kuiperi C, Nuyens D, Willems R, de Ravel T, et al. Lower than expected desmosomal gene mutation prevalence in endurance athletes with complex ventricular arrhythmias of right ventricular origin. Heart. 2010;96:1268-74.
20. Quarta G, Ward D, Tome Esteban MT, Pantazis A, Elliott PM, Volpe M, et al. Dynamic electrocardiographic changes in patients with arrhythmogenic right ventricular cardiomyopathy. Heart. 2010;96:516-22.
21. Hoedemaekers YM, Caliskan K, Michels M, Frohn-Mulder I, van der Smagt JJ, Phefferkorn JE, et al. The importance of genetic counseling, DNA diagnostics, and cardiologic family screening in left ventricular noncompaction cardiomyopathy. Circ Cardiovasc Genet. 2010;3:232-9.
22. Friedrich MG, Sechtem U, Schulz-Menger J, Holmvang G, Alakija P, Cooper LT, et al. Cardiovascular magnetic resonance in myocarditis: a JACC white paper. J Am Coll Cardiol. 2009;53:1475-87.
23. Assomull RG, Prasad SK, Lyne J, Smith G, Burman ED, Khan M, et al. Cardiovascular magnetic resonance, fibrosis, and prognosis in dilated cardiomyopathy. J Am Coll Cardiol. 2006;48:1977-85.
24. Alter P, Rupp H, Adams P, Stoll F, Figiel JH, Klose KJ, et al. Occurrence of late gadolinium enhancement is associated with increased left ventricular wall stress and mass in patients with non-ischaemic dilated cardiomyopathy. Eur J Heart Fail. 2011;13:937-44.
25. Monney PA, Sekhri N, Burchell T, Knight C, Davies C, Deaner A, et al. Acute myocarditis presenting as acute coronary syndrome: role of early cardiac magnetic resonance in its diagnosis. Heart. 2010;97:1312-18.
26. Leurent G, Langella B, Fougerou C, Lentz PA, Larralde A, Bedossa M, et al. Diagnostic contributions of cardiac magnetic resonance imaging in patients presenting with elevated troponin, acute chest pain syndrome and unobstructed coronary arteries. Arch Cardiovasc Dis. 2011;104:161-70.
27. Dickstein K, Vardas PE, Auricchio A, Daubert JC, Linde C, McMurray J, et al. 2010 focused update of esc guidelines on device therapy in heart failure: an update of the 2008 esc guidelines for the diagnosis and treatment of acute and chronic heart failure and the 2007 esc guidelines for cardiac and resynchronization therapy. Developed with the special contribution of the heart failure association and the European heart rhythm association. Eur Heart J. 2010;31:2677-87.
28. Verma A, Wulffhart Z, Lakkireddy D, Khaykin Y, Kaplan A, Sarak B, et al. Incidence of left ventricular function improvement after primary prevention icd implantation for non-ischaemic dilated cardiomyopathy: a multicentre experience. Heart. 2010;96:510-15.
29. Millat G, Bouvagnet P, Chevalier P, Sebbag L, Dulac A, Dauphin C, et al. Clinical and mutational spectrum in a cohort of 105 unrelated patients with dilated cardiomyopathy. Eur J Med Genet. 2011;54:e570-5.
30. Meune C, Van Berlo JH, Anselme F, Bonne G, Pinto YM, Duboc D. Primary prevention of sudden death in patients with lamin a/c gene mutations. N Engl J Med. 2006;354:209-10.
31. Merlini G, Westermark P. The systemic amyloidoses: clearer understanding of the molecular mechanisms offers hope for more effective therapies. J Intern Med. 2004;255:159-78.
32. Selkoe DJ. Folding proteins in fatal ways. Nature. 2003;426:900-4.
33. Selvanayagam JB, Hawkins PN, Paul B, Myerson SG, Neubauer S. Evaluation and management of the cardiac amyloidosis. J Am Coll Cardiol. 2007;50:2101-10.
34. Ishimaru S, Tsujino I, Takei T, Tsukamoto E, Sakaue S, Kamigaki M, et al. Focal uptake on 18F-fluoro-2-deoxyglucose positron emission tomography images indicates cardiac involvement of sarcoidosis. Eur Heart J. 2005;26:1538-43.
35. Langah R, Spicer K, Gebregziabher M, Gordon L. Effectiveness of prolonged fasting 18f-FDG PET-CT in the detection of cardiac sarcoidosis. J Nucl Cardiol. 2009;16:801-10.
36. Vignaux O, Dhote R, Duboc D, Blanche P, Dusser D, Weber S, et al. Clinical significance of myocardial magnetic resonance abnormalities in patients with sarcoidosis: a 1-year follow-up study. Chest. 2002;122:1895-901.
37. Kampmann C, Baehner F, Whybra C, Martin C, Wiethoff CM, Ries M, et al. Cardiac manifestations of Anderson-Fabry disease in heterozygous females. J Am Coll Cardiol. 2002;40:1668-74.
38. Chimenti C, Pieroni M, Morgante E, Antuzzi D, Russo A, Russo MA, et al. Prevalence of Fabry disease in female patients with late-onset hypertrophic cardiomyopathy. Circulation. 2004;110:1047-53.
39. Funabashi N, Toyozaki T, Matsumoto Y, Yonezawa M, Yanagawa N, Yoshida K, et al. Images in cardiovascular medicine. Myocardial fibrosis in Fabry disease demonstrated by multislice computed tomography: comparison with biopsy findings. Circulation. 2003;107:2519-20.

40. Moon JC, Sachdev B, Elkington AG, McKenna WJ, Mehta A, Pennell DJ, et al. Gadolinium enhanced cardiovascular magnetic resonance in Anderson-Fabry disease. Evidence for a disease specific abnormality of the myocardial interstitium. Eur Heart J. 2003;24:2151-5.
41. Imbriaco M, Spinelli L, Cuocolo A, Maurea S, Sica G, Quarantelli M, et al. MRI characterization of myocardial tissue in patients with Fabry's disease. Am J Roentgenol. 2007;188:850-3.
42. Weidemann F, Niemann M, Breunig F, Herrmann S, Beer M, Störk S, et al. Long-term effects of enzyme replacement therapy on Fabry cardiomyopathy: evidence for a better outcome with early treatment. Circulation. 2009;119:524-9.
43. Charron P, Arad M, Arbustini E, Basso C, Bilinska Z, Elliott P, et al. European Society of Cardiology Working Group on Myocardial and Pericardial Diseases. Genetic counselling and testing in cardiomyopathies: a position statement of the European Society of Cardiology Working Group on Myocardial and Pericardial Diseases. Eur Heart J. 2010;31:2715-26.
44. Hershberger RE, Lindenfeld J, Mestroni L, Seidman CE, Taylor MR, Towbin JA. Genetic evaluation of cardiomyopathy--a Heart Failure Society of America practice guideline. Heart Failure Society of America. J Card Fail. 2009;15:83-97.
45. Ingles J, Zodgekar PR, Yeates L, Macciocca I, Semsarian C, Fatkin D; CSANZ Cardiac Genetic Diseases Council Writing Group. Guidelines for genetic testing of inherited cardiac disorders. Cardiac Genetic Diseases Council Writing Group. Heart Lung Circ. 2011;20:681-7.
46. Ackerman MJ, Priori SG, Willems S, Berul C, Brugada R, Calkins H, et al. HRS/EHRA expert consensus statement on the state of genetic testing for the channelopathies and cardiomyopathies this document was developed as a partnership between the Heart Rhythm Society (HRS) and the European Heart Rhythm Association (EHRA). Heart Rhythm. 2011;8:1308-39.
47. Monserrat L, Mazzanti A, Ortiz-Genga M, Barriales-Villa R, Garcia-Giustiniani D, Gimeno-Blanes JR. The interpretation of genetic tests in inherited cardiovascular diseases. Cardiogenetics. 2011;1:e8.
48. Ingles J, McGaughran J, Scuffham PA, Atherton J, Semsarian C. A cost-effectiveness model of genetic testing for the evaluation of families with hypertrophic cardiomyopathy. Heart. 2012;98: 625-30.
49. Wordsworth S, Leal J, Blair E, Legood R, Thomson K, Seller A, et al. DNA testing for hypertrophic cardiomyopathy: a cost-effectiveness model. Eur Heart J. 2010;31:926-35.

34

Cardiac Tumors: A Story of Unbridled Excitement!

Biswajit Paul

INTRODUCTION

The excitement that engulfs an echo lab after a chance discovery of a cardiac mass would require skills of Tagore to describe in words. While the operator keeps viewing the mass in different planes with awe, amusement, or disbelief, the rest of the members ponder over several critical questions. Is this a vegetation or tumor or thrombus? If it is a tumor, is it primary or secondary? What next? Some smart fellows would open a textbook to come out with a superlative diagnosis. But therein lies the problem! Most books start with a classification on cardiac tumors, symptomatology and its causes, genetics to the very core, and then goes on to describe each primary tumor in detail to finally conclude with a few lines on treatment. Reading the chapter again and again hardly provides any clue to our awestruck, amused, or smart cardiologists. The reason is simple; books do not describe the clinical approach step by step nor do the review articles in journals that sometimes are discussed by pathologists. There are certain issues that need to be addressed by every cardiologist. For example, a physician who may have missed a diagnosis of cardiac tumor is justified in asking "when do I suspect cardiac tumors!" As cardiologists most of us have never thought about this question. The newer imaging techniques such as computed tomography (CT) and magnetic resonance imaging (MRI) offer a lot more than what is assumed. Why do we need to make a specific diagnosis if surgical removal is available as a form of treatment? What precautions need to be taken in follow-up visits? There are several small issues that need emphasis not because they are not known, but because they have lost relevance as "just surgical cases...referred to cardiac surgeons."

Cardiac tumors are extremely uncommon. Primary tumors have a necropsy incidence of 0.001–0.03%, while secondary tumors are seen in 1% of postmortem examinations.[1] This brings us to a relevant question "what are rare diseases and what its implications are?" In the United States, the "Rare Diseases Act of 2002" is based strictly according to prevalence of "any disease or condition that affects <2,00,000 persons in the United States" or about 1/5000 people. The European Commission on Public Health incorporates two important elements: (1) life-threatening or chronically debilitating disease and (2) low prevalence that is <1/2000 people. The legal definition in Japan is one that affects <50,000 people that is approximately 1/2500 people. The implications of "rare diseases" are many but suffice it to say that because of insufficient numbers, large-scale randomized studies are not possible and data in literature in the form of case studies are not truly representative of the population. This means standard guidelines are unavailable with regard to diagnosis and treatment of cardiac tumors.

This chapter highlights the issues that everyday are confronted by cardiologists as either a "bolt from the blue" or "surgical cases seeking cardiologists" opinion with regard to future course of action.

CASE VIGNETTE

A 64 years old Afghan woman was referred with the diagnosis of right atrial myxoma. Detailed clinical history revealed fever of over 3 months duration for which she was treated on the lines of urinary tract infection, malaria, pneumonitis, pulmonary tuberculosis, and pyrexia of unknown origin. She had a bout of palpitation that reverted after a while and the electrocardiogram (ECG) done as expected was normal. The next day she had another bout of palpitation and was rushed to the local clinic and this time the ECG showed the rhythm to be atrial fibrillation before reverting spontaneously. Subsequently echocardiography showed a mass in right atrium (RA) that was diagnosed as a "massive cardiac Myxoma." Echo was repeated in our institute that showed a large mass in inferior vena cava growing into the RA and across the tricuspid valve in the right ventricle. Further scanning showed the mass extending down into the left renal vein and an unusually enlarged and distorted left kidney.

The diagnosis of hypernephroma was made and further corroborated by contrast CT (Figs 34.1A and B).

WHEN TO SUSPECT CARDIAC TUMORS

Cardiac tumors have diverse clinical presentation and have been likened to the sea god "proteus" and hence said to have protean manifestations. Understanding the clinical features is likely to provide clues with regard to our problem. Certain features are common to all cardiac tumors:

1. *Systemic manifestations:* A number of systemic symptoms and signs are observed with cardiac tumors and notably with cardiac myxomas believed to be caused by interleukin-6 (IL-6) and other secretary products released by the tumor mass or as a result of tumor necrosis. These include fever, chills, malaise, weight loss, myalgia, arthralgia, and Raynaud phenomenon. These symptoms may mimic vasculitides and connective tissue diseases. Routine laboratory tests may reveal anemia, leukocytosis, leukopenia, polycythemia, thrombocytopenia, thrombocytosis, hypergammaglobulinemia, and increased ESR.
2. *Embolization:* There may be dislodgement of tumor or adherent thrombus that may lead to cerebrovascular events or may mimic vasculitis or endocarditis. Perceivably right-sided tumors would produce pleuritic symptoms or present with features of pulmonary embolism.
3. *Obstruction:* Tumors depending on their site of origin may produce obstruction of atrioventricular valves or semilunar valves. Hence, the clinical features are suggestive of valvular heart disease. Not surprisingly the symptoms and signs are position dependent as the mobile tumor mass is likely to assume several different positions. It is not uncommon to find a clinical diagnosis of mitral stenosis with its attendant opening snap (tumor plop!) and mid-diastolic murmur going all wrong the next

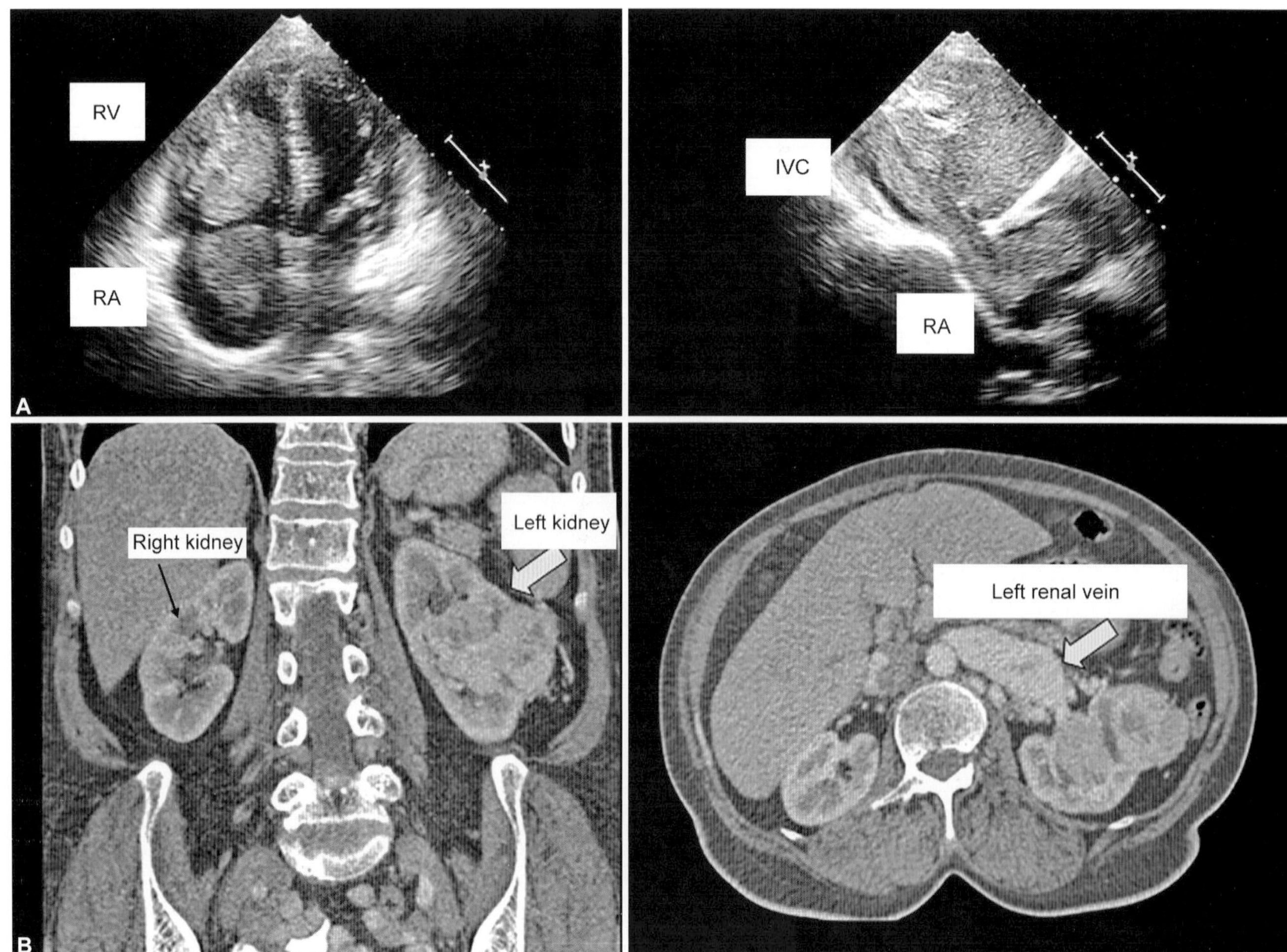

Figs 34.1A and B (A) Echocardiography shows a large mass, which is seen in right atrium and right ventricle in four-chamber view. The extension of the tumor mass seen in inferior vena cava in subcostal view. (B) Computed tomography shows an abnormally enlarged left kidney infiltrated by tumor (hypernephroma) and a dilated left renal vein with metastases

day when the prolapsing myxoma may have changed its position.

4. *Arrhythmias:* Tumors by means of direct infiltration of the conduction tissue or by irritating the myocardium may affect cardiac rhythm. This may range from bradycardia to complete heart blocks; or paroxysmal atrial fibrillation (as highlighted in our index case) to ventricular tachycardia.

It is therefore apparent that in our index case the patient was treated for so many different conditions till the time she manifested with palpitations. The numbers of differential diagnosis that may be assumed with manifestations of cardiac tumors are beyond the scope of this chapter. Therefore, arriving at the diagnosis would require views that are different and perhaps contradictory to the standard laws of clinical medicine. Remember that cardiac tumors are not only rare but unique! Such an entity cannot be expected to be diagnosed by the common logic "try to explain all symptoms with a single disease rather than multiple." Therefore, it may be said that when symptoms point to two different diseases or there is a reluctance for the diagnosed diseased to get cured think of cardiac tumors. For example, a tumor owing to multiple emboli may produce features of neurogenic nature along with polycythemia. In such cases, a differential diagnosis of cardiac tumors may not only be face saving but also be life saving!

APPROACH TO CARDIAC TUMORS: THE IFs AND BUTs!

The one important issue that comes to mind on discovering a cardiac tumor is "what next!" This is best highlighted in our index case where the cardiologist on discovering a large mass in the RA and RV did not stop to make a diagnosis but went on to study the entire extent of the tumor. It is not surprising that the initial mistaken diagnosis of "a massive cardiac myxoma" was made purely on the basis of the mass in RA and RV. It is important to study not only the entire extent of the mass in various views and planes but also other features. Whether it is homogeneous or heterogeneous? Is it cystic or solid? Does it suggest calcification? In our case, echo scanning did not stop at the level of the heart, but went on to scan the inferior vena cava, renal veins, and the kidneys as well! One may further confirm the findings by requesting an ultrasonologist (if needed) or supplement with another form of imaging such as CT scan as done in this case. But on no occasion should one quit echo scanning beyond the heart as transgression of territories is an accepted norm in the war arena!

Once a provisional diagnosis is made, a definitive tissue diagnosis is required. Now in our index case we have a large tumor burden. Should we treat the primary tumor and expect the secondary to resolve or remove the entire mass? Leaving the cardiac metastasis is fraught with danger of cardiac complications and ideally both the cardiac mass (inferior vena cava mass inclusive) and renal mass should be surgically removed in the same sitting. Later the subject may be taken up for chemotherapy and radiotherapy under the guidance of an oncologist. The value of an experienced cardiologist in such scenarios obviates unnecessary delay to treatment.

But all cases will not carry the clarity as our index case. There would be situations where arriving at a provisional diagnosis is difficult. For example, an incidentally diagnosed homogeneous mass in the ventricular wall in an asymptomatic individual needs attention. Sometimes even MRI fails to arrive at a diagnosis. Therefore, serial follow-up of a cardiac tumor is warranted in such cases to watch out for a progressive increase in size or onset of symptoms. Then there are myxomas that are found in the left atrial appendage and are likely to be mistaken for thrombus. In such cases, failure of appropriately instituted anticoagulation therapy requires surgical removal followed by pathological confirmation of the diagnosis. Some tumors such as myxomas are notorious as they are known to recur. The hazard of recurrence increases linearly for 4 years after resection. But after 4 years, the risk of recurrence is low. Hence, semiannual echocardiographic follow-up has been recommended 4 years after surgery.

A FEW WORDS ON IMAGING MODALITIES

The primary modality for imaging cardiac masses is echocardiography. It provides high-resolution, real-time images, whose quality has further improved with three-dimensional imaging. The newer modalities such as CT and MRI have made convincing inroads with faster image acquisition.[2] Nevertheless the spatial and temporal resolution is far lower with these modalities than with echocardiography. However, both CT and MRI are superior to that of echocardiography in terms of soft-tissue contrast, imaging the entire mediastinum and evaluation of extracardiac extent of disease. CT is able to detect calcium, besides easier operability and ease of procedure as compared to MRI. However, MRI has better soft-tissue contrast than CT and allows more flexibility in selection of imaging planes.

SECONDARY CARDIAC TUMORS

The cardiac tumors have been classified into primary and secondary as in all other tumor classification (Flow chart 34.1 and Table 34.1). This has been done to separately discuss the features of both as they are largely different with respect to their pathology, clinical presentation, and treatment. It needs to be mentioned that primary malignant cardiac tumors with metastases elsewhere are extremely rare.[3] In fact the malignant cardiac tumors constitute only 25% of cardiac tumors. As previously discussed, the metastatic deposits to heart are 20–30 times more common than primary tumors. However, metastases are rarely limited to heart. The development of arrhythmias, heart failure in a patient with

Flow chart 34.1 Classification of cardiac tumors

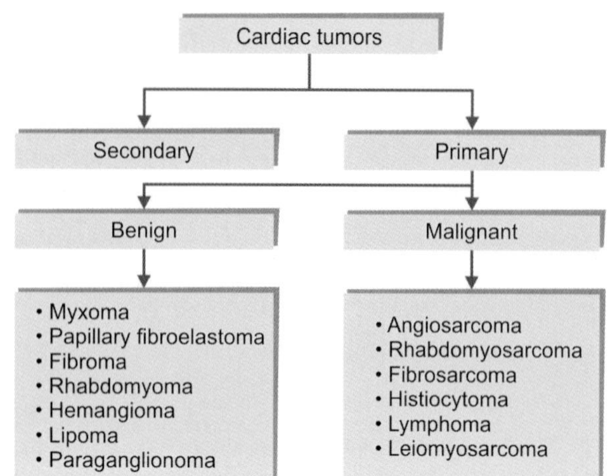

malignancy is suggestive of cardiac metastases. Rarely, cardiac involvement may be the first clinical feature of malignancy. The presentation is usually with a large pericardial effusion. Carcinoma of breast and lung is most common to invade the pericardium by local infiltration leading to pericardial effusion. The carcinoma of lung may invade the pulmonary veins and grow into the left atrium. Invasion of the inferior vena cava with subsequent spread to heart is seen with renal cell carcinoma and hepatoma. Besides malignant melanoma, primary gastrointestinal neoplasms, lymphoma, leukemia, and various sarcomas from extracardiac origin can secondarily involve the heart with melanoma having the highest propensity to spread. Most metastatic deposits are clinically silent and grow up to several centimeters before being apparent.

BENIGN PRIMARY CARDIAC TUMORS

Myxoma

These are the most common primary tumors of the heart (50%) with a slight female predisposition. They are typically seen in between 30 and 60 years age. They are seen both in the left atrium (LA) and RA. However, they are far more common in the left atrium and the fossa ovalis of the interatrial septum being the most common site. Most cardiac myxomas are sporadic, but may be familial and inherited as an autosomal dominant condition called Carney syndrome or complex.[4] It is associated with the development of extracardiac tumors (pituitary adenoma, breast fibroadenoma, psammomatous melanotic schwannoma) and hyperpigmented skin lesions (lentigines, ephelides, blue nevus). Patients with myxomas of the Carney syndrome are younger with equal sex predisposition. These tumors are likely to be multifocal and occur outside the left atrium with a propensity to recur after surgery. In contrast, sporadic myxomas are commonly of left atrial origin with a predilection to the fossa ovalis of the atrial septum. The most feared event with myxoma is embolism. Thrombus formed on the surface of tumor or actual embolisms of tumor fragments is common. The question that arises "is there any means of identifying myxomas which are likely to embolize?" There is no definite answer. But it is worth mentioning that these tumors are of two types: (a) Polypoid and (b) Villous. Polypoid varieties are compact and rarely undergo fragmentation, while those with villous extensions are fragile and likely to embolize. Nevertheless, thrombus formation on tumor surface leading to embolism cannot be predicted. They may grow up to several centimeters in size and depending upon their position may give rise to obstructive symptoms. Besides they are known to change their positions and accordingly have variable signs and symptoms.

They are easily distinguished at echocardiography by "a gelatinous mass with villous surface attached to the fossa ovalis of the atrial septum by a slender stalk," which is highly mobile and freely prolapse across the mitral valve in diastole producing a gradient. They may be homogeneous or heterogeneous, and may have origin outside the left atrium and may be sessile. They may have foci of hemorrhage, necrosis, and calcification. But the thin and delicate stalk may not be visible at CT or MRI.[5] A heterogeneous low attenuation at CT is due to its gelatinous nature. Calcification though is confidently picked up by CT. At MRI increased signal intensity on T2-weighted images is seen. Foci of calcification may give rise to decreased signal intensity. The treatment of choice is complete surgical resection with a sleeve of normal tissue. The risk of recurrence is 13% and more common with familial than sporadic tumors (22% vs 3%). A semiannual follow-up is recommended after surgery.

Papillary Fibroelastoma[6]

After myxoma, they are the most common benign primary cardiac tumor. They have a fibroelastic core and commonly seen on cardiac valves. Their size is usually <1 cm in diameter but large ones measuring 5 cm have also been reported. They are delicate, frond like, and attached to the endocardium by a short pedicle. They have been likened to a "sea anemone." No sex predisposition occurs and has been found in all age groups. Usually they are asymptomatic, but symptoms may be caused by embolization of tumor fragments or thrombi that collect over the tumor. They are more common on the aortic and mitral valves as compared to tricuspid and pulmonary valves. They are also known to arise from nonvalvular surfaces. At echocardiography, they produce a "shimmer" at the tumor–blood interface and have been used as a differentiating feature to distinguish a thrombus.

If they are small, immobile, and located in left heart, they may be left alone with periodic follow-up. But if they are large (≥ 1 cm), mobile, and produce symptoms due to embolism, they should be excised. Right-sided tumors require excision only if large and mobile. Usually they need a simple "shaving

Table 34.1 Features of benign primary cardiac tumors

Tumor Type	*Age of presentation*	*Associated syndromes*	*Most common location*	*Morphological characteristics*	*Echo features*	*CT features*	*MRI features*
Myxoma	30–60 years; younger if associated with Carney syndrome	Carney syndrome	Interatrial septum in region of fossa ovalis; LA more common than RA	Gelatinous; attached to a stalk. Calcification, hemorrhage, necrosis common	Mobile tumor attached to a stalk; may be sessile	Heterogeneous	Heterogeneous; bright on T2WI
Papillary fibroelastoma	Middle aged, elderly	None	Cardiac valves	Small (< 1 cm), narrow stalk; calcification, hemorrhage, necrosis rare	Shimmering edge	Usually not visible, if < 1 cm	Usually not seen
Fibroma	Infants, children, young adults	Gorlin syndrome	Ventricles	Intramural, large calcification common no hemorrhage or necrosis	Intramural; calcification seen	Low attenuation calcification seen	Isointense on T1WI bright on T2WI
Lipoma	Any age	Tuberous sclerosis (few cases)	Pericardial space or any cardiac chamber	Large, broad based no calcification, hemorrhage or necrosis	Hypoechoic in pericardial space; echogenic in cardiac chamber	Homogeneous low attenuation	Homogeneous fat signal intensity (increased T1) no enhancement
Rhabdomyoma	Infants, children < 4 years	Tuberous sclerosis	LV, RV in walls, on AV valves, outflow tract	Pedunculated, multiple, variable size, spontaneous regression	Brighter than surrounding myocardium	Hypodense on contrast CT	Isointense to myocardium T1WI; hyperintense to myocardium T2WI
Paraganglionoma	Young adults	Many possible, but sporadic	LA, coronary arteries aortic root	Broad-based, infiltrative; hemorrhage, necrosis common calcification rare	Echogenic, immobile	Low attenuation	Marked enhancement Isointense on T1WI Bright on T2WI
Lyphangioma	Infants, children	None	Pericardial space	Large, cystic no calcification, hemorrhage or necrosis	Heterogeneous, septate, hypoechoic	Low attenuation heterogeneous, septate	Heterogeneous, septated, bright on T2WI
Hemangioma (rare)	Any age	Kasabach–Merritt, may occur in extracardiac sites (GIT, skin, face	Any chamber	May contain fat, may derive blood supply from coronary arteries, may regress spontaneously, may recur	Hyperechoic	Heterogeneous, intense enhancement after contrast	Intermediate signal intensity on T1WI, hypointense on T2WI

Abbreviations: T1WI, T1 weighted images; T2WI, T2 weighted images

off" at the base of the tumor. An association has been noted with hypertrophic cardiomyopathy, surgical, radiation, and hemodynamic trauma.

Fibroma[7]

They are characteristically solitary, invariably located in the ventricle, well circumscribed, and show central calcification. They usually affect children and after rhabdomyomas are the most common cardiac tumors in children.[8] There is an increased prevalence of fibromas in association with Gorlin syndrome (autosomal dominant condition associated with basal cell carcinoma, jaw cysts, skeletal anomalies, and tendency to develop neoplasms in several organ systems). No sex predisposition is seen and the usual presentation is with arrhythmias, heart failure, and sudden death. The echo picture is a discrete, noncontractile mass ranging from 1 to 10 cm in diameter in a ventricular wall and often mimicking septal hypertrophy. Surgery is the treatment of choice in all symptomatic tumors that are respectable. For asymptomatic cases, fear of fatal arrhythmias may guide decision making in favor of surgery.

Rhabdomyoma[8]

These tumors are multiple, well-circumscribed masses that grow on the atrioventricular valves or in the ventricular walls. They are of variable size and may be pedunculated. An association with tuberous sclerosis has been observed. It is an autosomal dominant syndrome characterized by hamartomas, epilepsy, and skin lesions. They undergo spontaneous regression in most patients and rarely seen after 4 years of age. They are the most common benign cardiac tumors in children and often diagnosed in the first year of life. Rhabdomyomas are associated with pre-excitation and may increase the risk of arrhythmia. Because of spontaneous tumor regression, management is "watchful expectancy" and surgical option is rarely indicated.

Lipoma[9]

These are encapsulated tumors found in both male and female with equal predisposition. Usually they occur singly, but might be multiple in patients with tuberous sclerosis. Histologically, they consist of mature fat cells with occasional fibrous tissues with areas of calcification. Unlike lipomas of other areas, the genetic basis is not well elucidated. They are known to occur in both atrial and ventricular surfaces measuring about 1–8 cm in diameter. Depending on their location, they may or may not have symptoms. Those that grow subepicardially are largely asymptomatic except for pericardial effusion, which may occasionally be large. However, those with subendocardial location may produce obstructive symptoms, while those with intramyocardial location may produce arrhythmias. The imaging modality of choice is CT scan by virtue of better tissue characterization. If symptomatic, surgical excision gives excellent results.

Lipomatous hypertrophy of atrial septum is an entirely different entity. It is seen in elderly, obese individuals in whom there is fatty infiltration of the atrial septum with sparing of fossa ovalis giving rise to a dumbbell or hourglass appearance. Unlike lipomas, this is not capsulated and is thought to be of metabolic origin. They rarely produce symptoms so as to require surgical excision.

Hemangioma[10]

The vascular tumors of the heart include hemangioma, lymphangioma, and hemangioendothelioma. Hemangiomas are rare tumors (2% of cardiac tumors), while the other two are rarely seen. They assume importance as they have the potential for recurrence. They may be responsible for arrhythmias, pericardial effusion, heart failure, etc. They may be responsible for thrombosis, consumptive thrombocytopenia, and coagulopathy (Kasabach–Merritt syndrome). Cardiac hemangiomas may be associated with extracardiac hemangiomas such as those of gastrointestinal tract, skin, and face. They are more often seen in ventricles than atria and may be multiple in about 30% cases. Blood supply to the tumor may be demonstrated by coronary angiography. Echocardiographically they appear as hyper-echoic lesions. Contrast CT and CMR show intense enhance-ment. Conservative management is usually considered as spontaneous regression is known to occur and surgical excision may be hazardous. In view of recurrence, periodic echocardiography is recommended.

The above described tumors and some of their characteristics have been represented in Figures 34.2 and 34.3.

MALIGNANT PRIMARY CARDIAC TUMORS[11]

Of all primary malignant cardiac tumors, sarcomas are the most common followed by lymphomas. All sarcomas are highly aggressive and extremely lethal. Rather than the histologic type, aggression is based on high mitotic activity, extensive tumor necrosis, and lack of cell differentiation. The presence of metastases confers a poor prognosis. The presentation is variable and diagnosis is usually made by echocardiography and CT or CMR used for tissue characterization.

The angiosarcomas are the most common primary cardiac sarcomas in adults. They have a propensity to involve the pericardium. Hemorrhagic tamponade may be the presenting symptom. Stroke-like symptoms due to cerebral metastases are also known. They are typically large multilobular masses that protrude into most of the atrial cavity. About 90% angiosarcomas arise in the RA. They

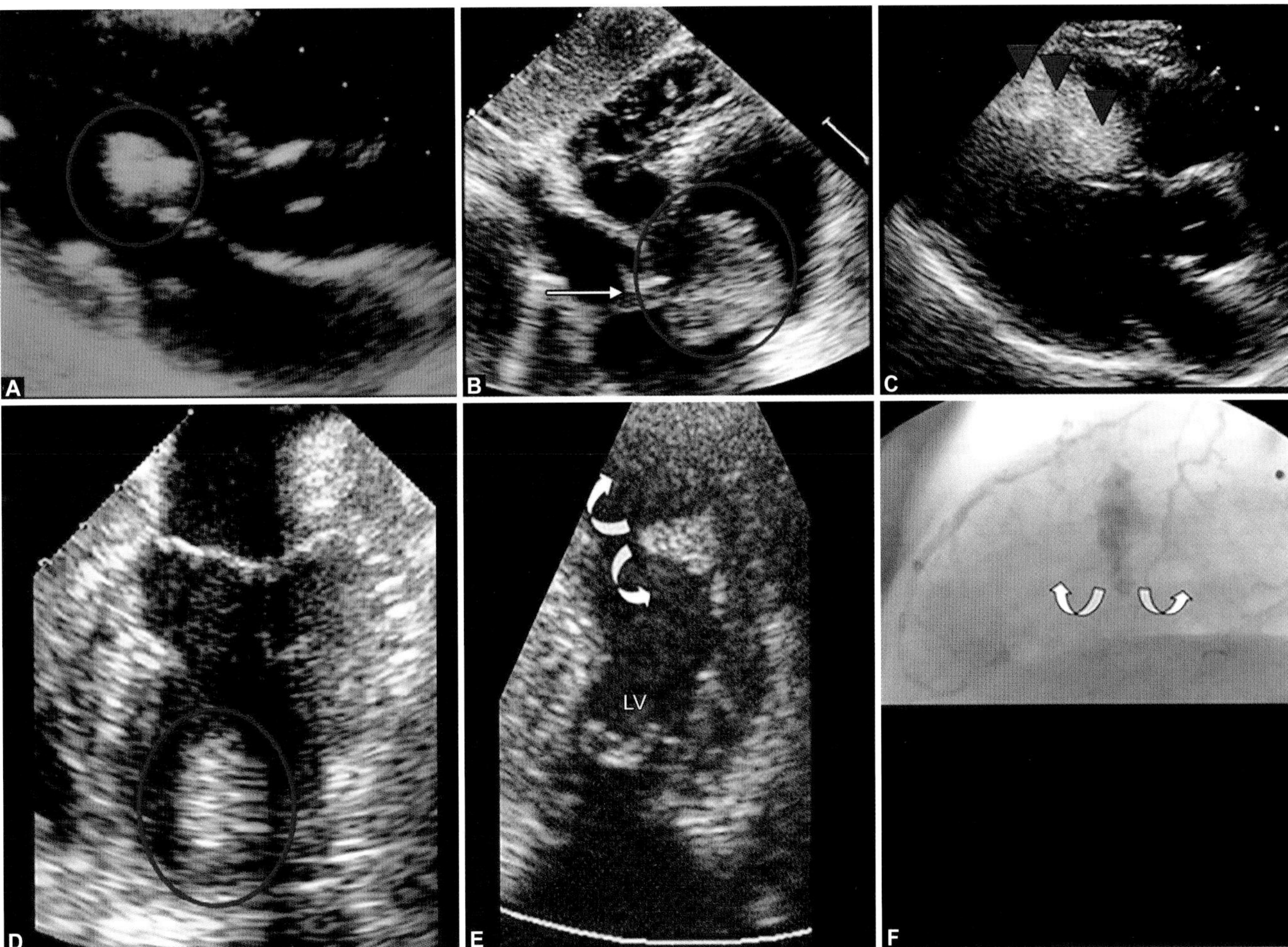

Figs 34.2A to F Album of cardiac tumors. (A) Papillary fibroelastoma attached to the anterior mitral leaflet. (B) Left atrium myxoma attached to the fossa ovalis region of interatrial septum. (C) Lipoma of the ventricular septum. (D) A mass at left ventricle (LV) apex was interpreted as clot and treated with anticoagulants for over a year. It was a dermoid and contained a (unbrushed) tooth! (E and F) Hemangioma of LV supplied by septal branches of left anterior descending artery

are highly aggressive neoplasms with a median survival of less than a year. Complete surgical excision along with radiation, neoadjuvant chemotherapy, and immunotherapy may improve survival. The use of heart transplantation is controversial.

Rhabdomyosarcomas are the most common primary cardiac malignant neoplasms of children. Like angiosarcomas, they have a varied presentation and carry a dismal prognosis. Surgical excision may be hindered by highly infiltrative nature of tumor. Response to chemotherapy and radiotherapy is poor. Leiomyosarcomas are malignant mesenchymal tumors with a large majority arising in the left atrium. The mean survival is 6 months after diagnosis. They have a tendency to recur. Palliative surgery may be considered in severely symptomatic patients. Other nonvascular sarcomas are highly aggressive tumors with little response to chemotherapy and radiotherapy.

Primary cardiac lymphomas are rare and have been recognized in association with HIV infection and post solid organ transplantation. They commonly involve the right side of the heart. Chemotherapy with or without radiotherapy is the treatment of choice. Radical surgical excision is discouraged. Recently "rituximab," a monoclonal antibody has shown promise in improving survival of patients.

CONCLUSION

Cardiac tumors because of their rarity provide a Herculean challenge to frame guidelines. Moreover, understanding tumor characteristic is also difficult because of myriad presentations. Notably the classification of sarcomas has been in a constant state of evolution. More data is required on cardiac tumors and an international consortium may provide

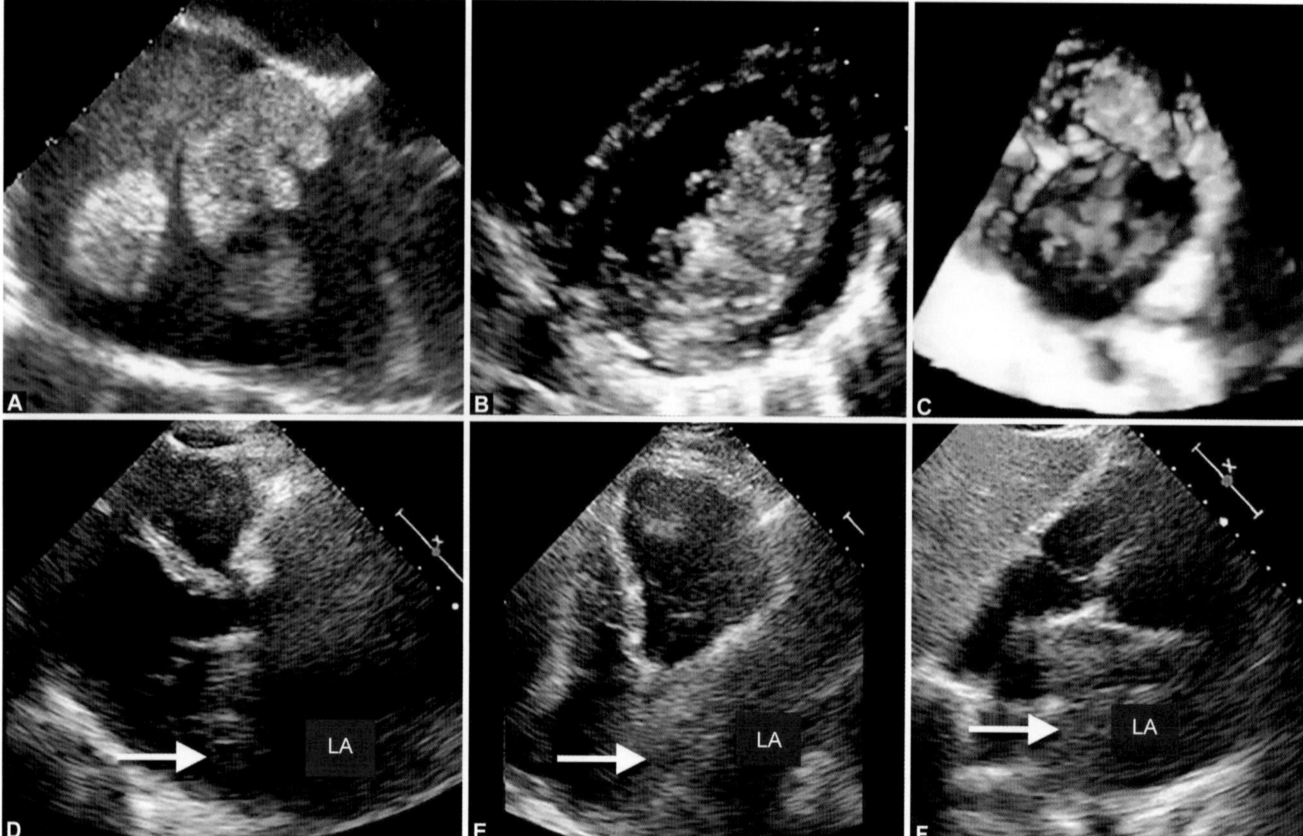

Figs 34.3A to F Album of cardiac tumors. (A) Right atrial myxoma. (B and C) A large tumor arising from and engulfing the posterior mitral leaflet. The anterior mitral leaflet is largely intact. ?Papillary fibroelastoma. It was a vegetation! (D to F) A mass diagnosed as a left atrial tumor from a PLAX, 4C and subcostal views turned out to be a "pericardial hemangioma"!

logical answers to the varying problem. Newer imaging modalities,[12] gene therapy, and understanding different apoptotic pathways for anticancer drug therapy[13] may provide better diagnostic and treatment approach for cardiac tumors.

REFERENCES

1. Reynen K. Frequency of primary tumours of heart. Am J Cardiol. 1996;77:107-13.
2. Araoz PA, Mulvagh SL, Tazehar HD, et al. CT and MR imaging of benign primary cardiac neoplasms with echocardiographic correlation. Radiographics. 2000;20:1303-19.
3. Simpson L, Kumar SK, Okurio SH, et al. Malignant primary cardiac tumours: review of a single institution experience. Cancer. 2008;112: 2440-6.
4. Carney JA, Gordon H, Carpenter PC, et al. The complex of myxomas, spotty pigmentation, and endocrine overactivity. Medicine (Baltimore). 1985;64:270-83.
5. Grebenc ML, Rosado-de-Christensen ML, Green LE, et al. Cardiac myxoma: imaging features in 83 patients. Radiographics. 2002;22:673-80.
6. Gowda RM, Khan IA, Nair CK, et al. Cardiac papillary fibroelastoma: a comprehensive analysis of 725 cases. Am Heart J. 2003;146:404-10.
7. Cho JM, Danielson GK, Paga FJ, et al. Surgical resection of ventricular cardiac fibromas: early and late results. Ann Thorac Surg. 2003;76:1929-34.
8. Beghetti M, Gow RM, Haney I, et al. Pediatric primary benign cardiac tumours: a 15-year review. Am Heart J. 1997;134:1107-13.
9. Piazza N, Chugtai T, Toledano K, et al. Primary cardiac tumours: eighteen years of surgical experience on 21 patients. Can J Cardiol. 2004;20:1443-8.
10. Lam KY, Dickens P, Chen AC, et al. Tumours of the heart. A 20 year experience with a review of 12,485 consecutive autopsies. Arch Pathol Lab Med. 1993;117:1027-31.
11. Burke A. Primary malignant cardiac tumours. Semin Diag Pathol. 2008;118(suppl14):s7-15.
12. Messa C, Di Muzio N, Picchi M, et al. PET/CT and radiotherapy. QJ Nucl Med Imaging. 2006;50:4-8.
13. Neragi- Miandoab S, Kim J, Vlahakes GJ, et al. Malignant tumours of the heart: a review of tumour type, diagnosis and therapy. Clin Oncol (R Coll Radiol). 2007;19:748-53.

35

Pregnancy and Heart Diseases: Advancement in Management

Smita Mishra, Seema Thakur

SECTION I
INTRODUCTION, EPIDEMIOLOGY, GENETICS, AND FETAL SCREENING

INTRODUCTION[1-7]

The population of the women with cardiovascular diseases (CVD) is growing worldwide with increasing facilities for cardiac interventions in congenital and acquired heart diseases. Furthermore, these women with treated or untreated CVD might be syndromic, or may be harboring residual defects. The cardiovascular status of these patients is often unknown, adding up to maternal mortality, morbidity, and fetal loss. The maternal factors such as cyanosis, systemic ventricular dysfunction, uncontrolled arrhythmias, pulmonary hypertension, use of fetotoxic drugs and fetal factors like fetal arrhythmias or complex congenital heart diseases (CHDs) contribute to adverse maternal/fetal outcome. The risk of acquired CVD in pregnancy has increased due to increasing age at first pregnancy and increasing prevalence of cardiovascular risk factors—diabetes mellitus, hypertension and obesity.

The pregnancy lays big hemodynamic challenges to a woman with the CVD. These horizons are still unexplored completely. Additionally, in India, pregnancy has been treated as ultimate attainment of womanhood socially and compels woman to take extra risk in midst of poor medical facilities. Up to 4% of pregnancies may have cardiovascular complications despite no known prior disease. Obstetric care in India, has to evolve to improve the outcome of this special group.

EPIDEMIOLOGY

Pregnancy with heart disease is not an uncommon complication in obstetrics with the incidence of 0.50–3.00%.[1-3] It is one of the most important reasons resulting in maternal and perinatal death. Heart disease in pregnancy is listed as the leading cause of non-obstetrical death in pregnant women. Congenital heart diseases dominate in developed countries and rheumatic heart diseases in developing countries.[6,7]

Bhatla et al. in Indian series, reported rheumatic heart diseases as the underlying cause of CVD in 88% women.[5] Expectedly, RHD is an important cause in >60% of pregnant women of CVD in developing countries, whereas in developed world, >70% cases are due to shunt lesions, are underlying CVD in >70% of cases in developed world.

GENETIC TESTING AND COUNSELING[8-11]

There is the risk of inheritance of cardiac defects in babies of mothers with CVD. Depending upon the etiological diagnosis of cardiac malformations risk of recurrence varies from 3% to 50%. Fesslova et al. reported high recurrence rate (RR) in their recently reported series. In this series, total RR of CHD was 3.98% (4.06% when risk factor was single, and 5% when risk factors were multiple.) Out of 22 cases with dextrocardia (with situs solitus or inversus) recurrent lesions occurred in two cases (total RR 8.7% and RR in siblings was 14.3%). Recurrence rate was 3.5% if one sibling was affected, 4.5% when two siblings are affected; reported risk to inherit CHD in baby is 5.2% when mother alone is affected, 7.5% when father alone affected, 3.5% when affected person is a distant relative.[12] In view of the current data, the genetic evaluation is a must. In India, the facilities for genetic testing and counseling are meager.

Group of Mothers who must Undergo Genetic Screening

- In mothers with family history of CHDs, cardiomyopathies, and channelopathies such as long QT syndromes.
- Unexplained deaths or when they themselves are affected.

- When the mother has dysmorphic features, develop mental delay/mental retardation, or when other noncardiac congenital abnormalities are present with or without syndromic associations, such as in Marfan, 22q11 deletion, Williams-Beuren, Alagille, Noonan, and Holt- Oram syndrome.
- History of recurrent abortions and stillbirths.

The modalities for screening are—chorionic villous biopsy at 12 weeks, ultrasound screening for the soft markers like nuchal fold thickness, as a part of screening for chromosomal disorders like Down's syndrome.

Westin et al. concluded that association of NT with cardiac defect is too weak to envisage a role for its measurement as single screening strategy for the prenatal detection of cardiac defects.[13] Fetal echocardiography between 18 and 20 weeks as a part of anomaly scan is best modality for fetal cardiac screening.

SECTION II
GENERAL CONSIDERATION OF PREGNANCY WITH CARDIOVASCULAR DISEASES

COMBATING STRESS ON CARDIOVASCULAR SYSTEM IN PREGNANCY AND PARTURITION[1-4,11]

The cardiovascular system is progressively stressed during the pregnancy and parturition. Most of the changes appear during the first trimester of pregnancy (Table 35.1), continue into the second and early third trimesters of pregnancy. The increase in cardiac output and oxygen consumption to meet the increased metabolic demand of growing fetus, is primarily a result of the increased stroke volume and the heart rate. Arterial blood pressure remains low during normal pregnancy because of a decrease in peripheral vascular resistance. Increased hormonal levels (estrogen, prostaglandins) cause the vasodilatation and therefore a decrease in systemic vascular resistance (SVR) and pulmonary vascular resistance. Decreased peripheral resistance causes a small decrease in systolic blood pressure and a more marked decrease in diastolic blood pressure resulting into compromised coronary circulation. Decrease in SVR is detrimental for mothers with cyanotic CHD or Eisenmenger syndrome because it increases right to left shunting and hypoxia.[11,14-16]

EVALUATION OF CARDIAC RESERVE AND RISK SCORING IN PREGNANCY WITH CVD[14-16] (TABLE 35.2)

Multiple risk scoring systems for prognostication of pregnancy outcome have been developed based on clinical and echocardiographic evidences (Tables 35.2 and 35.3). The adequacy of cardiac reserve in a woman with CVD must be assessed. The ESC Committee recommends to perform submaximal exercise tests to reach 80% of predicted maximal heart rate in asymptomatic pregnant patients with suspected CVD.[11] There is no evidence that it increases the risk of spontaneous abortion. Other modalities like semirecumbent cycle ergometry, treadmill walking, or upright cycle ergometry can also be used. Dobutamine stress should be avoided.

The exercise testing and stress echo can be very helpful in assessing functional reserve of myocardium in women who are taking preconception advice.

Barker et al. used maximal symptom-limited treadmill cardiopulmonary exercise testing to assess cardiac reserve and reported that direct measurement of cardiac functional reserve capacity can be performed by noninvasive assessment of mean/peak cardiac power output (PkCPO). This can be safely undertaken during pregnancy. A cutoff value of PkCPO was defined as 2.6 W, corresponding to that required for normal labor.[14]

Few other investigators recorded phonocardiogram of participants at resting status by exercise cardiac contractility monitor. They found that S1/S2 ratio, D/S ratio, and HR are useful in evaluating the cardiac reserve during abnormal pregnancy.[15]

The adequacy of cardiac reserve is the most important denominator of future outcome of pregnancy in a mother with CVD. The monitoring of New York Heart Association (NYHA) status, cardiac function, valvar obstruction, degree of cyanosis, and rhythm disturbances must be recommended to recognize high-risk patients. The patients with mechanical valves, need to be monitored closely for cardiac function, valve malfunction, arrhythmias and for thromboembolic events (Tables 35.2 and 35.3).

The lone presence of a CVD in a pregnant woman does not translate into a poor outcome. Overall outcome can be predicted applying a risk scoring system basis of a group of variables (Table 35.2).[16-18]

Table 35.1 Effect of pregnancy on cardiovascular parameters

Parameters	*Effect of pregnancy*
CO	Increased by 22% in first trimester and 30–40% above normal values in second and third trimesters
Oxygen consumption	Increased by 20%
SVR	Decreased by 30%
HR	Increased by 10–15 beats/min in second trimester
Blood volume	Increased up to 40–50% in third trimester
RBC volume	Increased to 30 mL/kg

Abbreviations: CO, cardiac output; SVR, systemic vascular resistance; HR, heart rate; RBC, red blood cell.

Table 35.2 Risk scoring system for pregnancy with CVD

	Scoring system	Variables	Grading	Proposed by
1.	Cardiac disease in pregnancy (CARPREG) risk score[16]	Untreated cyanotic CHD, history of prior cardiac event or arrhythmia, NYHA class, LVOT obstruction, LVEF <40%, PAH, Saturation (SaO_2) <90%,[2]	Depending on scored points, risks cardiac-complications are graded as 5%, 27%, and 75%	Siu et al.[12]
2.	ZAHARA predictors[17]	All of above and additional variables like presence of mechanical prosthesis and valvular regurgitation included		Drenthen et al.
	Khairy predictors[18]	All of above + Additional variables: history of smoking, RV dysfunction/ severe PR		Khairy P 2006
	WHO scoring	The risk scoring system is very elaborate and categorizes all the congenital and acquired CVDs operated or unoperated according to the severity and functional status	**Grades:** *Grade I:* Mild diseases like acyanotic CHD with low hemodynamic effect like small shunt or operated shunt without residual lesions, or mild PS; *Grade II:* The group contains unoperated shunts/operated TOF/arrhythmia; *Grade III:* Mechanical valves, unoperated cyanotic CHD, Marfan with borderline size of root, etc.; *Grade IV:* Severe diseases like Eisenmenger's syndrome, dilated cardiomyopathy. Marfan's syndrome with aortic root >50 mm, severe coarctation	Thorne et al.[35] (for details–see literature)

Abbreviations: CHD, congenital heart disease; CVD, cardiovascular diseases; NYHA, New York Heart Association; LVOT, left ventricular outflow tract; LVEF, left ventricular ejection fraction; PAH, polycyclic aromatic hydrocarbons; RV, right ventricle; TOF, tetralogy of Fallot.

Table 35.3 Changes in clinical features and electrocardiogram in pregnancy[26–27]

Clinical features
Apex beat: Shifted to the left due to elevated diaphragm in third trimester
Auscultation: First heart sound: loud; second heart sound: normal split
Murmurs: Soft systolic ejection murmur caused by increased blood flow and vasodilation
Electrocardiogram: QRS axis goes further left by 15%; Q waves may be present in leads III and AVF; inverted T waves may be seen in lead III; nonspecific ST, T, and Q wave changes and benign arrhythmias

CARDIAC FUNCTION IN PREGNANCY (TABLE 35.3)

Normally the ejection fraction, marker of systolic function goes up in early and mid-pregnancy and reduces marginally in the late pregnancy. Diastolic functions are also altered to some extent in normal pregnancy. However, in a woman with CVD, systolic as well as diastolic ventricular functions may be abnormal and may be cause of an adverse outcome.[19]

Normally, during pregnancy, the heart develops a reversible physiological hypertrophic growth or eccentric hypertrophy, in response to mechanical stress and increased cardiac output.

The rise of estrogen toward the end of pregnancy contributes to pregnancy-related heart hypertrophy by altering gene expression and provides a molecular correlate for the longer QT interval in pregnancy.[20]

Physiological Anemia and Pregnancy[21–24]

Anemia in pregnancy defined as hemoglobin (Hb) level of <10 g/dL. It is a qualitative or quantitative deficiency of Hb or red blood cells in circulation resulting in reduced oxygen (O_2)—carrying capacity of the blood. Maternal blood volume begins to increase early at sixth week and continues to rise by 45-50% till 34 weeks of gestation, returning to normal by 10-14 days, postpartum. Plasma volume increases up to 40% above of pre-pregnancy levels.[21] The different rate of increase in blood and plasma volume accounts for the relative anemia of pregnancy. The onset of relative anemia is compensated by several mechanisms like increase in cardiac output (CO), Pao_2, 2,3 diphosphoglycerate levels, rightward shift in the oxygen dissociation curve (ODC), decrease in blood viscosity and release of renal erythropoietin. Therefore, tissue oxygenation remains unaffected despite the relatively low arterial O_2 content.[21-24] The serious consequences like heart failure, angina or tissue hypoxemia may set-in, if decompensation takes place due to acute blood loss or secondary to a cardiac disease where oxygen supply is restricted like in mothers with polycythemia secondary to the cyanotic CHDs and Eisenmenger's syndrome. The basal low saturation and high level of hematocrit are the adverse factors for total pregnancy outcome. Neither the lower acceptable level of hemoglobin nor indication for RBC transfusion has been defined in the literature.[24]

Effect of Posture on Cardiac Output during Pregnancy

The cardiac output may be decreased in third trimester due to posture. In supine position, venous return reduces owing to compression of inferior vena cava (IVC) by the gravid uterus. This effect can be avoided by mother lying on lateral position.[25]

Effect of Pregnancy on Clinical Findings and ECG[11,26-27]

The cardiac diseases in pregnancy may be picked up for the first time. Usually, atrial septal defect or mitral stenosis may get unmasked because patients start having palpitation or dyspnea on exertion. Women with Eisenmenger syndrome may present with cyanosis during the pregnancy. The chest pain of cardiac origin must be differentiated from other mimicking conditions like pain of muscular or pulmonary origin. Chest pain secondary to acute coronary syndrome presents with discomfort, and hypotension. Classic symptoms of heart disease mimic common symptoms of late pregnancy, such as palpitations, shortness of breath with exertion, and occasional chest pain. Clinical findings are altered due to higher position of diaphragm as gravid uterus needs extra space. Accordingly, cardiac position and axis is changed that is reflected in clinical examination and electrocardiogram (Table 35.3). In order to detect pathologic changes in the electrocardiogram (ECG), one has to know about physiologic changes during pregnancy. Because of the leftward deviation, the heart may appear enlarged on the chest roentgenogram. The features pointing toward the significant heart disease are elaborated in Table 35.4.

Table 35.4 Signs of significant heart disease in the pregnant women[11,26,27]

- True cardiac enlargement
- Differential pulses
- Cyanosis
- Upper limb hypertension
- Severe arrhythmias
- Systolic murmur greater than grade III
- Significant diastolic murmur

EFFECT OF LABOR ON PREGNANCY WITH CVD

Onset of labor is translated into the increased cardiac work secondary to reverse transfusion from fetal to maternal circulation (autotransfusion), surge of catecholamine due to stress, apprehension and pain leading to rise in stroke volume and cardiac output by 45% of prelabor values.[25-26]

Immediate post-delivery, cardiac output increases due to relieved IVC compression and increased preload. As a result, there is a marked increase in cardiac output that predisposes for heart failure in these patients.

Conversely, 10% of pregnant patients near term develop signs of shock (hypotension, pallor, sweating, nausea, vomiting, changes in cerebration) when they assume supine position. Lee et al. reported additional mechanism of venous return through the paraspinal or azygos veins to overcome the IVC compression and maintain the cardiac output.[28]

Oron et al. found induction of labor safe and Advocated cesarean section only for specific indications.[29]

GENERAL RECOMMENDATIONS IN PREGNANCY WITH CVD (BOX 35.1)

Pregnancy with CVD needs special care. Symptomatic patients usually present with chest pain, dyspnea on exertion or palpitation. Sometimes they may come with critical hemodynamic disturbances. Preconception evaluation and counseling by an interdisciplinary team is essential. Special aspects of antenatal care, genetic factors of the cardiac disease and perinatal outcome should also be addressed. The enquiry must be made regarding recent evidence of infection, embolism, edema, recent onset breathlessness, syncope, drug intake, radiation exposure, bleeding events, drug history, and addiction. Routine laboratory examination must include complete blood count, platelet count, hemoglobin, kidney, and liver function test as well as routine urinary examination for proteinuria. Enquiry must be made for secondary rheumatic prophylaxis and dental problems.[11]

Box 35.1 Summary of general recommendations (based on Refs.[11,30])

1. Prepregnancy risk assessment and counseling must be done in all women with CVD.
2. Specialized institutional delivery is recommended for high-risk pregnancy.
3. Genetic counseling in patients with CVD where probability of inheritance exists like in hypertrophic cardiomyopathy.
4. Appropriate diagnostic procedures must be performed in each case. Echocardiography must be used to make exact diagnosis for risk scoring and follow-up for the deterioration of function secondary to affect pregnancy-related physiological changes.
5. Vaginal delivery is the mode of choice for most of elective deliveries. CS is reserved for mothers presenting with imminent threat to the mother or fetal life as mentioned above. The epidural anesthesia with instrumental delivery is one of choices for women with severe hypertension.
6. The aortic root >45 mm, severe AS, mother on oral anticoagulation are few of the indications for CS.
7. In case of premature induction of labor, corticosteroids must be administered to promote fetal lung maturation.
8. In presence of a shunt lesion, strict precautions must be taken to avoid any air in intravenous lines.
9. The cardiac interventions are preferred to the cardiac surgery and can be done by shielding the fetus. If cardiac surgery is essential near 28 weeks, fetus must be taken out before the surgery. Surgery is recommended in life-threatening condition of mother where medical therapy and catheter interventions are failed.
10. Deep vein thrombosis is much feared complication and meticulous prophylaxis is recommended. Low molecular weight heparin (LMWH) or heparin or oral anticoagulation must be done if required as in cases where prolonged bed rest is necessary.
11. Beta blockers are recommended antenatally and during the delivery for mothers with hypertrophic obstructive cardiomyopathy (HOCM) with moderate left ventricular outflow tract (LVOT) obstruction and wall thickness >1.5 cm.
12. The radiation to the fetus can be minimalized using a shield for abdomen of pregnant woman. The catheter procedures, X-ray of chests, CT scan must be avoided, but, if mandatory, can be done while protecting the fetus with shield.
13. The safety of gadolinium is not established hence MRI can be done without it.
14. The antibiotic IE prophylaxis is not recommended in recent guidelines during the delivery. In India, individual choices must be made according to the risk involved in the procedure.

The women operated for CVD with prosthetic material must be stratified for risk of thromboembolism according to the Royal College of Obstetricians and Gynaecologists (RCOG) guidelines.[30] Cardiac function should be optimized. Careful selection of drugs must be done and teratogenic drugs must be withdrawn before or just after the conception. The Individual follow-up schedules should be advised.[31]

Role of Echocardiography

Echocardiography is the main tool to evaluate structural and functional heart diseases. It can be done from transthoracic window or transesophageal route. Additionally, it can be utilized to evaluate fetal cardiac conditions. The ultrasound has been described to raise tissue temperature by the process known as acoustic cavitation and acoustic streaming secondary to gradient generated by moving ultrasound beams. The harmful effects on fetus have been contemplated in animal experiments but in human, no evidence has been seen.[32] Small increase in the frequency of nonright-handedness has been reported in male infants of mothers exposed to diagnostic ultrasound.[33]

The echocardiography must be done to make exact diagnosis of the cardiac lesions, evaluation of residual defects, size of cardiac chambers, systolic and diastolic functions of both the ventricles, valvar stenosis and regurgitation, size of the great vessels and aortic dimensions, presence or absence of clots and vegetation, IVC diameter. The echo evaluation helps in risk stratification, management, and pre- and post-conception counseling. Accordingly, follow-up echo-evaluation may be planned.[11]

Usually, fetal echo can be done accurately between 18 and 20 weeks by transthoracic route. A review of the accuracy of first trimester ultrasounds for detecting major fetal CHD showed a sensitivity and specificity of 85% and 99%, respectively.[34] Early fetal echo (within 20 weeks of pregnancy) allows parents to consider all options, including termination of pregnancy, when fetus has a severe cardiac disease, noncompatible with normal life.

An abnormal fetal echo must be further investigated to find out other fetal anomalies including chromosomal defects, chronic medical disorders, and viral illnesses in mother. Screening for deletion in 22q11.2 is recommended when conotruncal anomalies are present in fetus. History of intake of teratogenic drugs, must be taken.

MODIFIED WHO CLASSIFICATION OF MATERNAL CARDIOVASCULAR PREGNANCY RISK[35]

The women suffering from CVD needs preconception advice that includes to be allowed to conceive with acceptable risks or high risk. If required, they also should be advised about pre-pregnancy intervention for their cardiac problems. The WHO classification of risk for contraception in women with CVD was developed to create some guidelines to understand issues involved in this group. Thorne et al. adopted it to provide a classification of risk for cardiac lesions and to bring out more information about contraception, pre-pregnancy assessment and antenatal management of individual cardiac lesions, depending on type and severity of lesions (Table 35.2).

ANESTHESIA IN PREGNANCY WITH CVD (BOX 35.2)[11,21,25,29,36–38]

The pregnancy in woman with CVD requires "state-of-art" anesthetic management. Box 35.2 shows the point of considerations in choosing anesthetic drugs and basic principles anesthesia. Different modes of anesthesia can be used during procedures and delivery as discussed below:

1. *Regional analgesia* has been considered a substantial risk because of the potential for both venodilation leading to decreased preload, and arterial dilation resulting in decreased SVR.
2. *Segmental lumbar epidural anesthesia* avoids sudden changes in hemodynamic parameters and helps in achieving desired result.[37] Additionally, the opioids, such as fentanyl can be added to synergize the analgesia. Adequate segmental and perineal anesthesia removes anxiety and reduces catecholamine-induced tachycardia. It also prevents unwanted urge to push, allowing the fetal descent with natural uterine contractions and thus avoids inadvertent Valsalva maneuver by the parturient.
3. *Low-spinal anesthesia* may be used during second stage of labor. If patients develop hypotension, the metaraminol or phenylephrine can be used to restore the blood pressure.[11,35–38]
4. *Caudal anesthesia* is another reasonable option. Pudendal nerve block can provide adequate anesthesia.
5. *General anesthesia (GA) is expected to* provide a very stable hemodynamic course. However, the endotracheal intubation can be difficult due to relative smaller lumen of airways and sympathetic stimulation. Depending on the severity of the disease, the need to blunt the hemodynamic response to endotracheal intubation may necessitate the use of a high-dose narcotic-based technique. This also serves to avoid myocardial depression and the fall in SVR that may occur with commonly employed short-acting barbiturates. Anesthesia is maintained with narcotics, muscle relaxants, nitrous oxide, and oxygen. Emergence from anesthesia must be carefully controlled to ensure return of protective reflexes and avoidance of tachycardia.

Box 35.2 Pregnancy with CVD: management goals for anesthesia[11,21,25,29,36–38]

Special hemodynamic features affecting the choice of anesthesia:

1. Patient's tolerance to pain during labor or surgery will affect the catecholamine secretion.
2. The uterine contraction-induced autotransfusion will increase total blood volume and increased load on maternal heart.
3. The hemodynamics after delivery will change because of relief of vena caval obstruction.
4. There are factors that can promote postpartum hemorrhage.
5. Use of uterine oxytocic agents may put extra hemodynamic burden of compromised cardiovascular system.

Basic principles of anesthesia management pregnancy with CVD:[11,21,25,29,36–38]

1. Maintenance of uteroplacental perfusion by avoiding aortocaval compression.
2. Control the heart rate according to cardiac lesions—like tachycardia in MS and bradycardia in MR/AR.
3. Minimize sympathetic blockade in case of valvar stenosis coupled with intravascular volume and preload optimization.
4. Specialized monitoring of parturient and fetus maintaining hemodynamic parameters within a narrow therapeutic window.
5. Aspiration prophylaxis.

Goals of Managing Pregnancy with CVD

The common belief that CS and GA are the best options to manage delivery in a woman with CVD, has been confronted by various studies. Goals of management can be defined as discussed below:

1. *Minimize hemodynamic stress:* Theoretically, cesarean section may be preferred because it avoids prolonged and unpredictable labor, ability to time the delivery, and prepare equipment and personnel, hemodynamic control, and eliminating stress of labor. Nonetheless, the preference of CS over normal vaginal delivery has been challenged by the reports showing higher mortality in CS in comparison to NVD.[39] The Valsalva maneuver and maternal pushing can be avoided by assisting delivery with low forceps or vacuum extraction.[11,39] The cesarean delivery is indicated for patients with dilated aortic root (>4 mm), significant ventricular dysfunction, severe left ventricular (LV) outflow obstruction, severe pulmonary hypertension, patient on oral anticoagulants, preterm delivery, and patients presenting with cardiac arrest.[38-40]
2. *Prevent sudden change in cardiac output and blood volume:* As mentioned above, the anesthetic management helps in smooth changes in hemodynamic status. The tocolytic and oxytocic drugs may be harmful. β-Adrenergic drugs may cause tachycardia, arrhythmia, myocardial ischemia and pulmonary edema, hyperglycemia, lactic, and ketoacidosis. IV Magnesium is used as tocolytic and neuroprotective reagent. The calcium channel blockers (CCB) may precipitate cardiac failure in susceptible mother with CVD.

3. *Prevent aortocaval compression and ensure adequate venous return:* Aortocaval compression should be avoided during labor by keeping the lateral position, tilting the table or by raising the right buttock with the help of pillow. The uterus can be shifted manually also if one plans to resuscitate in supine. Otherwise the cardiac output may fail to rise.[41] Maternal safety is important till the fetus reaches to the age of viability. Later fetal wellbeing becomes equally important.[11,41]
4. *Avoid complications related to hypercoagulable state of pregnancy:* The pregnant woman at term, is in a hypercoagulable state, due to increased levels of factors VII, VIII, X, plasma fibrinogen as well as decreased capacity of fibrinolysis. In addition, stasis caused by compression of inferior vena cavae by gravid uterus may contribute in the intravascular thrombosis. Consequently, the women with CVD are predisposed for life-threatening thromboembolism and acute coronary events.[11,30]

Imaging in Pregnancy with CVD

Radiation[42–48]

This is an established fact that exposure to radiation may be associated with adverse fetal outcome. Conversely, radiation in pregnancy may have dose-dependent damaging effect letting cell depletion known as deterministic effects, leading to malformation of a developing organ or dose-independent stochastic effects that may induce changes in single cell, at any miniscule dose and can potentially result in neoplasia or in changes to reproductive genes.

As shown in animal and insect studies in preconception period, ovum is vulnerable to stochastic effect of radiation and can carry the genomic changes. But in human no such effects have been demonstrated. Exposure to radiation in first 15 days post-conception, can lead to spontaneous abortion. After 25 weeks of pregnancy, radiation may not have any significant effect. In the embryonic stage, beginning near the end of the second post-conception week and extending through the eighth week post-conception (about 4–10 weeks menstrual age), major organogenesis occurs. This period might be a subject of cell depletion in fetus and may lead to the radiation-mediated growth retardation and malformation of the organs.

The assumed radiation exposure in fetus is as follows: For an X-ray of chest -<0.01 mGy; CT scan of chest -0.3 mGy; coronary angiography-1.5 mGy; and radiofrequency catheter ablation -3 mGy. Evidently, the amount of radiation is usually below the threshold for damaging deterministic effects (>50–100 mGy). The radiation doses above 100 mGy can be associated with problems in the age-related manner, like spontaneous abortion (1–14 days of conception), possible malformations (15–56 day postconception), risk of diminished IQ or of mental retardation (57–105 days of postconception), possible IQ deficit (106–175 postconception), and possible no effect (beyond 175 days).

As a general rule, according to the principle "as low as reasonably achievable" (ALARA), all radiation doses due to medical exposures must be kept as low as reasonably achievable and modality like X-ray chest should be used only if essential absolutely.

Magnetic Resonance Imaging and Computed Tomography[11,49,50]

Magnetic resonance imaging (MRI) is probably a safe modality for cardiac diagnosis. MRI is also being used for fetal cardiac imaging with good results. However, safety of its use between 15 and 56 days (period of organogenesis) is not yet established. Similarly, there are concerns regarding the long-term safety with the use of gadolinium ions. The CT scan is not to be used unless major diagnostic dilemma has to be sorted out like in patients presenting with suspected pulmonary embolism. Radiation dose must be reduced in such a situation.[11,49,50]

Cardiac Catheterization[42,44–46,48]

As discussed above, during angiography, fetal exposure to ionized radiation is much less and unlikely to cause harm. Furthermore, in women with pregnancy, there might be multiple reasons to have angiography or intervention. In older mothers diagnostic and therapeutic coronary angiography may be needed. During coronary angiography, fluoroscopic time must be low. The expected radiation to fetus is 20% of total radiation, which can be prevented to a great extent by shielding the abdomen. The electrophysiological studies and ablation procedures are not recommended until they are causing major hemodynamic compromise. Electroanatomical mapping may help in reducing the radiation doses.

Interventions in the Mother during Pregnancy

Percutaneous Therapy

After the period of organogenesis (15–56 days post-conception), a percutaneous catheter intervention can be planned if absolutely necessary.[11,44,48,51]

The second trimester is targeted as fetal size is still small and abdominal shielding can be prohibitive. For mother, during this period of pregnancy, lying on table is not so uncomfortable. The mitral stenosis secondary to RHD, one of the most common valvular abnormality in our country, has been treated successfully with percutaneous balloon mitral valvotomy. Furthermore, important precaution during the cardiac interventions is administration of heparin to keep activated clotting time (ACT) just around 200. Heparin is given in smaller doses (40–70 U/kg).[11] Recently, Orchard et al. suggested the use of echocardiography along with low frame rate during the fluoroscopy to reduce the dose of ionized radiation in a modified protocol.[51]

Cardiac Surgery

The cardiac surgery is the last option in the pregnant woman with CVD. Moreover, the neonatal critical care has evolved to achieve excellent intact survival. Therefore, the CS before cardiac surgery is a better option if pregnancy can be extended up to 26–28 weeks. The cardiac surgery can be done between 13 and 28 weeks with reasonably good results. With the evolving understanding about cardiac anesthesia and surgery, maternal morbidity and mortality is better controlled. The problem still remains with the response of the uteroplacental unit to the cardiopulmonary bypass and fetal morbidity and mortality.[52,53] The fetal mortality rate during maternal cardiac surgery with CPB ranges from 16% to 33%.[54–56] The sustained uterine contractions are attributed to the adverse fetal outcome.[57] Off-pump antenatal surgeries like closed mitral valvotomy and coronary bypass have shown better fetomaternal outcome.[58]

In summary, the chief concerns in the optimal management of pregnant patients who are undergoing CPB are the control of temperature, perfusion pressure, and the nature of the bypass flow. Pump flow 2.5 L/min/m^2 (60–80 mL/kg/min, arterial flow should essentially be 20–40% higher than flows used for routine CPB in non-pregnant patients) and perfusion pressure >70 mm Hg, high FiO_2 to produce an arterial pO_2 of at least 200 mm Hg, is recommended. Current evidence favors maintaining normothermic CPB, avoiding the use of vasoconstrictors (which may have a profound effect on the placental unit), and maintaining both high hematocrit (>28%) and high flow rates. Fetal hypoperfusion and hypoxia may also be ameliorated by the use of pulsatile perfusion.[11,58–60]

Fine management of pH is preferred to avoid hypocapnia responsible for uteroplacental vasoconstriction and fetal hypoxia. CPB time should also be minimized.[60]

Cardiac Arrest in Pregnancy[11,41,61]

Cardiac arrest is rare and occurs in 1 of 30,000 pregnancies. Survival after such an event is exceptional unless it occurs during anesthesia.[62] The reported survival rate is as low as of 6.9%. The algorithm for CPR in parturient must be modified from non-pregnant woman, because of fetal dependence on maternal survival (Box 35.3).

Pre-empting cardiac arrest and start life-saving support early is the best strategy. Maternal hypotension that warrants therapy has been defined as a systolic blood pressure <100 mm Hg or <80% of baseline. One should alarm anesthesia and obstetric team to perform emergency CS in cases when CPR is not successful in 3–4 minutes. The CPR done in supine posture may get compromised due to reduced venous return because of aortocaval compression. This can be avoided by tilting the patient in left lateral position (15–30°). The CPR must be started with in the few minutes of arrest. In a case of failed CPR and nonsurvival of mother, delivery of fetus must be done within the 10 minutes for best results. Sometimes, extracting the fetus leads to better chances of survival to the mother. The electrical cardioversion can be done as it is neither contraindicated nor has been proven harmful to the fetus.

Box 35.3 Management of maternal cardiac arrest

- The time of arrest must be recorded because failed resuscitation for 4 minutes is an indication for CS.
  - Keep the patient supine (Remember it may cause cavo-aortic compression)
  - Place a hand little above on sternum than usual for chest compression
- Maternal intervention:
  - Defibrillate if required (effect on fetus not known)
  - Drugs as per protocol
  - Ventilation 100% oxygen
  - Monitor waveform capnography/CPR quality
  - Appropriate postarrest care
- Maternal medication:
  - Start IV line above diaphragm
  - Correct hypovolemia with fluid bolus
  - Advanced airway management
  - If patient is receiving n/10 magnesium stop and start with $CaCl_2$ 10 mL/10% saline or calcium gluconate 30 mL in 10% solution
  - Continue defibrillator, fluid, drugs, positioning if required
- Obstetric consideration

Gravid uterus may cause aortocaval compression

- Positioning: left uterine displacement
- Keep obstetric/neonatal team ready
- If nonresponse in 4 minutes, go for CS

Adapted from reference.[41,61]

Timing and Mode of Delivery: Risk for Mother and Child High-Risk Delivery

The peripartum management of patient requires a highly specialized team of doctors that includes cardiologist, neonatologist in addition to obstetrician, anesthetist, experienced nurse and paramedical staff. The delivery must be done in a well-equipped maternal-fetal medicine unit.

Timing of Delivery

Timing of delivery to be customized according to the individual patient based on her cardiac status and Bishop scoring. As discussed above, the surgical interventions for cardiac disease in a pregnant woman, are better to be delayed till the 26 weeks of pregnancy and CS must be conducted before the surgery. The full extent of fetal compromise is best identified by the combination of fetal biometry, biophysical profile scoring, nonstress testing and Doppler ultrasound evaluation of fetal arterial and venous blood flow (Box 35.4).[62-67]

Induction of Labor

There are various methods of induction of labor and decision to be taken based on Bishop score for the patient and according to the ESC guideline. The long induction time must be avoided. Prostaglandins may not be very suitable drugs and may cause adverse effect on coronary circulation and blood pressure. Some apparently safe physical methods can also be applied in place of pharmacological methods.[11,68,69]

Cesarean Delivery in Patients with Cardiac Disease[11,70-74]

The cesarean section is not preferred mode of delivery due to the risks of aspiration, venous thrombosis, and thromboembolism.[11,76] However, it is the preferred mode of delivery in conditions like dilated aortic root and fear of dissection, prosthetic valve dysfunction, severe hypertension secondary to pre-eclampsia, severe valvar stenosis. The outcome of CS in such a challenging situation needs (1) advanced airway management, (2) achieving stable hemodynamics, (3) optimizing fluid status, and (4) preventing seizures. New York Heart Association status of these patients correlates best with the maternal outcome. Mortality rate of <1% is reported in classes I and II, while in classes III and IV, it is between 5% and 15%.[11,72-74]

Box 35.4 Ultrasound evaluation of fetal arterial and venous blood flow[62-67]

1. Doppler waveforms in the umbilical arteries (UAs), either in the form of absent or reversed end diastolic flow.
2. Increase in diastolic flow to cerebral vessels.
3. Abnormal umbilicalcerebral or placentalcerebral index.
4. An increased distribution of flow to the ductus venosus rather than the fetal liver (shown in hepatic veins velocity). Decrease of the late diastolic flow component in the ductus venosus waveform.
5. Flow reversal in fetal IVC and abnormal umbilical venous pulsation s/o possible myocardial dysfunction in fetuses with severe growth restriction. Abnormal umbilical venous flow volume (s/o abnormal total cardiac output of the fetus).
6. Increased uterine artery pulsatility and resistance indices with or without notching of the waveform.

Termination of Pregnancy[11,75-79]

The termination of pregnancy is one of the options when there is threat to the life of mother. The pharmacological termination of pregnancy is possible with the help of mifepristone. The prostaglandins are another drugs used often to induce abortion. However, the PGE1 congeners may cause sudden hypotension hence strict monitoring of saturation and vitals is recommended. To maintain the SVR and diastolic BP, norepinephrine infusion may be started at low doses. The PGF compounds are more risky, as they can cause coronary compromise as well as may increase the PA pressure.[74-77] Abortion, using saline, may have adverse effects for women with a borderline hemodynamics. Probably safest method of abortion in first or second trimester is the surgical procedure—dilatation and evacuation.[78] There is chance of 5%, to have bacteremia after a surgical termination. The antibiotic prophylaxis is controversial after the publication of new guidelines lately.[79] Gynecologists routinely advise antibiotic prophylaxis to prevent postabortal endometritis, which occurs in 5–20% of women not given antibiotics.

Anticoagulation and Thrombolysis in Pregnancy with CVD[80-82]

As discussed above, pregnancy can be considered as a prothrombotic state for a woman with CVD. Both venous and arterial thromboembolisms have higher incidences. The estimated risk of arterial thromboembolism (strokes and heart attacks) and venous thromboembolism (VTE) are increased by three- to fourfold and four- to fivefold, respectively, when compared with nonpregnant woman.[11,80-82]

There are additional risk for thrombosis when pregnancy is associated with complications like the pre-eclampsia, multiple gestation, hyperemesis, disorders of fluid, electrolyte and acid-base balance, antepartum hemorrhage, cesarean delivery, mid-cavity forceps, prolonged second stage of labor postpartum infection, postpartum hemorrhage, hemoglobinopathies, and transfusion. The risks for thromboembolism has been categorized and integrated in RCOG and ESC guidelines.[11,30] One of the most serious complication may be pulmonary thromboembolism (PTE). In Western world, PTE is the chief cause for maternal mortality.[11,84]

Clinically, the patient with PTE present with breathlessness, hemoptysis, chest pain, desaturation, and syncope. Patients with PTE present with classical ECG finding of right ventricular (RV) strain and right bundle branch block pattern.

S1QT3 pattern is also known as McGinn-White sign, is the classical ECG findings. There are prominent S wave in lead I; prominent Q in lead III; inverted T in lead III. Usually, arterial blood gas analysis shows metabolic acidosis. Blood biochemistry suggests abnormal level of troponine I and D-dimer concentration. According to updated algorithm for treatment of PTE, strong clinical suspicion is enough to start with low molecular weight heparin (LMWH) and only after definitive exclusion of DVT/PTE, the treatment must be withdrawn (see Table 35.5 for dosage of LMWH). The MRI and spiral CT can be used with all precautions (see above). The ventilation-perfusion lung scanning is another diagnostic tool, though radiation dose to fetus may be higher.[11,84]

All pregnant women with suspected DVT should undergo screening-like pretest probability, D-dimer testing, and compression ultrasonography. If DVT is confirmed, appropriate treatment must be started. MRI venography can also be done.

Anticoagulation

Heparin[11,85,86]

Heparin is a sulfated polysaccharide with a molecular weight range of 3,000–30,000 Da (mean, 15,000 Da). It produces its major anticoagulant effect by inactivating thrombin and activated factor X (factor Xa) through an antithrombin (AT)-dependent mechanism. Its effect is measured by the activated thromboplastin time or, when very high doses are used, by the ACT. Heparin is administered in infusion form, may have variable anticoagulant response, secondary to its AT independent binding to plasma and other proteins, released by blood cells. It cannot act upon factor Xa in prothrombinase complex and thrombin attached to endothelium/fibrin. It can cause platelet depletion and osteopenia.[85]

Low molecular weight heparin[11,30,87-89]

LMWHs have a mean molecular weight of 4,500–5,000 Da (one third of size of heparin molecule) and are obtained from heparin after depolymerization of the molecule. They have low affinity to plasma proteins; therefore, have longer duration of action and more predictable anticoagulation response. The low molecular weight heparin does not cross placenta and is the drug of choice for thromboprophylaxis particularly in period of organogenesis. To ensure adequate anticoagulation throughout pregnancy, dosing options include (1) adjusting the dose in proportion to the actual weight change or (2) performing anti-factor Xa activity monitoring (as 4-hour peak levels after steady state has been achieved) and adjusting the LMWH dose to achieve a therapeutic anti- Factor Xa activity of approximately 0.5–1.0 IU/mL (Table 35.5). The suggested LMW heparin doses by RCOG guideline has been accommodated in ESC guideline.[11] This has been clearly mentioned in RCOG guideline that doses of LMWH for obese mothers and puerperium are not evidence based due to lack of appropriate data in literature. Therefore, the thromboprophylactic doses in Table 35.5 are only suggestions.[30]

Furthermore, the monitoring guidelines to ensure stable and safe therapeutic blood levels of anticoagulants are not established. Anti-Xa levels provide only a rough guide of the concentration of heparin present and levels provide little or no evidence on the efficacy in relation to prevention of thrombosis. In most of the studies, routine monitoring of anti-Xa levels in patients getting LMWH is not recommended.

Warfarin in pregnancy[91-93]

The use of warfarin during the period of organogenesis has been associated with a risk for embryopathy in up to 5% cases. It is also reported to cause stillbirth miscarriages neurological problems and maternal as well as fetal hemorrhage.[93,94]

Table 35.5 Thromboprophylactic doses of low molecular weight heparin[11,102]

Weight (kg)	Enoxaparin**	Dalteparin**	Tinzaparin** (75 unit/kg/day)
<50	20 mg/day	2,500 unit/day	3,500 unit/day
50–90	40 mg/day	5,000 unit/day	4,500 unit/day
90–130	60 mg/day*	7,500 unit/day*	7,000 unit/day*
131–170	80 mg/day*	10,000 unit/day*	9,000 unit/day*
>170	0.6 mg/kg/day*	75 unit/kg/day	75 unit/kg/day*
50–90 kg High prophylactic doses	40 mg/12-hourly	5,000 units 12-hourly	4,500 units 12-hourly
Treatment dose	1 mg/kg/12-hourly antenatal/1.5 mg/kg/daily postnatal	100 unit/kg/12-hourly antenatal/200 units/kg/daily postnatal	or 175 unit/kg/daily antenatal or postnatal

*May be given in two divided doses.

**Monitor anti-Xa values especially when given for mechanical valve.

Although the absolute incidence is unknown, but drug has been transferred in pregnancy drug category (FDA) "D" from "X." The risk does appear to be dose-related, with a very low incidence in patients taking 5 mg per day or less.[95] Most safe and practical alternative LWMH is difficult to get monitored and multiple studies have shown that LWMH therapy is associated with a higher incidence of thrombotic complications during the pregnancy.[93-96] The low-dose warfarin used throughout pregnancy is probably the safe approach from the maternal perspective, in country like India. Preconception counseling is important about the risk or benefit of drug regimen. The current recommendations suggest use of subcutaneous unfractionated heparin before the sixth week of gestation and to discontinue warfarin for a while. The warfarin can be restarted after 12th weeks of gestation.[11,94-97] Heparin should be restarted at the 36th week of gestation to minimize the risk of fetal intracranial hemorrhage during delivery. Alternatively, elective CS can be planned after 36 weeks and heparin infusion can be started till the 4 hours before of surgery.

Low-dose aspirin[97-99]

There are meta-analysis trials supporting usefulness of aspirin in VTE and pulmonary embolism prevention.[11,30,97,98]

American College of Chest Physicians (ACCP) guideline does not recommends its use.[97] Aspirin is appropriate for women with antiphospholipid syndrome to improve fetal outcomes.[11,30,98,99] There were no adverse fetal outcomes reported in meta-analysis of large randomized control trials of low-dose aspirin for prevention of pre-eclampsia in pregnancy.[99]

Other oral anticoagulant drugs: see Box 35.5.

Thrombolysis in Pregnancy[100-102]

Thrombolysis is a relative contraindication unless patient is having life-threatening hypotension and shock.

It carries 8% chance of maternal-hemorrhage and 6% of risk for fetus; although thrombolytic agents like streptokinase or recombinant tissue plasminogen activator have poor ability to cross placental barrier. The results of fibrinolysis during the pregnancy are not studied properly. In a review, the results of use of the recombinant tissue plasminogen activator for the fibrinolysis on 28 pregnant patients where 7 women had thrombosis of prosthetic valve, were analyzed by Leonhardt et al. In this series, 7% maternal mortality, 11% therapeutic failure and 24% fetal and peripartum mortality were reported.[100] Fasullo et al. thrombolyzed a 26-year-old woman with massive pulmonary embolism, with tPA, successfully. They concluded that disadvantages of fibrinolysis have to be weighed against the mortality benefit to the patient.[101] Surgery may be better choice in the management of thrombosis of mitral valve (MV) prosthesis during the pregnancy.

The thromboprophylaxis and prophylactic antiplatelet agents are recommended in pregnant women with history of Kawasaki disease and coronary artery aneurysm.[102]

Box 35.5 Other oral anticoagulant drugs

- *Danaparoid* a heparinoid, can be used in pregnant women with heparin intolerance; it has both anti-IIa and anti-Xa effects and is given IV or SC injections.[89-91]
- *Fondaparinux* is a synthetic pentasaccharide that functions through specific inhibition of factor Xa via antithrombin. It has a broadly similar efficacy to LMWH. No placental passage of fondaparinux was found in a human cotyledon model.[89-90]
- *Lepirudin* is a direct thrombin inhibitor is used in the management of patients with heparin-induced thrombocytopenia. It may cross placenta and may cause embryopathy.[87]
- *Oral thrombin and Xa inhibitors* rivaroxaban, apixaban and edoxaban, and the thrombin inhibitor—dabigatran etexilate (dabigatran) have gained approval for use in several indications, most notably for the prevention and treatment of VTE and for the prevention of stroke in patients with atrial fibrillation. Hepatic impairment can affect the disposition. Its pharmacokinetics in pregnancy is not known.[92]

SECTION III
CARDIAC DISEASES IN PREGNANCY

PREGNANCY IN PATIENTS WITH PRE-EXISTING CARDIOMYOPATHIES

The presence of pre-existing cardiomyopathy (CMP) compromises the cardiac reserve of the patient and there is a chance of cardiac decompensation during labor resulting into arrhythmias, ventricular dysfunction, low output heart failure and occasionally may culminate into maternal death. A highly experienced and well-equipped multidisciplinary center must be available. Preconception counseling to explain the risks and outcome of pregnancy for both mother and fetus, must be explained to the family. Genetic counseling must be done in appropriate cases where genetic etiology is suspected. Diagnosis of onset of heart failure sometimes may be indistinguishable from that of usual physiological changes associated with pregnancy. Although limited clinical data are available, measuring BNP or NT-proBNP levels seems to have clinical utility when the diagnosis of heart failure is in question.[11,103]

Dilated Cardiomyopathy and Peripartum Cardiomyoathy[104–110]

The women with dilated cardiomyopathy (DCM) and peripartum cardiomyopathy (PPCM) present with low ejection fraction and dilated heart and need similar line of management but relative outcome is better for DCM patients.

In pregnant women with DCM, the risk of adverse cardiac events is considerable, and pre-pregnancy characteristics can identify women at the highest risk. Pregnancy seems to have a short-term negative impact on the clinical course in women with DCM.[11,17]

Peripartum cardiomyopathy is defined as a dilated cardiomyopathy with congestive heart failure within the last month of pregnancy or within 5 months of delivery. This condition occurs at a rate of 1 in 2,289 live births and risk factors are multiparity, advanced maternal age, pre- eclampsia, gestational hypertension, and African descent. Some studies show a 75% recovery rate to normal ventricular function. Although the cause is not well understood, the treatment remains similar to that for congestive heart failure in general. Recent research papers have shown that a 16 kDa subform that is derived from proteolytic cleavage of prolactin hormone, probably secondary to peripartal oxidative stress, may be responsible for PPCM. This subform is a potent anti- angiogenic, proapoptotic and proinflammatory in nature. Therefore, there is hope that therapy with bromocriptine, a dopamine D2 receptor agonist can be used to prevent the occurrence as well as recurrence of PPCM in susceptible patients.[104]

Bernstein et al. showed that women with stable DCM may do well during pregnancy without significant deterioration in their cardiac status. They compared 23 mothers with PPCM to 8 expectant mothers with DCM. In DCM group cardiac status remained stable in all but one case where LVEF was <15% from the beginning. Whereas PPCM group had three maternal deaths while four other women needed the heart transplant. Infants born to mothers from both the groups, had comparable good outcome. Authors concluded that over-all outcome of mothers varies in two groups. In view of this fact, counseling of the patient and family must be done accordingly.[105] The treatment of PPCM and DCM is similar which includes judicious use of diuretics, digoxin, β-blockers and vasodilators like oral hydralazine. The Angiotensin-Converting Enzyme (ACE) inhibitors are contraindicated. Anticoagulants have a role when clot is detected or when EF is low predisposing the patient for intracardiac thrombosis. Mortality for PPCM is between 25% and 50%.[11,106] The normal vaginal delivery is preferred. Basic principles for labor induction and anesthetic management are discussed above. The future pregnancy must be avoided in those whose LV function fails to recover.[107-110]

Idiopathic Hypertrophic Subaortic Stenosis[11,111]

Idiopathic hypertrophic subaortic stenosis (IHSS) is a form of LV hypertrophy, usually presenting with left ventricular outflow tract (LVOT) obstruction. Unlike other form of AS, the hemodynamic limitations of IHSS are produced as the ventricle contracts. The hypertrophied walls narrow the outflow region during systole. There is systolic anterior motion of anterior mitral leaflet to increase LVOT obstruction. The severity of obstruction is directly proportional to the contractility of ventricle, inversely proportion to the preload, and SVR. The patient, therefore, requires a high preload in order to maintain a full left ventricle, a reduced contractile force in order to minimize outflow tract narrowing, and a high SVR to maintain distension of the left ventricle during systole. Optimization of volume therapy and β-blockers are the main therapeutic agents. In HCM, cardioversion should be considered for persistent atrial fibrillation.

HYPERTENSION IN PREGNANCY

Hypertension in pregnancy needs special definition, as the normal values differ from that of pre-pregnancy values. It is diagnosed if there is an absolute rise of SBP above 140 mm Hg and DBP above 90 mm Hg. The elevation must be recorded at least in two different occasions. The relative rise of BP from the first reading taken on booking may also be considered to be potential hypertensive. The reading must be taken in sitting position and with appropriate cuff size. If BP is low on lying down position, the woman must be lying on side.

Korotkoff phases I and V (disappearance) must be used to record BP. Phase IV is recorded when phase V is not present.[112]

Hypertension during pregnancy can be classified into three main categories—chronic hypertension, gestational hypertension, and pre-eclampsia, with or without pre-existing hypertension. There are additional group of patients who are included in a separate group under "other" category. In general, hypertensive disorders can complicate 12–22% of pregnancies and are a major cause of maternal morbidity and mortality. The reported recurrence risk in literature was 19%, 32%, and 46% for gestational hypertension, pre-eclampsia, and pre-eclampsia superimposed on pre-existing chronic hypertension, respectively. In addition, severe isolated intrauterine growth restriction (IUGR) is also a risk factor for developing hypertension in a subsequent pregnancy.[11,112-116]

Table 35.6 Features associated with severe preeclampsia

Features	Findings in severe pre-eclampsia[117]
Gestational age	<35 weeks
Diastolic BP	>110 mm Hg
Headache	Present
Visual disturbances	Present
Abdominal pain	Present
Oliguria	Present
$S_{Creatinine}$ (GFR)	Elevated
LDH, AST	Elevated
Proteinuria	Nephrotic range (>3 g/24 h)
Nonreassuring fetal testing	Present

Types of Hypertension in Pregnancy[11,116-118]

Pre-existing Hypertension

If preconception or before 20 weeks of gestation BP is ≥140/90 mm Hg, it is most likely to persist after the pregnancy. About 1–5% cases may fall in this category. There might be associated proteinuria.

Gestational Hypertension

The onset of hypertension after 20 weeks of gestation that is likely to resolve within the 42 days postpartum, is called as gestational hypertension and is not associated with abnormal proteinuria. The women have a risk to develop essential hypertension in later life.

Pre-eclampsia (Table 35.6)

Pre-eclampsia is a pregnancy-specific syndrome that occurs after mid-gestation, defined by the de novo appearance of hypertension, accompanied by new-onset of significant proteinuria 0.3 g/24 h.

It is a systemic disorder with both maternal and fetal manifestations. Edema is no longer considered part of the diagnostic criteria, as it occurs in up to 60% of normal pregnancies. Pre-eclampsia is characterized by proteinuria, usually presenting late. The suggestive findings in early stage are—onset of de novo HT, headache, visual disturbance abdominal pain, abnormal laboratory test, specifically low platelet counts, and abnormal liver enzymes. Table 35.6 lists features associated with severe pre-eclampsia.

Combination of Pre-existing HT with Superimposed Gestational HT and Proteinuria

When pre-existing hypertension is associated with further worsening of BP and protein excretion ≥3 g/day in 24-hour urine collection after 20 weeks of gestation.

Antenatal Unclassifiable Hypertension

The first abnormal blood pressure is recorded after 20 weeks of gestation. These patients must be treated according to guidelines for hypertension in pregnancy. The follow-up must be done 42 weeks postpartum, to know the long-term prognosis of it.

Chronic Hypertension

The BP persisting equal or above the 140/90 mm Hg from preconception time and remains same beyond the 42nd postpartum day. The treatment regime must be changed to safer antihypertensive drugs for the fetus during the pregnancy.

Late Postpartum Hypertension

Late postpartum hypertension is usually mild, appears several weeks to 6 months of postpartum period and then normalizes by the end of first postpartum year.[118]

Managing Hypertension in Pregnancy: Key Points[11,113–126]

A. *Criteria to start pharmacological management:*
   1. SBP (systolic blood pressure) of 150 mm Hg and a DBP (diastolic blood pressure) of 95 mm Hg (any circumstances).
   2. SBP of 140 mm Hg or a DBP of 90 mm Hg (for gestational hypertension ± proteinuria, pre-existing hypertension with the superimposition of gestational hypertension, hypertension with subclinical organ damage or symptoms at any time during pregnancy).

B. *Nonpharmacological management of borderline systemic hypertension (SBP of 140–150 mm Hg or DBP of 90–99 mm Hg, or both):* It includes bed rest if required, hospitalization, lateral position, salt restriction, calcium (1 g/day) and fish oil, micronutrients, low-dose asprin.[116,123-124]

C. *Choice of drug (Table 35.7)*[11,117,118]
   1. *First-line antihypertensive drug during pregnancy:* Methyldopa.
   2. *First-line antihypertensive postpartum:* Atenolol.
   3. Angiotensin enzyme inhibitors reported as fetotoxic capable of producing oligohydramnios, IUGR, joint contracture, pulmonary hypoplasia, hypocalvaria (incomplete ossification of the fetal skull), fetal renal tubular dysplasia and neonatal renal failure, and must not be used. They are not teratogenic.

D. *Management of hypertensive emergency (hospitalization is required)*
   - *SBP ≥170 mm Hg or DBP ≥110 mm Hg:* A pregnant woman with these values must be treated as an emergency. Pharmacological treatment with IV labetalol or oral methyldopa or nifedipine should be initiated. The drug of choice in hypertensive crises is sodium nitroprusside given as an IV infusion at 0.25-5.0 mg/kg/min.
   - The drug of choice in pre-eclampsia associated with pulmonary edema, is nitroglycerin (glyceryl trinitrate) given as an IV infusion of 5 mg/min and gradually increased every 3-5 minutes to a maximum dose of 100 mg/min.
   - *Indication-induction of labor:* Induction of labor is indicated if gestational HT is associated with proteinuria, visual disturbances coagulation abnormalities or fetal distress.

The women having hypertension during pregnancy have potential to become hypertensive in later life when compared with nulliparous counterpart. Pregnancy may offer a glimpse of future cardiovascular health of a woman. Conversely there is no such opportunity to have a glance in future cardiovascular health of men.[126]

Table 35.7 Drug therapy of hypertension in pregnancy[11,113,115–119]

First line drugs
1. *Alpha methyldopa (Per oral route, PO):* 0.5–3.0 g/day in two divided doses. Drug of choice according to NHBEP working group;
2. *Labetolol (PO):* 200–1200 mg/day in two to three divided
Second line drugs
1. *Hydralazine (PO):* 50–300 mg/day in two to four divided doses
2. *Nifedipine (PO):* 30–120 mg/day of a slow release pre paration
3. *β-Blockers (PO):* Depends on specific agent
Contraindicated drugs
1. Angiotensin converting enzyme inhibitors (PO)
2. Angiotensin receptor blockers (PO)
3. Aldosterone antagonists (PO)
Drugs to be avoided
1. Thiazide diuretics
Severe hypertensive urgency or emergency first line drugs
1. *Labetalol (Intravenous route—IV):* 20 mg IV, then 20–80 mg every 20–30 minutes, up to a maximum of 300 mg; or constant infusion of 1–2 mg/min
2. β-Blockers (IV)
3. Nifedipine (PO) tablets recommended only; 10–30 mg orally, repeat in 45 minutes if needed
4. Hydralazine IV (not recommended in ESC guidelines 2013; it can be considered in mothers with positive cocaine use. 5 mg, IV or IM, then 5–10 mg every 20–40 minutes; or constant infusion of 0.5–10 mg/h)
5. Nitroprusside (IV) constant infusion of 0.5–10 g/kg/min there is positive evidence of human fetal risk, but the benefits of use in pregnant women may be acceptable despite the risk (e.g. if the drug is needed in a life-threatening situation or for a serious disease for which safer drugs cannot be used or are ineffective)

Primary Pulmonary Hypertension

According to definition, primary pulmonary hypertension (PPH) exists when mean pulmonary artery pressure remains elevated above the 25 mm Hg mean at rest, and no demonstrable primary etiology is found. The reason for the elevation is the permanent changes in pulmonary vasculature leading to medial hypertrophy, intimal changes, thrombosis, pulmonary vasoconstriction, dysfunctional pulmonary vascular endothelium.[127] Pregnancy in these patients can be lethal. The patients with PPH develop right heart failure and eventually LV output also goes down. The management goals for the woman with PPH are, to reduce the pulmonary pressure as much down as can be possible by using targeted pulmonary vasodilators. The fluid to be restricted to optimize preload and vasopressors must be used cautiously, as and when required. The anticoagulation is recommended to avoid pulmonary embolism. The intravenous prostaglandins (epoprostenol, treprostinil) and PDE 5 inhibitor sildenafil are kept in category "B" in WHO list of drug in pregnancy. The endothelin inhibitors and inhaled NO are categorized as "X." The patients with proven reactive pulmonary vasculature can be prescribed calcium channel blocker (category "C") drugs. The preferred mode of delivery is elective cesarean section either under regional and general anesthesia. The vaginal delivery can be preferred in less severe cases. Slow induction epidural anesthesia is advised for regional anesthesia. The use of nitric oxide (NO), a potent vasodilator during the labor in patients with PPH, has been reported recently.[127–130]

Coronary Artery Disease

Burden of Disease and Prevalence of Risk Factors

Although rare but pregnancy may lead to coronary artery dissection and acute myocardial infarction at relatively younger age in the peripartum period.

The overall reported incidence of AMI in pregnancy varies from 1 in 16,129 deliveries to 1 in 35,700. Roth et al. reported in a literature review that though AMI may occur in any stage of pregnancy, it is the most common in multiparous pregnant women of age group above 30 years, during the third trimester. Up to 78% of patients presenting with acute coronary syndrome (ACS) had anterior wall MI.[131–134]

In their second publication in 2008, Roth et al. reported an increasing incidence of known risk factors for AMI in this group of patients despite their young age. Forty-five percent mothers with AMI were smokers, 24% had hyperlipidemia, 22% had family histories of myocardial infarction (MI), 15% had hypertension, and 11% had DM. The other risk factors associated with ACS were pre-eclampsia, multiple parity, cocaine abuse, age over 35 years, coronary artery disease in the family history, previous MI or ischemic heart disease, pulmonary hypertension, shunts, and valvular diseases of the heart. Kawasaki disease may also be potential predictor of coronary event.[131–138] Pregnancy itself can boost chances to have coronary events, secondary to hypercoagulable state that predisposes for thrombosis. The degenerative effect of pregnancy on blood vessels stressed with increased blood flow and consequent intimal shear stress may lead to spontaneous coronary dissections. Coronary dissection, a rare cause of AMI in the nonpregnant population, was reported in 28 patients (27%) who had 41 dissected coronary arteries.[136] Coronary dissection was the primary cause of infarction in the peripartum period (50%) and was found more commonly in postpartum compared with antepartum cases (34% vs. 11%).[136]

Coronary artery morphology was studied (angiographically or at autopsy) in 93% (96/103) patients of the women included in a review. Atherosclerosis, with or without, intracoronary thrombus was found in 40%, and coronary thrombus without evidence of atherosclerotic disease was present in 8%. They found atherosclerotic disease in 54% of patients in antepartum period, 27% in peripartum and 29% in postpartum period.[136] This data suggests that patients having atherosclerotic changes in coronary arteries are more prone ACS, in antenatal period.

Management Plan (Box 35.6)

The management plan depends on the severity of symptom. Antenatal revascularization can be done, if needed. As mentioned above, normal vaginal delivery under epidural anesthesia is first choice unless the life-threatening situation demands CS. Shivering which is common during labor and administration of regional anesthesia should be strictly avoided. The oxytocin and ergot alkaloids both may cause coronary vasospasm. Oxytocin must be given in a diluted infusion form, whereas ergots alkaloids better not to be used. Use of small doses of phenylephrine rather than ephedrine is recommended to counter hypotension. Ephedrine may cause tachycardia.[11,132–136]

Myocardial ischemia during pregnancy must be treated conservatively unless there are compelling reasons to intervene. It includes bed-rest oxygen mask, avoidance of supine posture, and supportive pharmacological therapy which may be adequate in most of the patients. Thrombolysis has been used successfully for complex conditions like PE. The women with acute coronary events may also benefit from it though no guidelines are available. Thrombolysis with urokinase or tissue plasminogen activator can be done with caution. The placental transfer of these drugs may be minimal and they are not teratogenic.[11,134–136]

Percutaneous Transluminal Coronary Angioplasty

Severely symptomatic women with ACS may need catheter or surgical intervention for revascularization. Catheter procedures are reasonably safe and radiation exposure to fetus is prevented by shielding the abdomen.[11,135–138] The successful percutaneous transluminal coronary angioplasty and stenting procedure have been reported in literature.[11,135–138]

Box 35.6 CAD in pregnancy: recommendations for the management of coronary artery disease[11]

- ECG and troponin levels should be performed in the case of chest pain in a pregnant woman (IC).
- Coronary angioplasty is the preferred reperfusion therapy for STEMI during pregnancy (IC).
- A conservative management should be considered for non-ST elevation ACS without risk criteria (IIaC).
- An invasive management should be considered for non-ST elevation ACS with risk criteria (including NSTEMI) (IIaC).

Coronary Artery Bypass Grafting

More than 100 cardiac surgeries during pregnancy have been reported since 1959. However, fetal complications are common than maternal complication. The poor maternal outcome after coronary artery bypass grafting (CABG) can be due to patient characteristics. The chances of having cardiac surgery are more when coronary or coronary-aortic dissection is noticed; hence, surgery becomes more challenging in such a situation. However, avoidance of CPB by doing beating heart surgery can be safer than conventional surgery.[139] There are specific guidelines for CPB in a pregnant women and must be followed to avoid fetal complications.[57,58,61]

VALVULAR HEART DISEASES (BOX 35.7)

Valvular diseases are the most common form of CVD during the pregnancy in developing countries, due to high prevalence of rheumatic heart disease. A summary of management plan for valvular heart disease is given Box 35.7. These patients may present either with native or prosthetic valves with or

Box 35.7 Management of the valvar heart diseases[11,30,140,141,144,147,152-155]

- Mitral stenosis
  - Selective β-blockers (IC) are recommended for symptomatic MS with PAH
  - Additional diuretics (IB) to be added if CHF persist despite the β-blockers
  - Preconception intervention for severe MS (IC)
  - Therapeutic anticoagulation (IC) is advised to the cases of atrial fibrillation, LA thrombosis, or prior embolism
  - The pregnant women with severe MS who are symptomatic and have SPAP >50 mm Hg must go for balloon mitral valvoplasty (IIaC)
- Stenosis of aortic valve
  - Preconception aortic valvuloplasty is recommended for
  - Presence of symptom (IB)
  - LVEF is <50% (IC)
  - Severe AS, asymptomatic at rest but are symptomatic on exercise test (IC) or have fall in BP during the exercise (IIB)
- Regurgitation of valves
  - Those patients with severe AR and MR must undergo surgery, who are symptomatic or they have impaired ventricular function or significant LV dilatation should be treated surgically preconception (IC)
  - Medical management must be done for symptomatic MR/AR patients (IC)
- Mechanical valve
  - Oral anticoagulants are recommended 12–36 weeks of gestation (IC)
  - Change in anticoagulation protocol must be done after the hospitalization (IC)
  - If labor starts on oral anticoagulants, the CS is preferred (IC)
  - In routine, the OAC must be discontinued by 36 weeks and ultrafractionated heparin (aPTT) more than 2X control)/LMWH (anti-Xa level 4–6 hours postdose 0.8–1.2 unit/mL and then assess weekly (IC)
  - At least 36 hours before planned labor, UFH must be started and LMWH must be stopped (IC). IV heparin must continue before 4–6 hours of planned labor and then must be restarted after the delivery of baby if there is no bleeding problems
  - Sudden onset of arrhythmia or embolic event in a pregnant woman must be investigated with echocardiography
  - The first trimester use of OAC may be allowed (IIaC) with written consent if therapeutic doses are low (<5 mg/day warfarin <3 mg/day for phenprocoumon <2 mg/day acenocoumarol), LMWH should only be used if anti-Xa levels can be monitored (IIIC)

Abbreviations: aPTT, activated partial thromboplastin activated partial thromboplastin time; AS, aortic stenosis; LMWH, low molecular weight heparin; LVEF, left ventricular ejection fraction; MS, mitral stenosis; OAC, oral anticoagulants; UFH, ¼ unfractionated heparin.

Class I: are indicated; IIa, can be considered; IIb, can be considered; III, cannot be recommended.

Level of evidence: A, evidence from multiple randomized clinical trial or meta-analysis; B, evidence from a single randomized clinical trial or large non-randomized studies from a single randomized clinical trial or large non-randomized studies; C, consensus opinion of experts. Consensus of opinion of the experts and or retrospective studies.

without additional complications. They can be acquired or congenital like bicuspid aortic valve. A diseases heart valve can be obstructive or regurgitant. The hemodynamic effects may be same in congenital or acquired variety but severity and management as well as response to management may differ (Table 35.8). Specific problems, mainly related to anticoagulant therapy, are present in women with mechanical valve prostheses.

The evaluation of valvular heart disease is based on transthoracic echo or transesophageal echo (Table 35.8). There are well-defined criteria in literature to grade the severity. In few patients, exercise testing can be useful to understand the severity of valvular obstruction or myocardial capacity to cope with stress.

Rheumatic Heart Disease and Pregnancy

In 1936, Henderson et al. reported a series of 35 pregnant women with RHD.[141] They also reported less number of CS (46% in previous series vs. 2.8% in this series) and successful outcome of vaginal delivery, when compared to previous series. It led to shift of the protocol towards either the normal labor or forceps assisted delivery. Only one death occurred in the study population that too after 27 days of forceps delivery, whereas previous series where CS was the preferential mode for delivery showed maternal mortality of 5–8%.

Mitral valve is the most common valve to be involved in rheumatic process. The incidence of MS is around 90% and MR 7%. The second most common valve involved is aortic valve (AS = 1%; AR = 2.5%). In RHD patients, involvement of tricuspid and pulmonary valve is never in isolation and such involvement is always combined with mitral or aortic disease.[142–145]

Irrespective of etiology, the stenotic valve diseases carry a higher pregnancy risk than regurgitant lesions, and left-sided valve diseases have a higher complication rate than right-sided valve lesions. Table 35.8 elaborates on the predictors of poor prognosis.

Table 35.8 Valvular heart lesions associated with high maternal and/or fetal risk during pregnancy[11,16–18]

- Severe aortic stenosis with or without symptoms
- Aortic regurgitation with NYHA functional class III–IV symptoms
- Mitral stenosis with NYHA functional class II–IV symptoms
- Mitral regurgitation with NYHA functional class III–IV symptoms
- AV and/or MV disease resulting in severe PAH (PAP >75% of systemic pressures)
- AV/MV disease with severe LV dysfunction (LVEF <40%)
- Mechanical prosthetic valve requiring anticoagulation
- Marfan's syndrome with or without aortic regurgitation

Abbreviations: LV, left ventricular; LVEF, LV ejection fraction; NYHA, New York Heart Association; AV, aortic valve; MV, mitral valve; PAH, polycyclic aromatic hydrocarbons.

In recent publications, high incidence RHD and its presentation with complications have been reported. The rheumatic heart disease accounted for 88% of pregnant women with CVD.[5] The rheumatic heart disease was present in 44% of pregnant women presenting with the stroke.[145]

Mitral Stenosis

In presence of moderate-to-severe fixed obstruction at MV, the capacity of body to upsurge cardiac output is limited. Restricted forward flow at MV, MS augments LA pressure and pulmonary venous hypertension. The RHD with the MS is the most common variety of CVD in pregnancy. Data regarding the association of congenital MS with the pregnancy are lacking. Probably, the patients with significant obstruction are being treated in childhood and may present in adulthood with repaired or replaced MV.

Heart failure in MS depends on severity of lesion and often is progressive. Atrial fibrillation can further hasten hemodynamic decompensation leading to pulmonary edema. AF also contributes to the thrombosis and may cause thromboembolism in 15% cases. The reported mortality is 0–3% in severe cases. Risk to fetus is well correlated with NYHA class and grades of pulmonary edema. The fetal complications are prematurity 20–30%, intrauterine growth retardation 5–20%, and stillbirth 1–3%.[146]

Preconception assessment of patients must be done to grade the severity of MS. The diagnosis is based on echocardiographic findings. Usually, pressure half time, direct planimetry, mean gradient across MV and PAP are the indicators used in non-pregnant mothers to evaluate severity. However, except MVA all other parameters may be fallacious during the pregnancy. The medical management with diuretics, β-blockers and anticoagulants are recommended if required. Anesthetic management is oriented toward the avoidance of tachycardia, as the time required for LV diastolic filling is prolonged. Activity must be restricted in symptomatic patients. Percutaneous balloon valvoplasty can also be undertaken beyond 20 weeks of pregnancy in presence of significant dyspnea (NYHA III, IV) and pulmonary hypertension (PAP > 50 mm Hg) with adequate shielding of abdomen. BMV increases cardiac output without a need for anticoagulation. BMV is contraindicated in presence of mitral regurgitation (MR), AF, or clots. Preferred mode of delivery is not CS unless absolutely needed.[11,141]

Aortic Stenosis

The isolated aortic stenosis (AS) is caused by unicuspid or bicuspid aortic valve. Usually, bicuspid aortic valve is associated with pathological aortic dilatation that is a substrate for the aortic dissection. The recommendations are to keep a close watch on aortic dimensions pre- and postpregnancy, and surgery should be considered when the aortic diameter is 50 mm. A careful evaluation to rule out coarctation of aorta must be done.[147-151]

Yap et al. recognized 35 women with congenital aortic stenosis who had a total of 58 pregnancies, of which 53 were successful. The outcome of pregnancy depends upon the degree of hypertrophy of LV and its systolic and diastolic functional capacity. The cardiac output is fixed for these mothers. The complication of AS reported in 9.4% cases in this study, the most common were the heart failure and atrial arrhythmias. Obstetric and perinatal complications were 22.6% and 24.5%, respectively. The premature delivery was 13.2% and small-for-gestational age births were also common. Severe aortic stenosis is an incremental risk factor for heart failure and premature labor.[149]

Pregnancy is contraindicated in all symptomatic patients with severe AS or asymptomatic patients with impaired LV function, significant LV hypertrophy (posterior wall ≥15 mm), the echo-evidence of recent progression of gradient, recent evidence of arrhythmia, or a pathological exercise test. The patient should be counseled to get pre-pregnancy valvuloplasty or surgery.[11,152,153] Pregnancy is allowed in asymptomatic patients with severe AS but normal LVEF and normal exercise test (Table 35.8).[11,154,155] Heart failure occurs in 10% of patients with severe AS and arrhythmias in 3–25%. Maternal mortality is now rare in mothers with VHD if careful management is provided.[11,150-155]

The conservative management with restricted activities is indicated for patients with heart failure. The tachycardia in patients presenting with AF can be avoided by prescribing the β-blocker or a nondihydropyridine CCB. Digoxin is an alternative choice in patients who are not tolerating or responding to beta blockers or CCB drugs.[152] Catheter intervention and balloon valvuloplasty can be tried in unstable patients with isolated AS.[153-155]

Valve replacement should be considered if all other methods fail. Preferably, baby can be delivered through CS before going for CPB. In severe AS, CS done with intubation and GA is preferred method of delivery.[153-155] In nonsevere AS, vaginal delivery is preferred as discussed above.

Regurgitant Lesions: Mitral and Aortic Regurgitation

The regurgitant aortic and MV at childbearing age can be of rheumatic, congenital, or degenerative in origin. The RHD is usual culprit when multiple valves are involved. Previous valvulotomy and infective endocarditis may also be causative factors.[11,153,154] The cardiologic complications like left-sided regurgitant lesions that might be hemodynamically significant are also common in antiphospholipid syndrome.[156] These patients may also have acute MI, pericardial effusion, and pulmonary hypertension.

Left-sided regurgitant valve lesions with preserved LV function are well-tolerated than stenotic lesions, since decreased SVR decreases the afterload of LV. However, the decreased systolic function of LV is not tolerated well. Likewise, acute regurgitant lesions have bad prognosis. Sudden deterioration in the asymptomatic women with preserved LV function must be investigated for the presence of the arrhythmias. As narrated above, preconception risk stratification must be done before making a management plan.[153,154,157]

Conversely, the hemodynamic implications of MR and AR are not exactly same. Hemodynamics of MR differs with that of aortic regurgitation. In MR, the LV has a low pressure chamber to offload its volume hence true contractility is masked until lesion is corrected. In MR, myocardial function is overestimated.[158] In a recently published study, echocardiographic evaluation of pregnant women with MR was done. The LV wall was relatively thinner than control, suggesting further chamber dilatation as an effect of pregnancy that may be secondary to increased blood volume.[159] Therefore, the tailored management is warranted for either of lesions.

Maternal cardiovascular risk depends on severity of regurgitation, symptoms, and degree of heart failure. Maternal and fetal risks are closely associated with severity of lesions, ventricular function, and presence arrhythmias. The normal or assisted vaginal delivery is preferable if patient is otherwise stable.[11,153,154,157]

The goals for anesthesia are specific in patients with left-sided regurgitant lesions: (1) to keep the SVR low by minimizing pain; (2) decrease the regurgitation time by avoiding bradycardia; and (3) myocardial suppressant must be avoided. Preconception repair of valve can be planned. Follow-up plans need to be adapted according to clinical status and symptoms.

Symptoms must be managed with rest, fluid restriction, and decongestives. Acute severe regurgitation may need surgery, and if surgery is done when fetus has crossed the age of viability, baby must be delivered before cardiac surgery.

Selection of Valve Prosthesis

An ideal valve must have following features:
1. Long durability and low thrombogenicity.
2. Low prosthesis patient mismatch and low postoperative transprosthetic gradient.
3. Should have largest valve effective orifice area in relation to the annulus of the patient.[160]

The mechanical valves are durable and perform excellently in relation to hemodynamics. Major issue with them is thrombosis.[11,154,160-165] Bioprosthetic valves offer good hemodynamic performance and low thrombogenicity but degenerate early and there is a definite chance for reoperation with the mortality risk of 0.5%.[163] Pregnancy may accelerate the degenerative process.[11,154,162] Ross procedure is alternative surgery for young population. In this procedure, the pulmonary valve is transferred to the aortic valve position and a homo- or heterograft is placed in RVOT position.[164,165]

The operation is technically demanding and has significant reoperation rate after 10 years. It provides growth potential to aortic valve and root and no chance of aortic thrombosis.[165]

Mechanical Prosthesis and Anticoagulation

Mechanical valves carry the increased risk of valve thrombosis and neurological complications, secondary to thromboembolism, during pregnancy. There are controversies regarding the strategy for thromboprophylaxis during pregnancy.[160-163-,166] Anticoagulation can be prescribed in three possible approaches[11,166-169]: (1) low-molecular-weight (LMW) heparin administered subcutaneously twice daily throughout pregnancy, (2) unfractionated heparin administered subcutaneously twice daily throughout pregnancy, or (3) unfractionated or LMW heparin administered subcutaneously twice daily until gestational week 13, followed by warfarin from weeks 13–35, followed by a return to unfractionated or LMW heparin administered subcutaneously twice daily until delivery takes place. The UFH and LMWH are safe drugs as they do not cross placenta and are free from risk of embryopathy. But they can be used only by parenteral route. LMWH are effective, more easy to use and their pharmacokinetics is such that they can be given without regular monitoring of antiFactor Xa activity.[85,86] Chan et al. in a large series reviewed the risk for valve-thrombosis in three recommended regimes. The risk for valve-thrombosis was 3.9% with OACs throughout pregnancy, 9.2% when UFH was used in the first trimester, and OACs in the second and third trimester, and 33% with UFH throughout pregnancy. Maternal death occurred in these groups in 2%, 4%, and 15%, respectively, and was usually related to valve thrombosis.[166]

Nevertheless, in rural India where RHD is more prevalent, OACs have distinct advantage. There are evidence in literature that warfarin can be safe throughout the pregnancy. Cotrufo et al. found no abortions or malformations in a group of patients whose warfarin requirement was <5 mg/day.[168]

Meschengieser et al. found no such correlation. They found warfarin as a safe anticoagulants in patients with prosthetic valve and pregnancy.[163] The fetus of the mothers on OACs are in increased risk for intracranial bleed during the forceps assisted delivery.

Despite the evidence from literature about the safety of OACs in pregnancy when INR is under strict control, dilemma exists because adequate randomized studies that compare different regimens are not available. The superiority of either UFH or LMWH in the first trimester is unproven, though a recent review suggests higher efficacy of LMWH.[167]

CONGENITAL HEART DISEASE

Several recent studies have addressed congenital heart disease (CHD) in pregnancy. In general, the acyanotic shunt or regurgitant lesions are well tolerated, whereas acyanotic obstructive or cyanotic lesions are poorly tolerated. Accordingly, the acyanotic shunt lesions are safer during the pregnancy. The results are analogous between the atrial and ventricular septal defects, atrioventricular septal defects (AVSDs). The cyanotic CHDs [tetralogy of Fallot (TOF) or other complex CHD] with NYHA class I or II where saturation and systemic ventricular function are good, pregnancy is tolerated well.

Agrawal et al. reported better maternal and perinatal outcome in pregnant woman with acyanotic heart disease in analysis of 196 pregnancies with CHD.[170] When compared with acyanotic patients, cyanotic group showed high incidence of cardiac complications. The incidence of pregnancy induced hypertension (16.6% vs. 5.2%) prematurity (25% vs. 11.6%)/IUGR (50% vs. 15.1%) abortion (4.1% vs. 2.1%) were higher. In CCHD group, there were four cases of maternal mortality; of which two women had Eisenmenger's syndrome. In acyanotic group, two mortality happened—one before the delivery and other one after the delivery. Recently, Baliant et al. highlighted incidence of late cardiac events (LCE) appearing after 6 months of pregnancy in 50 out of 405 (12%) cases in a series.[151] Occurrence of LCE was correlated with adverse cardiac events during the pregnancy. Those women who had dyspnea, cyanosis, subaortic ventricular dysfunction, subpulmonary ventricular dysfunction, significant PR, LVF, and cardiac events before or during pregnancy were at higher risk.[151] Presbitero et al. reported relatively better outcome for mothers with CCHD but high chances of adverse fetal outcome.[171]

Atrial Septal Defect

Atrial septal defect (ASD) is a shunt lesion between the two atria that can be classified in four groups. ASDs are common and can present at any age. Females constitute 65–75% of patients with secundum ASDs, but the gender distribution is equal for sinus venosus and ostium primum ASDs. It usually manifests late and patient may present with dyspnea on exertion, palpitation, paradoxical embolism, or intractable atrial arrhythmias. About 10–15% patients may have high PA pressure.[172-174]

Literature shows significant disproportion between systemic and pulmonary circulation in presence of ASD. There were evidence of RV strain pattern and increased episodes of atrial tachycardia.[173] Asymptomatic women with ASD or those who are in NYHA class I or II are likely to have uneventful pregnancy. Symptomatic women with NYHA class >II, severe hemodynamic compromise, history of recurrent stroke prior to or during pregnancy, can be considered for catheter or surgical closure of ASD in the second trimester. According to one study, incidence of stillbirths, recurrence of congenital heart defect in the offspring, or long-term cardiac complications were similar when the mothers with repaired ASD were compared with those who had unrepaired ASDs. However, incidence of miscarriage, preterm delivery, and cardiac symptoms during pregnancy were higher in women who had unrepaired ASD.[175]

Normal vaginal delivery as a rule is preferred mode as mentioned above.

Post-tricuspid Shunt Lesions

Ventricular Septal Defect, Patent Ductus Arteriosus and Aortopulmonary Window

The incidence of ventricular septal defect (VSD) is approximately 3.0–3.5 infants per 1,000 live births. The VSD may exist as isolated lesion or as an integral part of complex anatomy. Other acyanotic lesions associated with VSD are left-sided obstructive or regurgitant lesions, ASD, patent ductus arteriosus (PDA), etc. The VSD is prototype of post-tricuspid shunt lesions. Patent ductus arteriosus and A-P window are other disorders that manifest either with volume and pressure or in late stage, only pressure overload of lungs.

Women with small VSDs, no PAH, and no associated lesions have no increased cardiovascular risk for pregnancy. Pregnancy is generally well tolerated in the absence of pulmonary obstructive vascular disease (POVD), with no maternal mortality and no significant maternal or fetal morbidity. Although the left-to-right shunt may increase with the increase in cardiac output during pregnancy, this is counterbalanced by the decrease in peripheral resistance. Women with large shunts and PAH may experience arrhythmias, ventricular dysfunction, and progression of PAH. Pre-eclampsia may occur more often in these women than in the normal population.[164,176]

Women having post-tricuspid shunt lesions (VSD, PDA, AP window) with Eisenmenger's syndrome (POVD with shunt reversal) should be counseled against pregnancy. Pregnancy in these patients is associated with excessive maternal and fetal mortality. The management plan for them remains on same principles as for VSD. AP window rarely present in adulthood without established obstructive pulmonary vascular disease.

Atrioventricular Septal Defect

The terms atrioventricular septal defect (AVSD), atrioventricular (AV) canal defect, and endocardial cushion defect can be used interchangeably to describe this group of defects. The defect has panorama of clinical presentation. In general, the isolated partial AVSD has similar perspective as with ASD. The complete AVSD with good ventricular size and nonobstructive RVOT/LVOT will behave like a nonrestrictive VSD. These patients may present with early Eisenmenger's syndrome. The AVSD may be associated with severe RVOT obstruction (TOF), LVOT obstruction, and heterotaxy syndrome. It can be complicated by arrhythmia, AV valve regurgitation and ventricular dysfunction during the course of pregnancy. The increased PAP and paradoxical embolism are additional risk factors. In a stable patient, normal vaginal delivery can be appropriate. Offspring mortality has been reported in 6%, primarily due to the occurrence of complex CHD. The possibility of recurrence in fetus and association with syndromes are specific issues related to the AVSD.[11,154,176,177]

All women with a history of AVSD should be evaluated before conception to ensure that there are no significant residual hemodynamic lesions that might complicate the management of pregnancy. The issue of pregnancy risk and preventive measures should be discussed with women with Down's syndrome. In noncomplicated AVSD, the principles of intrapartum management remain same as for VSD.

The operated patients with AVSD may present with de novo AV valve regurgitation.

Coarctation of Aorta

Coarctation of aorta is characterized by narrowing of the aorta at or near the insertion of ductus arteriosus. Upper limb hypertension, systolic and diastolic LV dysfunction, heart failure, renal dysfunction, pulmonary venous/arterial hypertension, and pulmonary edema in critical patients are principal concern. There may be associated aortic valve and aortic root disease in sizeable number of cases. During the pregnancy, the risk of rupture and dissection of aorta considerably increases. Furthermore, these patients have poor postcoarct perfusion and have high fetal mortality rate (up to 20%). β-blockers are helpful for maternal benefit, but they may have negative impact on fetal growth. The anesthetic management must focus on maintaining near normal heart rate and SVR and adequate intravascular volume. The paradox of coarctation of aorta is such that upper part of body keep on struggling to prevent complications secondary to the systemic hypertension, while lower part of body remains hypotensive and hypoperfused. Hence, pregnancy with coarctation has significant maternal mortality (3–9%) and high fetal loss (up to 20%). If correction is not possible, close BP monitoring and regular follow-up to see the fetal well-being are recommended.[176–180]

Vriend et al. reviewed the CONCOR national registry on CHD (Netherlands) and reported miscarriage rate of 18% in 54 women with repaired coarctation of aorta who had 126 pregnancy.[180] Total 26 episodes of pregnancy were complicated by hypertension and five mothers had pre-eclampsia. Five women had increase in gradient across the repaired coarct gradient. Only one of them needed intervention after the delivery.[180]

Management of hypertension, while maintaining good perfusion of fetoplacental unit is required. Percutaneous intervention for re-CoA is possible during pregnancy. The use of covered stents may lower the risk of dissection. The risk of dissection is higher during a procedure in the pregnancy. Spontaneous vaginal delivery is preferred with use of epidural anesthesia particularly in hypertensive patients if there is no imminent danger to fetus and mother.[11,178–180]

Pulmonary Valve Stenosis and Regurgitation

Valvular pulmonary stenosis is usually tolerated well unless the RV pressures are systemic or suprasystemic leading to RV failure.[11,176,181] The ballooning procedure can be undertaken in second trimester with adequate shielding of the abdomen. There is a risk of recurrence in fetus. Usually, according to convention normal vaginal delivery with epidural anesthesia remains the best choice.[11,176] The severe pulmonary regurgitation is an independent risk factor for maternal complication. Preconception relief of stenosis (usually by balloon valvulotomy) is recommended for severe pulmonary valve stenosis if peak Doppler gradient is >64 mm Hg. Likewise, preconception pulmonary valve implantation is recommended if criteria for pulmonary valve implantation with bio-prosthesis are fulfilled in patients with previous corrective surgery and severe PR.[11] However, Greutmann et al. reported good outcome of pregnancy operated for CHD and who had residual RVOT lesions. Thirty-nine percent patients (30/76) had moderate-to-severe PR and 16% had RVOT obstruction ≥30 mm Hg. The right heart failure was more likely if there was moderate-to-severe PR in combination with at least one additional risk factor like twin pregnancy, peripheral pulmonary stenosis, right ventricular systolic dysfunction, and RV hypertrophy. They concluded that a careful antenatal medical follow-up and treatment with the diuretics yielded good outcome.[182]

Tetralogy of Fallot

Tetralogy of Fallot (TOF) is the CHD with a VSD and severe obstruction to right ventricular outflow letting direct entry of significant portion of systemic venous return into LV, and hence, cyanosis is conspicuous presenting feature. In unrepaired patients, surgical repair is indicated before pregnancy. Women with repaired TOF usually tolerate pregnancy well (WHO risk class II). Cardiac complications during pregnancy includes arrhythmias, heart failure, thromboembolism, and endocarditis. Like in patients with Marfan's syndrome, TOF patients may also have cystic medial necrosis, progressive aortic root dilatation and share risk of dissection.[182]

Kaur et al. reported in a retrospective analysis of perinatal outcome of mother and fetus in a mixed cohort of women with corrected and uncorrected TOF during the 1996–2008.[183]

Uncorrected TOF group had more obstetric and cardiac complications (70% vs. 40% and 40% vs. nil, respectively). The abortions and preterm birth were more in the unoperated group (37.5% and 25%, respectively, in uncorrected group vs. nil in corrected group). The incidence of IUGR or small for date baby, was more in uncorrected group (40% vs. 20%). Therefore, overall better maternal–fetal outcomes were expected for patients underwent correction before pregnancy. Right ventricular dysfunction and dilatation in presence of pulmonary regurgitation are the risk factors for adverse outcome of pregnancy. Preconception valve replacement is one of the preventive procedure.[184]

However, Greutmann et al. preferred close medical follow-up over the valve replacement.[185] Medical management includes cardiac evaluation with echocardiography, treatment with diuretics should be started and bed rest advised. Antenatal evaluation for presence of fetal CHD must be done and recurrence risk must also be explained to family.[186] The delivery must be planned as discussed in general principles of managing pregnancy in mothers with CVD.

Transposition of Great Vessels (VA Discordance)

The discordant ventriculoarterial connection needs early arterial or atrial switch operation. Arterial switch is anatomical correction, an ideal surgery with relatively event free survival. Atrial switch or Senning operation is a physiological correction where systemic ventricle is RV. Considerable number-of-late presenting patients are still undergoing atrial switch operation. Systemic RV is un-natural choice that eventually dilates, often develops tricuspid regurgitation leading to dysfunction in long run. Atrial arrhythmias are common in this subset of pregnant women (WHO risk class III). However, many women can tolerate pregnancy well. Those with atrial tachycardia or junctional rhythm can have further deterioration in functional status. β-Blockers may not be tolerated well. Ten percent women may have irreversible fall in RVEF. Patients with moderate-to-severe RV dysfunction and TR may be advised against carrying the pregnancy.[11,16,187]

The obstetric complications like pre-eclampsia and pregnancy-induced hypertension can be seen often. The rhythm disturbances, RV dysfunction, and systemic AV valve regurgitation are other complications seen in pregnant mothers with atrial switch.[11,187] In asymptomatic patients with moderate or good ventricular function, vaginal delivery is advised. If ventricular function deteriorates, an early cesarean delivery should be planned to avoid the development or worsening of heart failure.[187] Postarterial switch patient may have coronary insufficiency or supravalvar obstruction. Theoretically, they carry less risk and normal vaginal delivery must be preferred in these patients.[188]

Tricuspid Regurgitation

Tricuspid regurgitation can be primary, due to organic diseases of TV or secondary to annular dilatation in presence of volume or pressure overload of RV. The tricuspid regurgitation of any form can be treated conservatively. Surgical intervention can be done in adjunct to left-sided valve surgery pre- or postconception.[11,153] In symptomatic patients with severe TR tricuspid, valve repair can be done prepregnancy. As mentioned above, vaginal delivery is recommended in most of cases.

Ebstein's Anomaly

The Ebstein's anomaly per se does not cause sterility even if it is associated with cyanosis. In women with mild-to-moderate symptoms usually pregnancy is well tolerated. The patients with apparent heart failure and significant dyspnea and cyanosis preconception surgery can be performed or counseling must be done to avoid pregnancy. The problems seen during pregnancy depend primarily on the severity of the TR. The paradoxical emboli and arrhythmias pose additional risk for morbidity and mortality. Preferable mode of delivery is normal or forceps assisted vaginal delivery.[11,153,189]

Fontan Surgery

Women with Fontan palliation have low fertility but may have good outcome in absence of pulmonary hypertension, ventricular dysfunction, and arrhythmias.

Fontan repair or cavopulmonary anastomosis is a surgical procedure to direct deoxygenated systemic venous blood directly into the pulmonary artery. In this surgery, the systemic venous blood flows into the pulmonary artery continuously under the small pressure gradient between systemic veins and PA evading the need for a pumping chamber (RV). Hence, mean systemic venous pressure are high relatively. Several hemodynamic changes related to the pregnancy may have adverse effect on Fontan circulation. These physiological happenings may potentially threaten the health of both the mother with a Fontan circuit and the fetus. Moreover, the post-Fontan patients are prone for atrial arrhythmias as well as effusion in body cavities and edema. Mostly fertility also goes down in this group of patients.[190–192]

Pregnancy must be avoided for those Fontan patients who have atrial arrhythmias and NYHA class deterioration, low resting oxygen saturation, low ventricular ejection fraction, and have moderate-to-severe AV valve regurgitation. In principle, vaginal delivery is the first choice for relatively asymptomatic patients. However, if ventricular function is deteriorating, early CS can be done in an experienced center. Fetal death is reported up to 50% of cases. Also, there may be premature birth and neonate may be small for gestational age needing NICU care. However, the experience regarding the outcome of pregnancy in patients with TCPC (total cavopulmonary connection) is limited.

Canabbio et al. reported 15 (45%) live birth from 14 mothers out of total 33 pregnancies after Fontan operation.[191] There were 13 spontaneous abortions and 5 elective terminations. Reported pre-pregnancy problems in these gravidas were—atrial flutter, supraventricular tachycardia, ventricular dysfunction, aortic regurgitation, and atrioventricular valve regurgitation. No maternal cardiac complications were reported during labor, delivery, or the immediate puerperium. There were six female and nine male infants (mean gestational age 36.5 weeks; median weight 2,344 g). One infant had an atrial septal defect. At follow-up, mothers and infants were alive and well. Hoare et al. reported four fontan patients who underwent successful pregnancy completion but had premature births.[192]

Eisenmenger's Syndrome

Severe hypoxemia, severe polycythemia, LV dysfunction, presence of arrhythmias, low SVR, renal dysfunction, low hemoglobin, and coagulation abnormalities are markers of poor outcome in pregnancy with Eisenmenger's syndrome.

Eisenmenger's syndrome is a hemodynamic consequence of chronic volume and/or pressure overload secondary to a shunt lesion, resulting into systemic PA pressure, raised pulmonary vascular resistance, which eventually leads to flow reversal, systemic hypoxemia, and central cyanosis. The cyanotic CHD with increased pulmonary blood flow also may have similar changes in lungs in long run. Congenital heart defects that can lead to Eisenmenger's syndrome include atrial septal defects, ventricular septal defects, persistent arterial ducts, as well as more complex defects such as atrioventricular septal defects, truncus arteriosus, aortopulmonary window, complex CHD-like TGA with VSD, TAPVC, and the univentricular heart.[193] When pregnancy occurs in women with Eisenmenger's syndrome, medical termination is considered safer than any mode of delivery.[11]

Acute arrhythmias are particularly dangerous, as these patients have little or no cardiac reserve and need a normal sinus rhythm to keep up with the increased workload. Maternal mortality rate is estimated at 30–50%.[193–195] Cardiac complications include supraventricular and ventricular arrhythmias, CHF, valvar regurgitation, and sudden death. Noncardiac complications are bleeding (lung, GI, cerebral), ischemic episodes (thromboembolic events, paradoxic emboli, air embolism) kidney dysfunction, symptoms related to hyperviscosity (headache, dizziness, visual disturbances, altered sensorium, fatigue) iron deficiency, infections (infective endocarditis, cerebral abscess), and gout.[193–195]

Eisenmenger's syndrome poses great challenges to anesthetists. Careful vital monitoring, fluid optimization, infection control, maintaining SVR to certain level are the goals to be achieved during anesthetic management. Delivery must be conducted under multidisciplinary supervision in an expert center.[196] The Bosentan, an endothelin receptor antagonist, was found to be teratogenic in animal experiments. However, medical modulation of nitric oxide pathway, by the drugs like sildenafil/l-arginine, have been successfully used to control PA pressure for uncomplicated completion of pregnancy in mothers with ES.[197]

The hypotension must be essentially avoided that may lead to compromised pulmonary blood flow resulting in sudden life-threatening hypoxia. Prior knowledge of medication including anticoagulants must be provided to anesthetist. The regional or general anesthesia can be used and vaginal or CS delivery can be performed according to the situation. A dilutes solution of phenylephrine can be used to maintain the SVR.[198] The blood transfusion or crystalloid infusion must be given if blood loss is suspected.

Aortopathy in Pregnancy

There are group of congenital defects that may cause aortic root dilatation making it vulnerable for dissection, aneurysmal dilatation, and rupture. They may also cause annular dilatation and AR. The conditions included in this group are Marfan's syndrome, Ehlar-Danlos syndrome (vascular type 4), Turner's syndrome, Loeys-Dietz syndrome, and bicuspid aortic valve.[199-205] The echocardiographic evaluation of root dimension is recommended during the pregnancy. The features of these syndrome, their genetic inheritance, cardiovascular features, and maternal risk are given in Box 35.8.

Box 35.8 Feature of congenital syndromes causing aortic root dilatation

Syndrome	*Genetic inheritance*	*Cardiovascular features*	*Preferred mode of delivery*	*Maternal fetal risk*
Marfan's syndrome[11,191,200]	Marfan's syndrome is an inherited connective tissue disorder transmitted as an autosomal dominant (AD) trait	Aortic root dilatation, dissection, regurgitant lesions of MV/AV	Preferable vaginal delivery. CS in patients who have significant root dilatation. Preconception surgery is more appropriate	If aortic diameter is normal (<4 cm) <1% maternal risk, 4–4.5: risk is increased. >4.5 cm: Counseling against pregnancy. The patient must go for surgery though risk of dissection remains in remaining aorta
Ehlar–Danlos syndrome[11,201]	AD Inheritance: arthrochalasia, classic, hypermobility, and vascular forms of the disorder; Autosomal Recessive (AR): Other types of EDS	Mild MR, Mild TR or AR TR, Mild AR Seen in 25% of Cases Aortic root dilatation in 10.8%	Preferable vaginal delivery. Unless significant valvar leak or Significant valvar leak or Aortic root dilatation Preconception cardiac surgery is preferred	Increased M-F risks because of (i) hypotension facilitated by dysautonomia, (ii) meningeal fragility complicating in cerebrospinal fluid hypotension in case of EPI/peridural anesthesia, (iii) proneness to pelvic prolapse after episiotomy, and (iv) an apparently increased rate of suture dehiscence and minor hemorrhages after surgery, (v) aortopathy
Turner's syndrome[202,203]	One of X chromosome is missing	Bicuspid aortic valve, CoA, and/or systemic hypertension	CS/normal delivery if there are no aortic complications	The treatment will depend on size of aorta and gestational age
Bicuspid AV[11,204]	Prevalence of BAV of 9.1% among the first degree relatives. An autosomal dominant inheritance with reduced penetrance	Aortic dilation, dissection, coarctation	All women with bicuspid AV must be monitored closely	If aortic root >50 mm, surgery is recommended
Loeys–Dietz syndrome[205]	Autosomal dominant genetic syndrome caused by mutant genes encoding transforming growth factor β-receptor 1	Bicuspid aortic valve, aortic dilatation; PDA	Close monitoring CS/normal delivery if there are no aortic complications	Principle of management of aortic complication remains same as for other patients with aortopathy

SECTION IV
RHYTHM DISORDER IN PREGNANCY (TABLE 35.9)

The arrhythmias can ensue during pregnancy as a primary rhythm disorder or may be in conjunction with structural heart disease. The arrhythmias are one of the important causes for the sudden cardiac death in antenatal period. In women with known structural heart disease, however, arrhythmia is one of the five independent predictors of having a cardiac event during the pregnancy and should, therefore, be treated seriously.[16-18] Incidence of sustained tachycardia in pregnancy is around 2–3/1,000.[206] Pathological bradycardia in pregnant women is rare and usually secondary to congenital heart block, with an incidence of 1:20,000 women.[207]

The management of arrhythmias needs an exact etiopathological diagnosis. Echo-screening is recommended to rule out underlying cardiac disease. Patient must be investigated for the presence of predisposing factors like the abnormalities of thyroid function, hemorrhage, pulmonary embolism, infections, and inflammatory states. The old ECG records must be viewed to recognize pattern of basic rhythm. The Holter monitoring is advised for the patients presenting with occasional palpitation or history of syncope. An operated patient for congenital defect like TAPVC repair, atrial switch, Fontan repair may present with atrial tachycardia.[11] A patient of Ebstein's anomaly may have accessory pathway-dependent re-entrant tachycardia. The adults with TOF surgery or post-valve replacement surgery may present with intractable ventricular tachyarrhythmia.[208]

The patient with arrhythmia may present clinically with the mild symptoms like the palpitation or may have the life-threatening hemodynamic compromise. After making a diagnosis of the tachy or bradyarrhythmias, appropriate emergency management must be done. The electrical cardioversion under the general anesthesia and intubation is not contraindicated in the pregnancy and does not harm the fetus. For the bradyarrhythmias, pacing can be done.[11,209]

The antiarrhythmic drugs can be selected according to the need. WHO has released the list of drugs with FDA category

Table 35.9 Recommended therapy for management of arrhythmias[11]

Acute conversion of paroxysmal SVT	Vagal maneuver/IV adenosine (I C) IV metoprolol or propranolol (IIaC) IV verapamil may be considered (IIbC)
Tachycardia with hemodynamic instability	Electrical cardioversion (IC)
Long-term management of SVT	Oral digoxin or metoprolol (IC) or sotalol or flecainide (IIaC) Oral propafenone or procainamide (IIbC) Oral verapamil (IIbC) (contraindication: atenolol III)
Pre- or postconception whenever needed	Implantable cardioverter defibrillators (I)
Congenital long QT syndrome	Blocking agents are recommended during pregnancy and also postpartum when they have a major benefit (IC)
Long-term management of idiopathic sustained VT	Oral metoprolol, propranolol or verapamil (IC)
Sustained, unstable and stable VT	Immediate electrical cardioversion (IC)
Sustained, hemodynamically stable and monomorphic VT	IV sotalol or procainamide (IIaC)
Bradycardia and complete AV block	Implantation of permanent pacemakers or ICDs (preferably one chamber) under echoguidance if fetus is beyond 8 weeks (IIaC)
Sustained, monomorphic, hemodynamically unstable, refractory to electrical cardioversion or not responding to other drugs VT	IV amiodarone should be considered (IIaC)
For long-term management of idiopathic sustained VT	Oral sotalol, flecainide, propafenone should be considered if other drugs fail (IIaC)
Drug refractory and poorly tolerated tachycardias	Catheter ablation (IIbC)

Digoxin (c); metoprolol (c); propranolol (c); atenolol (d); sotalol (c); amiodarone (d); flecainide (c); propafenone (c)

of pregnancy. Most of the antiarrhythmic drugs can cross the placental barrier so much so that the maternal drug therapy is done routinely for fetal arrhythmias. The pharmacokinetics of drugs is altered in the pregnancy and the blood levels need to be checked to ensure maximum efficacy and avoid the toxicity.[206] Patient must be kept in ICU and must be given appropriate cardiac resuscitation if required, airway management, and circulatory support. For those pregnant women with on-going malignant arrhythmias despite the pharmacological treatment, an implantable cardioverter defibrillator may be a safe alternative.[210]

RESTING ELECTROCARDIOGRAPHY

The resting ECG is different in the pregnancy. First of all, there is shifting of heart upward and left which changes the axis of heart without a change in amplitude of waves and inferior leads may show Q and inverted T waves. Second, the physiological tachycardia leads to decreased PR, QRS, and QT intervals; ectopics (premature atrial/ventricular beats) are common during pregnancy.[11,26,27,211] There may be a Q-wave and inverted T-wave in the inferior leads. Third, in a mother with CVD, one must try to identify basal patterns as there might be evidence of the accessory pathways and changes related to the underlying structural heart disease or previous interventions may also be seen.[11,211]

The intrauterine growth retardation has been associated with β-blockers, particularly with the Atenolol. Atenolol may cause IUGR if administered in periconception period.[212]

However, more or less they are harmless. Essentially β-blockers are needed for many serious conditions arrhythmias, mitral stenosis, Marfan's syndrome, thyrotoxicosis, and can be recommended according to the current guideline.

DIRECT CURRENT CARDIOVERSION[213]

When drugs fail or in case of shock or pulmonary edema, DC cardioversion is indicated. Tromp et al. analyzed 44 case reports from literature, which describe the use of electrical cardioversion (ECV) during pregnancy. They found considerable variation in specific arrhythmias for which ECV was applied and required energy varied from 50 to 400 J. Successful ECV after one or more attempts was reported in 41 pregnant women (93.2%).[213,214]

ECV in the nonpregnant population was reported to be successful in 42–92%.[214,215]

IMPLANTABLE CARDIOVERTER DEFIBRILLATORS

The mothers with implantable cardioverter defibrillators have been reported to have uneventful pregnancy and normal fetal outcome.[11] The studies done on women with the implantable cardioverter defibrillator (ICD) implant in situ found it safe and there was no increase in either device or treatment complications, nor any increase in the number of shocks (that women received), when compared to preconception.[216] It is postulated that the exposure to electrical field for fetus is not much to cause harm. However, it is recommended that after each shock therapy, fetal well-being must be checked. The fetus may be harmed because of hypotension and decreased placental flow during the episodes of arrhythmias. ICD is particularly helpful for the mothers who have malignant recurrent arrhythmias, difficult to control with drugs. ICD implantation can be echo-guided and radiation can be avoided.[11,216]

MANAGEMENT OF SPECIFIC ARRHYTHMIAS

Bradycardia

The pregnant women may have physiological bradycardia, commonly in second trimester, and may become hypotensive due to presence of pregnancy induced low SVR. Symptomatic bradycardia may manifest due to aortocaval compression. Moreover, conduction defect may also present with bradycardia needing temporary pacing. Permanent pacemaker can be implanted during the pregnancy with low risk.[11,216,217]

Types of Bradyarrhythmias[11,206–211]

1. *Sinus node dysfunction:* Usually associated with posture or Valsalva maneuver.
2. *Atrioventricular blocks:* First-degree AV block: the first-degree heart block is often seen and is usually due to delay at the level of bundle of His. It is nonprogressive in absence of underlying cardiac disease Wenckebach block or type I second-degree AV block is asymptomatic but type II second-degree HB usually presents in associated with the structural heart disease like the tetralogy of Fallot, AVSD, VSD, or drug therapy. Complete heart block undetected till adulthood due to adequate chronotropy and narrow QRS complex escape rhythm from high up His bundle are expected to have normal pregnancy outcome.[11,206–211] These patients can be treated on routine line with or without pacing, without any extra risk.[217–220]

Supraventricular Tachycardia[11,206,209,221]

These can be classified as:

1. *Atrioventricular nodal re-entry tachycardia and atrioventricular re-entry tachycardia:* On surface ECG, it manifests as narrow complex tachycardia with long-PR and short-RP interval tachycardia. In AV nodal re-entry tachycardia, P-wave may be difficult to appreciate.

2. *Focal atrial ectopic tachycardia:* This is a short PR, long PR interval narrow complex tachycardia with or without changed P-wave axis.
3. *Atrial flutter and fibrillation:* Atrial flutter is an atrial re-entry tachycardia with saw tooth appearance of P-wave. P-waves are more than QRS complexes numerically, as P-waves are conducted with fixed or varying second-degree block. Atrial fibrillation is characterized by ill-defined fibrillatory waves that are conducted irregularly with slow or fast heart rates.

The exact diagnosis of SVT can be made based on ECG by the analysis of P-wave morphology and its relationship with QRS complex. To abort an episode of SVT, physical methods like carotid sinus massage can be first applied by attending doctor or by patient can also learn to self-administer it. The adenosine remains the first line of drug to abort the arrhythmia. The half-life of adenosine is so short, it does not affect the fetus.[221–223]

Canlorbe et al. reported onset of premature labor in patient who received up to 20 mg of IV adenosine.[223] The maximum dose up to 18–24 mg is allowed, though mostly doses in the range of 6–12 mg are effective because degradation of adenosine is reduced during the pregnancy. The β-blockers other than atenolol and CCB are the second line of drugs. IV verapamil is an effective second line for the treatment of SVTs and can be used in doses up to 10 mg without affecting the fetal heart rate. However, fetal distress has been associated with verapamil-induced maternal hypotension.[11,221,223] Before the use of digoxin or CCB one must rule-out presence of accessory pathways on surface ECG. These agents delay AV nodal conduction, hence, may lead to accelerated conduction through accessory pathways. β-Blockers are the drugs of choice for controlling rate in women with known WPW syndrome.[11,221,223]

Atrial fibrillation and flutter are usually associated with conditions like VHDs particularly MS, HOCM, thyrotoxicosis, or electrolyte imbalance. They can lead to serious hemodynamic consequences for both the mother and the fetus due to loss of atrial kick that is required for late diastolic filling of ventricles. AF leads to stasis of blood in atrium. The atrial stasis imposes risk of thrombosis. The pharmacological conversion to sinus rhythm must be tried with drugs like sotalol, flecainide, procainamide, mexiletine, or amiodarone. Restoration of sinus rhythm is beneficial in a prothrombotic state like pregnancy with CVD. When restoration of sinus rhythm is not possible, rate control can be accomplished by drugs like β-blockers, verapamil, and digoxin. They must be combined with the adequate anticoagulation.[11,224,225] Electrical cardioversion should be performed in the case of hemodynamic instability. The DC shock is safe modality.[11,224,225]

Before the cardioversion of atrial flutter and AF, one has to rule out atrial clot. Anticoagulation is required appropriately. Warfarin is avoided in first and last trimester and heparin UFH or LMWH must be used instead, for at least 3–4 weeks prior to cardioversion, because of the risk of thromboembolism related to so-called atrial stunning. However, for high-risk for recurrence patients anticoagulation must be given life-long. Either single or dual antiplatelet therapy (clopidogrel and acetylsalicylic acid) were not as effective as warfarin in high-risk patients with atrial fibrillation.[11,224,225]

Ventricular Tachycardia

Life-threatening ventricular arrhythmias during pregnancy may set-in, in patients with corrected or uncorrected structural heart diseases. The presence of inherited arrhythmogenic disorders should always be considered by family history and appropriate diagnostic tests during or after pregnancy.

Idiopathic Ventricular Tachycardia

Idiopathic RVOT: Ventricular tachycardia (right ventricular outflow) is the most common form in this group. Patient may not have instant hemodynamic instability and may manifest either with self-abortive episodes of nonsustained VT or only with ectopic beats. The ECG is diagnostic in such cases showing persistent left bundle branch block pattern of QRS complexes with an inferior axis. β-blockers are recommended for these patients who are expected to respond it well. Another less common variety of idiopathic ventricular tachycardia (IVT) may present with right branch block pattern. Usually, it is treated with verapamil.[11,206,226,227]

Monomorphic ventricular tachycardia in the mothers with CVD: Rapid VT may present with severe hypotension and has propensity to degenerate into ventricular fibrillation. Treatment should be with intravenous lignocaine, amiodarone, DC cardioversion, or overdrive pacing. In women with non-long QT-related sustained VT and a stable hemodynamic situation, IV sotalol acutely can be considered to terminate the tachycardia. IV procainamide may be considered. IV amiodarone should be avoided until absolutely necessary is not ideal for early conversion of stable monomorphic VT. Close monitoring of BP is recommended in the presence of LV dysfunction.[11,206,226–229]

Prophylactic therapy with oral sotalol or a cardioselective β-blocking agent such as metoprolol can be continued. In cases with resistant VT amiodarone and/or ICD implantation should be considered for protection of maternal life.[11,205,207,225–229]

Polymorphic Ventricular Tachycardia

Polymorphic VT can degenerate into the ventricular fibrillation. The emergency treatment requires correction of electrolyte disturbance including magnesium, removal of precipitating drugs, particularly class I and III antiarrhythmic drugs, macrolide antibiotics, nonsedating antihistamines, antidepressants and some antipsychotics, and potentially temporary overdrive pacing.[11,216,225-228]

Prognosis

Prognosis of arrhythmia-management will depend on (1) Type of arrhythmia and (2) Type of underlying heart disease, and (3) Degree of hemodynamic compromise of the patient.

In isolated cases of arrhythmia, prognosis usually points to a benign condition, responding favorably to antiarrhythmic drugs. Treatment remains a challenge though, as clinical decision must be tackled with appropriate consideration of both maternal and fetal factors. The FDA classification for pregnancy risk drug categories must be consulted while choosing a drug. Finally, for the refractory arrhythmias options are few that includes ECV and ICD. Many relatively newer drugs may be beneficial but needs to be investigated before inclusion in recommendations.

CONCLUSION

Cardiovascular diseases when present in a pregnant women pose special hemodynamic challenges. Cardiac dilatation and altered thrombogenicity are the normal physiological changes that may synergize the cardiac dysfunction and thrombosis in a predisposed mother with CVD. The question may be raised about the benefits of evolution in obstetrics sciences for this subgroup of patients. Can methods for assisted fertilization, like in-vitro conception and surrogacy be recommended for these patients regularly with borderline hemodynamics? A meticulous approach, review of records, preconception counseling, Holter monitoring, pulse oxymetry, echocardiography, MRI, stress testing must be done to stratify risk. For example, an Eisenmenger pregnancy has chances of adverse outcome up to 30–50% of cases. But if saturation is above 90 and patient is not overtly polycythemic or anemic and has good functional capacity on exercise testing will have the better chance of uneventful outcome. So instead of blanket opinion, one has to customize the risk for individual patient in a group. The appropriate medicines must be started and converted to safe drugs for fetus during the period of organogenesis. The article has given all evidences from the literature for individual conditions. There are detailed guidelines issued by ESC and RCOG expert committees. Accordingly institutional guidelines must be prepared and followed. The safety of drugs has been evaluated by FDA and categorized according to the level of evidence. List is given in the appendix and Table 35.10.

Table 35.10 List of drugs with FDA category for pregnancy

Drug/FDA[11,229]	Categories
Abciximab	C
Acenocoumarol	D
Acetylsalicylic acid (low dose)	B
Adenosine	C
Amiodarone	D
Amlodipine	C
Atenolol	D
Bisoprolol	C
Candesartan	D
ACE inhibitors (captopril, enalapril ramipril)	D
Clopidogrel	C
Danaparoid	B
Digoxin	C
Diltiazem	C
Disopyramide	C
Eplerenone	Unknown
Flecainide	C
Furosemide	C
Glyceryl trinitrate	B
Heparin (low molecular weight)	B
Heparin (unfractionated)	B
Hydralazine	C
Hydrochlorothiazide	B
Isradipine	C
Irbesartan and telmisartan	D
Labetalol	C
Lidocaine	C
Methyldopa	B
Metoprolol	C
Mexiletine	C
Nifedipine	C
Phenprocoumon	D
Procainamide	C
Propranolol	C
Quinidine	C
Sotalol	B
Spironolactone	D
Statins	X
Ticlopidine	C
Valsartan	D
Verapamil	C
Warfarin	D

APPENDIX

DRUGS DURING PREGNANCY AND BREASTFEEDING

General Principles

General principles of drug administration cannot be translated into definite protocol due to inadequate evidences and conflicting opinion in literature. ESC guidelines recommend customized approach to individual patients. Since the drug treatment in pregnancy is targeted at mother and fetus the task of drug selection becomes difficult. ESC guidelines states "use of drug must be based on emergency of situation and not on recommendation of pharmaceutical industry. The potential risk of a drug and the possible benefit of the therapy must be weighed against each other."[11]

Drugs which can be Secreted in Breast Milk

Anticoagulant (acenocoumarol, warfarin up to 10% of ingested dose); antiplatelets—salicylates (status of antiplatelet agents—clopidogrel and ticlopidine is not known); ACE inhibitors—captopril, enalapril, ramipril (status is not known for angiotensin II receptor blockers); the antiarrhythmic agents—quinidine, mexiletine, disopyramide (status for propafenone not known); β-blockers—atenolol, metoprolol, propranolol; diuretics—furosemide, chlorothiazide, spironolactone; calcium channel blockers—verapamil nifedipine, diltiazem; antihypertensive (hydralazine, labetalol, methyl dopa), (Status not known for glyceryl trinitrate); others, digoxin. These drugs may have a pharmacological effect on the infants. The approach to continue drug or breastfeeding, must be individualized according to the estimated risks.

US FOOD AND DRUG ADMINISTRATION CLASSIFICATION

This classification has been taken from article published by Bonow et al.[226]

The following categories are used for safe drugs in pregnancy and breastfeeding:

- *Category A:* Safety for fetus in first trimester is proven based on adequate and well-controlled trials (and no risk was demonstrated in second trimester).
- *Category B:* The safety was established in animal reproduction studies but no controlled study in human fetus is available. Or animal experiments shown some side effects not proven in controlled human trials.
- *Category C:* Animal studies showed adverse effects on fetus, but no controlled human study or no animal or human studies are available. Drug is administered when potential benefit justifies the use.
- *Category D:* There are studies to show human fetal risk, but benefit from using it in pregnancy is such that risk is acceptable. Like drugs used for treatment of life-threatening conditions.
- *Category X:* Studies in animals and human subjects showed fetal anomaly and its use in pregnancy is totally contraindicated because risk overweigh possible benefits.

"Final Rule": New Statement by US Food and Administration (2014)

With the release of this statement, it is stated that old letter category system was too simplistic. The 'final rule' sets new standard regarding the labeling of prescription drugs to expectant/lactating mothers. This divided in three groups:

1. Pregnancy;
2. Lacation;
3. Females and males of reproductive age.[230] There are subsections for each categories.

FDA also releases guidelines for industry for clinical lactation studies—design, data collection, analysis.[231]

REFERENCES

1. Weissgerber TL, Wolfe LA. Physiological adaptation in early human pregnancy: adaptation to balance maternal-fetal demands. Appl Physiol Nutr Metab. 2006;31(1):1-11.
2. Arafeh JM, Baird SM. Cardiac disease in pregnancy. Crit Care Nurs Q. 2006;29:32-52.
3. Ueland K. Intrapartum management of the cardiac patient. I Clin Perinatol. 1988;8:155-64.
4. Kuczkowski KM, Review: Anesthesia for the parturient with cardiovascular disease; Southern African Journal of Anaesthesia & Analgesia; 2003.
5. Bhatla N, Lal S, Behera G, Kriplani A, Mittal S, Agarwal N, Talwar KK. Cardiac disease in pregnancy. Int J Gynaecol Obstet. 2003;82:153-9.
6. Peters RM, Flack JM. Hypertensive disorders of pregnancy. J Obstet Gynecol Neonatal Nurs. 2004;33:209-20.
7. Stangl V, Schad J, Gossing G, Borges A, Baumann G, Stangl K. Maternal heart disease and pregnancy outcome: a single-centre experience. Eur J Heart Fail. 2008;10:855-60.
8. Burn J, Brennan P, Little J, Holloway S, Coffey R, Somerville J, et al. Recurrence risks in offspring of adults with major heart defects: results from first cohort of British collaborative study. Lancet. 1998;351:311-6.
9. Pierpont ME, Basson CT, Benson DW Jr., Gelb BD, Giglia TM, Goldmuntz E, et al. Genetic basis for congenital heart defects:

current knowledge: a scientific statement from the American Heart Association Congenital Cardiac Defects Committee, Council on Cardiovascular Disease in the Young: endorsed by the American Academy of Pediatrics. Circulation. 2007;115: 3015-38.

10. Hyett J, Perdu M, Sharland G, Snijders R, Nicolaides KH. Using fetal nuchal translucency to screen for major congenital cardiac defects at 10–14 weeks of gestation: population based cohort study. BMJ. 1999;318:81-5.
11. Regitz-Zagrosek V, Blomstrom Lundqvist Borghi C, Cifkova R, Ferreira R, Foidart JM, Gibbs JSR, et al. ESC Guidelines on the management of cardiovascular diseases during pregnancy. The Task Force on the Management of Cardiovascular Diseases during Pregnancy of the European Society of Cardiology (ESC). European Heart Journal. 2011;32:3147-97.
12. Fesslova V, Brankovic J, Lalatta F, Villa L, Meli V, Piazza L, et al. Recurrence of congenital heart disease in cases with familial risk screened prenatally by echocardiography. Journal of Pregnancy Volume 2011 (2011), Article ID 368067.
13. Westin M, Saltvedt S, Bergman G, Almström H, Grunewald C, Valentin L. Is measurement of nuchal translucency thickness a useful screening tool for heart defects? A study of 16,383 fetuses. Ultrasound Obstet Gynecol. 2006;27(6):632-9.
14. Barker D, Lewis N, Mason, Tan LB. A generic method to assess the adequacy of individual maternal cardiac reserve to tolerate the demands of pregnancy and labour. Heart. 2011;97:A97 doi: 10.1136/heartjnl-2011-300198.173.
15. Xing-ming G, Li-sha Z, Dong W, Feng-zhi Y, Shou-zhong X. Change of cardiac reserve during abnormal pregnancy and its evaluation. Zhongguo Yi Xue Ke Xue Yuan Xue Bao. 2011; 33(1):58-61.
16. Siu SC, Sermer M, Colman JM, Alvarez AN, Mercier LA, Morton BC, et al. Prospective multicenter study of pregnancy outcomes in women with heart disease. Circulation. 2001; 104(5):515-21.
17. Drenthen W, Boersma E, Balci A, Moons P, Roos-Hesselink JW, Mulder BJ, et al. Predictors of pregnancy complications in women with congenital heart disease. Eur Heart J. 2010;31: 2124-32.
18. Khairy P, Ouyang DW, Fernandes SM, Lee-Parritz A, Economy KE, Landzberg MJ. Pregnancy outcomes in women with congenital heart disease. Circulation. 2006;113:517-24.
19. Dominica Zentner D, Du Plessis M, Brennecke M, Wong J, Grigg L, Harra S. Deterioration in cardiac systolic and diastolic function late in normal human pregnancy. Clinical Science. 2009;116:599-606.
20. Eghbali M, Deva R, Alioua A, Minosyan TY, Ruan H, Wang Y, et al. Molecular and functional signature of heart hypertrophy during pregnancy. Circulation Research. 2005;96:1208-16.
21. Greval A. Anaemia and pregnancy: anaesthetic implications. Indian J Anaesth. 2010;54(5):380-6.
22. Lund CJ, Donovan JC. Blood volume during pregnancy: significance of plasma and red cell volumes. Am J Obstet Gynecol. 1967;98:394-403.
23. Duvekot JJ, Cheriex EC, Pieters FA, Menheere PP, Peeters LH. Early pregnancy changes in hemodynamics and volume homeostasis are consecutive adjustments triggered by a primary fall in systemic vascular tone. Am J Obstet Gynecol. 1993;169:1382-92.
24. Rutter TW, Tremper KK. The physiology of oxygen transport and red cell transfusion. In: Thomas EJ, Healy, Knight PR (Eds). Wylie and Churchill-Davidson's Anesthesia, 7th edn. London: Arnold; 2003.pp.167-83.
25. Malinow AM, Ostheimer GW. Anesthesia for the high-risk parturient. Obstet Gynecol. 1987;69:951-64.
26. Colman JM, et al. Cardiac monitoring during pregnancy. In: Steer P, Gatzoulis M, Baker P (Eds). Heart Disease and Pregnancy. London: RCOG Press, 2006. pp.67-77.
27. Nihoyannopoulos P. Cardiovascular examination in pregnancy and the approach to diagnosis of cardiac disorder. In: Oakley C, Warnes CA (Eds). Heart Disease in Pregnancy. Blackwell Publishing. Malden, Massachusetts; 2007.pp.18-28.
28. Lee SWY, Khaw KS, Ngan Kee WD, Leung TY, Critchley LAH. Haemodynamic effects from aortocaval compression at different angles of lateral tilt in non-labouring term pregnant women. Br J Anaesth. Page 1 of 7 doi:10.1093/bja/aes349.
29. Oron G, Hirsch R, Ben-Haroush A, Hod M, Gilboa Y, Davidi O, Bar J. Pregnancy outcome in women with heart disease undergoing induction of labour. BJOG. 2004;111(7):669-75.
30. RCOG guideline-reducing the risk of thrombosis and embolism during pregnancy and the puerperium;*http://www.vtepreventionnhsengland.org.uk/nnmnweb/index.php/component/k2/item/89-rcog-guideline-reducing-the-risk-of-thrombosis-and-embolism-during-preganancy-and-the-puerperium.*
31. Merz WM, Gembruch U. Preconception and contraceptive counselling of women with cardiovascular diseases. Z Geburtshilfe Neonatol. 2012;216(2):45-53.
32. Abramowicz, JS. Is this hot technology too hot? JUM. 2002; 21(12):1327-33.
33. Kieler H, Cnattingius S, Haglund B, Palmgren J, Axelsson O. Sinistrality, a side-effect of prenatal sonography: a comparative study of young men. Epidemiology. 2001;12:618-23.
34. Rasiah SV, Publicover M, Ewer AK, Khan KS, Kilby MD, Zamora J. A systematic review of the accuracy of first-trimester ultrasound examination for detecting major congenital heart disease. Ultrasound Obstet Gynecol. 2006;28:110-6.
35. Thorne S, MacGregor A, Nelson-Piercy C. Risks of contraception and pregnancy in heart disease. Heart. 2006;92:1520-5.
36. Malinow AM, Ostheimer GW. Anesthesia for the high-risk parturient. Obstet Gynecol. 1987;69:951-64.
37. Ziskind S, Etchin A, Frenkel Y, et al. Epidural anesthesia with the Trendelenburg position for cesarean section with or without a cardiac surgical procedure in patients with severe mitral stenosis:a hemodynamic study. J Cardiothorac Anesth. 1990;3:354-9.
38. Kuczkowski KMA. Anesthesia for the parturient with cardiovascular disease. Southern African Journal of Anaesthesia & Analgesia; 2003.
39. Deneux-Tharaux C, Carmona E, Bouvier-Colle MH, Bréart G. Postpartum maternal mortality and cesarean delivery. Obstet Gynecol. 2006;108(3 Pt 1):541-8.
40. Elkayam U, Ostrzega E, Shotan A, Mehra A. Cardiovascular problems in pregnant women with the Marfan syndrome. Ann Intern Med. 1995;123:117-22.
41. 2005 American Heart Association Guidelines for Cardiopulmonary Resuscitation and Emergency Cardiovascular Care: Circulation. 2005;112: IV-150-IV-153.
42. ACR–SPR practice guideline for imaging pregnant or potentially pregnant adolescents and women with ionizing radiation: *http://www.acr.org/~/media/9E2ED55531FC4B4FA53EF3B6D3B25DF8.pdf*

43. Brent RL. The effect of embryonic and fetal exposure to X-ray, microwaves, and ultrasound: counseling the pregnant and nonpregnant patient about these risks. Semin Oncol. 1989; 16:347-68.
44. ACOG Committee Opinion. Number 299, September 2004 (replaces No. 158, September 1995). Guidelines for diagnostic imaging during pregnancy. Obstet Gynecol. 2004;104:647-51.
45. Bourguignon MH. Implications of ICRP 60 and the patient directive 97/43 Euratom for nuclear medicine. Q J Nucl Med. 2000;44:301-9.
46. Damilakis J, Theocharopoulos N, Perisinakis K, Manios E, Dimitriou P, Vardas P, Gourtsoyiannis N. Conceptus radiation dose and risk from cardiac catheter ablation procedures. Circulation. 2001;104:893-7.
47. Osei EK, Faulkner K. Fetal doses from radiological examinations. Br J Radiol; 1999.
48. Patel SJ, Reede DL, Katz DS, Subramaniam R, Amorosa JK. Imaging the pregnant patient for nonobstetric conditions: algorithms and radiation dose considerations. Radiographics. 2007;27:1705-22.
49. Shellock FG, Crues JV. MR procedures: biologic effects, safety, and patient care. Radiology. 2004;232:635-52.
50. De Wilde JP, Rivers AW, Price DL. A review of the current use of magnetic resonance imaging in pregnancy and safety implications for the fetus. Prog Biophys Mol Biol. 2005;87:335-3.
51. Orchard E, Dix S, Wilson N , Mackillop L, Ormerod,O. Reducing ionizing radiation doses during cardiac interventions in pregnant women. Obstet Med. 2012;5(3):108-11.
52. Vedrinne C, Tronc F, Martinot S, Robin J, Allevard AM, Vincent M, et al. Better preservation of endothelial function and decreased activation of the fetal renin-angiotensin pathway with the use of pulsatile flow during experimental fetal bypass. J Thorac Cardiovasc Surg. 2000;120(4):770-7.
53. Reddy VM, McElhinney DB, Rajasinghe HA, Liddicoat JR, Hendricks-Munoz K, Fineman JR, Hanley FL. Role of the endothelium in placental dysfunction after fetal cardiac bypass. J Thorac Cardiovasc Surg. 1999;117(2):343-51.
54. Becker RM. Intracardiac surgery in pregnant women. Ann Thorac Surg. 1983;36(4):453-8.
55. Chambers CE, Clark SL. Cardiac surgery during pregnancy. Clin Obstet Gynecol. 1994;37(2):316-23.
56. Bernal JM, Miralles PJ. Cardiac surgery with cardiopulmonary bypass during pregnancy. Obstet Gynecol Surv. 1986;41(1):1-6.
57. Pomini F, Mercogliano D, Cavalletti C, Caruso A, Pomini P. Cardiopulmonary bypass in pregnancy. Ann Thorac Surg. 1996; 61(1):259-68.
58. Patel A, Asopa S, Ohri SK. Cardiac surgery during pregnancy. Tex Heart Inst J. 2008;35(3):307-12.
59. Talwar S, Kale SC, Kumar L, Sabu R, Sampath AK. Open heart surgery during pregnancy. Indian J Thorac Cardiovasc Surg. 2003;19(4):184-5.
60. Chandrasekhar S, Cook CR, Collard CD. Cardiac surgery in the parturient. Anesth Analg. 2009;108:777-85.
61. Maria HLS, Elias DO. Guidelines for cardiopulmonary bypass during pregnancy *http://perfline.com/index.php? option= com_content&view=article&id=172&Itemid=289#*
62. Westergaard HB, Langerhoff-Roos J, Lingman G, et al. A critical appraisal of the use of umbilical artery Doppler ultrasound in high-risk pregnancies: use of meta-analysis in evidence-based obstetrics. Ultrasound Obstet Gynecol. 2001;17:466-76.
63. Valcamonico A, Danti L, Frusca T, et al. Absent end diastolic velocity in umbilical artery: risk of neonatal morbidity and brain damage. Am J Obstet Gynecol. 1994;170:796-801.
64. Fong FW, Ohlsson A, Hannah ME, et al. Prediction of perinatal outcome in fetuses suspected to have intrauterine growth restriction: Doppler US study of cerebral,renal, and umbilical arteries. Radiology. 1999;213:681-9.
65. Baschat AA, Gembruch U, Reiss I, et al. Relationship between arterial and venous Doppler and perinatal outcome in fetal growth restriction. Ultrasound Obstet Gynecol. 2000;16:407-13.
66. Kiserud T, Kessler J, Ebbing C, Rasmussen S. Ductus venosus shunting in growth-restricted fetuses and the effect of umbilical circulatory compromise. Ultrasound in Obstetrics and Gynecology. 2006;28(2):143-9.
67. Huisman TW. Doppler assessment of the fetal venous system. Semin Perinatol. 2001;25:21-31.
68. Jozwiak M, Bloemenkamp KW, Kelly AJ, et al. Mechanical methods for induction of labour. Cochrane Database Syst Rev. 2012;3:CD001233. doi: 10.1002/14651858.CD001233.pub2.
69. Nanda S, Nelson-Piercy C, Mackillop L. Cardiac disease in pregnancy. Clin Med. 2012;12(6):553-60.
70. Hibbard LT. Maternal mortality due to cardiac disease. Clin Obstet Gyencol. 1975;18:27-36.
71. S, Maurtua MA, Cywinski JB. Anaesthetic management for emergency caesarean section in a patient with severe valvular disease and preeclampsia. Int J Obstet Anesth. 2006;15:250-3.
72. Bonanno C, Gaddipati S. Mechanisms of hemostasis at cesarean delivery. Clin Perinatol. 2008;35:531-47, xi.
73. James AH, Bushnell CD, Jamison MG, Myers ER. Incidence and risk factors for stroke in pregnancy and the puerperium. Obstet Gynecol. 2005;106:509-16.
74. Dodd JM , Crowther CA. Misoprostol for induction of labour to terminate pregnancy in the second or third trimester for women with a fetal anomaly or after intrauterine fetal death, *http://apps.who.int/rhl/reviews/CD004901.pdf1998.*
75. Jain JK, Mishell DR Jr. A comparison of intravaginal misoprostol with prostaglandin E2 for termination of second trimester pregnancy. N Engl J Med. 1994;331:290-3.
76. Secher NJ, Thayssen P, Arnsbo P, Olsen J. Effect of prostaglandin E2 and F2 alphaon the systemic and pulmonary circulation in pregnant anesthetized women. Acta Obstet Gynecol Scand. 1982;61:213-8.
77. Kulier R, Fekih A, Hofmeyr GJ, et al. Surgical methods for first trimester termination of pregnancy. Cochrane Database Syst Rev. 2001;(4).
78. World Health Organization Special Programme of Research. Vaginal administration of 15-methyl-PGF2a methyl ester for preoperative cervical dilation. Contraception. 1981;23:251-9.
79. Wilson W. Prevention of infective endocarditis: guidelines from the American Heart Association: a guideline from the American Heart Association Rheumatic Fever, Endocarditis and Kawasaki Disease Committee, Council on Cardiovascular Disease in the Young, and the Council on Clinical Cardiology, Council on Cardiovascular Surgery and Anesthesia, and the Quality of Care and Outcomes Research Interdisciplinary Working Group. J Am Dent Assoc. 2007;138(6):739-45,747-60.
80. Heit JA, Kobbervig CE, James AH, Petterson TM, Bailey KR, Melton LJ, III. Trends in the incidence of venous thrombo-embolism during pregnancy or postpartum: a 30-year population-based study. Ann Intern Med. 2005;143: 697-706.

81. James AH, Jamison MG, Brancazio LR, Myers ER. Venous thromboembolism during pregnancy and the postpartum period: incidence, risk factors, and mortality. Am J Obstet Gynecol. 2006;194:1311-5.
82. Fontaine P, Leeman L, King Vj. Venous thromboembolism during pregnancy. Am Fam Physician. 2008;77(12):1709-16.
83. Ahearn GS, Hadjiliadis D, Govert JA, et al. Massive pulmonary embolism during pregnancy successfully treated with recombinant tissue plasminogen activator. Arch Int Med. 2002;162:1221-7.
84. Leung AN, Bull TM, Jaeschke R, Lockwood CJ, Boiselle PM, Hurwitz LM, et al. An Official American Thoracic Society/Society of Thoracic Radiology Clinical Practice Guideline: Evaluation of Suspected Pulmonary Embolism In Pregnancy *http://www.thoracic.org/statements/resources/pvd/evaluation-of-suspected-pulmonary-embolism-in-pregnancy.pdf*
85. Hirsh J, Anand S, Halperin JL, Fuster V. Mechanism of action and pharmacology of unfractionated heparin. Arterioscler Thromb Vasc Biol. 2001;21:1094-6.
86. Baglin T, Barrowcliffe TW, Cohen A, Greaves M, for the British Committee for Standards in Haematology. Guidelines on the use and monitoring of heparin. Br J Haematol. 2006;133:19-34.
87. Warkentin TE, Greinacher A, Koster A, Lincoff AM. Treatment and prevention of heparin-induced thrombocytopenia. American College of Chest Physicians Evidence-Based Clinical Practice Guidelines, 8th edn. Chest. 2008;133:340S-80S.
88. Salazar E, Izaguirre R, Verdejo J, Mutchinick O. Failure of adjusted doses of subcutaneous heparin to prevent thromboembolic phenomena in pregnant patients with mechanical cardiac valve prostheses. J Am Coll Cardiol. 1996; 27(7):1698-703.
89. Hanania G. Management of anticoagulants during pregnancy. Heart. 2001;86(2):125-6. PMCID: 1729872.
90. Mazzolai L, Hohlfeld P, Spertini F, Hayoz D, Schapira M, Duchosal MA. Fondaparinux is a safe alternative in case of heparin intolerance during pregnancy. Blood. 2006;108: 1569-70.
91. Lagrange F, Vergnes C, Brun JL, Paolucci F, Nadal T, Leng JJ, et al. Absence of placental transfer of pentasaccharide (fondaparinux, Arixtra®) in the dually perfused human cotyledon in vitro. Thromb Haemost. 2002,87:831-5.
92. Graff J, Harder S. Anticoagulant therapy with the oral direct factor Xa inhibitors rivaroxaban, apixaban and edoxaban and the thrombin inhibitor dabigatran etexilate in patients with hepatic impairment. Clin Pharmacokinet. 2013;52(4):243-54. doi: 10.1007/s40262-013-0034-0.
93. Holzgreve W, Carey JC, Hall BD. Warfarin-induced fetal abnormalities. Lancet. 1976;2:914-15.
94. Wesseling J, Van Driel D, Heymans HS, Rosendaal FR, GevenBoere LM, Smrkovsky M, et al. Coumarins during pregnancy: long-term effects on growth and development of school-age children. Thromb Haemost. 2001;85:609-13.
95. Vitale N, De Feo M, De Santo LS, Pollice A, Tedesco N, Cotrufo M. Dose-dependent fetal complications of warfarin in pregnant women with mechanical heart valves. J Am Coll Cardiol. 1999;33(6):1637-41.
96. Geerts WH, Bergqvist D, Pineo GF, Heit JA, Samama CM, Lassen MR, et al. Prevention of venous thromboembolism. American College of Chest Physicians Evidence-Based Clinical Practice Guidelines, 8th edn. Chest. 2008;133:381-453.
97. Gherman RB, Goodwin TM, Leung B, Byrne JD, Hethumumi R, Montoro M. Incidence, clinical characteristics, and timing of objectively diagnosed venous thromboembolism during pregnancy. Obstet Gynecol. 1999;94:730.
98. Antiplatelet Trialists' Collaboration. Collaborative overview of randomised trials of antiplatelet therapy III: reduction in venous thrombosis and pulmonary embolism by antiplatelet prophylaxis among surgical and medical patients. BMJ. 1994;308:235-46.
99. 122 CLASP (Collaborative Low-dose Aspirin Study in Pregnancy) Collaborative Group. CLASP: a randomised trial of low-dose aspirin for the prevention and treatment of pre-eclampsia among 9364 pregnant women. Lancet. 1994;343:619-29.
100. Leonhardt G, Gaul C, Nietsc HH, Buerke M, Scleussner E. Thrombolytic therapy in pregnancy. J Thromb Thrombolysis. 2006;21:271-6.w 9x
101. Fasullo S, Maringhini G, TerrazzinoGanci F, Paterna S, Pasquale PD. Thrombolysis for massive pulmonary embolism in pregnancy: a case report. Int J Emerg Med. 2011;4:69.
102. RCOG guideline. Reducing the risk of thrombosis and embolism during pregnancy and the puerperium; *http://www.vteprevention-nhsengland.org.uk/nnmnweb/index.php/component/k2/item/89-rcog-guideline-reducing-the-risk-of-thrombosis-and-embolism-during-preganancy-and-the-puerperium III*
103. Tanous D, Siu SC, Mason J, Greutmann M, Wald RM , Parker JD, et al., B-type natriuretic peptide in pregnant women with heart disease. JACC. 2010;56(15).
104. Bernstein PS, Magriples U. Cardiomyopathy in pregnancy: a retrospective study. Am J Perinatol. 2001;18(3):163-8.
105. Yamac H, Bultmann I, Sliwa K, Hilfiker-Kleiner D. Prolactin: a new therapeutic target in peripartum cardiomyopathy. Heart. 2010;96:1352-7.
106. Beus E, Mook WNKA, Ramsay G, Stappers JLM, Putten HWHM. Peripartum cardiomyopathy: a condition intensivists should be aware of. Intensive Care Med. 2003;29:167-74.
107. Bowater SE, Thorne SA. Management of pregnancy in women with acquired and congenital heart disease. Postgrad Med J. 2010;86(1012):100-5. [PubMed]
108. Demakis JG, Rahimtoola SH. Peripartum cardiomyopathy. Circulation. 1971;44(5):964-8.
109. Amos AM, Jaber WA, Russell SD. Improved outcomes in peripartum cardiomyopathy with contemporary. Am Heart J. 2006;152(3):509-13.
110. Pyatt JR, Dubey G. Peripartum cardiomyopathy: current understanding, comprehensive management review and new developments. Postgrad Med J. 2011;87(1023):34-9.
111. Boccio RV, Chung JH, Harrison DM. Anesthetic management of caesarean section in a patient with idiopathic hypertrophic subaortic stenosis. Anesthesiology. 1986;65:663-5.
112. Shennan A, Gupta M, Halligan A, et al. Lack of reproducibility in pregnancy of Korotkoff phase IV measured by mercury sphygmomanometry. Lancet 1996;347:139-42.
113. Brown MA, Hague WM, Higgins J, et al. The detection, investigation and management of hypertension in pregnancy: full consensus statement. Aust N Z J Obstet Gynaecol. 2000; 40:139-55.
114. Zhang J, Troendle JF, Levine RJ. Risks of hypertensive disorders in the second pregnancy. Paediatr Perinat Epidemiol. 2001;15: 226-31.

115. James PR, Nelson-Piercy C. Management of hypertension before, during, and after pregnancy. Heart. 2004;90:1499-504.
116. Mancia G, De Backer G, Dominiczak A, Cifkova R, Fagard R, Germano G, et al. 2007 ESH-ESC Practice Guidelines for the Management of Arterial Hypertension: ESH-ESC Task Force on the Management of Arterial Hypertension. J Hypertens. 2007;25:1751-62.
117. Report of the National High Blood Pressure Education Program Working Group on High Blood in Pregnancy. Am J Obstet Gynecol 2000;183:S1-22.
118. Lindheimer MD, Conrad KP, Karumanchi SA. Renal physiology and disease in pregnancy. In: Alpern RJ, Hebert SC, (eds). Seldin and Giebisch's The Kidney; Physiology and Pathophysiology, 4th edn. San Diego, California: Academic Press, Elsevier; 2008.pp.2339-98.
119. Rachael J P, Nelson-Piercy C. Management of hypertension before during and after pregnancy. Heart. 2004;90(12):1490-504.
120. Lindheimer MD, Taler SJ, Cunningham FG. Hypertension in pregnancy (ASH Position Article). Journal of the American Society of Hypertension. 2008;2(6):484-94.
121. Steegers EA, von Dadelszen P, Duvekot JJ, Pijnenborg R. Pre-eclampsia. Lancet. 2010;376:631-44.
122. Hiett AK, Brown HL, Britton KA. Outcome of infants delivered between 24 and 28 weeks' gestation in women with severe pre-eclampsia. J Matern Fetal Med. 2001;10:301-4.
123. Hofmeyr GJ, Atallah AN, Duley L. Calcium supplementation during pregnancy for preventing hypertensive disorders and related problems. Cochrane Database Syst Rev. 2006;3: CD001059.
124. Olsen SF, Osterdal ML, Salvig JD, Weber T, Tabor A, Secher NJ. Duration of pregnancy in relation to fish oil supplementation and habitual fish intake: a randomised clinical trial with fish oil. Eur J Clin Nutr. 2007;61:976-85.
125. Duley L, Henderson-Smart DJ, Meher S, King JF. Antiplatelet agents for preventingpre-eclampsia and its complications. Cochrane Database Syst Rev. 2007;2:CD004659.
126. Seely EW. Hypertension in pregnancy: a potential window into long-term cardiovascular risk in women. Clin Endo Metab. 1999;84:1858-61.
127. Lewis J, Rubin MD. Primary pulmonary hypertension. New Engl J Med. 1997;336:111-17.
128. Goland S, Tsai F, Habib M, Janmohamed M, Goodwin T M, Elkayam U. Favorable outcome of pregnancy with an elective use of epoprostenol and sildenafil in women with severe pulmonary hypertension. Cardiology. 2010;115(3):205-8.
129. Huang S, DeSantis ERH. Treatment of pulmonary arterial hypertension in pregnancy. Am J Health-System Pharma. 2007;64(18):1922-6.
130. Bassily-Marcus AM, Yuan C, Oropello J, Manasia A, Seth RK, Benjamin E. Pulmonary hypertension in pregnancy: critical care management. Pulmonary Medicine. 2012; Article ID 709407.
131. Roth A, Elkayam U. Acute myocardial infarction associated with pregnancy. Ann Intern Med. 1996;125:751-62.
132. Kealey AJ. Coronary artery disease and myocardial infarction in pregnancy: A review of epidemiology, diagnosis and medical and surgical management. Can J Cardiol. 2010;26(6): e185-e189.
133. Kealey AJ. Coronary artery disease and myocardial infarction in pregnancy: a review of epidemiology, diagnosis, and medical and surgical management. Can J Cardiol. 2010;26(6):e185-e9.
134. Tsuda E, Kawamata K, Neki R, Echigo S, Chiba Y. Nationwide survey of pregnancy and delivery in patients with coronary arterial lesions caused by Kawasaki disease in Japan. Cardiol Young. 2006;16:173-8.
135. Hankins GD, Wendel GD Jr, Leveno KJ, Stoneham J. Myocardial infarction during pregnancy: a review. Obstet Gynecol. 1985; 65:139-46.
136. Roth A, Elkayam U. Acute myocardial infarction associated with pregnancy. J Am Coll Cardiol. 2008;52(3):171-80.
137. Ladner HE, Danielson B, Gilbert WM. Acute myocardial infarction in pregnancy and the puerperium: a population-based study. Obstet Gynecol. 2005;105:480-4.
138. James AH, Jamison MG, Biswas MS. Acute myocardial infarction in pregnancy: a United States population-based study. Circulation. 2006;113:1564-71.
139. Silberman S, Fink D, Berko RS, Mendzelevski B, Bitran D. Coronary artery bypass surgery during pregnancy. Eur J Cardiothorac Surg. 1996;10(10):925-6.
140. Bonow RO, Carabello BA, Chatterjee K, et al. 2008 Focused update incorporated into the ACC/AHA 2006 guidelines for the management of patients with valvular heart disease: a report of the American College of Cardiology/American Heart Association Task Force on Practice Guidelines (Writing Committee to Develop Guidelines for the Management of Patients With ValvularHeart Disease). Circulation. 2008;118: e523-e661.
141. Henderson N. Pregnancy complicated by rheumatic heart disease. Med Assoc J. 1936;35(4):394-8.
142. Szekely P, Turner R, Snaith L. Pregnancy and the changing pattern of rheumatic heart disease. Br Heart J. 1973;35:1293-303.
143. Robbins SL, Cotran RS, Kumar V. Robbin's Pathologic Basis of Disease, 4th ed. Philadelphia: WB Saunders. 1989:597.
144. Hess DB, Hess LW. Management of cardiovascular disease in pregnancy. Obstet Gynecol Clin North Am. 1992;19:679-95.
145. Jeng JS, Tang SC, Yip PK. Incidence and etiologies of stroke during pregnancy and puerperium as evidenced in Taiwanese women. Cerebrovasc Dis. 2004;18:290-5.
146. Silversides CK, Colman JM, Sermer M, Siu SC. Cardiac risk in pregnant women with rheumatic mitral stenosis. Am J Cardiol. 2003;91:1382-5.
147. Bonow RO, Carabello BA, Chatterjee K, de Leon AC Jr, Faxon DP, Freed MD, et al. 2008 Focused update incorporated into the ACC/AHA 2006 guidelines for the management of patients with valvular heart disease: a report of the American College of Cardiology/American Heart Association Task Force on Practice Guidelines (Writing Committee to Revise the 1998 Guidelines for the Management of Patients With Valvular Heart Disease): endorsed by the Society of Cardiovascular Anesthesiologists, Societyfor Cardiovascular Angiography and Interventions, and Society of Thoracic Surgeon. J Am Coll Cardiol. 2008;52(13):e1-142. doi: 10.1016/j.jacc.2008.05.007.
148. Harris IS. Management of pregnancy in patients with congenital heart disease. Prog Cardiovasc Dis. 2011;53(4):305-11.
149. Yap SC, Drenthen W, Pieper PG, Moons P, Mulder BJ, Mostert B, et al. Risk of complications during pregnancy in women with congenital aortic stenosis. Int J Cardiol. 2008;126(2):240-6.
150. Silversides CK, Colman JM, Sermer M, Farine D, Siu SC. Early and intermediate term outcomes of pregnancy with congenital aortic stenosis. Am J Cardiol. 2003;91:1386-9.
151. Balint OH, Siu SC, Mason J, Grewal J, Wald R, Oechslin EN, et al. Cardiac outcomes after pregnancy in women with congenital heart disease. Heart. 2010;96:1656-61.

152. Camm AJ, Kirchho FP, Lip GY, Schotten U, Savelieva I, Ernst S, et al. Guidelines for the management of atrial fibrillation: the Task Force for the Management of Atrial Fibrillation of the European Society of Cardiology (ESC). Eur Heart J. 2010;31: 2369-429.
153. Vahanian A, Baumgartner H, Bax J, Butchart E, Dion R, Filippatos G, et al. Guidelines on the management of valvular heart disease: the Task Force on the Management of Valvular Heart Disease of the European Society of Cardiology. Eur Heart J. 2007;28:230-68.
154. Baumgartner H, Bonhoeffer P, De Groot NM, de Haan F, Deanfield JE, Galie N, et al. ESC Guidelines for the management of grown-up congenital heart disease (new version 2010). Eur Heart J. 2010;31:2915-57.
155. Bhargava B, Agarwal R, Yadav R, Bahl VK, Manchanda SC. Percutaneous balloon aortic valvuloplasty during pregnancy: use of the Inoue balloon and the physiologic antegrade approach. Cathet Cardiovasc Diagn. 1998;45:422-5.
156. Badui E, Solorio S, Martinez E, Bravo G, Enciso R, Barile L, Gutierrez-Vogel S, Miranda J. The heart in the primary anti-phospholipid syndrome. Arch Med Res. 1995;26(2):115-20.
157. Lesniak-Sobelga A, TraczW, KostKiewicz M, Podolec P, Pasowicz M. Clinical and echocardiographic assessment of pregnant women with valvular heart diseases—maternal and fetal outcome. Int J Cardiol. 2004;94:15-23.
158. Borer JS, Bonow RO. Review: clinical cardiology: new frontiers: contemporary approach to aortic and mitral regurgitation. Circulation. 2003;108:2432-8.
159. Borges VTM, Matsubara IBB, Magalhães CG, Peraçoli JC, RudgeI MVC. Effect of physiological overload on pregnancy in women with mitral regurgitation; Clinics (Sao Paulo). 2011; 66(1):47-50.
160. Pibarot P, Dumesnil JG. Valvular heart disease: changing concepts in disease management, prosthetic heart valves. Circulation. 2009;119:1034-48.
161. Elkayam U, Bitar F. Valvular heart disease and pregnancy: part II: prostheticvalves. J Am Coll Cardiol. 2005;46:403-10.
162. Meschengieser SS, Fondevila CG, Santarelli MT, Lazzari MA. Anticoagulation in pregnant women with mechanical heart valve prostheses. Heart. 1999;82:23-6.
163. Avila WS, Rossi EG, Grinberg M, Ramires JA. Influence of pregnancy after bioprosthetic valve replacement in young women: a prospective five year study. J Heart Valve Dis. 2002; 11:864-9.
164. Yap SC, Drenthen W, Pieper PG, Moons P, Mulder BJ, Klieverik LM, et al. Outcome of pregnancy in women after pulmonary autograft valve replacement for congenital aortic valve disease. J Heart Valve Dis. 2007;16:398-403.
165. Bowater SE, Thorne SA. Management of pregnancy in women with acquired and congenital heart disease. Postgrad Med J. 2010;86(1012):100-5.
166. Chan WS, Anand S, Ginsberg JS. Anticoagulation of pregnant women with mechanical heart valves: a systematic review of the literature. Arch Intern Med. 2000;160:191-6.
167. Cotrufo M, de Luca TS, Calabro R,et al. Coumarin anti-coagulation during pregnancy in patients with mechanical valve prostheses. Eur J Cardiothorac Surg. 1991;5:300-5.
168. Abildgaard U, Sandset PM, Hammerstrom J, Gjestvang FT, Tveit A. Management of pregnant women with mechanical heart valve prosthesis: thromboprophylaxis with low molecular weight heparin. Thromb Res. 2009;124:262-7.
169. Goldhaber SZ, Editorials. "Bridging" and mechanical heart valves perils, promises, and predictions. Circulation. 2006; 113:470-2.
170. Aggarwal N, Suri V, Kaur H, Chopra S, Rohila M, Vijayvergiya R. Retrospective analysis of outcome of pregnancy in women with congenital heart disease: single-centre experience from North India. Aust N Z J Obstet Gynaecol. 2009;49(4):376-81.
171. Presbitero P, Somerville J, Stone S, et al. Pregnancy in cyanotic congenital heart disease: outcome of mother and fetus. Circulation. 1994;89:2673-6.
172. Webb G, Gatzoulis MA. Congenital heart disease for the adult cardiologist atrial septal defects in the adult recent progress and overview. Circulation. 2006;114:1645-53.
173. Peisiewicz, W, Goch A. Blinikowski, Z, et al. Changes in the cardiovascular system during pregnancy in women with secumdum atrial septal defect. Kardiol Pol. 2004;60:218-28.
174. Balaguru D; Pregnancy Issues in Women with Atrial Septal Defect; *http://cdn.intechopen.com/pdfs/35792/InTech Pregnancy_issues_in_women_with_atrial_septal_defect.pdf*
175. Actis Dato GM, Rinaudo P, Revelli A, et al. Atrial septal defect and pregnancy: a retrospective analysis of obstetrical outcome before and after surgical correction. Minerva Cardioangiol. 1998;46:63-8.
176. Drenthen W, Pieper PG, Roos-Hesselink JW, van Lottum WA, Voors AA, Mulder BJ, et al. Outcome of pregnancy in women with congenital heart disease: a literature review. J Am Coll Cardiol. 2007;49(24):2303-11.
177. Drenthen W, Pieper PG, van der Tuuk K, Roos-Hesselink JW, Voors AA, Mostert B, et al. Cardiac complications relating to pregnancy and recurrence of disease in the offspring of women with atrioventricular septal defects. Eur Heart J. 2005; 26:2581-7.
178. Yentis S, Malhotra S. Chapter 89 - Coarctation of the aorta in Analgesia, Anaesthesia and Pregnancy-A Practical Guide; Publisher: Cambridge University Press; Publication Year: 2012c. pp. 223-224.
179. Beauchesne LM, Connolly HM, Ammash NM, Warnes CA. Coarctation of the aorta: outcome of pregnancy. J Am Coll Cardiol. 2001;38:1728-33.
180. Vriend JW, Drenthen W, Pieper PG, Roos-Hesselink JW, Zwinderman AH, van Veldhuisen DJ, Mulder BJ. Outcome of pregnancy in patients after repair of aortic coarctation. Eur Heart J. 2005;26:2173-8.
181. Hameed, AB, Goodwin TM , Elkayam U. Effect of pulmonary stenosis on pregnancy outcomes—A case-control study. Am Heart J. 2007;154(5):852-4.
182. Niwa K, Perloff JK, Bhuta SM, et al. Structural abnormalities of great arterial walls in congenital heart disease: light and electron microscopic analyses. Circulation. 2001;103:393-400.
183. Kaur H, Suri V, Aggarwal N, Chopra S, Vijayvergiya R, Talwar KK. Pregnancy in patients with tetralogy of Fallot: outcome and management. World J Ped Congen Heart Surg. 2010;1:170-4.
184. Veldtman GR, Connolly HM, Grogan M, Ammash NM, Warnes CA. Outcomes of pregnancy in women with tetralogy of Fallot. J Am Coll Cardiol. 2004;44:174-80.
185. Greutmann M, Klemperer KV, Brooks R , Peebles D, O'Brien P, Walker F. Pregnancy outcome in women with congenital heart disease and residual haemodynamic lesions of the right ventricular outflow tract. Eur Heart J. 2010;31:1764-70.
186. Meijer JM, Pieper , van Veldhuisen DJ. Pregnancy, fertility, and recurrence risk in corrected tetralogy of Fallot. Heart. 2005; 91(6):801-5.

187. Guedes A, Mercier LA, Leduc L, Berube L, Marcotte F, Dore A. Impact of pregnancy on the systemic right ventricle after a Mustard operation for transposition of the great arteries. J Am Coll Cardiol. 2004;44:433-7.
188. Ploeg M, Drenthen W, van Dijk A, Pieper PG. Successful pregnancy after an arterial switch procedure for complete transposition of the great arteries. BJOG. 2006;113(2):243-4.
189. Chopra S, Suri V, Aggarwal N, Rohilla M, Vijayvergiya R, Keepanasseril A. Ebstein's anomaly in pregnancy: maternal and neonatal outcomes. J Obstet Gynaecol Res. 2010;36(2):278-83. doi: 10.1111/j.1447-0756.2009.01130.x.
190. Drenthen W, Pieper PG, van Veldhuisen DJ. Pregnancy and delivery in women after Fontan palliation. Heart. 2006;92(9):1290-4.
191. Canobbio MM, Mair DD, van der Velde M, Koos BJ. Pregnancy outcomes after the Fontan repair. J Am Coll Cardiol. 1996;28(3):763-7.
192. Hoare JV, Radford D. Pregnancy after Fontan repair of complex congenital heart disease. Aust N Z J Obstet Gynaecol. 2001;41(4):464-8.
193. Weiss BM, Zemp L, Seifert B, Hess OM. Outcome of pulmonary vascular disease in pregnancy: a systematic overview from 1978 through 1996. J Am Coll Cardiol. 1998;31:1650-7.
194. Kiely DG, Condliffe R, Webster V, Mills GH, Wrench I, Gandhi SV, et al. Improved survival in pregnancy and pulmonary hypertension using a multiprofessional approach. BJOG. 2010;117(5):565-74. doi: 10.1111/j.1471-0528.2009.02492.x.
195. Bendayan D, Hod M, Oron G, Sagie A, Eidelman L, Shitrit D, et al. Pregnancy outcome in patients with pulmonary arterial hypertension receiving prostacyclin therapy. Obstet Gynecol 2005;106 (5Pt2):1206-10.
196. Galie N, Manes A, Palazzini M, Negro L, Marinelli A, Gambetti S, et al. Management of pulmonary arterial hypertension associated with congenital systemic-to-pulmonary shunts and Eisenmenger's syndrome. Drugs. 2008;68(8):1049-66.
197. Lacassie HJ, Germain AM, Valdes G, et al. Management of Eisenmenger syndrome in pregnancy with sildenafil and l-arginine. Obstet Gynecol. 2004;103:1118-20. doi: 10.1097/01.AOG.0000125148.82698.65.
198. Maitra G, Sengupta S, Rudra A, Debnath S. Pregnancy and non-valvular heart disease - Anesthetic considerations. Annals Cardiac Anesthesia. 2010;13(2):102-9.
199. Meijboom LJ, Vos FE, Timmermans J, Boers GH, Zwinderman AH, Mulder BJ. Pregnancy and aortic root growth in the Marfan syndrome: a prospective study. Eur Heart J. 26 2005:914-20.
200. Marfan's syndrome and other aortopathies in pregnancy Obstet Med. 2013;6(3):112-9.
201. Yen JL, Shuan-Pei L, Chen MR, Niu DM. Clinical features of Ehlers-Danlos syndrome. J Formos Med Assoc. 2006;105(6):475.
202. Hovatta O. Pregnancies in women with Turner's Syndrome. Ann Med. 1999;31:106-10.
203. Lin AE, Lippe B, Rosenfeld RG. Further delineation of aortic dilation, dissection and rupture in patients with Turner syndrome. Pediatrics. 1998;102:12-20.
204. Fedak PW, de Sa MP, Verma S, Nili N, Kazemian P, Butany J, et al. Vascular matrix remodeling in patients with bicuspid aortic valve malformations: implications for aortic dilatation. J Thorac Cardiovasc Surg. 2003;126:797-806.
205. Gutman G, Baris HN, Hirsch R, Mandel D, Yaron Y, Lessing JB, Kuperminc MJ. Loeys-Dietz syndrome in pregnancy: a case description and report of a novel mutation. Fetal Diagn Ther. 2009;26:35-7.
206. Shotan A, Ostrzega E, Mehra A. et al. Incidence of arrhythmias in normal pregnancy and relation to palpitations, dizziness, and syncope. Am J Cardiol. 1997;79:1061-4.
207. Michaelson M, Jonzon A, Riesenfeld T. Isolated congenital complete atrioventricular block in adult life: a prospective study. Circulation. 1995;92:442-9.
208. Niwa K., Tateno S, Akagi T, et al. Arrhythmia and reduced heart rate variability during pregnancy in women with congenital heart disease and previous reparative surgery. Int J Cardiol. 2007;122:143-8.
209. Avila WS, Rossi EG, Ramires JA, Grinberg Mg, Bortolotto MR, Zugaib M, da Luz PL. Pregnancy in patients with heart disease: experience with 1,000 cases. Clin Cardiol. 2003;26:135-42.
210. Rotmensch HH, Elkayam U, Frishman W. Antiarrhythmic drug therapy during pregnancy. Ann Intern Med. 1983;98:h487-97.
211. Carruth JE, Mivis SB, Brogan DR, et al. The electrocardiogram in normal pregnancy. Am Heart J. 1981;102:1075-8.
212. Lydakis C, Lip GY, Beevers M, Beevers DG. Atenolol and fetal growth in pregnancies complicated by hypertension. Am J Hypertens. 1999;12(6):541-7.
213. Tromp CHN, Nanne ACM, Bolte AC. Electrical cardioversion during pregnancy: safe or not? Neth Heart J. 2011;19(3):134-6.
214. Barnes EJ, Eben F, Patterson D. Direct current cardioversion during pregnancy should be performed with facilities available for fetal monitoring and emergency caesarean section. BJOG. 2002;109:1406-7.
215. Boodhoo L, Mitchell AR, Bordoli G, et al. DC cardioversion of persistent atrial fibrillation: a comparison of two protocols. Int J Cardiol. 2007;114:16-21. doi: 10.1016/j.ijcard.2005.11.108.
216. Natale A, Davidson T, Geiger MJ, Newby K. Implantable cardioverter-defibrillators and pregnancy: a safe combination? Circulation. 1997;96:2808-12.
217. Hidaka N, Chiba Y, Kurita T, et al. Is intrapartum temporary pacing required for women with complete atrioventricular block? An analysis of seven cases. BJOG. 2006;113:605.
218. Güdal M, Kervancioğlu C, Oral D, et al. Permanent pacemaker implantation in a pregnant woman with the guidance of ECG and two-dimensional echocardiography. Pacing Clin Electrophysiol. 1987;10:543.
219. Dalvi BV, Chaudhuri A, Kulkarni HL, Kale PA. Therapeutic guidelines for congenital complete heart block presenting in pregnancy. Obstet Gynecol. 1992;79:802-4.
220. Suri V, Keepanasseril A, Aggarwal N, Vijayvergiya R, Chopra S, Rohilla M. Maternal complete heart block in pregnancy: analysis of four cases and review of management. J Obstet Gynaecol Res. 2009;35:434-7.
221. Blomstrom-Lundqvist C, Scheinman MM, Aliot EM, Alpert JS, Calkins H, Camm AJ, et al. ACC/AHA/ESC guidelines for the management of patients with supraventricular arrhythmias—executive summary—a report of the American college of cardiology/American heart association task force on practice guidelines and the European society of cardiology committee for practice guidelines (writing committee to develop guidelines for the management of patients with supraventricular arrhythmias) developed in collaboration with NASPE-Heart Rhythm Society. J Am Coll Cardiol. 2003;42:1493-531.

222. Ghosh N, Luk A, Derzko C, Dorian P, Chow CM. The acute treatment of maternal supraventricular tachycardias during pregnancy: a review of the literature. J Obstet Gynaecol Can. 2011;33:17-23.
223. Canlorbe G, Azria E, Michel D, Iung B, Mahieu-Caputo D. Preterm labour after adenosine treatment for paroxysmal supraventricular tachycardia during pregnancy: a case report. Ann Fr Anesth Reanim. 2011;30:372-4.
224. Camm AJ, KirchhoFP, Lip GY, Schotten U, Savelieva I, Ernst S, et al. Guidelines for the management of atrial fibrillation: the Task Force for the Management of Atrial Fibrillation of the European Society of Cardiology (ESC). Eur Heart J. 2010;31:2369-429.
225. Fuster V, Ryden LE, Cannom DS, Crijns HJ, Curtis AB, Ellenbogen KA, et al. ACC/AHA/ESC 2006 guidelines for the management of patients with atrial fibrillation-executive summary: a report of the American College of Cardiology/American Heart Association Task Force on Practice Guidelines and the European Society of Cardiology Committee for Practice Guidelines (Writing Committee to Revise the 2001 Guidelines for the Management of Patients with Atrial Fibrillation). Eur Heart J. 2006;27:1979-2030.
226. Zipes DP, Camm AJ, Borggrefe M, Buxton AE, Chaitman B, Fromer M, et al. ACC/AHA/ESC 2006 guidelines for management of patients with ventricular arrhythmias and the prevention of sudden cardiac death—executive summary: a report of the American College of Cardiology/American Heart Association Task Force and the European Society of Cardiology Committee for Practice Guidelines (Writing Committee to Develop Guidelines for Management of Patients with Ventricular Arrhythmias and the Prevention of Sudden Cardiac Death) Developed in collaboration with the European Heart Rhythm Association and the Heart Rhythm Society. Eur Heart J. 2006;27:2099-140.
227. Kotchetkov R, Patel A, Salehian O. Ventricular tachycardia in pregnant patients. Clin Med Insights Cardiol. 2010;4:39-44.
228. Heart Disease and Pregnancy - study group (RCOG) statement Consensus views arising from the 51st Study Group: Heart Disease and Pregnancy Overarching consensus views. *http://www.rcog.org.uk/womenshealth/clinical-guidance/heart-disease-and-pregnancy-study-group-statement.*
229. Buhimschi CS, Weiner CP. Medications in pregnancy and lactation. Obstet Gynecol. 2009;113:417-32.
230. FDA issues final rule on changes to pregnancy and lactation labeling information for prescription drug and biological products. *http://www.fda.gov/NewsEvents/Newsroom/Press Announcements/ucm425317.htm*
231. Guidance for Industry, Clinical Lactation Studies–Study Design, Data Analysis, and Recommendations for Labeling. *http://www.fda.gov/downloads/Drugs/Guidance Compliance Regulatory Information/Guidances/UCM072097. pdf*

36

Fluid and Electrolyte Management in Critically Ill Cardiac Patients

Amit Varma, Rajat Agrawal, Pradyut Bag

FLUID RESUSCITATION AND MANAGEMENT

Fluid resuscitation with crystalloid and colloid solutions is a necessary intervention in acute medicine. The selection and use of resuscitation fluids is based on physiological principles, but clinical practice is determined largely by clinician preference, with marked individual variation. We believe that there is no ideal resuscitation fluid!!!

In cardiac critically ill patients, while the resuscitation goals are same as any other disease process, the type of fluid, the volume and rate of infusion is very dependent on the baseline cardiac status. Adjunctive therapies to fluid resuscitation, such as the use of catecholamine's to augment cardiac contraction and venous return, need to be considered early to support the failing circulation.

Intravenous (IV) fluid therapy has evolved significantly overtime. From the initial report of the first IV administration of sodium chloride-based solution to the development of goal-directed fluid therapy using novel dynamic indices, efforts have focused on improving patient outcomes. The goal of this review is to provide a brief overview of evidence based current concepts for IV fluid administration in the intensive care unit (ICU).

HISTORY OF FLUID RESUSCITATION

In 1832, Robert Lewins described the effects of the IV administration of an alkalinized salt solution in treating patients during the cholera pandemic. He observed that "the quantity necessary to be injected will probably be found to depend upon on the quantity of serum lost. The observations of Lewins are as relevant today as they were nearly 200 years ago.

Proponents of colloid solutions have argued that colloids are more effective in expanding intravascular volume because they are retained within the intravascular space and maintain colloid oncotic pressure. The volume-sparing effect of colloids, as compared with crystalloids, is considered to be an advantage, which is conventionally described in a 1:3 ratio of colloids to crystalloids to maintain intravascular volume.

Semisynthetic colloids have a shorter duration of effect than human albumin solutions but are actively metabolized and excreted. Proponents of crystalloid solutions have argued that colloids, in particular human albumin, are expensive and impractical to use as resuscitation fluids, particularly under field-type conditions. Crystalloids are inexpensive and widely available and have an established, although unproven, role as first-line resuscitation fluids. However, the use of crystalloids has classically been associated with the development of clinically significant interstitial edema (Table 36.1).

COLLOID VERSUS CRYSTALLOID: CLINICAL STUDIES

Mortality in Critically Ill Patients

The clinical relevance of the theoretical advantages of colloids was questioned as early as the late 1970s. After three decades, clinicians got some definitive conclusion from the landmark study "Saline versus Albumin Fluid Evaluation (SAFE) trial". The SAFE trial compared the effects of 4% albumin versus normal saline in 7,000 critically ill patients and they found no difference in the primary outcome (all-cause mortality at 28 days). Subgroup analysis revealed a possible association between resuscitation with albumin and increased mortality at 2 years in patients with traumatic brain injury.

Table 36.1 Types of resuscitation fluids

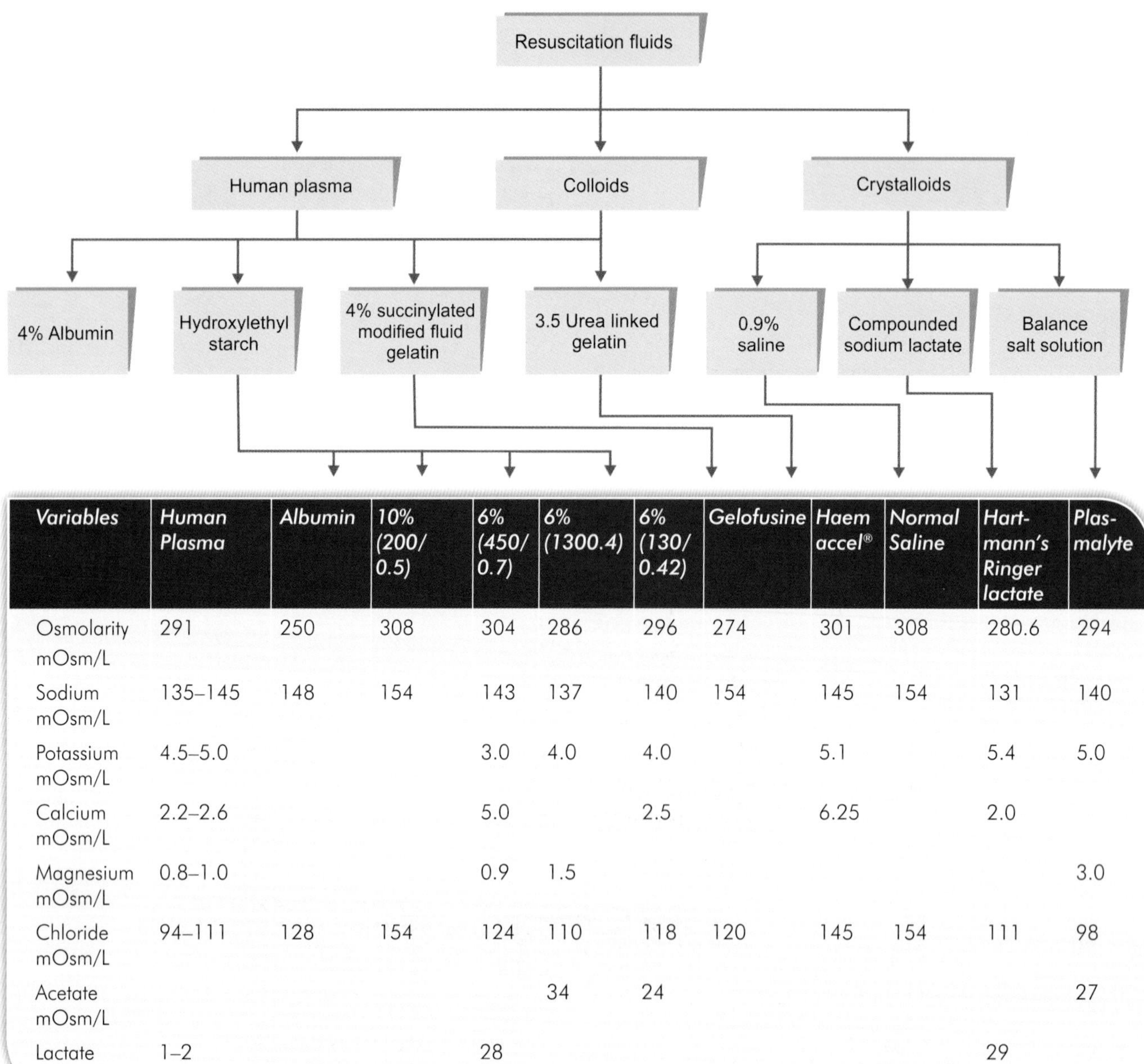

Variables	*Human Plasma*	*Albumin*	*10% (200/ 0.5)*	*6% (450/ 0.7)*	*6% (1300.4)*	*6% (130/ 0.42)*	*Gelofusine*	*Haem accel®*	*Normal Saline*	*Hart-mann's Ringer lactate*	*Plas-malyte*
Osmolarity mOsm/L	291	250	308	304	286	296	274	301	308	280.6	294
Sodium mOsm/L	135–145	148	154	143	137	140	154	145	154	131	140
Potassium mOsm/L	4.5–5.0			3.0	4.0	4.0		5.1		5.4	5.0
Calcium mOsm/L	2.2–2.6			5.0		2.5		6.25		2.0	
Magnesium mOsm/L	0.8–1.0			0.9	1.5						3.0
Chloride mOsm/L	94–111	128	154	124	110	118	120	145	154	111	98
Acetate mOsm/L					34	24					27
Lactate mOsm/L	1–2			28						29	

In recent Scandinavian 6S trial compared low molecular hydroxyethyl starch (HES) 130/0.42 versus Ringer's acetate in the resuscitation of 804 septic ICU patients. This multicenter, randomized, blinded clinical trial reported that the use of 6% HES (130/0.42), as compared with Ringer's acetate, was associated with a significant increase in the rate of death at 90 days and a significant 35% relative increase in the rate of renal-replacement therapy.

Another recent blinded, randomized, controlled trial, named "Hydroxyethyl starch or saline for fluid resuscitation in intensive care" by CHEST Investigators involving 7000 adults in the ICU, the use of 6% HES (130/0.4), as compared with saline, was not associated with a significant difference in the rate of death at 90 days. However, the use of HES was associated with a significant 21% relative increase in the rate of renal replacement therapy.

In summary, HES (130/0.4) did not provide any substantial advantages to ICU patients requiring IV fluid resuscitation and the analysis of secondary endpoints confirmed an association of its use with renal injury.

Goal-directed Fluid Therapy

Last few decades, attempts at answering the question "how much fluid do I give?" focused on the volume of fluid given and neglected the timing of fluid administration. Approach involves adjustments of cardiac preload, afterload, and contractility to balance oxygen delivery with oxygen demand by manipulating hemodynamics and designed to achieve specific targets for mean arterial pressure, urine output, central venous pressure (CVP) and central venous oxygen saturation in septic patients. Rivers and colleagues showed that mortality could be improved by achieving hemodynamic goals beyond simply maintaining adequate blood pressure (Flow chart 36.1).

A recent trial conducted by protocolized care for early septic shock (ProCESS) investigators to determine whether these findings were generalizable and whether all aspects of the protocol were necessary. They concluded in this multicenter trial conducted in the tertiary care setting, patients were identified early in the emergency department as having septic shock and received antibiotics and other nonresuscitation aspects of care promptly, no significant advantage with respect to mortality or morbidity, of protocol-based resuscitation over bedside care that was provided according to the treating physician's judgment. They also found no significant benefit of the mandated use of central venous catheterization and CVP monitoring in all patients.

Dynamic variables attempt to predict the hemodynamic response to volume administration, i.e. change in cardiac output after a standardized fluid bolus and are based on the interaction between intrathoracic pressure changes and left ventricular end-diastolic volume and cardiac output. These new modalities seem to better answer the question "what will happen to oxygen delivery if I administer fluids?" Common variants available in clinical practice include systolic pressure variation, pulse pressure variation, stroke volume variation, and pleth variability index.

Flow chart 36.1 Algorithm of early goal-directed fluid therapy

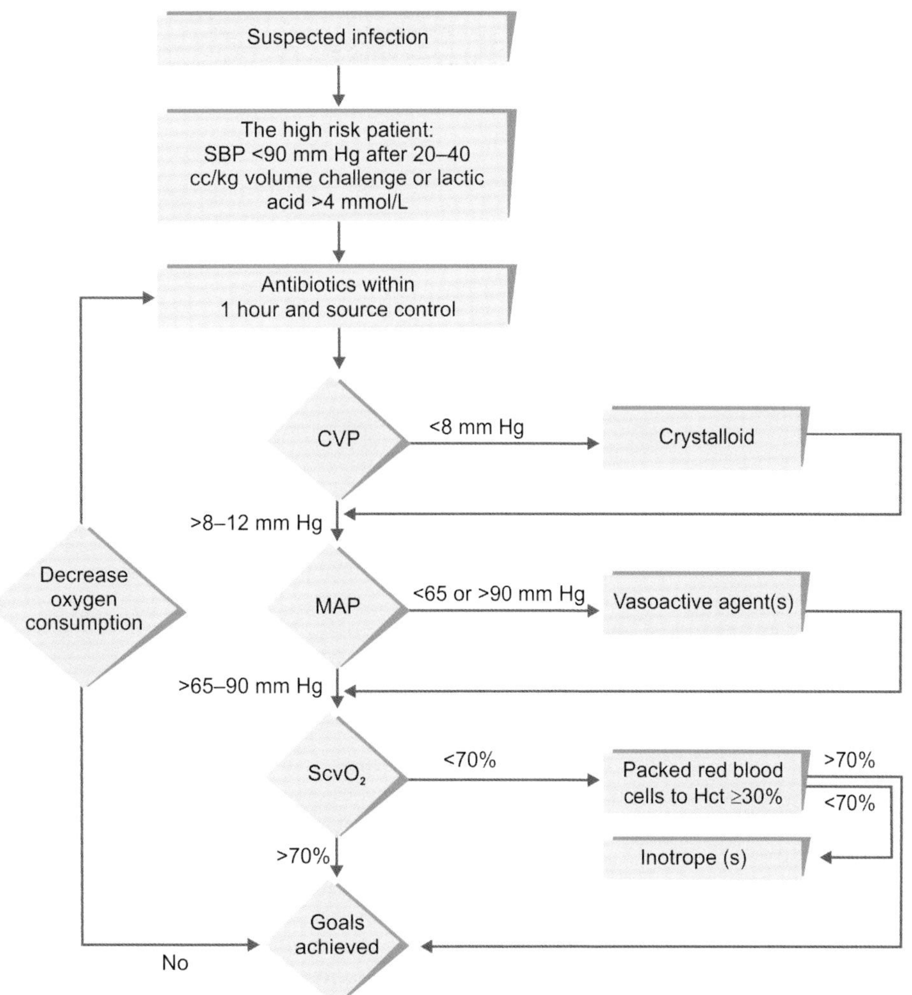

Abbreviations: CVP, central venous pressure; SBP, systolic blood pressure; MAP, mean arterial pressure

Key Messages

- In appropriate time and adequate amount of fluid administration is most important.
- Consider early goal-directed fluid therapy in critically ill patient.
- Consider the type, dose, indications, contraindications, potential for toxicity, and cost.
- Consider serum sodium, osmolarity, and acid-base status when selecting a resuscitation fluid.
- Consider cumulative fluid balance and actual body weight when selecting the dose of resuscitation fluid.
- Consider the early use of catecholamines as concomitant treatment of shock.
- Fluid requirements change over time in critically ill patients.
- HES appear to cause harm and should not be used in sever sepsis and septic shock patients, who are at risk for kidney injury.
- New modalities for assessment of dynamic indices to guide fluid therapy and assess the likely hemodynamic response to volume administration may helpful.

Conclusion

The selection, timing, and doses of IV fluids should be evaluated as carefully as they are in the case of any other IV drug, with the aim of maximizing efficacy and minimizing iatrogenic toxicity.

COMMON ELECTROLYTE DISORDERS

Hyponatremia

The serum sodium concentration and serum osmolality are closely controlled by water homeostasis, which is mediated by thirst, arginine vasopressin, and the kidneys. A disruption in the water balance is manifested as an abnormality in the serum sodium concentration—hypernatremia or hyponatremia. Hyponatremia is defined as a decrease in the serum sodium concentration to a level below 136 mmol/L. Hyponatremia can be associated with low, normal, or high tonicity, effective osmolality or tonicity refers to the contribution to osmolality of solutes, such as sodium and glucose, that cannot move freely across cell membranes, thereby inducing transcellular shifts in water. Dilutional hyponatremia, by farthermost common form of the disorder, is caused by water retention (Table 36.2 and Flow chart 36.2).

Table 36.2 Causes of hypotonic hyponatremia irrigating

Renal sodium loss	Central nervous system disorders
Diuretic agents	Acute psychosis
Osmotic diuresis (glucose, urea, mannitol)	Mass lesions
Adrenal insufficiency	Inflammatory and demyelinating diseases
Salt-wasting nephropathy	Stroke
Diarrhea	Hemorrhage
Vomiting	Trauma
Blood loss	*Excessive water intake*
Excessive sweating (e.g. in marathon runners)	Sodium-free irrigant solutions (used in hysteroscopy, laparoscopy, or transurethral resection of the prostate)
Fluid sequestration in "third space" bowel obstruction	
Increased volume of extra-cellular fluid	*Drugs*
Congestive heart failure	Tricyclics
Cirrhosis	Serotonin-reuptake inhibitors
Nephrotic syndrome	Opiate derivatives
Renal failure (acute or chronic)	Chlorpropamide
Pregnancy	Clofibrate
Thiazide diuretics	Carbamazepine
Hypothyroidism	*Miscellaneous*
Adrenal insufficiency	Postoperative state
Syndrome of inappropriate secretion of antidiuretic hormone	Pain
Cancer	Infection with the human immunodeficiency virus
Pulmonary tumors	Decreased intake of solutes
Mediastinal tumors	
Extrathoracic tumors	

Management

The optimal treatment of hypotonic hyponatremia requires balancing the risks of hypotonicity against those of therapy. The presence of symptoms and their severity largely determine the pace of correction.

Hypernatremia

Hypernatremia, defined as a rise in the serum sodium concentration to a value exceeding 145 mmol/L. Hypernatremia invariably denotes hypertonic hyperosmolality and always causes cellular dehydration, at least transiently. The resultant morbidity may be inconsequential, serious, or even life-threatening. Hypernatremia frequently develops in hospitalized patients as an iatrogenic condition, and some of its most serious complications result not from the disorder itself but from inappropriate treatment of it (Table 36.3).

Flow chart 36.2 Evaluation of hyponatremia

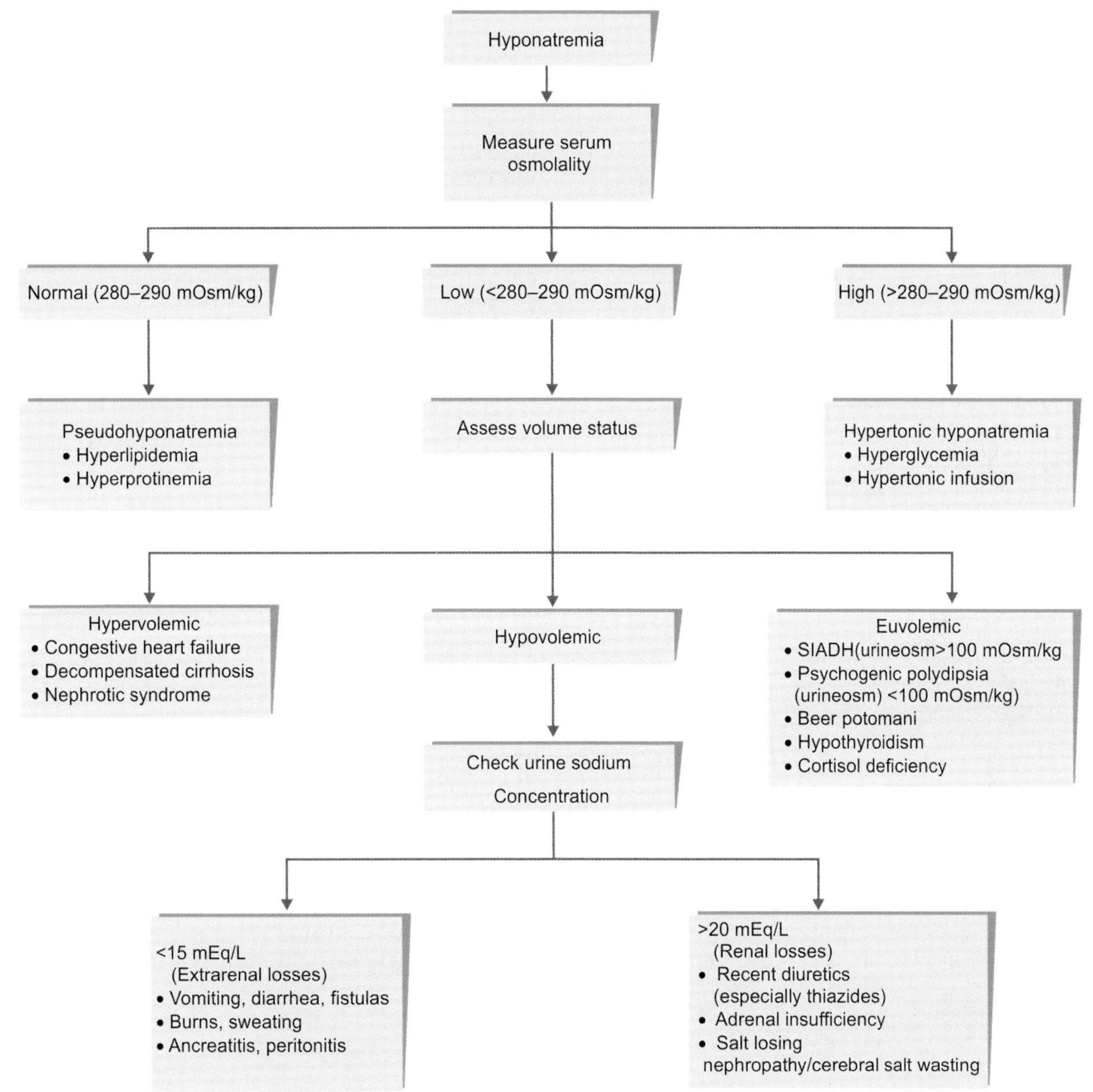

Clinical Manifestation

Signs and symptoms of hypernatremia largely reflect central nervous system dysfunction and are prominent when the increase in the serum sodium concentration is large or occurs rapidly (i.e. over a period of hours). Unlike infants, elderly patients generally have few symptoms until the serum sodium concentration exceeds 160 mmol/L. Intense thirst may be present initially, but it dissipates as the disorder progresses and is absent in patients with hypodipsia. Muscle weakness, confusion, and coma are sometimes manifestations of coexisting disorders rather than of the hypernatremia itself. As in children, rapid sodium loading in adults can cause convulsions and coma. In patients of all ages, orthostatic hypotension and tachycardia reflect marked hypovolemia. Brain shrinkage induced by hypernatremia can cause vascular rupture, with cerebral bleeding, subarachnoid hemorrhage, and permanent neurologic damage or death.

Management

The goals of treatment of hypernatremia are correcting hypertonicity, diagnosis and treatment of underlying cause. Managing the underlying cause such as stopping gastro-

Table 36.3 Causes of hypernatremia

Net water loss	*Renal causes*
Pure water Intake	Loop diuretics
Unreplaced insensible losses (dermal and respiratory)	Osmotic diuresis (glucose, urea, mannitol)
Hypodipsia	Postobstructive diuresis
Neurogenic diabetes insipidus	Polyuric phase of acute tubular necrosis
Post-traumatic	Intrinsic renal disease
Caused by tumors, cysts, histiocytosis, tuberculosis,	*Gastrointestinal causes*
Sarcoidosis	Vomiting
Idiopathic	Nasogastric drainage
Caused by aneurysms, meningitis, encephalitis,	*Hypertonic sodium gain*
Guillain-Barré syndrome	Hypertonic sodium bicarbonate infusion
Congenital nephrogenic diabetes insipidus	Hypertonic feeding preparation
	Primary hyperaldosteronism
Acquired nephrogenic diabetes insipidus	Cushing's syndrome
Caused by renal disease (e.g. medullary cystic disease)	
Caused by hypercalcemia or hypokalemia	
Caused by drugs (lithium, demeclocycline, foscarnet, methoxyflurane, amphotericin B, vasopressin V_2–receptor antagonists)	
Hypotonic fluid	

intestinal fluid losses, controlling pyrexia, hyperglycemia, and glucosuria, withholding lactulose and diuretics, correcting hypercalcemia and hypokalemia; moderating lithium-induced polyuria; or correcting the feeding preparation. In patients with hypernatremia that has developed rapid (over a period of hours) rapid correction improves the prognosis without increasing the risk of cerebral edema. In such patients sodium concentration by 1 mmol/L/hr is appropriate. A slower pace of correction is prudent in patients with hypernatremia of longer or unknown duration, because the full dissipation of accumulated brain solutes occurs over a period of several days. In such patients, reducing the serum sodium concentration at a maximal rate of 0.5 mmol/L/hr prevents cerebral edema and convulsions. Consequently, we recommend a targeted fall in the serum sodium concentration of 10 mmol per liter per day for all patients with hypernatremia except those in whom the disorder has developed over a period of hours. The goal of serum sodium correction is 145 mmol/L.

Calculation of fluid requirements:

$$\textbf{Water deficit (L)} = \textbf{TBW} \times [(\textbf{serum } [Na^+] \ (\textbf{mmol/L})/145) - 1]$$

This is the amount of free water required to return the serum sodium to normal and can be estimated by the formula.

Hypokalemia

A low serum potassium concentration is perhaps the most common electrolyte abnormality encountered in clinical practice. Hypokalemia defined as decrease in the serum potassium concentration to a level below 3.6 mmol/L. Hypokalemia is usually well tolerated in otherwise healthy people, but it can be life-threatening when severe. Even mild or moderate hypokalemia increases the risks of morbidity and mortality in patients with cardiovascular disease.

Clinical Spectrum

Patients with mild hypokalemia (serum potassium, 3.0–3.5 mmol/L) often have no symptoms. Patients with moderate hypokalemia, nonspecific symptoms such as generalized weakness, lassitude, and constipation are more common. In more severe hypokalemia (less than 2.5 mmol/L) muscle necrosis, abdominal distention can occur, and at serum concentrations of less than 2.0 mmol/L, an ascending paralysis can develop, with impairment of respiratory muscles function. In patients without underlying heart disease, arrhythmia unusual, even when the serum potassium concentration is below 3.0 mmol/L. In patients with cardiac disease, even mild-to-moderate hypokalemia increases the risk of cardiac arrhythmias. We will focus on common causes pertaining to cardiac patients (Table 36.4).

Drug-induced Causes

***β_2-sympathomimetic drugs*:** A wide range of drugs have β_2-sympathomimetic activity, including decongestants, bronchodilators. A standard dose of nebulized albuterol reduces serum potassium by 0.2–0.4 mmol/L, and a second dose taken within 1 hour reduces it by almost 1 mmol/L. The hypokalemia caused by these drugs is sustained for up to 4 hours.

***Diuretics*:** The most common cause of hypokalemia is diuretic therapy. Both the thiazide and loop diuretics block chloride-associated sodium reabsorption and, as a result, increase delivery of sodium to the collecting tubules, where its reabsorption creates a favorable electrochemical gradient for potassium secretion. Diuretic-induced hypokalemia is

Table 36.4 Drug-induced hypokalemia

Hypokalemia due to transcellular potassium shift	Hypokalemia due to increased renal potassium loss
β_2-adrenergic agonists	*Diuretics*
Epinephrine	Acetazolamide
Decongestants	Thiazides
Pseudoephedrine	Indapamide
Phenylpropanolamine	Metolazone
Bronchodilators	Bumetanide
Albuterol	Furosemide
Terbutaline	Torsemide
Isoetharine	Mineralocorticoids
Tocolytic agents	Fludrocortisone
Ritodrine	High-dose glucocorticoids
Nylidrin	High-dose antibiotics
Theophylline	Penicillin
	Nafcillin
	Ampicillin
	Carbenicillin
	Drugs associated with magnesium depletion
	Aminoglycosides
	Cisplatin
	Foscarnet
	Amphotericin B

usually but not always associated with a mild-to-moderate metabolic alkalosis.

Non-drug Causes due to Transcellular Shifts

Patients with hyperthyroidism rarely present with severe hypokalemia, resulting in a sudden onset of severe muscle weakness and paralysis. This presentation has occurring in 2–8% of patients with hyperthyroidism in Asian countries.

Non-drug Causes due to Abnormal Losses of Potassium

***Gastrointestinal loss*:** The concentration of potassium in stool is 80–90 mmol/L. In diarrheal states, large quantities of potassium can be lost as the volume of stool increases.

***Loss through the kidney*:** Large amounts of potassium are lost through the kidney in patients with a variety of disorders. These disorders are categorized according to acid-base status.

***Metabolic alkalosis*:** In metabolic alkalosis, most of the time hypokalemia occurs due intracellular shift of potassium. Most common causes of this disorder, induced by selective chloride depletion due to vomiting or nasogastric drainage, hypokalemia develops during the induction of alkalosis as a result of increased renal potassium loss. In the chloride-sensitive form of metabolic alkalosis, the administration of chloride corrects the alkalosis and body conserve potassium, correct the potassium level.

***Metabolic acidosis*:** Hypokalemia is a cardinal feature of type I (distal) renal tubular acidosis. The degree of hypokalemia in this disorder is not directly correlated to the degree of acidosis but more likely reflects dietary sodium and potassium intake and serum aldosterone concentrations. In type I renal tubular acidosis, administration of sodium bicarbonate ameliorates the hypokalemia. Potassium supplementation is usually required on a long-term basis. In cases of type II (proximal) renal tubular acidosis, hypokalemia often develops when sodium bicarbonate is administered.

***Magnesium deficiency*:** Magnesium depletion decreases the intracellular potassium concentration and causes renal potassium wasting. The mechanism by which magnesium depletion causes renal potassium loss is unclear. Magnesium depletion often coexists with potassium depletion as a result of drugs (e.g. diuretics and amphotericin B) or disease processes (e.g. hyperaldosteronism and diarrhea) that cause loss of both potassium and magnesium, making it difficult to assess whether the hypokalemia is caused by the hypomagnesemia or is an independent effect. Regardless of the cause, the ability to correct potassium deficiency is impaired when magnesium deficiency is present, particularly when the serum magnesium concentration is less than 0.5 mmol/L.

PRINCIPLES OF POTASSIUM REPLACEMENT

Potassium replacement is the mainstay of therapy for hypokalemia. In asymptomatic mild hypokalemia oral preparations are prefer. Three salts are available for repletion of body potassium stores—potassium chloride (KCl), potassium phosphate, and potassium bicarbonate. Potassium phosphate is used to replace phosphate losses, and potassium combined with bicarbonate or organic anion is only recommended when potassium depletion occurs in the setting of metabolic acidosis. In all other settings, KCl should be used. When potassium is given intravenously, the rate should not be more than 20 mEq/hr, and the patient's cardiac rhythm should be monitored. The peripheral intravenous dose is usually 20–40 mmol of KCl per liter; higher concentrations can cause localized pain from chemical phlebitis, irritation, and sclerosis. If hypokalemia is severe (< 2.5 mmol/L) and/or critically symptomatic, IV KCl can be administered through a central vein with cardiac monitoring in an intensive care setting at rates of 10–20 mmol/hr. Patients receiving diuretics, typically, 40–100 mmol of supplemental KCl is needed each day to maintain normal serum potassium concentrations and hypokalemia persists despite aggressive potassium replacement in approximately 10% of such patients. A more effective way to correct serum potassium to normal concentrations is to use a potassium-sparing diuretic such as amiloride, triamterene, or spironolactone. Patients treated with one of these potassium-sparing diuretics should have their renal function and serum potassium concentrations monitored frequently. The target potassium serum level should be 4–4.5 mmol/L in cardiac patients.

Hyperkalemia

Hyperkalemia can be a life-threatening condition in cardiac critically patients due to arrhythmias.

Etiology (Table 36.5)

The net release of potassium from the cells, either due to enhanced release or decreased entry, can also cause hyperkalemia. As with exogenous potassium loading, the elevation is typically transient because the excess potassium is excreted in the urine. Because persistent hyperkalemia requires impairment in urinary potassium excretion, it may be inferred that this problem is generally associated with a reduction in either aldosterone effect or in the delivery of sodium and water to the distal secretory site.

Increased Potassium Release from Cells

Pseudohyperkalemia

Pseudohyperkalemia refers to conditions in which the elevation in the measured plasma potassium concentration is due to potassium movement out of the cells during or after the blood specimen has been drawn. The major cause of this problem is mechanical trauma during venipuncture, resulting in hemolysis.

Table 36.5 Major causes of hyperkalemia

Increased potassium release	*Reduced urinary potassium excretion*
Pseudohyperkalemia	Hypoaldosteronism
Metabolic acidosis	Renal disease
Insulin deficiency	Medications
Increased tissue catabolism (Burns)	Nonsteroidal anti-inflammatory drugs
β-adrenergic blockade	Angiotensin-converting enzyme inhibitors
Digitalis overdose	Heparin
Succinylcholine	Potassium-sparing diuretics

Metabolic Acidosis

The buffering of excess hydrogen ions in the cells can lead to potassium movement into the extracellular fluid; this transcellular shift is necessitated, in part, by the need to maintain electroneutrality. This phenomenon is less likely to occur in the organic acidosis, ketoacidosis, and lactic acidosis.

Insulin Deficiency, Hyperglycemia, and Hyperosmolality

Insulin promotes potassium entry into cells; thus, the ingestion of glucose (which stimulates endogenous insulin secretion) minimizes the rise in the plasma potassium concentration induced by concurrent potassium intake. Inpatients with uncontrolled diabetes mellitus, the combination of insulin deficiency and the hyperosmolality induced by hyperglycemia frequently leads to hyperkalemia.

Increased Tissue Breakdown

Any cause of increased tissue breakdown can result in the release of potassium into the extracellular fluid. Hyperkalemia is particularly likely to develop in this setting if renal impairment is also present. Clinical examples include breakdown of a large hematoma, gastrointestinal hemorrhage, rhabdomyolysis, patients receiving cytotoxic or radiation therapy for lymphoma or leukemia (the tumor lysis syndrome).

β-adrenergic Blockade

β-adrenergic blockers interfere with the β_2-adrenergic facilitation of potassium uptake by the cells. This effect is associated with only a minor elevation in the plasma potassium concentration in healthy subjects (< 0.5 mEq/L).

Reduced Urinary Potassium Excretion

Impaired urinary potassium excretion generally requires an abnormality in one or both of the two major factors required for adequate renal potassium handling: aldosterone and distal nephron sodium and water delivery.

Hypoaldosteronism

Any cause of decreased aldosterone release or effect diminishes the efficiency of potassium secretion and can lead to hyperkalemia. The resulting rise in the plasma potassium concentration directly stimulates potassium secretion, partially overcoming the relative absence of aldosterone. As a consequence, the rise in the plasma potassium concentration is small in patients with normal renal function, but it can be clinically important in the presence of underlying renal insufficiency or a high potassium intake. Major causes of hypoaldosteronism are hyporeninemic hypoaldosteronism, renal disease, most often diabetic nephropathy; nonsteroidal anti-inflammatory drugs, angiotensin-converting-enzyme (ACE) inhibitors, Addison's disease, potassium-sparing diuretics, heparin, etc.

Potassium-sparing Diuretics

Potassium-sparing diuretics are probably the most common cause of hyperkalemia due to impairment of aldosterone function. These drugs antagonize the action of aldosterone on the collecting tubule cells: spironolactone and eplerenone by competing for the aldosterone receptor, and amiloride and triamterene by closing the sodium channels in the luminal membrane.

Heparin

Commercial heparin preparations exert a direct toxic effect on the zona glomerulosa cells of the adrenal cortex. Even low-dose heparin can lead to a 75% reduction in plasma aldosterone levels. The mechanism appears to involve a reduction in the number and affinity of adrenal angiotensin II receptors involved in aldosterone synthesis and release.

CHRONIC KIDNEY DISEASE

The ability to maintain potassium excretion at near-normal levels is generally maintained in patients with renal disease as long as both aldosterone secretion and distal tubular urine flow are maintained. Patients who are oliguric or who have an additional problem such as a high-potassium intake, increased tissue breakdown, or hypoaldosteronism are more predisposed to hyperkalemia.

Clinical Manifestations

In general, severe symptoms of hyperkalemia do not occur until the plasma potassium concentration is more than 7.5 mEq/L. There is, however, substantial interpatient variability because factors such as hypocalcemia and metabolic acidosis can increase the toxicity of excess potassium. Thus, careful monitoring of the electrocardiogram (ECG) and muscle strength is indicated to assess the functional consequences of the hyperkalemia. A plasma potassium concentration of more than 7.5–8.0 mEq/L, severe muscle weakness, or marked electrocardiographic changes are potentially life-threatening and require immediate treatment. The earliest ECG abnormality is symmetric peaking of T waves, followed by reduced P-wave voltage and widening of QRS complexes. If untreated, severe hyperkalemia can deteriorates into a sinusoidal ECG form, with one oscillation representing a wide QRS complex and the complementary oscillation representing an abnormal T wave. ECG changes usually do not appear until the plasma K^+ concentration exceeds 6.5 mEq/L, and are more likely to develop when the rise in K^+ occurs rapidly (Fig. 36.1).

Treatment (Table 36.6)

Specific treatment of severe or symptomatic hyperkalemia is directed at antagonizing the membrane effects of potassium,

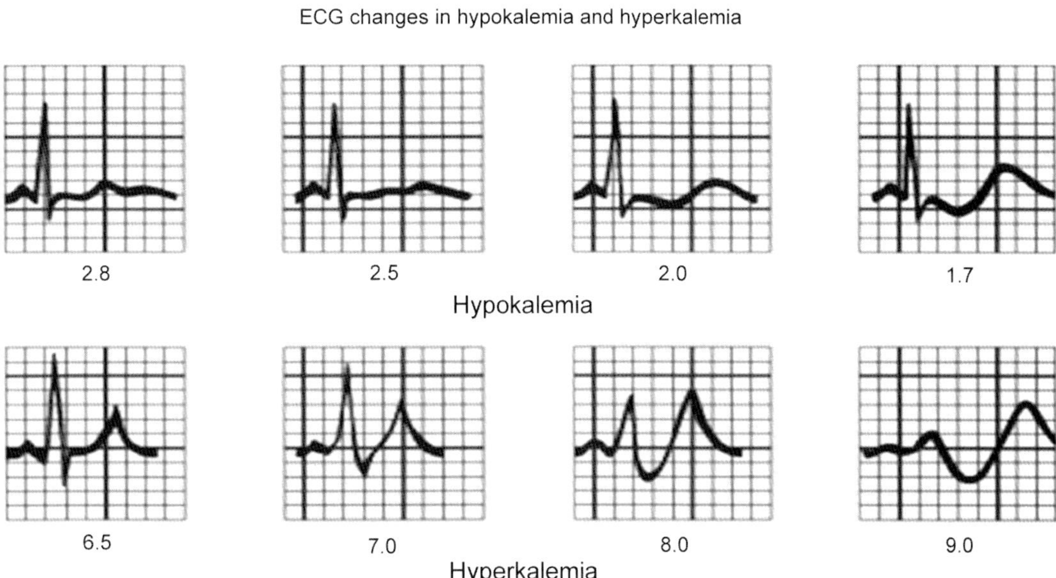

Fig. 36.1 Electrocardiogram (ECG) changes in hypokalemia and hyperkalemia

Table 36.6 Treatment of hyperkalemia

Treatment	Glucose and insulin	Salbutamol	Kayexalate and sorbitol	Loop diuretics	Hemodialysis	Sodium bicarbonate
Mechanism	Shift k to cell	Shift k to cell	Removes k from body	Removes k from body	Removes k from body	Shift k to cell
Dose	10 IU and 50 g	10 mg nebulization	15–30 g oral, 30–50 g retention enema	IV, varies by drug and renal function		45 mEq over 5 min
Onset	15–30 min	20–30 min	1 hours	1 hours	Immediate	15–30 min
Duration	2–4 hours	2–3 hours	–	–	–	–

driving extracellular potassium into the cells, or removing excess potassium from the body. The following modalities may be beneficial.

Calcium

Calcium directly antagonizes the membrane actions of hyperkalemia. Hyperkalemia-induced depolarization of the resting membrane potential leads to inactivation of sodium channels and decreased membrane excitability. Calcium antagonizes this membrane effect of hyperkalemia, although how this is achieved is not well understood. The usual dose is 10 mL of a 10% calcium gluconate solution infused slowly during 2-3 minutes with constant cardiac monitoring. This dose can be repeated after 5 minutes if the ECG changes persist. Calcium should not be given in bicarbonate-containing solutions because this can lead to its precipitation as calcium carbonate.

Insulin and Glucose

Increasing the availability of insulin lowers the plasma potassium concentration by driving potassium into the cells, apparently by enhancing the activity of the Na^+/K^+-ATPase pump in skeletal muscle.

Sodium Bicarbonate

Raising the systemic pH with sodium bicarbonate promotes hydrogen ion release from the cells and a reciprocal movement of potassium into the cells. The elevation in the plasma bicarbonate concentration appears to have another direct, albeit not delineated, effect on lowering the plasma potassium concentration that is independent of pH. The potassium-lowering action of sodium bicarbonate is most prominent in patients with metabolic acidosis. Sodium bicarbonate appears to be less effective in correcting hyperkalemia in patients with renal failure. Insulin plus glucose or a β_2-agonist is more predictably effective in this setting.

β_2-adrenergic Agonists

Like insulin, β_2-adrenergic agonists drive potassium into the cells by increasing Na^+/K^+-ATPase activity. Salbutamol 10 mg in 4 mL of saline by nebulization for 10 minutes can lower the plasma potassium concentration by 0.5-1.5 mEq/L. Furthermore, the effect of these agents is additive to that of insulin plus glucose.

Loop or Thiazide Diuretics

Loop and thiazide diuretics can be used when hyperkalemia is present in an individual with hypertension or volume overload. However, the effectiveness of diuretic therapy is frequently limited by moderate-to-severe renal insufficiency.

Cation Exchange Resin

In the gut, this resin takes up potassium, calcium and magnesium to lesser degrees, and releases sodium. Each gram of resin may bind as much as 1 mEq of potassium and release 1-2 mEq of sodium.

Dialysis

Dialysis can be used if the conservative measures listed in the preceding sections are ineffective, if the hyperkalemia is severe, if the patient has marked tissue breakdown and is releasing large amounts of potassium from the injured cells, or, of course, if the patient has hyperkalemia in the setting of renal failure.

ACE Inhibitors and Spironolactone

ACE inhibitors and spironolactone in the settings of chronic kidney disease should be administered with caution with regular potassium monitoring. The benefits in heart failure patients should be weighed against risk of hyperkalemia.

SUMMARY

The field continues to evolve with newer measurement techniques coming to the fore. What is important is to realize that the fundamentals do not change.

BIBLIOGRAPHY

1. Albert K, van Vlymen J, James P, et al. Ringer's lactate is compatible with the rapid infusion of AS-3 preserved packed red blood cells. Can J Anaesth. 2009;56:352-6.
2. Anderson RJ. Hospital-associated hyponatremia. Kidney Int. 1986;29:1237-47.
3. Arieff AI, Llach F, Massry SG. Neurological manifestations and morbidity of hyponatremia: correlation with brain water and electrolytes. Medicine (Baltimore). 1976;55:121-9.
4. Barsoum N, Kleeman C. Now and then, the history of parenteral fluid administration. Am J Nephrol. 2002;22:284-9.
5. Bartels K, Thiele R, Gan T. Rational fluid management in today's ICU practice. Critical Care. 2013;17(Suppl 1):S6.
6. Bayer O, Reinhart K, Sakr Y, Kabisch B, Kohl M, Riedemann NC, et al. Renal effects of synthetic colloids and crystalloids in patients with severe sepsis: a prospective sequential comparison. Crit Care Med. 2011;39:1335-42.
7. Brunkhorst FM, Engel C, Bloos F, Meier-Hellmann A, Ragaller M, Weiler N, et al. German Competence Network Sepsis (SepNet): intensive insulin therapy and pentastarch resuscitation in severe sepsis. N Engl J Med. 2008;358:125-39.
8. Challand C, Struthers R, Sneyd JR, Erasmus PD, Mellor N, Hosie KB, et al. Randomized controlled trial of intraoperative goal-directed fluid therapy in aerobically fit and unfit patients having major colorectal surgery. Br J Anaesth. 2012;108:53-62.
9. Christidis C, Mal F, Ramos J, Senejoux A, Callard P, Navarro R, et al. Worsening of hepatic dysfunction as a consequence of repeated hydroxyethyl starch infusions. J Hepatol. 2001;35:726-32.
10. Cope JT, Banks D, Mauney MC, Lucktong T, Shockey KS, Kron IL, et al. Intraoperative hetastarch infusion impairs hemostasis after cardiac operations. Ann Thorac Surg. 1997;63:78-83.
11. Cosnett JE. The origins of intravenous fluid therapy. Lancet. 1989;1:768-71.
12. Feig PU, McCurdy DK. The hypertonic state. N Engl J Med. 1977;297:1444-54.
13. Finfer S, Bellomo R, Boyce N, French J, Myburgh J, Norton R. A comparison of albumin and saline for fluid resuscitation in the intensive care unit. N Engl J Med. 2004;350:2247-56.
14. Gan TJ, Soppitt A, Maroof M, el-Moalem H, Robertson KM, Moretti E, et al. Goal-directed intraoperative fluid administration reduces length of hospital stay after major surgery. Anesthesiology. 2002;97:820-6.
15. Gattas DJ, Dan A, Myburgh J, Billot L, Lo S, Finfer S. Fluid resuscitation with 6% hydroxyethyl starch (130/0.4) in acutely ill patients: an updated systematic review and meta-analysis. Anesth Analg. 2012;114:159-69.
16. Gennari FJ. Hypohypernatraemia: disorders of water balance. In: Davison AM, Cameron JS, Grünfeld JP, Kerr DNS, Ritz E, Winearls CG (Eds). Oxford textbook of clinical nephrology, 2nd edition. Oxford, England: Oxford University Press; 1998. pp. 175-200.
17. Gennari FJ. Serum osmolality: uses and limitations. N Engl J Med. 1984;310:102-5.
18. Grocott MP, Mythen MG, Gan TJ. Perioperative fluid management and clinical outcomes in adults. Anesth Analg. 2005;100:1093-106.
19. Guidet B, Martinet O, Boulain T, Philippart F, Poussel JF, Maizel J, et al. Assessment of hemodynamic efficacy and safety of 6% hydroxyethyl starch 130/0.4 vs. 0.9% NaCl fluid replacement in patients with severe sepsis: the CRYSTMAS study. Crit Care. 2012;16:R94.
20. Gurgel ST, do Nascimento P. Maintaining tissue perfusion in high-risk surgical patients: a systematic review of randomized clinical trials. Anesth Analg. 2011;112:1384-91.
21. Hamilton MA, Cecconi M, Rhodes A. A systematic review and meta-analysis on the use of preemptive hemodynamic intervention to improve postoperative outcomes in moderate and high-risk surgical patients. Anesth Analg. 2011;112:1392-402.
22. Hartog CS, Bauer M, Reinhart K. The efficacy and safety of colloid resuscitation in the critically ill. Anesth Analg. 2011;112:156-64.
23. Hoffmann JN, Vollmar B, Laschke MW, Inthorn D, Schildberg FW, Menger MD. Hydroxyethyl starch (130 kD), but not crystalloid volume support, improves microcirculation during normotensive endotoxemia. Anesthesiology. 2002;97:460-70.
24. Hyponatremia and hypernatremia. In: Adrogué HJ, Wesson DE. Salt & Water. Boston: Blackwell Scientific; 1994. pp.205-84.
25. Hypoosmolal states—hyponatremia. In: Rose BD. Clinical physiology of acid-base and electrolyte disorders, 4th edition. NewYork: McGraw-Hill; 1994. pp.651-94.
26. Kellum JA. Determinants of blood pH in health and disease. Crit Care. 2000;4:6-14.
27. Kozek-Langenecker SA. Effects of hydroxyethyl starch solutions on hemostasis. Anesthesiology. 2005;103:654-60.
28. Lang JD, Figueroa M, Chumley P, Aslan M, Hurt J, Tarpey MM, et al. Albumin and hydroxyethyl starch modulate oxidative inflammatory injury to vascular endothelium. Anesthesiology. 2004;100:51-8.
29. Latta T. Malignant cholera. Documents communicated by the Central Board of Health, London, relative to the treatment of cholera by the copious injection of aqueous and saline fluids into the veins. Lancet. 1832;18:274-80.
30. Lobo SM, Ronchi LS, Oliveira NE, Brandao PG, Froes A, Cunrath GS, et al. Restrictive strategy of intraoperative fluid maintenance during optimization of oxygen delivery decreases major complications after high-risk surgery. Crit Care. 2011;15:R226.
31. Maas AH, Siggaard-Andersen O, Weisberg HF, Zijlstra WG. Ion-selective electrodes for sodium and potassium: a new problem of what is measured and what should be reported. Clin Chem. 1985;31:482-5.
32. Maitland K, Kiguli S, Opoka RO, Engoru C, Olupot-Olupot P, Akech SO, et al. FEAST Trial Group: Mortality after fluid bolus in African children with severe infection. N Engl J Med. 2011;364:2483-95.
33. Marik PE, Cavallazzi R, Vasu T, Hirani A. Dynamic changes in arterial waveform derived variables and fluid responsiveness in mechanically ventilated patients: a systematic review of the literature. Crit Care Med. 2009;37:2642-7.
34. Massa DJ, Lundy JS, Faulconer A, et al. A plastic needle. Proc Staff Meet Mayo Clin. 1950;25(14):413-5.
35. Myburgh J, Cooper DJ, Finfer S, Bellomo R, Norton R, Bishop N, et al. Saline or albumin for fluid resuscitation in patients with traumatic brain injury. N Engl J Med. 2007;357:874-84.

36. Myburgh JA, Finfer S, Bellomo R, Billot L, Cass A, Gattas D, et al. Hydroxyethyl starch or saline for fluid resuscitation in intensive care. N Engl J Med. 2012;367:1901-11.
37. Natalini G, Rosano A, Taranto M, Faggian B, Vittorielli E, Bernardini A. Arterial versus plethysmographic dynamic indices to test responsiveness for testing fluid administration in hypotensive patients: a clinical trial. Anesth Analg. 2006;103:1478-84.
38. Neuhaus W, Schick MA, Bruno RR, Schneiker B, Forster CY, Roewer N, et al. The effects of colloid solutions on renal proximal tubular cells in vitro. Anesth Analg. 2012;114:371-4.
39. Perner A, Haase N, Guttormsen AB, Tenhunen J, Klemenzson G, Aneman A, et al. Hydroxyethyl starch 130/0.42 versus Ringer's acetate in severe sepsis. N Engl J Med. 2012;367:124-34.
40. Perner A, Haase N, Guttormsen AB, Tenhunen J, Klemenzson G, Aneman A, et al. Hydroxyethyl starch 130/0.4 versus Ringer's acetate in severe sepsis. N Engl J Med. 2012;367:124-34.
41. Reinhart K, Perner A, Sprung CL, Jaeschke R, Schortgen F, Johan Groeneveld AB, et al. Consensus statement of the ESICM task force on colloid volume therapy in critically ill patients. Intensive Care Med. 2012;38:368-83.
42. Reinhart K, Takala J. Hydroxyethyl starches: what do we still know? Anesth Analg. 2011;112:507-11.
43. Rhodes A, Cecconi M, Hamilton M, Poloniecki J, Woods J, Boyd O, et al. Goal-directed therapy in high-risk surgical patients: a 15-year follow-up study. Intensive Care Med. 2010;36: 1327-32.
44. Rioux JP, Lessard M, De Bortoli B, Roy P, Albert M, Verdant C, et al. Pentastarch 10% (250 kDa/0.45) is an independent risk factor of acute kidney injury following cardiac surgery. Crit Care Med. 2009;37:1293-8.
45. Rivers E, Nguyen B, Havstad S, Ressler J, Muzzin A, Knoblich B, et al. Early goal-directed therapy in the treatment of severe sepsis and septic shock. N Engl J Med. 2001;345:1368-77.
46. Rose BD. New approach to disturbances in the plasma sodium concentration. Am J Med. 1986;81:1033-40.
47. Ross EJ, Christie SB. Hypernatremia. Medicine (Baltimore). 1969;48:441-73.
48. Schortgen F, Girou E, Deye N, et al. The risk associated with hyperoncotic colloids in patients with shock. Intensive Care Med. 2008;34:2157-68.
49. Shafer SL. Shadow of doubt. Anesth Analg. 2011;112:498-500.
50. Snyder NA, Feigal DW, Arieff AI. Hypernatremia in elderly patients: a heterogeneous, morbid, and iatrogenic entity. Ann Intern Med. 1987;107:309-19.
51. The ProCESS Investigators. A Randomized Trial of Protocol-Based Care for Early Septic Shock. N Engl J Med. 2014;370: 1683-93.
52. Virgilio RW, Rice CL, Smith DE, James DR, Zarins CK, Hobelmann CF, et al. Crystalloid vs. colloid resuscitation: is one better? A randomized clinical study. Surgery. 1979;85:129-39.

37

Transcatheter Aortic Valve Implantation: Status for Low Risk Group

Vijay Kumar, Ashok Seth

INTRODUCTION

Transcatheter aortic valve replacement (TAVR) is a very good option of treatment for the very high surgical risk patients of severe aortic stenosis who are deemed unsuitable for surgical aortic valve replacement (SAVR) due to various comorbidities. Transcatheter aortic valve replacement has been used as an alternative to relieve symptoms and extend life in these patients. Almost one lakh patients have been treated worldwide with one of the two commercially approved TAVR devices, including the balloon-expandable Edwards SAPIEN Transcatheter Heart Valve (Edwards Life Sciences, Irvine, CA, USA) and the self-expanding Core Valve Revalving System (Medtronic, Minneapolis, MN, USA). Several trials and observational studies have come up with good data in support. With the noninferiority and definitive significant mortality benefits of TAVR demonstrated in patients at high-risk for SAVR, there is general interest in expanding the clinical trial portfolio to include lower risk patients. Outcomes of TAVR in low surgical risk patients show impressive results according to the available retrospective and prospective data and there appears to be an optimism about the consistency of its results and the possibility of becoming an established option over SAVR in the next decade.

RISK STRATIFICATION IN TRANSCATHETER AORTIC VALVE REPLACEMENT

Risk stratification plays a decisive role in the optimal selection of therapeutic strategies for severe aortic stenosis patients. The accuracy of contemporary surgical risk algorithms for severe aortic stenosis patients has spiraled a significant debate especially in the higher risk patient population as well as the intermediate- and low-risk patients.

Risk stratification in patients referred for TAVR evaluation remains challenging, as there is no specified risk scoring system validated for TAVR patients in particular, and the currently used surgical risk scores may over- or underestimate the actual risk incurred. The Society for Thoracic Surgery Predicted Risk of Mortality (STS-PROM) has been used to estimate 30-day mortality operative risk. An STS-PROM >4 comprises the highest 25% risk of patients currently undergoing SAVR, and an STS-PROM >3 identifies the highest 33% risk (Fig. 37.1).[1] Other surgical risk scores, such as the logistic EuroSCORE, while correlated with overall prediction of risk, are poorly calibrated to estimate precise SAVR mortality rates. The logistic EuroSCORE widely used in Europe has a cutoff value of 20% considered as high risk. As the experience is increasing with regards to patient selection and performing the procedure, it is being now seen that the logistic EuroSCORE overestimates risk for adverse clinical outcomes. A large number of patients undergoing TAVR in contemporary times are at high risk when calculated based on the logistic EuroSCORE but only at intermediate risk when applying the STS score. This quandary has led to inconsistent inclusion criteria across different studies. The role of a dedicated heart team is helpful to in-patient selection and

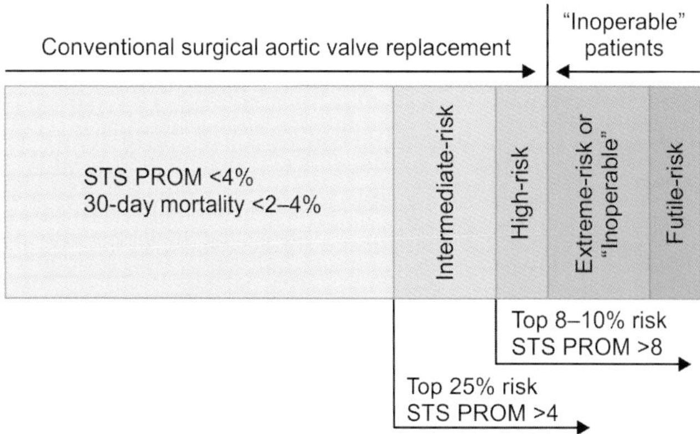

Fig. 37.1 Spectrum of surgical risk in patients with aortic stenosis

Source: Raheem S, Popma JJ. Clinical studies assessing transcatheter aortic valve replacement. Cardiovasc J. 2012;8(2):13-8.

treatment decision. There is a difference between "Calculated Risk" versus "Clinical Risk." The current surgical risk scoring methods are poor at predicting outcomes post-TAVR. The "Heart Team" model, with individualized, holistic, patient centered "clinical risk" scoring is the ideal way to identify suitable TAVR candidates. Many patients who were presumed to be at increased risk for SAVR during the Heart Team discussion were found to be at an intermediate risk when applying the STS score. Important comorbidities and high-risk features that were not considered in the STS risk and EuroSCORE contribute to this difference. This implies that patient selection based on risk score calculation alone is not adequate to define the "true" risk of a patient undergoing SAVR.

Low-risk patients constitute the low STS score patients, are often less sick and have younger age, good renal function, favorable vascular access anatomy, lesser tortuous aorta, lesser aortic atheroma and generally not high on the frailty index, lesser comorbidities, and constitute an interesting set of population to assess results of TAVR. Factors like the general health condition and frailty of the patient influence the modality of treatment decision selection, beyond the estimated surgical risk as assessed by available risk scores. It is an established fact now that patients at high risk according to the STS score have worse clinical outcome after SAVR compared with patients with lower STS risk. The clinical results among cautiously chosen patients considered at low- or intermediate-risk based on the STS score are favorable fair well when compared with high-risk patients.

STUDIES ON TRANSCATHETER AORTIC VALVE REPLACEMENT FOR LOW- AND INTERMEDIATE-RISK PATIENTS

Single and multicenter studies from different parts of Europe, namely Rouen, Bern, Munich, Milan and Rotterdam, all throw light on the favorable results of TAVR in low- to intermediate-risk patients. The comparisons with high-risk patients and challenges of TAVR in low- and intermediate-risk patients have also been observed. The surgical replacement and transcatheter aortic valve implantation (SURTAVI) trial and ongoing placement of aortic transcatheter valves trial (PARTNER) II will further throw light on the data of this subset of low- and intermediate-risk patients.

Godin and his colleagues examined TAVI outcomes in both low- and high-risk patients who had contraindications to surgery.[2] The analysis included 177 consecutive patients who were implanted with the Edwards Sapien or Sapien XT valve at their center from 2006 to 2011. About one-third of the patients had a EuroSCORE >20% (mean 11.9%). The average EuroSCORE in patients at high-risk was 32.2%. The procedural success rate did not differ between the low-risk group (100%) and the high-risk group (95.3%). There was no difference in major vascular complications (5% vs. 6%), major stroke (1.7% vs. 0.9%), or permanent pacemaker implantation (5% vs. 6%) between the low- and high-risk groups, although patients with low-risk had a shorter hospital stay and less life-threatening bleeding. None of the low-risk patients died within 30 days, compared with 11.1% of high-risk patients ($p = 0.009$). The survival benefit was sustained at 1 year.

Another single center study by Anke Opitz of the German Heart Center in Munich provided 3-year data on the durability of Medtronic's CoreValve.[3] The analysis included 393 patients (mean age 80, mean EuroSCORE 19.1%) who underwent a successful TAVR procedure from June 2007 to June 2011. The effective orifice area increased significantly in all patients from 0.7 to 1.5 cm^2 ($p < 0.001$) and peak and mean aortic valve gradients decreased significantly in all patients ($p < 0.001$ for both). Left ventricular ejection fraction improved without a change the size of the left ventricle. About two-thirds of patients had paravalvular aortic regurgitation after TAVI, although it was mostly trivial with no impact on clinical outcome. The changes persisted through 3 years.

In SURTAVI study, a prospective three-center comparison of 1-year mortality between November 2006 and January 2010, 3,666 consecutive patients of severe aortic stenosis was done who underwent either TAVR (n = 782) or SAVR (n = 2,884).[4] Propensity-score matched pairs of TAVR and SAVR patients with Society of Thoracic Surgeons (STS) scores between 3% and 8% made up the study population. Primary end point was all-cause mortality at 1 year. The patients were categorized into three different risk groups comparing TAVR with SAVR among intermediate-risk patients (low-risk STS score, <3%, intermediate risk 3–8%, high risk as >8%). Four hundred five TAVR patients were matched to 405 SAVR patients. Of matched TAVI patients, 99 (24%) patients had STS scores <3%, 255 (63%) had scores between 3% and 8%, and 51 (13%) had scores >8%. Cumulative all-cause mortality at 30 days and 1 year was similar among propensity-score matched TAVI and SAVR patients at intermediate surgical risk.[4]

In a study between 2007 and 2011, 389 serial patients underwent TAVR and were classified according to the STS score into low (STS < 3%; n = 41, 10.5%), intermediate (STS ≥ 3% and ≤8%, n = 254, 65.3%), and high risk (STS > 8%; n = 94, 24.2%). The all-cause mortality at 30 days (2.4 vs. 3.9 vs. 14.9%, $p = 0.001$), and at 1 year (10.1 vs. 16.1 vs. 34.5%, $p = 0.0003$). There was no difference observed with respect to cerebrovascular accidents and myocardial infarction during 1-year follow-up.[5] The low or intermediate risk had significantly lower rates of major bleeding, major vascular complications, and deterioration of renal function. The rates of access site and bleeding complications after TAVR have been a matter of argument and several measures have been devised to reduce these risks. Important advances in the pre-TAVR workup, including semi-automated, CT-scan-based, post-processing software to assist in device and access site selection, a further reduction in vascular delivery sheath diameter, and refinements in suture-based vascular closure devices have led to the favorable results. A serious concern has been the high rate of permanent pacemaker implantation and paravalvular aortic regurgitation after TAVR, which is not described after SAVR. Recent data suggest that the need for permanent pacemaker implantation after TAVR is not associated with bad clinical outcomes, post TAVR aortic regurgitation ≥2 is said to affect mortality. Newer generation TAVR prosthesis with improved frame and valve designs as well as more precision in implantation and positioning methodology might reduce the need of a permanent pacemaker implantation and reduce the rate of significant residual aortic regurgitation. The future data are going to throw light on these aspects. In a subgroup analysis, transfemoral TAVR patients, the 30-day complication rate was very low. Low-risk patients undergoing transfemoral TAVR had best results with no events in terms of all-cause mortality, cerebrovascular accidents, myocardial infarction, major access site complications, and acute renal failure at 30 days of TAVR. The small patient number as well as the primary motive to treat patients with the transfemoral route needs to be kept in mind when analyzing these findings. In any case transfemoral access is thought to be the least invasive route to perform TAVR, and can be performed as fully percutaneous procedure under local anesthesia with conscious sedation in experienced centers.

Low- and intermediate-risk patients have low rates of periprocedural complications which are appealing; the issue of cerebrovascular adverse events has been a matter of concern. Atrial fibrillation, concomitant cerebrovascular disease, and aortic arch atheroma may increase the risk of stroke independent of the procedure among elderly patients undergoing TAVR. The procedure itself is associated with a certain risk of thromboembolic complications. Several causes have been found to increase the risk of cerebral injury including the retrograde passage of bulky catheter delivery system across the calcified aortic valve, aortic arch, and the ascending aorta as well as the balloon aortic valvuloplasty, and the deployment of the prosthesis or the postdilatation done to oppose a partially unexpanded valve.

The present data show promising short- and mid-term clinical outcomes of low- and intermediate-risk patients as compared with the high-risk group. When STS score was compared, all-cause and cardiovascular mortality correlated well with the predicted risk. Mortality had a linear function at 30 days and 1 year for cardiovascular and all-cause death in favor of low- and intermediate-risk patients. By the valve academic research consortium (VARC) combined safety end point, the low-risk group had a 59% and the intermediate-risk group a 45% lower risk to reach this end point compared with the high-risk group. The improved clinical outcome for lower risk patients was maintained over time, showing a sustained 71% and 59% relative risk reduction, respectively.

The UK TAVI Registry investigators[6,7] have inclusion of lower risk patients and the results further substantiate the promising results in these patients. Using the logistic EuroSCORE, the authors report an estimated perioperative risk of 18.5% (11.7–27.9), which is comparable with the intermediate-risk group [logistic EuroSCORE 19.6% (12.8–28.7)] of the present patient population.

In an observational study of patients undergoing TAVR and SAVR for severe aortic stenosis, the relatively low-risk propensity-matched population analyzed and was found that 30-day mortality and procedural mortality rate were same for both TAVR and SAVR, but SAVR was associated with a higher risk for blood transfusion, whereas TAVR showed a significantly higher vascular damage, permanent AV block and residual aortic valve regurgitation.[7]

The PARTNER II trial randomly assigns patients at intermediate surgical risk to undergo either SAVR or TAVI with the Edwards Sapien XT bioprosthesis. The enrolment till 2013 November and its 5-year follow-up will give results to compare the low- and intermediate-risk patients with the high-risk patients.

CONCLUSION

Currently, TAVR procedure is indicated in patients with severe symptomatic aortic stenosis who are judged by the "heart team" to be unsuitable for surgery but have sufficient life expectancy. In contemporary practice, TAVR is not restricted just to inoperable or STS-defined high-risk patients and should be guided by the decision of an interdisciplinary Heart Team. Compared with patients at calculated high-risk, well-selected patients with STS-defined intermediate or low risk appear to have favorable clinical outcomes.

Rapid advances are occurring in prosthesis design, catheter delivery system, imaging, and the hybrid operating room and would increase the possibility of choosing more and more TAVR cases over SAVR in lower risk patients.

Trials like the SURTAVI model[8] propose for a pragmatic risk stratification for patients with severe aortic stenosis rather than the existing conventional surgical risk scoring systems.[8] SURTAVI and PARTNER II will give more data about this population in their long-term follow-up.

Future trials will explore more about TAVR in patients at intermediate and low operative risk. The presently available data may be the first step toward a broader assessment of percutaneous techniques in populations at lower surgical risk, but without forgetting that the SAVR is currently the gold standard. Europe has already largely moved to "intermediate risk" in clinical practice.

REFERENCES

1. Raheem S, Popma JJ. Clinical studies assessing transcatheter aortic valve replacement. Cardiovasc J. 2012;8(2):13-8.
2. European Society of Cardiology Source reference: Godin M, et al. Transcatheter aortic valve implantation with the Edwards valve prosthesis in patients with low (<20%) logistic EuroSCORE: results of a prospective single—center registry, ESC 2011; Abstract P4994.

3. European Society of Cardiology Source reference: Opitz A, et al. Hemodynamic results after TAVI: up to three years follow-up of 338 patients after CoreValve implantation. ESC 2011; Abstract P4973.
4. Piazza N, Kalesan B, van Mieghem N, et al. A 3-center comparison of 1-year mortality outcomes between transcatheter aortic valve implantation and surgical aortic valve replacement on the basis of propensity score matching among intermediate-risk surgical patients. JACC Cardiovasc Interv. 2013;6(5):443-51.
5. Wenaweser P, Stortecky S, Schwander S, et al. Clinical outcomes of patients with estimated low or intermediate surgical risk undergoing transcatheter aortic valve implantation. Eur Heart J. 2013;34(25):1894-905.
6. Moat NE, Ludman P, de Belder MA, et al. Long-term outcomes after transcatheter aortic valve implantation in high-risk patients with severe aortic stenosis: the U.K. TAVI (United Kingdom Transcather Aortic Valve Implantation) Registry. J Am Coll Cardiol. 2011;58:2130-38.
7. D'Errigo P, Barbanti M, Ranucci M, et al. Transcatheter aortic valve implantation versus surgical aortic valve replacement for severe aortic stenosis: results from an intermediate risk propensity-matched population of the Italian OBSERVANT study. Int J Cardiol. 2013;167(5):1945-52.
8. van Mieghem NM, Head SJ, van der Boon RM, et al. The SURTAVI model: proposal for a pragmatic risk stratification for patients with severe aortic stenosis. EuroIntervention. 2012;8(2):258-66.

38

Approach to Acyanotic Congenital Heart Diseases

Neeraj Awasthy, S Radhakrishnan

Congenital heart disease (CHD) occurs in approximately 1% of live births, considering the population and the birth rate in India it is apparent that we have a considerable load of CHD patients in our country. Classically, the CHD have been classified into acyanotic congenital heart disease (ACHD), cyanotic congenital heart diseases, and admixture lesions. The present chapter would concentrate on acyanotic CHD. The topic will be discussed under the following headings:

1. Classification of ACHD
2. Pathophysiology of ACHD
3. How to suspect ACHD
4. Clinical features of ACHD
5. Chest X-ray and electrocardiographic features of ACHD
6. Echocardiography including specific ACHD
7. Plan of management and timing of intervention for ACHD.

CLASSIFICATION OF ACYANOTIC CONGENITAL HEART DISEASE

The acyanotic congenital heart defects can be classified into the lesions that increase the volume load of the heart, i.e. those that increase pulmonary blood flow and those that increase the pressure load on the heart (obstructive) (Table 38.1).

Table 38.1 The classification of acyanotic congenital heart disease

Left-to-right shunt lesions
Pretricuspid shunt lesions
Atrial level
Post-tricuspid shunt lesions
Ventricular level
Great artery level
Obstructive lesions
Left-sided obstructive lesions
Right-sided obstructive lesions

PATHOPHYSIOLOGY OF ACYANOTIC CONGENITAL HEART DISEASE (FIG. 38.1)

Pathophysiology of Left-to-Right Shunts

- Shunt at any level leads to volume overloading of the heart as well as lungs.
- Increased flow across lung leads to increased interstitial fluid which facilitates bacterial growth (frequent chest infections). These take longer to resolve too.
- The increased respiratory efforts causes in drawing of the soft ribs at diaphragmatic attachment leading to precordial bulge.
- When there is a defect in the partition between left and right heart structures, the oxygenated blood is shunted from left to right because of generally lower pressure and/or resistance in the right heart pulmonary vascular bed than in the left side.
- Volume load results in increased heart size as well as hyperkinetic precordium and congestive heart failure (CHF). Congestive heart failure manifests itself as sweating, failure to thrive, and slow weight gain.
- These patients have shunt murmurs and flow murmurs. Shunt murmurs is because of the flow through the abnormal communication [generally absent in atrial septal defect (ASD) as the pressure difference is too small]. Flow murmur is because of the flow through the normal valve. Flow murmur can be systolic or diastolic.
- The volume overloading of the lungs results in changes in pulmonary vasculature, overall increase in pulmonary vascular markings, and pulmonary vascular obstructive disease at a later stage.
- Since the overall impact is on pulmonary vasculature and chamber size and does not lead to significant myocardial hypertrophy, roentgenogram is a better modality then electrocardiogram in shunt lesions.
- The physical findings are either a manifestation of flow across the defects or due to effects of excessive flow across

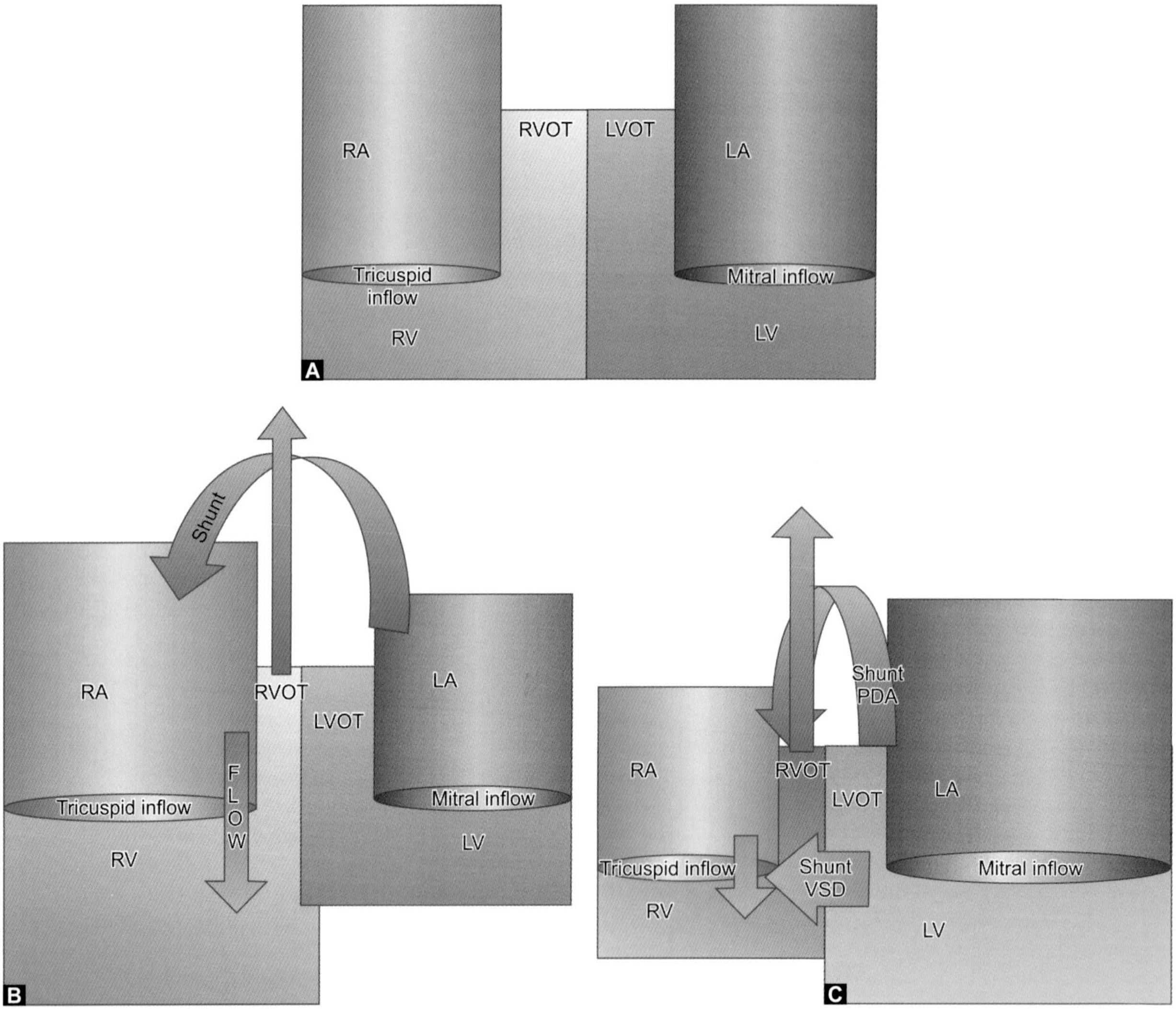

Figs 38.1A to C (A) Schematic diagrams showing the hemodynamics. (B) Schematic diagram in a case of pretricuspid shunt showing left-to-right shunt at the atrial level with dilated right-sided structures (right atrium and right ventricle). There is increased flow across the right ventricular outflow tract and across the tricuspid valve (which produces flow murmur). (C) Schematic diagram in a case of post-tricuspid shunt showing left-to-right shunt at the ventricular level (VSD) and at great arteries level (PDA) with dilated left-sided structures (left atrium and left ventricle)

the cardiac chambers (volume overload) and valves or both. The magnitude of the shunt determines the clinical presentation and symptoms. These finds are emphasized by classical shunt lesions as below.

Pretricuspid Shunt: ASD (Figs 38.1A and B)

- Magnitude of the left-to-right shunt is determined by the size of the defect and the relative compliance of the left (LV) and the right ventricle (RV).
- The magnitude of the shunt is determined by the enlargement of the right-sided structures: right atrium (RA), RV, and pulmonary arteries.
- Absence of the enlargement of the left-sided structures: left atrium (LA) and left ventricle (LV) (as LA gets decompressed).
- The dilated RV prolongs the time required for RV depolarization producing right bundle branch block (RBBB).
- The shunt murmur does not produce any findings. Increased flow across pulmonary valve produces pulmonary ejection systolic murmur. Increased flow across the tricuspid valve produces the diastolic murmur across tricuspid valve. The widely split S2 results from the partial RBBB and compliance of the pulmonary vascular bed, delayed pulmonary component because of delayed

P2 and remains fixed as large atrial shunt tends to abolish respiratory related variation in systemic venous return to right side of the heart, thus making the S2 fixed.
- There is no direct transmission of systemic pressures to pulmonary artery pressures and because of the large compliance of the pulmonary vascular bed PA pressures do not generally increase until late.

Post-tricuspid Shunt (Figs 38.1A and C)

Ventricular septal defect

- The magnitude of the shunt is determined by the size (not the location) of the defect and the level of pulmonary vascular resistance.
- The shunt of the ventricular septal defect (VSD) occurs in systole when RV is contracting and hence the blood goes to the PA rather than remaining in the RV, thus no RV volume overload.
- Left-sided structures dilate (LA, LV) leading to cardiomegaly.
- Increased flow across the mitral valve produces flow (diastolic) murmur across mitral valve. There is wide and variable S2.
- *Large VSD*: Defect offers no resistance and hence the PA pressures and systemic pressures are the same. The magnitude of the shunt flow is determined by the pulmonary vascular resistance across the pulmonary bed.
- *Moderate VSD*: PA pressures are less then systemic pressures (30–50% of systemic pressures). There may be left-sided volume overload with dilated LA and LV.
- *Small (restricted) VSD*: PA pressure is 25–30% of systemic and magnitude of shunt, not significant enough to dilate left-sided structures.

Patent Ductus Arteriosus

The pathophysiology is similar to VSD except for an enlarged aorta, which also handles increased amount of blood flow.

Obstructive Lesions

- Obstruction to the flow of blood is compensated by an increase in pressure proximal to the obstruction in order to maintain forward flow.
- The increased pressure is possible through muscular hypertrophy (pressure overload).
- This leads to concentric myocardial hypertrophy without increase in ventricular cavity thus no cardiomegaly.
- Precordial impulse is forcible or heaving depending on severity, hence ventricular hypertrophy.
- Flow through obstruction leads to turbulence hence ejection systolic murmur, palpable as thrill.
- Ejection period gets prolonged, thus duration of systole increases that is proportional to the degree of obstruction as long as ventricular muscle is not failing.
- This leads to delayed closure of the corresponding component of second heart sound (A2 in left-sided obstruction and P2 in right-sided obstruction).
- These are generally acyanotic in the absence of associated shunt lesion, do not have history of frequent chest infection, do not have precordial deformity or cardiomegaly unless the obstructive lesion results in failing ventricle.

HOW TO SUSPECT ACYANOTIC CONGENITAL HEART DISEASE

How to Suspect Left-to-Right Shunts (Tables 38.2 and 38.3)

Classically left-to-right shunts present with CHF manifested in terms of feeding difficulty. This may be seen as suck rest suck cycle in the neonates. The decreased intake and congestive symptoms leads to decreased weight gain and hence may manifest itself as failure to thrive. Typical clinical features of a patient of shunt lesion are classified in Table 38.2.

Table 38.2 Increased pulmonary blood flow is suspected in the presence of one or more of the following features on physical examination

Recurrent lower respiratory tract infection (LRTI)
Feeding difficulty
Excessive sweating
Hyperdynamic precordium
Failure to thrive
Respiratory distress in the form of tachypnea, tachycardia, and retractions

Table 38.3 Problems associated with left-to-right shunt lesions

Respiratory complications
Pulmonary hypertension
Myocardial dysfunction
Congestive heart failure
Bacterial endocarditis
Chest deformities
Malnutrition

Presenting Features and Age of Presentation

Ventricular Septal Defect

Large or moderate VSD: Features of increased pulmonary blood flow like history of recurrent lower respiratory tract infection, feeding difficulty, and failure to gain weight. The presentation is generally in infancy. Restricted VSD or moderate-sized VSDs may present at any age and get referred generally on account of presence of murmur.

Atrial Septal Defect

Atrial septal defects generally present beyond infancy and mostly on account of a coincidental detection of a flow-related ejection murmur of the right ventricular outflow. These rarely present with features of increase pulmonary blood flow. Less than 10% of the patients present with CHF. Most commonly, they present in later decade with the onset of arrhythmias and acute deterioration.

Patent Ductus Arteriosus

The manifestations depend on the degree of shunt and are similar to VSD. Restricted VSDs present with murmur at a later date similar to VSD.

Obstructive Lesions

Critical lesions present with dyspnea on exertion, chest pain, and palpitations. Others get referred in view of murmur. These may present in early newborn period with severe obstruction with ventricular dysfunction in CHF, and are generally the earliest lesions to manifest.

CLINICAL EXAMINATION

Pulse and Blood Pressure

Femoral pulses are important as they particulary in obstructive lesions such coarctation of aorta. Bounding pulses are present in a child with patent ductus arteriosus (PDA) or aortopulmonary window. These may have a large pulse pressure on taking a blood pressure (BP). Blood pressure with difference of the upper and lower limb BP is a feature of coarctation of aorta.

Saturation

This is particularly relevant to differentiate a cyanotic CHD especially when the cyanosis may not be very apparent to the examiner (generally saturation above 85% is not well appreciated by clinical examination). The presence of lower limb desaturation may point toward a duct dependent lower limb circulation seen in severe coarctation or interrupted aortic arch particulary when PDA feeds the lower limb.

General Physical Examination

It is essential to look for the associated stigmata of shunt lesions such as other midline defects like cleft palate, neural tube defect. The presence of limb deformities (e.g. presence of absence radii in Holt-Oram syndrome) (Figs 38.2A and B) and syndromic associations should always be looked for [William's syndrome for aortic stenosis (AS) and peripheral pulmonary stenosis (PS)] (Fig. 38.3). There may be failure to thrive because of persistent CHF (hence the need for anthropometry in small children). ASD patients are known to be thin and asthenic although these are soft signs.

Precordial Activity

In post-tricuspid large shunt lesions such as VSD, PDA, or AP window the precordium is hyperdynamic. Hyperkinetic LV apex is also a feature in these patients. Forceful LV apex is a feature of left-sided obstructive lesions. RV (parasternal heave) is a finding in moderate-to-severe PS.

Second Heart Sound (S2)

Second heart sound is an important deciding factor for the diagnosis and differentiation of CHDs.

- Wide and fixed heart S2 is a feature of ASD (also observed in total anomalous systemic venous drainage, WPW type A and RBBB due to delayed P2).
- Wide and variable split S2 with normal intensity of P2 is usually a feature of moderate VSD. P2 component gets accentuated depending upon the degree of pulmonary artery hypertension.
- Closely split S2 with loud P2 is a feature of large post-tricuspid shunt (like VSD).
- Second heart sound may be normal in patients with small shunt lesions and mild obstructive lesions.
- S2 is normally split with mild PS, wide and variably split with moderately severe or severe PS. The width of splitting of the S2 is directly proportional to the severity of PS (Table 38.4).
- S2 is normally split with mild AS and single or paradoxically split with increasing severity due to delay in the aortic component of S2.

Murmur

Pansystolic murmur: A murmur starting with the first heart sound (partially masking it) and ending with the second heart sound without change in character is a pansystolic murmur.

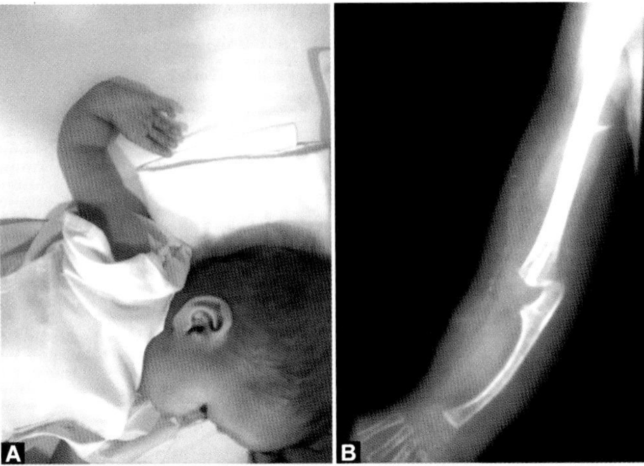

Figs 38.2A and B A case of ASD with absent radii (Holt–Oram syndrome). (A) Shows the physical defect with upper limb deformity. (B) X-ray of the right upper limb showing the absent radii in the same patient

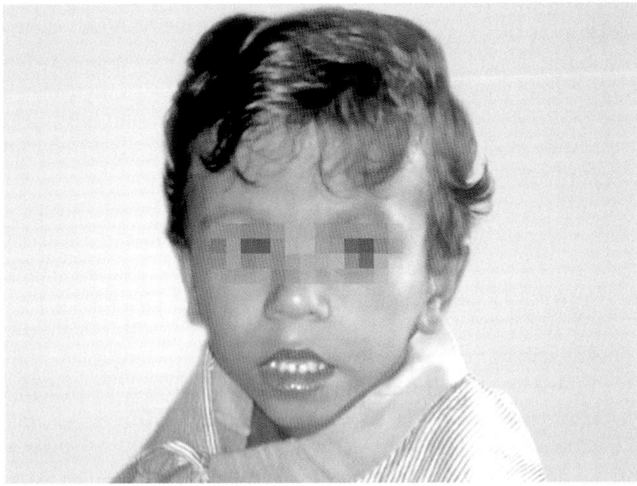

Fig. 38.3 A case of aortic stenosis in a 5-year-old child. Note the characteristic features of William's syndrome (commonly called "Elfin facies") this includes sunken nasal bridge, mild puffiness around the eyes, epicantal fold, long upper lip length (long philtrum), small and widely spaced teeth, wide mouth, prominent lower lip, and small chin

There are three differential diagnosis of a pansystolic murmur: VSD, mitral regurgitation, and tricuspid regurgitation. This indicates the presence of pressure gradient throughout the systole:

1. *VSD*: Pansystolic murmur is seen in moderate and small VSD. This is best heard at left parasternal border.
2. *Mitral regurgitation*: This may be seen in patients of large shunts with dilated annulus (in the presence of post-tricuspid shunt lesions). The features of large shunt must be present. The murmur is present at the apex and radiates to axilla.
3. *Tricuspid regurgitation*: This murmur is present in the parasternal area (tricuspid area) and increases on inspiration. May be present with annular dilatation in pretricuspid shunt lesions like ASD.

***Ejection systolic murmur*:** Murmur audible during the phase of ejection, i.e. after the first heart sound and ending with or before the second heart sound, is called ejection murmur. The ejection murmurs are crescendo and decrescendo the peak may in be in the middle of systole giving a diamond shape to the murmur. The ejection murmur could be pulmonary or aortic being produced at the respective valves either due to obstruction to the flow or increased flow across the normal valve. A murmur starting with the first heart sound and ending before mid-systole is early systolic murmur and a murmur starting late in systole ending with the second heart sound is late systolic murmur. This generally indicates the murmur across the outflow tract and may be heard in following circumstances in ACHD:

1. *Aortic stenosis*: Heard best is right and left upper parasternal area (especially aortic area) and may radiate to carotids. Delayed peaking indicates severity of the AS.
2. *Pulmonary stenosis*: This is generally present in pulmonary area and its peaking indicates the severity of the lesion.
3. *VSD*: This is generally heard in left upper parasternal area because of the large flow across a large VSD. This may also be seen in doubly committed or outlet VSD when the blood flow gets directed to right ventricular outflow tract.

***Continuous murmur*:** A continuous murmur begins in systole and continues without interruption or change in character through the second heart sound into diastole. It may occupy whole or part of diastole:

1. Heard in the left infraclavicular area indicates the restricted PDA (small or moderate size).
2. Continuous murmur of peripheral PS may be heard in bilateral lung fields.

Auscultation in Individual ACHD

Left-to-right Shunts

Left-to-right shunts at atrial, ventricular, or pulmonary artery level can be diagnosed with fair degree of certainty by auscultation, if uncomplicated. A pulmonary ejection and delayed diastolic flow murmurs are heard in left-to-right shunts if the pulmonary to systemic flow ratio is more than 2:1. The longer the flow murmur the larger the shunt. In general, the size of left-to-right shunt can be judged by the presence and length of the flow murmur across the tricuspid valve in atrial shunts and mitral valve in VSD and PDA. The loudness of the pulmonary component of the second heart sound reflects the degree of pulmonary hypertension except in atrial shunts where it could be loud in the absence of pulmonary hypertension due to dilatation and rotation of the pulmonary artery. The classical findings are modified with the development of pulmonary arterial hypertension (PAH). The flow murmurs become less and disappear, the shunt murmurs become attenuated and pulmonary component of the second sound becomes louder.

Atrial Septal Defect

The diagnostic features consist of a loud first heart sound, wide split "fixed," or mobile second heart sound with pulmonary ejection and tricuspid delayed diastolic murmurs. The common associated lesions with ASD are mitral regurgitation. Apical pansystolic murmur is heard in addition to findings of ASD. The mitral regurgitation could be secondary to rheumatic heart disease, myxomatous mitral valve, or endocardial cushion defect. Presence of a dynamic mid systolic click if present at the apex will point to an associated mitral valve prolapse. If the ejection click is pulmonary (inconstant) and the pulmonary ejection systolic murmur is louder in proportion to the left-to-right shunt, associated pulmonary valvular stenosis should be suspected.

Ventricular Septal Defect

Ventricular septal defect can be diagnosed by a pansystolic murmur masking the first and second heart sounds at the lower left sternal border. At the upper left sternal border a normally split or wide split, mobile second heart sound can be heard depending on the size of shunt. A mitral delayed diastolic murmur is heard at the apex if the shunt is large. Sometimes the pansystolic murmur has a mid-systolic accentuation with large shunts due to the superimposition of the pulmonary flow murmur. If the VSD is very small the murmur is of high frequency, early systolic, decrescendo ending in mid-systole at the third of fourth left interspace.

***Left ventricle to right atrial communication*:** The murmur is like that of VSD but has a more rightward location. Both tricuspid and mitral delayed diastolic murmurs are audible. The second sound is widely split, mobile.

While following patients with VSD a lot of information regarding hemodynamic alterations can be obtained by careful auscultation. Development of aortic regurgitation murmur will point to the onset of prolapse of the aortic valve and will be a definite indication for closure of the defect even though the left-to-right shunt is small. Some patients of VSD develop infundibular PS. The ejection murmur becomes louder, and the flow murmur across the mitral valve becomes attenuated and later disappears. The pulmonary component of the second sound becomes soft and delayed. In spontaneous closure of VSD, a sharp clicking sound 100–130 ms after the first sound may appear and represents the aneurysm formation of the interventricular septum. The systolic murmur gradually disappears. The second sound remains normal. With increase in pulmonary vascular resistance, the murmur of VSD and the flow murmur become attenuated and later disappear. The pulmonary component of the second sound becomes loud and the split becomes narrower and disappears with the onset of right-to-left shunt. Later, a pulmonary regurgitation murmur may appear.

Patent Ductus Arteriosus

The first heart should is accentuated. The second heart sound mostly masked by the murmur varies from normal split to paradoxically split depending on the size of the left-to-right shunt. The hallmark of the diagnosis is the continuous murmur best heard at second left intercostal space and radiating to below the left clavicle. The murmur is soft and of high frequency with a small PDA and loud noisy, machinery like with a late systolic accentuation with a moderate size PDA. Super-added systolic eddy sounds are heard with a large ductus, giving the systolic component a very rough character. Mitral delayed diastolic murmur may be heard if the size of the left-to-right shunt is large. Classically, the continuous murmur of PDA is best heard at the second left intercostal space and just below the left clavicle. One may also hear continuous murmurs in patients with rupture of sinus of Valsalva into the right-sided chambers and coronary arteriovenous fistulae. The location of the maximum intensity of the murmur is, however, different. A continuous murmur in pulmonary area could also be heard in patients with anomalous left coronary from pulmonary artery (ALCAPA). Mitral regurgitation murmur may be associated and the electrocardiogram show infarction or ischemic pattern in ALCAPA. Venous hum, bronchial collaterals, peripheral PS, and systemic arteriovenous fistulae over the chest wall should also be considered in the differential diagnosis of a continuous murmur. Sometimes a combination of a systolic and an early diastolic murmur as in VSD with aortic regurgitation, mitral regurgitation with aortic regurgitation, AS and regurgitation, tricuspid regurgitation with aortic regurgitation may give a superficial impression of a continuous murmur. Careful analysis of murmurs will, however, separate the true continuous murmur from a combination of systolic with a diastolic murmur. The classical continuous murmur of PDA gets modified with the development of PAH. The diastolic component becomes smaller and later disappears. The pulmonary component of the second sound becomes louder. The mitral delayed diastolic murmur becomes attenuated and later disappears. With the development of severe PAH the only audible murmur may be a pulmonary regurgitation murmur. Since the pulmonary regurgitation murmur is produced at a high pressure, it is high pitched and starts with the pulmonary component of the second sound. It is a classical decrescendo murmur. In contrast, the pulmonary regurgitation murmur heard with normal pulmonary artery pressures as in absent pulmonary valve syndrome, dysplastic pulmonary valve, and idiopathic dilation of pulmonary artery with pulmonary regurgitation, is low pitched and may have an early build up. It is short in duration as well. The pulmonary second sound is either absent, soft, or normal.

Obstructive Lesions (Tables 38.4 and 38.5)

The obstruction could to the right or left ventricular outflow. Obstructive lesions on either side produce ejection systolic murmurs at the respective valve areas and delays in the corresponding component of the second sound. If the obstruction is at the valvular level an ejection click is heard. The ejection click is constant with AS and inconstant with PS. Increasing severity of obstruction results in movement of the ejection click closure to the first sound, increase in the loudness of the murmur with delayed peaking, and increasing delay in the corresponding component of second heart sound with the appearance of a fourth heart sound on the respective side. In very critical obstruction if the forward output gets reduced due to ventricular failure the murmur may become soft. In subvalvular obstructions clicks are not heard. In subvalvular AS, an early diastolic murmur may be heard due to leaking of the blood trapped in the subvalvar area or associated valvular regurgitation. The severity of obstruction may be graded from the auscultatory findings (Table 38.4).

CHEST X-RAY

Combination of cardiac enlargement and increased vascularity indicates increased pulmonary blood flow. The magnitude of changes depends on the degree of shunt. If the shunt is small the chest X-ray could be normal. The larger the shunt the bigger is the heart and more prominent pulmonary vascularity.

ASD (Fig. 38.4)

- Cardiomegaly
- Increased pulmonary vascular markings
- Right atrial enlargement
- Dilated main pulmonary artery

VSD (Fig. 38.5)

- Increased pulmonary vascular markings
- Cardiomegaly
- Left atrial and left ventricular enlargement

PDA (Fig. 38.6)

- Increased pulmonary vascular markings
- Cardiomegaly
- Left atrial and left ventricular enlargement
- Prominent aorta

AP Window

- Increased pulmonary vascular markings
- Cardiomegaly
- Left atrial and left ventricular enlargement
- Prominent ascending aorta

Table 38.4 Pulmonary stenosis: severity

S2 splitting directly proportional to severity
Right ventricular hypertrophy and decreased distensibility of RV leads to audible S4 and a wave in jugular venous pulse (JVP)
In valvular pulmonary stenosis closer the click to S1, more severe the stenosis (may even merge with S1 (S1 appears louder in expiration)
Peak of the murmur gets delayed and length increases with increasing severity

Table 38.5 Characteristic clinical features of aortic stenosis

A narrow pulse pressure
Presence of LVH
A systolic thrill at the base
Delayed aortic component of the second heart sound
An ejection systolic murmur radiating to carotids

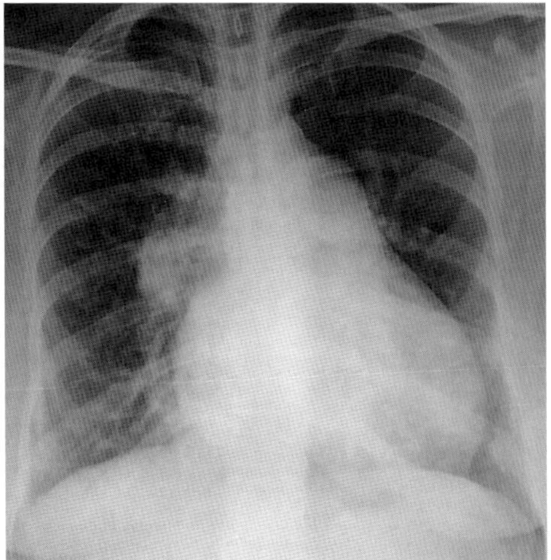

Fig. 38.4 Chest X-ray posterioanterior (PA) view in a case of atrial septal defect. Features show increased pulmonary blood flow with dilated right atrium and prominent pulmonary artery segment

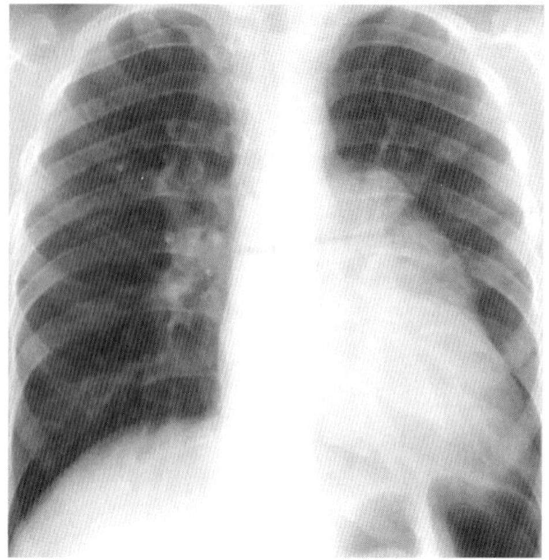

Fig. 38.5 X-ray chest shows cardiomegaly (left ventricular type apex) with enlargement of main pulmonary artery (MPA) segment. Pulmonary vasculature is markedly increased. The aortic shadow is not prominent. It is indicative of large shunt at ventricular level

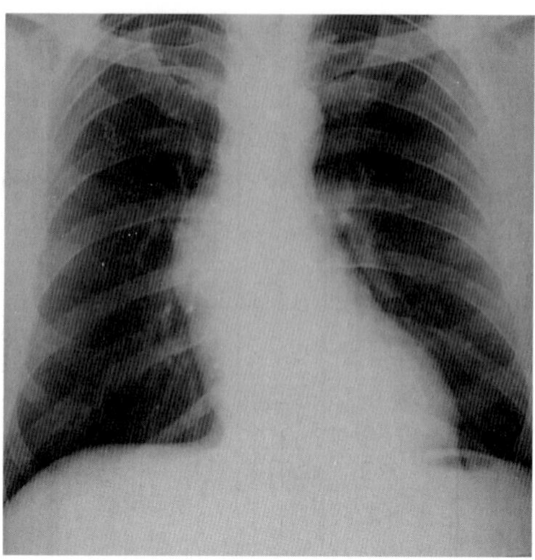

Fig. 38.7 Characteristic X-ray findings in patient with valvular aortic stenosis with preserved left ventricular function. Note the presence of normal heart size with dilated ascending aorta suggestive of the diagnosis

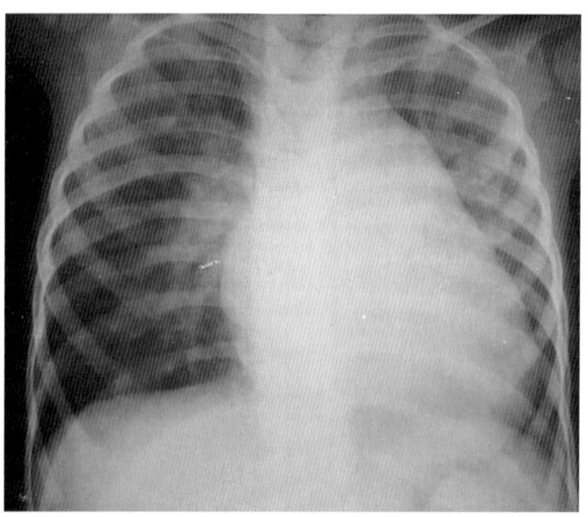

Fig. 38.6 X-ray chest shows cardiomegaly (left ventricular type apex) with enlargement of MPA segment. Pulmonary vasculature is markedly increased. The aortic shadow is prominent. It is indicative of large shunt at great arterial level

Obstructive Lesions

Aortic Valvular Stenosis (Fig. 38.7)

- The ascending aorta is dilated.
- The X-ray chest is of no value in assessing the severity of AS. Only in late stage with the development of CHF the cardiac enlargement occurs.

Coarctation of Aorta

- The X-ray chest beyond infancy may show a dilated left subclavian artery with a notch at the site of coarctation giving three sign.
- After the age of 5 years. The X-ray chest shows rib notching at the lower ends of third to eight ribs.
- The Barium swallow shows typical "E" sign due to dilated pre- and postcoarctation segments causing deviation on the barium filled esophagus.

Pulmonary Valvular Stenosis (Fig. 38.8)

- Prominent main and left pulmonary artery with normal vasculature is the hall mark of the diagnosis of valvular PS.
- The X-ray chest does not give any help in assessing the severity of the stenosis.
- In very severe obstruction, there is cardiomegaly, right atrial enlargement, and thinned pulmonary vessels.

ELECTROCARDIOGRAM

Given a choice between electrocardiogram (ECG) and X-ray for the evaluation of CHD in a case of acyanotic CHD, a commonly asked question in any examination one would rather choose a X-ray whenever suspecting a shunt lesion and an ECG when suspecting a obstructive lesion. In general, ECG has to be interpreted along with clinical and radiologic data.

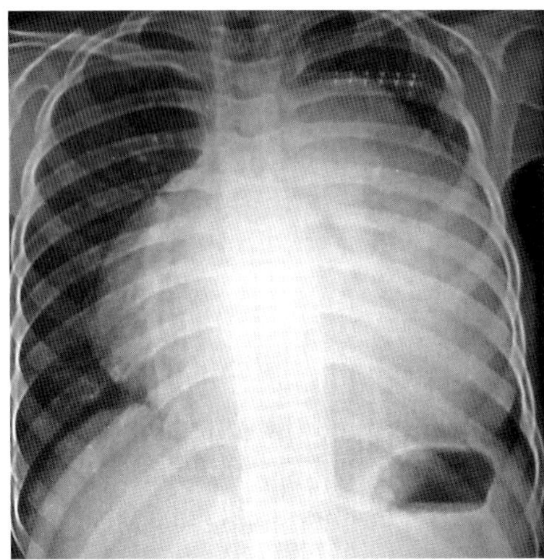

Fig. 38.8 Characteristic X-ray findings in patient with valvular pulmonary stenosis with severe TR. Note the presence of cardiomegaly with dilated main pulmonary artery segment

Left-to-Right (L–R) Shunts

Pretricuspid L→R Shunts (Fig. 38.9)

- L-R shunts occurring at the atrial level produce volume overload of the RA and RV, which manifests in the form of RSR, Rsr, rsr, or RsR, patterns in right-sided chest leads (V$_4$R, V1). These are mentioned as incomplete RBBB patterns. So an ECG showing incomplete RBBB in patients with L-R shunt suggests that the shunt is at the atrial level. This could be an ASD or partial anomalous pulmonary venous drainage (PAPVD).
- The associated presence of right axis deviation (RAD) or a normal axis will suggest secundum ASD or PAPVD. However, the presence of left axis deviation (LAD) of -30° to -60° will suggest ostium primum ASD, and an axis to the left of >60° suggests a complete atrioventricular canal defect.
- The presence of significant right ventricular hypertrophy (RVH) suggests associated PAH or pulmonic stenosis (PS).
- On the other hand, if the ECG shows additional left ventricular hypertrophy (LVH) one should carefully evaluate for mitral regurgitation that could be caused by an associated mitral valve prolapse, rheumatic mitral valve disease, or cleft mitral leaflet. Associated LVH is also seen in unusual types of atrial shunts like LV to right atrial communication or rupture of the sinus of Valsalva into the RA.

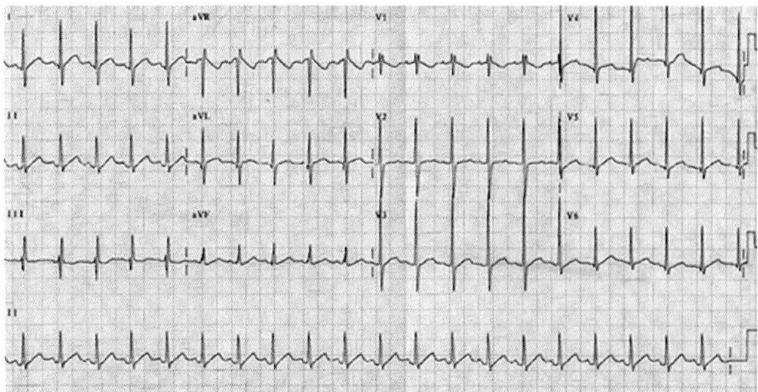

Fig. 38.9 ECG in a case of ASD showing right axis deviation with features of right ventricular volume overload in the form of incomplete right bundle branch block pattern

Abbreviations: ECG, electrocardiogram; ASD, atrial septal defect

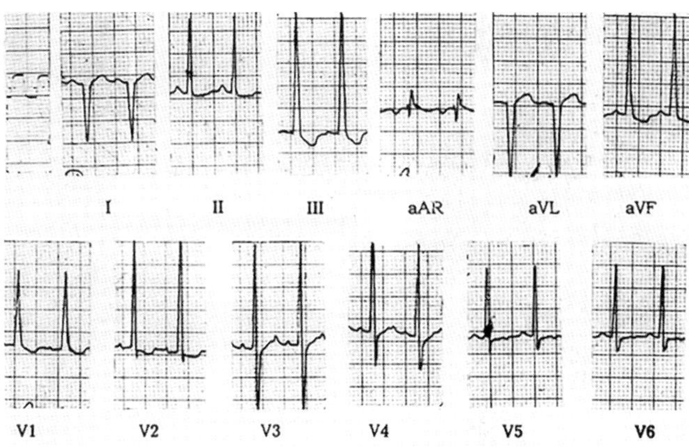

Fig. 38.10 ECG in a case of VSD showing the left axis deviation with left ventricular volume overload pattern

Abbreviations: ECG, electrocardiogram; VSD, ventricular septal defect

Post-tricuspid L–R Shunts (Fig. 38.10)

- A small PDA or VSD may have a normal ECG because the volume overload is not severe enough to produce ECG changes.
- Larger shunts produce left ventricular and left atrial overload patterns in the ECG. Hyperkinetic PAH with large shunts is associated with biventricular hypertrophy. Severe obstructive pulmonary vascular disease results in severe RVH.
- The ECG is very useful in the follow-up of patients with VSD. If the ECG normalizes it indicates that VSD is becoming smaller. If it shows progressive increase in

RVH, it suggests that the child is either developing PAH or PS. Both these developments require prompt workup for surgical consideration. If during follow-up there is progressive increase in LVH a careful evaluation for aortic regurgitation is required.

Obstructive Lesions

Right Ventricular Outflow Obstruction (Fig. 38.11)

- In valvular PS the ECG has been found to be a useful predictor of its severity.
  - In mild PS, ECG may be normal.
  - In moderate PS, normal ECG is uncommon (10%), mean QRS axis is usually between +90° and +120°, rR, or RS complexes (with R/S >4) are seen in V1 and R in V1 may be up to 20 mm in amplitude.
  - QRS axis of +110° to +150° or more, pure R or qR in V1 with R wave of 20 mm or more, right atrial overload and deeply inverted T waves indicate severe PS. The height of the pure R wave in V1 or VR correlates well with the right ventricular systolic pressure (RVSP) in pure valvular PS.
  - R wave magnitude in mm in V1 or VR multiplied by 5 or R wave in millimeter multiplied by 3+47 indicates the approximate RVSP.
- Infants with critical PS and hypoplastic RV may show RAD with LVH in the ECG.
- Presence of abnormal quadrant axis in a patient with RV outflow obstruction suggests dysplastic pulmonary valve that may be associated with the rubella syndrome or the Noonan's syndrome.
- The ECG in pure infundibular PS, obstructing anomalous muscle bundles of RV, supravalvular PS or peripheral PS are essentially similar to those in valvular PS.
- In obstructing muscle bundles of RV an upright T wave in V3 R may be the only evidence of RVH in up to 40% of the patients.

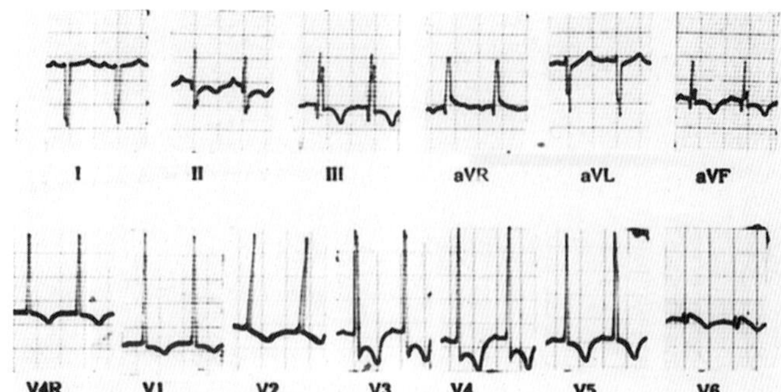

Fig. 38.11 ECG from a child with severe valvar pulmonary stenosis (suprasystemic RV pressure) with intact interventricular septum. ECG shows normal sinus rhythm; normal "P" wave axis; RA enlargement (tall "P" wave), right axis deviation (frontal QRS axis +100°); RVH, presence of RV strain pattern (q wave in lead V1, T wave inversion in V1–V6), absence of transition.
Abbreviations: ECG, electrocardiogram; RV, right ventricular

Left Ventricular Outflow Obstruction (Fig. 38.12)

- The ECG will show varying grades of LVH depending upon the severity of obstruction.
- Electrocardiographic prediction of severity of AS is not as accurate as in PS. Deeply inverted T waves with ST depression in left-sided leads indicate severe AS, though their absence does not exclude severe AS. In some cases, ECG may be normal even in severe AS.
- Supravalvular and discrete subvalvular AS are electrocardiographically indistinguishable from valvular AS.
- Associated peripheral PS in supravalvular AS may produce RVH in the ECG.
- The ECG in coarctation of aorta in the first year of life may show RVH often with a strain pattern in V1 or V3R.

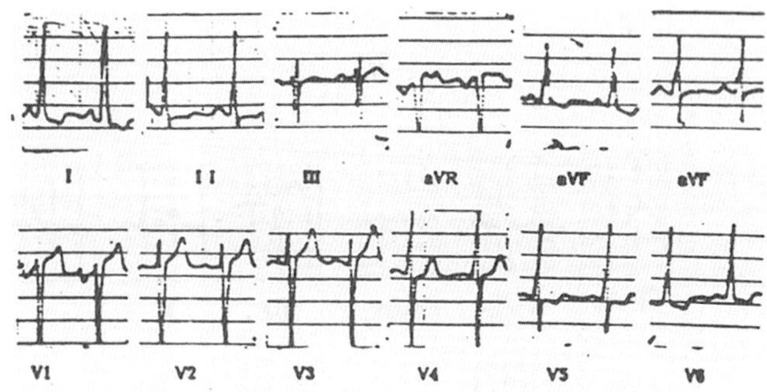

Fig. 38.12 ECG from a 25-year-old patient with subaortic membrane, critical aortic stenosis. ECG shows sinus rhythm; normal "P" wave axis; QRS axis +40°; LVH, inverted "T" wave in V4, V5, and V6

- LVH develops in most patients with hemodynamically significant aortic coarctation by 2 years of age.
- Strain pattern (ST depression and T inversion) in left-sided leads is rare in uncomplicated coarctation of aorta and suggests associated endocardial fibroelastosis, severe AS, or mitral regurgitation.

It is important to know of certain characteristic ECG patterns of patients of cardiomyopathy who may present in CHF and thus one may keep a differential diagnosis of these while evaluating a child of suspected ACHD.

Anomalous Left Coronary Artery from Pulmonary Artery (ALCAPA) (Fig. 38.13)

- Characteristic ECG pattern in this condition is one of anterolateral myocardial infarction with deep Q waves in

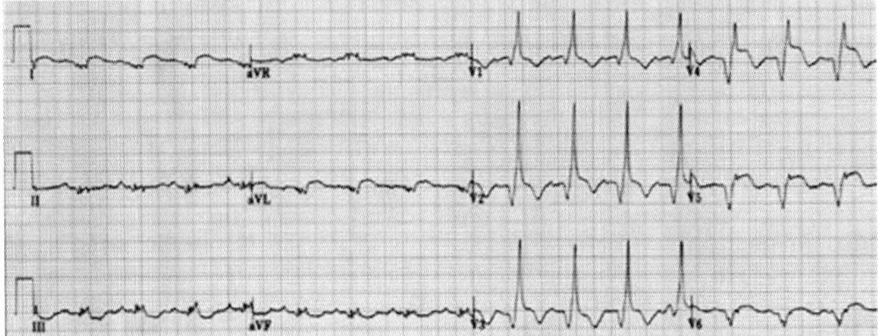

Fig. 38.13 ECG in a case of ALCAPA. ECG shows deep q waves in left-sided precordial leads with evidence of ischemic pattern
Abbreviations: ALCAPA, anomalous left coronary artery from pulmonary artery; ECG, electrocardiogram

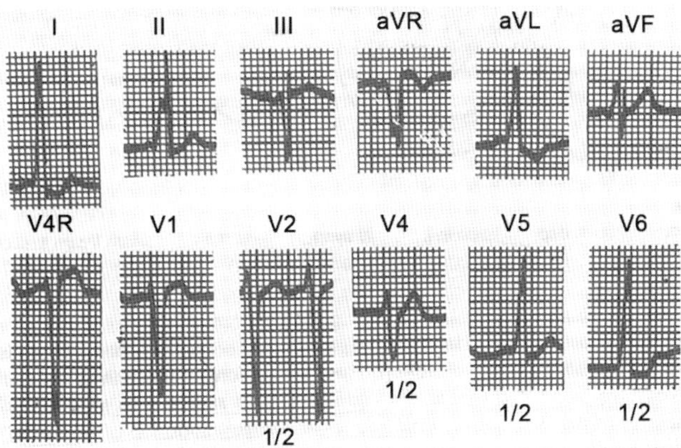

Fig. 38.14 ECG in a case of Pompe's disease. ECG shows tall QRS complexes with short PR interval

1, aVL and V4–V6 with ST segment elevation and T wave inversion.

- As the child grows older, if he survives (80–90% die within the first year if untreated), ST and T wave changes may disappear and Q waves diminish in size.
- ECG features of LVH and LAD are common especially in older patients. This represents true cardiac hypertrophy especially of the posterobasal portion of the LV. Left atrial overload pattern may also be present.

Pompe's Disease (Fig. 38.14)

- The ECG typically shows a short PR interval (0.05–0.09 s) and huge QRS complexes (LVH). The QRS voltages being one of the highest recorded in any disease.
- The QRS axis may be shifted leftward and left atrial overload pattern may be present.
- A short PR interval with marked LVH suggests Pompe's disease.

ECHOCARDIOGRAPHY

Echocardiography (echo) has revolutionized the practice of pediatric cardiology. The pediatric cardiologist now refers patients for surgical treatment without cardiac catheterization especially in neonate and infants.

General Features: Shunt Lesions

There are a few salient features of all the shunt lesions:

- The shunt would lead to volume overloads of the chambers it feeds (particularly in relation to the tricuspid valves), e.g. while a shunt proximal to the tricuspid valve would lead to volume overloading of the RA and RV and further (Fig. 38.1). A lesion beyond the tricuspid valve would lead to the volume overloading of the LA and LV.
- The magnitude of the chamber enlargement depends upon the magnitude of the shunt. Thus, significant RA and RV enlargement would be a feature of pretricuspid shunt, while a significant LA and LV enlargement would be a feature of post-tricuspid shunt.
- The pressure of the investigated chamber would rise not only on account of distal obstruction (obstruction of the outflow of the chamber) or it would be because of the transmitted pressures from the adjacent chambers on account of the shunt.
  - Increase in RV pressures may be because of distal PS, obstruction in branch pulmonary arteries, or obstruction in pulmonary vascular bed (as in PAH).
  - Increase in pressures in RV and beyond may be seen in large VSD, similarly a large PDA would lead to significant increase in PA pressures.
- The magnitude of the gradient from a chamber outflow would be dependent on the magnitude of shunt into the chamber.
  - This may lead to exaggerated gradients even in hemodynamically scuttle lesions, namely, exaggerated PS gradients in associated pretricuspid shunts (like ASD), exaggerated mitral and aortic valve gradients in associated post-tricuspid shunts like VSD or PDA in absence of significant stenosis. For example, gradients up to 60 mmHg have been reported across pulmonary valve in patients of ASD in absence of PS.
- The secondary manifestations of the shunt lesions may themselves lead to exaggerated secondary effects, e.g. the mitral annular dilatation on account of post-tricuspid shunt may lead to mitral regurgitation and this may further lead to mitral valve dilatation and LV dilatation.
- Since a shunt lesion almost always signifies a communication between two chambers, the gradient between the two chambers can guide as to the magnitude of the shunt lesion or the size of the defect.

- The size of the defect in two dimensions may be a useful guide in deciding the degree of shunt. It also is useful to help the interventional modality.
  - The size of the VSD may be compared to the size of the aortic root for classifying the size of the VSD.
  - The size of defects like ASD, coronary AV fistulae, VSD, RSOV, etc. would help in deciding the size of the device that may be used.
- Echocardiography should focus not only on the characteristics of the primary lesion but also on the adjacent structures of the defect, e.g. distances from the adjoining valves:
  - VSD, it is important to note the distances from the aortic valve when considering for device closure. It is also important from the surgical point of view.
  - For ASD, the rims are seen not only for their adequacy but also the adjoining structures being encroached upon, whenever contemplating a device closure.
  - For AP window, the distance from coronaries and valves becomes important.
  - The post-tricuspid shunt is known to mask the manifestations of ALCAPA, and thus one should keenly look at the two-dimensional anatomy and origin of the coronary arteries whenever investigating an associated shunt lesion.
- Whenever investigating a shunt at multiple sites or an associated lesions, one must remember that the shunt flow may be modified by the presence of distal obstruction and also by the associated shunt:
  - The associated post-tricuspid shunt may lead to exaggerated manifestations of pretricuspid shunt lesions (namely, ASD). Thus, RA and RV may be unduly dilated even in the presence of small ASD, with the associated presence of post-tricuspid shunt (VSD or PDA) or associated presence of mitral stenosis.
  - The associated AS or coarctation of aorta may exaggerate the shunt across the VSD.
- The associated lesions being drained off by the shunt lesions may become masked and may manifest themselves only after the shunt lesion is closed:
  - Mitral stenosis may not manifest itself in the presence of ASD (although it may exaggerate the shunt flow across it) (Figs 38.15A to C)
  - The manifestations of significant mitral regurgitation may get unmasked after ASD closure.
  - High LV end diastolic pressure (LVedp), secondary to various causes may not only exaggerate ASD shunt, they may manifest themselves as pulmonary edema after ASD closure.
  - VSD or PDA may mask the gradients across the AS or coarctation of aorta and this may manifest itself after the treatment of the underlying shunt lesion.
- Systemic disorders and conditions may exaggerate or confound the features and even echocardiographic features of a shunt lesion:
  - Anemia may exaggerate the gradients across any shunt lesion or across valves. Anemia may lead to LV dilatation thus confounding the assessment of associated post-tricuspid shunt lesion.
  - Systemic hypertension may not only lead to exaggerated shunt gradients, it may also lead to secondary ventricular hypertrophy thus leading to high LVedp and exaggerating ASD shunt.
  - Hyperdynamic states such as fever, anemia, and thyroid disorders may exaggerate the shunt gradients.

Thus, an assessment of a patient with shunt lesion does not mean an isolated evaluation by echocardiography, it refers to complete clinical evaluation of the individual. Now, we will discuss individually the assessment of certain shunt lesions seen commonly.

Also any assessment of shunt lesions must be preceded by a complete clinical information, chest X-ray and electrocardiogram. There would be a situation when information gained by these investigations will lead to clinical decision when echocardiographic findings are equivocal.

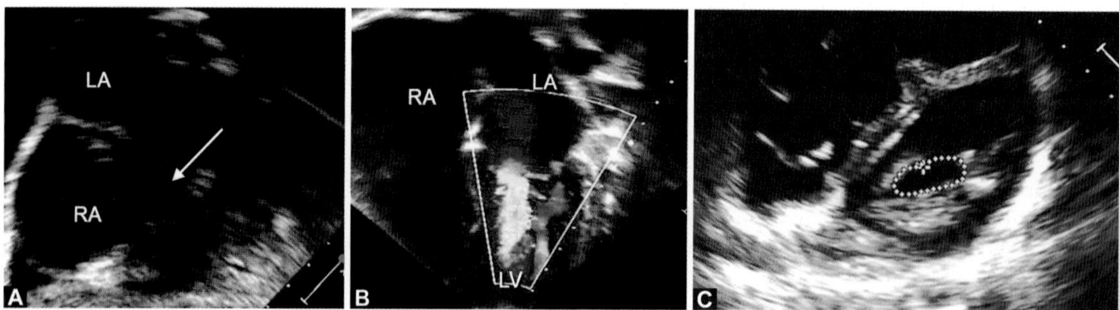

Figs 38.15A to C Echogardigraphic imaging in a case of coronary sinus type of ASD with severe mitral stenosis. (A) 2D echo with subcostal coronal view shows the coronary sinus type of defect marked by arrow. (B) 2D echocardiography with color flow mapping shows the flow across the mitral valve in the same patient. (C) 2D echo with parasternal short axis view and planimetry of the mitral valve shows the severe mitral stenosis with mitral valve area being measured by 2D plainmetry

The essential approach to any lesion should not be directed at the shunt lesion, rather it should be a standardized sequential analysis, as it is not the shunt lesion in isolation that exist and one needs to evaluate all the structural heart defects. A few salient features of the important shunt lesions—ASD, VSD, PDA, and AP window are illustrated here.

Atrial Septal Defects

Objectives on echocardiography:
1. To diagnose ASD, asses its anatomical site and size.
2. To assess the direction and quantum of flow.
3. To assess the degree of PAH.
4. To assess atrioventricular valve anomalies, pulmonary veins and pulmonary valve stenosis.

ASD Classification

Echocardiography plays a major role in the management of ASD, both in their diagnosis and in decision making. With a combination of imaging (transthoracic, transesophageal) and color flow the sensitivity and specificity of diagnosis of ASD approaches 100%. False positive and negative can occur in inexperienced hands. Defects of atrial septum are classified into five types:
1. *Patent foramen ovale (PFO)*: In most individuals, the foramen ovale is functionally closed shortly after birth; however, patency of a competent foramen ovale has been found in 25% of normal heart on autopsy. A PFO can stretch to manifest as small ASD in certain hemodynamic conditions (e.g. high left atrial pressures). However, if a true flap is seen then it would be defined as PFO. The pattern of shunting across foramen ovale is dependent on hemodynamic factors. Thus, a PFO can shunt left to right only, right to left only, or bidirectionally.
2. *Fossa ovalis ASD (Fig. 38.16)*: These are the most common of the ASDs (69%) with varied sizes. This type of defect occupies the central part of atrial septum involving in part or whole flap valve of the foramen ovale. Septum ovale defects are bounded on either side by the limbic bands (superior and inferior limbic bands). These limbic bands separate the defect from atrial wall.
3. *Sinus venosus defect (Fig. 38.17)*: These defects are beyond the boundaries of the embryological septum and thus more appropriately called defects rather than "ASDs." Hallmark of all of these defects is that the border of the fossa ovalis should be intact, the defect is overlapped by either superior vena cava (SVC) (SVC type of defect) or inferior vena cava (IVC) (IVC type of defect) and there may or may not be an anomalous drainage of the pulmonary vein. Defects extending from the fossa ovalis superiorly or inferiorly should not be classified as a sinus venosus defect.
4. *Coronary sinus atrial septa defect*: Coronary sinus defect is a rare anomaly. It is located in the inferior most part of the atrial septum at the anticipated site of the coronary sinus ostium. The clue to the diagnosis of such defect may be the presence of a persistent left SVC with evidence of RV volume overload.
5. *Ostium primum ASD (Fig. 38.18)*: This type of defect is part of atrio-VSD and is characterized by the absence in part or whole of the atrioventricular septum. This defect is present in the lower most part of the atrial septum and there is absence of normal offsetting of atrioventricular valves.

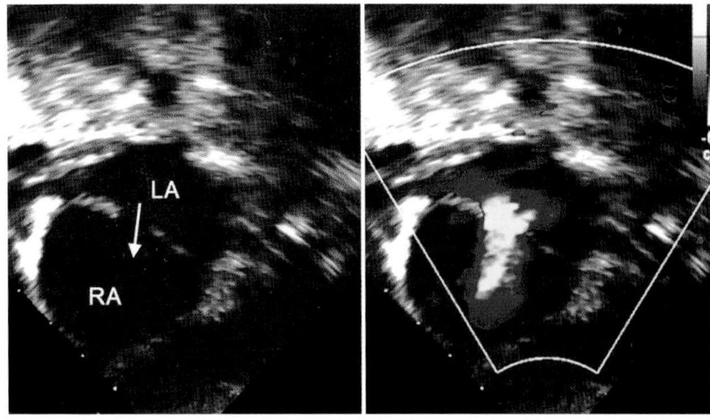

Fig. 38.16 Two-dimentional echocardiography with color compare in subcostal coronal view showing fossa ovalis ASD with left-to-right shunt

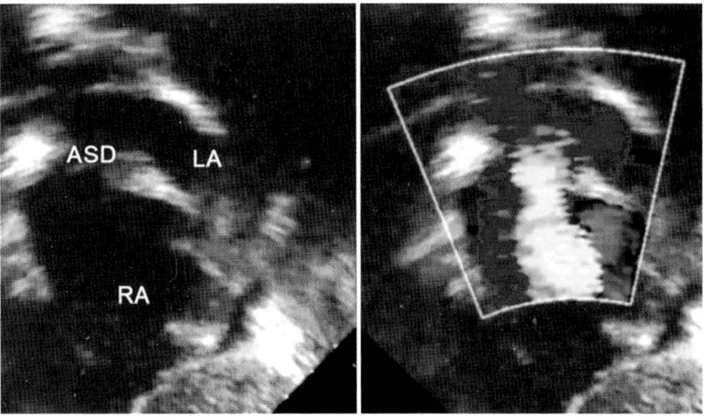

Fig. 38.17 2D echo with subcostal coronal view in a case of sinus venosus ASD showing the over-riding of the SVC over the ASD

Abbreviations: ASD, atrial septal defect; RA, right atrium; LA, left atrium; SVC, superior vena cava

Echoevaluation

- The abnormal interventricular septal motion and enlarged RA and RV are indirect evidence of left-to-right shunt at atrial level.
- The best views to directly visualize the ASD is subcostal coronal and sagittal views. Atrial septal defect will be

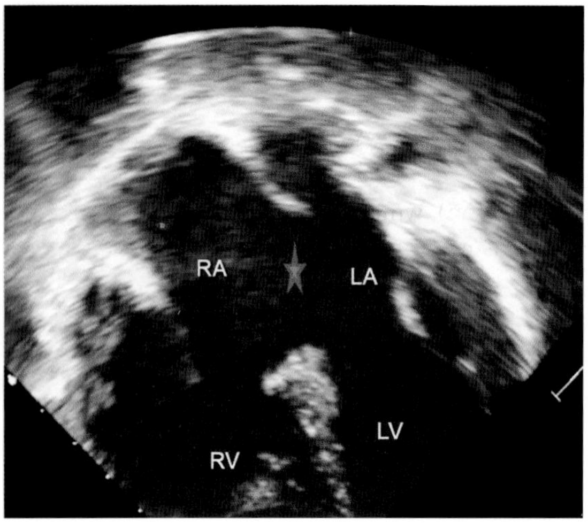

Fig. 38.18 2D echo with apical four-chamber view showing large ostium primum ASD defect in lower part of the interatrial septum marked by the star (*)

Abbreviations: RA, right atrium; RV, right ventricle; LA, left atrium; LV, left ventricle

diagnosed by a dropout in the interatrial septum with flow across the defect on Doppler interrogation.

- When the defect is visualized, its relationship to the SVC and IVC should be evaluated. If the SVC forms the roof of the defect, the defect is SVC sinus venous type. If the IVC straddles the defect, it is IVC type. The defects in the center of the atrial septum involving the fossa ovalis area are fossa ovalis defects. The defect in the lower most part of the interatrial septum with atrioventricular valves attached at the same level are designated as ostium primum defects.
- It should also be viewed in apical four chamber and short-axis views. The four-chamber view will also show the attachments of the atrioventricular valves. These will be at the same level in ostium primum defect.
- The color flow mapping across the defect will show the direction of flow and also presence or absence of any regurgitation. Doppler velocities across all valves should be taken in particular the pulmonary valve to look for any PS.
- The inflow velocities of the AV valves should be seen to rule out any mitral valve obstruction. The associated mitral obstruction may get missed unless specifically seen on two-dimensional echocardiography, as there may not be significant gradient across the mitral valve even with significant obstruction because of associated ASD (true for all Lutembacher cases) (Figs 38.15A to C).
- All pulmonary veins should be specifically imaged to see if they are abnormally connected or not and to look for any pulmonary vein stenosis. The pulmonary veins are best seen in subcostal coronal and sagittal, apical four chamber and short-axis and suprasternal short-axis views.

Indication of Cardiac Catheterization

Diagnostic cardiac catheterization in ASDs is:

- For evaluation of pulmonary artery pressure, where it is not possible by Doppler and pulmonary hypertension is suspected.
- When pulmonary vascular resistance is required in decision making.

Ventricular Septal Defect

In most centers for pediatric cardiology, cardiac catheterization is not routinely undertaken for infants and children with an isolated VSD routinely. The combination of transthoracic cross-sectional imaging and Doppler techniques is sufficient for clinical decision making and if needed surgical correction.

Objectives of Echocardiography

- Confirm VSD
- Determine the size and morphological location of VSDs.
- Rule out associated lesions.
- Assessment of chamber size and wall thickness.
- Estimation of shunt size (pulmonary/systemic flow ratio).
- Estimate right ventricular and pulmonary arterial pressures.

Classification of VSD (Fig. 38.19)

Ventricular septal defects should be imaged from several planes. Artifactual dropouts may confuse the viewer using single plane imaging about the presence or absence of a VSD, particularly if it is small. In addition, color flow Doppler imaging is useful to reconfirm the presence of VSDs. Color flow imaging of VSDs has also radically improved the ability to detect unusually located and very small VSDs.

Morphological location of VSD is described as viewed from the RV. Ventricular septal defects can be classified into four types:

1. Perimembranous VSD
2. Muscular VSD
   a. Muscular inlet
   b. Muscular outlet
   c. Trabecular defect
3. Doubly committed VSD
4. Inlet VSD

Doppler Evaluation of VSD

***Color Doppler*:** It has added to the evaluation of a VSD in the following ways:

1. The location of VSD especially smaller VSDs and multiple muscular VSDs can be determined using Doppler color flow mapping techniques

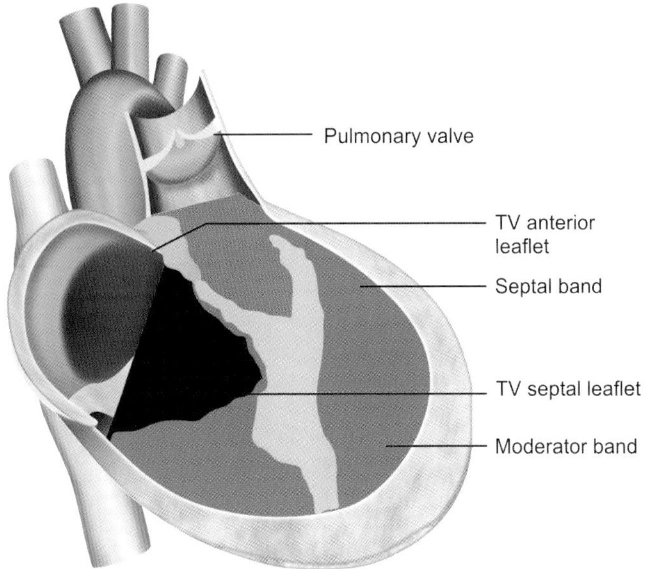

Fig. 38.19 Schematic diagram of the interventricular septum with removed RV cavity from the RV side. Various parts of the septum are profiled. Blue muscular septum forms the region of the muscular VSD. The muscular septum can further be classified with respect to the muscular moderator and septal band. Yellow region signifies the perimembranous region; purple color signifies the inlet septum, and the green color the outlet septum

2. Size of VSD
3. Determination of shunt direction across the VSD
4. For Doppler evaluation of velocities color flow mapping is used for proper alignment of jet flow.

Patterns of Shunting Across VSD

With isolated nonrestrictive VSD with high pulmonary vascular resistance, direction of flow can be bidirectional or dominantly right to left depending upon the severity of pulmonary vascular obstructive disease. With associated PS, there may be isolated right to left shunt depending upon the severity of PS. With severe right ventricular outflow obstruction, if VSD is small, one can get a turbulent jet of right to left shunt with suprasystemic RV systolic pressure.

With the use of color flow mapping with careful interrogation, one should also look for any LV to right atrial shunt as high velocity of LV to right atrial jet can be misinterpreted as elevated RV pressure. This can happen particularly with VSD which are getting smaller by septal leaflet of tricuspid valve.

Pressure Gradient Across VSD

While taking continuous wave Doppler across VSD, the cursor should be well aligned with VSD jet on color flow mapping. The velocity of the VSD shunt can be determined using the Bernoulli's equation, $p = 4v^2$ where p is the pressure difference and v is of the maximum recorded velocity. This will give the difference between the left and right ventricular systolic pressure. The left ventricular systolic pressure is derived from the systolic BP (provided there is no left ventricular out flow obstruction), which should be recorded at the time of Doppler study using appropriate sized BP cuffs.

Right ventricular pressure = Systolic blood pressure – VSD jet peak gradient ($4\ v^2$)

M-mode Echocardiography

M-mode echocardiography is used to assess the left atrial and left ventricular size to quantitate shunt across VSD and right ventricular size and wall thickness, which will reflect elevated right ventricular systolic pressure. For direction of shunt, this is rarely used in daily practice but depicts best the direction of shunting during the various phases of a cardiac cycle.

Interrogation of the Atrioventricular and Semilunar Valves for Regurgitation and Stenosis

The tricuspid regurgitation velocity should always be obtained to predict the right ventricular systolic pressure and hence indirectly the pulmonary artery pressure if there is no PS. Presence of PS and aortic regurgitation should be evaluated. The velocities of both atrioventricular valves and semilunar valves should be taken to rule out any associated abnormality. The mitral valve gradients may get exaggerated in the presence of VSD.

Pulmonary Blood Flow to Systemic Blood Flow Ratio

As regards quantifying pulmonary and systemic shunt flow using Doppler echocardiography several methods currently exists, although none is widely used due to variable results.

Assessment of Suitability for Device Closure

Percutaneous closure for mid muscular VSD and perimembranous VSD can be done. While assessing the child for device closure of muscular defect, the defect should have sufficient margin and should not encroach upon the surrounding structures such as atrioventricular valves and semilunar valves and there should not be associated other defects requiring cardiopulmonary bypass.

Patent Ductus Arteriosus

The ductus arteriosus is a normal fetal structure, allowing blood to bypass circulation to the lungs. The high level of oxygen that is exposed to after birth causes it to close in most cases within 24 hours. Persistence of this fetal structure beyond 10 days of life in a term baby is considered abnormal.

Anatomy: The ductus arteriosus is the portion of the sixth aortic arch that connects the left pulmonary artery with the descending portion of the aortic arch. The pulmonary artery end of the PDA is usually immediately to the left of the pulmonary artery bifurcation. The aortic connection is just distal to the origin of the left subclavian artery. The normal direction of flow in the ductus determines its orientation, and its size (along with pressure differences) determines the amount of flow. Closure of the PDA usually starts at the pulmonary end, accounting for the funnel-shaped configuration seen in approximately two-thirds of patients.

Objectives of Echocardiography

- The presence of a duct
- Detailed definition of ductus
  - Size of the duct
  - Type of duct
- The hemodynamic significance of a duct
  - Direction of shunt
  - Pulmonary arterial pressure
  - Quantification of shunt
- Associated defects

Detailed description of the echocardiographic view is essential in order to characterize accurately the morphology of the duct. There are basically four views to do this:

1. *Ductal view (Fig. 38.20)*: This uses the high parasternal window just beneath the left clavicle. After obtaining the short axis cut of the great vessel visualizing the pulmonary artery bifurcation the transducer is rotated anticlockwise in gradual motion. At one point, the left pulmonary artery goes away from view and the duct with adjacent descending aorta opens. This view in neonates and infants also visualizes the origin of the left subclavian artery. In patients with associated coarctation the posterior shelf is also well visualized.
2. *Suprasternal view*: There are three views to visualize the duct.
   a. *Suprasternal long-axis view*: This view can never open up the usual ductus, which arises from the lateral wall of the descending aorta. However, this is the best view for visualizing the vertical duct arising from the undersurface of the transverse arch in patients with pulmonary atresia. The origin of such ducti is well seen but the insertion point at the pulmonary artery required further anterior tilt. This is because of the tortuous nature of such ducti.

      In patients with discordant ventriculoarterial connection (e.g. transposition of great vessels), the duct can be visualized very well in its entire length in this view.

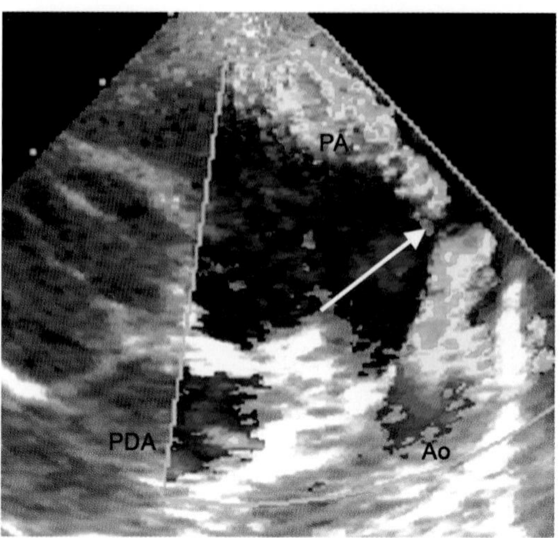

Fig. 38.20 Two-dimensional echocardiography with color flow mapping in a high parasternal view (ductal view) showed the PDA with left-to-right shunt across. There is a good ampulla of the ductus with narrowing of the ductus before its insertion into the pulmonary artery

   b. *Suprasternal short-axis view*: This is the classical short-axis arch view and can visualize those rare ducti that arise from the base of the left subclavian artery and descend straight down to insert into the left pulmonary artery. If aortic arch is right sided and the patient has PS physiology. The entire length of the duct can be seen in one view because unlike in those patients with vertical duct it does not follow a tortuous course.
   c. *Modified ductal view*: This is a less well-described view to visualize the usual duct. It has the advantage of visualizing the duct in its entire length and most closely mimics the lateral angiogram performed during cardiac catheterization. From the usual suprasternal long-axis view the transducer is rotated anticlockwise. A slight anterior tilt then shows the duct from its ampullary part to its insertion and accurate measurements can be made.

***Hemodynamic significance*:** Hemodynamic significance of ductus arteriosus can be assessed by evidence of volume overload of LA and LV, direction of shunt, and pulmonary arterial pressure.

***Chamber dimensions*:** Left atrial enlargement signifies increased pulmonary venous return because of left-to-right ductal shunting.

- The reference measure is the ratio of the left atria to aorta at the level of the aortic valve (the LA:Ao ratio) by M-mode echocardiography in parasternal long-axis view. The aortic root does not enlarge significantly with even extremely large PDA. In general, a LA:Ao ratio >1.3:1 indicates a significant shunt.

- Left ventricle will enlarge as cardiac output increases with both increased pulmonary venous return and with increased diastolic runoff from the systemic circulation. The best method to determine the presence of volume overload of LV is M-mode measurement of LV diastolic dimensions and compare with normal values for the patient's age and weight.

DIRECTION OF SHUNT AND PULMONARY ARTERIAL PRESSURE

Color Doppler imaging of duct:

- On color flow mapping, small duct with normal pulmonary artery pressure is displayed as a mosaic flow from descending aorta to pulmonary artery.
- With large duct, and low pulmonary vascular resistance, the duct jet appears as predominantly red flow with minimal aliasing.
- In patients with severe PAH, on color flow mapping, there will be bidirectional shunt.
- With suprasystemic pulmonary artery pressure as in obstructed total anomalous pulmonary venous connection a restrictive duct will show turbulent high velocity right-to-left flow in systole and diastole in the descending aorta. This can give signals very similar to coarctation of aorta.

***Continuous wave Doppler examination of ductus arteriosus (Fig. 38.21)*:** By the use of continuous wave Doppler, direction of shunt in relation to cardiac cycle and pulmonary arterial pressure (systolic blood pressure minus pressure gradient cross duct = systolic pulmonary arterial pressure) can be detected accurately.

- With isolated left-to-right shunt, with small-to-moderate sized PDA and normal or mildly elevated pulmonary artery pressure, Doppler examination of duct shows continuous flow toward the transducer with peak in late systole.
- In large duct with PAH, there will be bidirectional shunting on Doppler imaging of duct, right to left in systole and left to right in diastole.
- With increasing pulmonary vascular resistance as with no step up in oxygen saturation above and below the duct, peak of right-to-left shunt appear early in systole.
- With further rise in pulmonary vascular resistance, right-to-left shunt begins in diastole extending to systole and right-to-left shunt if present occurs only in late systole to early diastole.
- With duct dependent systemic circulation and severe PAH, there will be isolated right-to-left shunting across the duct.

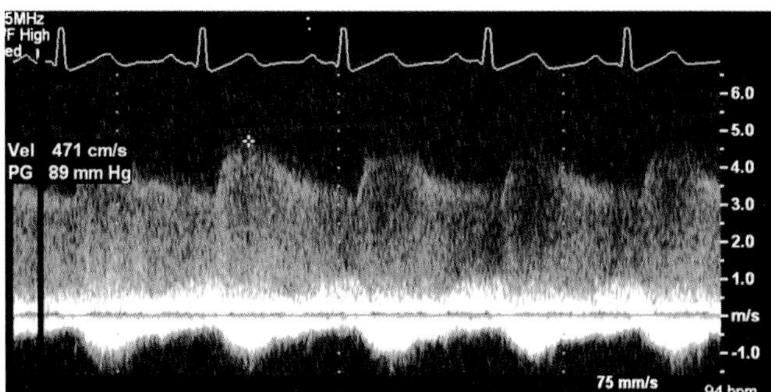

Fig. 38.21 Echocardiographic imaging with continuous wave Doppler gradient across the patent ductus arteriosus (PDA), showing the PDA gradient of 89 mm Hg against systemic pressures of 100 mm Hg. The pulmonary artery (PA) pressures from the gradient is systemic pressures (100 mm Hg)—PDA gradient (89 mm Hg) = 11 mm Hg

Evidence of aortic runoff:

- Color flow mapping shows flow reversal in descending aorta in diastole up to the level of ductus arteriosus.
- On continuous wave Doppler examination of the descending aorta in suprasternal long-axis view below the ductus, there will be forward flow signal in systole (below the baseline) and reverse signal in diastole (above the baseline). The reverse signal indicates flow from descending aorta to pulmonary artery. With Doppler sample volume above the level of duct, the signal will be forward in both systole and diastole. Here the diastolic signal is away from the transducer toward the ductus arteriosus.
- M-mode of descending aorta to detect the aortic runoff, after color flow mapping, M-mode cursor is placed over descending aorta in suprasternal long-axis view. The flow pattern in systole and diastole can be detected accurately.

OBSTRUCTIVE LESIONS

Aortic Stenosis (Figs 38.22A to C)

Valvar AS is the most common type of left ventricular outflow tract obstruction accounting for 70–91% of aortic obstructions.

- The echocardiographic study of valvular AS should include:
  - Morphology of the stenotic valve
  - Dimensions of the aortic root
  - Severity of valvar obstruction
  - Left ventricular function
  - Associated anomalies.
- Direct quantitative assessment of the severity of aortic valvar stenosis can be obtained using Doppler echocardiography (Table 38.6). At the same time one should also look for indirect measures of aortic valve stenosis and hemodynamic consequences.
- Normal aortic valve blood flow is laminar and peak systolic velocity of blood flow across the valve rarely exceeds 1.5 m/s. In aortic valve stenosis, the LV generates

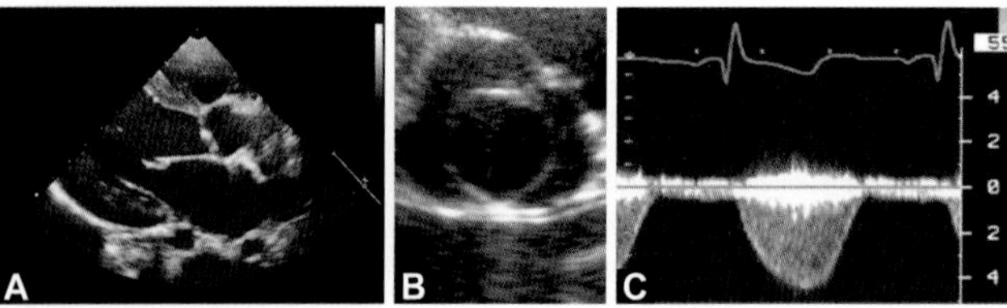

Figs 38.22A to C 2D echocardiography in a case of valvular aortic stenosis. (A) Shows parasternal long-axis view showing domed aortic valve. (B) Parasternal short-axis view with fused noncoronary cusp and left coronary cusp showing fish mouth opening of the bicuspid aortic valve. (C) Doppler gradient across the aortic valve sowing the gradient across the valve

Table 38.6 Severity of aortic stenosis

	Mild	*Moderate*	*Severe*
Peak velocity (m/s)	<3.0	3.0–4.0	>4.0
Mean gradient (mm Hg)	< 25	25–40	>40
Ao valve area (cm^2/m^2)	1.5–0.8	0.8–0.5	<0.5
Absolute value (cm^2)	1.5	1.0–1.5	<1.0

high pressures to overcome the obstruction, resulting in both turbulent flow and increased velocity across the valve. The pulse wave (PW) Doppler helps in localizing the site of obstruction by demonstrating low velocity in the LV outflow and increased velocity across the aortic valve. However, velocities above 1.5 m/s exceed the Nyquist limit of the pulse-Doppler and, continuous wave Doppler is required to quantitate the valvar obstruction.

- The jet velocities distal to the stenotic aortic valve orifice are recorded from multiple views; subcostal, apical, right parasternal and suprasternal transducer locations.
- The velocity of the AS jet is defined as the highest continuous wave Doppler signal obtained from any window. Only well-defined envelopes should be used for quantification of velocities to obviate significant errors.
- The ultrasound beam must be aligned parallel to the flow for accurate velocity recording guided by two-dimensional image and color flow.
- Angle correction should be avoided. Underestimation of stenosis severity can occur due to a non-parallel intercept angle. At higher velocities, a small error may lead to significant underestimation of gradients because of the quadratic relation between velocity and pressure gradient.
- The usual cause of overestimation of AS is if one interrogates the mitral regurgitation signal mistakenly. Both jets occur in systole and in the same direction. A difference in timing may be helpful as the mitral regurgitation signal velocity starts during isovolumic contraction and continues through isovolumic relaxation.
- The velocity determination across the aortic valve is flow related. Hence, conditions causing increased flow such as aortic regurgitation, elevated cardiac output as seen in anemia, anxiety, pregnancy and exercise will increase the flow velocity across the aortic valve. Hence, it is necessary to determine the velocity proximal to the aortic valve and do the necessary correction in Bernoulli's formula. Conditions associated with low cardiac output such as in left ventricular failure commonly seen in neonatal or elderly AS or elderly preclude the use of valve gradient as an indicator of valvar stenosis.
- Another physiologic issue that needs to be considered in the Doppler assessment of pressure gradients in patients with AS is the phenomenon of distal pressure recovery. The fluid dynamics of valvular AS are characterized by a laminar high-velocity jet in the narrowed orifice, with the narrowed segment of the flow stream (the vena contracta) occurring downstream from the anatomic valve orifice. As the jet expands and decelerates beyond the vena contracta, the associated turbulence results in an increase in aortic pressure "pressure recovery" such that when aortic pressure is measured in the distal ascending aorta, the left ventricular to aortic pressure difference is less than if aortic pressure is measured in the vena contracta. Clinically recovery accounts for an observed magnitude of pressure recovery is only 5–10 mm Hg.
- *Pressure gradient*: Doppler measured peak gradient corresponds to the catheter measured peak instantaneous pressure gradient, which is fundamentally different from the peak-to-peak catheter "gradient."
- *Critical neonatal AS*: Echocardiographic features include the following:
  - The aortic valve leaflets are thickened and domed. In many cases, the leaflets are immobile and a clear systolic opening cannot be visualized. The annulus usually measures 5–8 mm.
  - Usually, there is poststenotic dilatation of the ascending aorta and the ratio of the ascending aorta to the annulus is >1.0. This phenomenon characterizes a LV generating a pressure gradient across the aortic valve leading to release of energy in the ascending aorta and poststenotic dilatation.
  - The LV is thickened and has an end-diastolic cross-sectional area in the parasternal long-axis view of 1.7 cm^2 or greater with critical AS.
  - Increased echogenicity of the mitral valve papillary muscles is seen in parasternal short-axis, parasternal long-axis, and apical four-chamber views.
  - Redirection of fetal flow patterns results in the RV and the main pulmonary artery being enlarged.

Pulmonary Stenosis (Figs 38.23A and B)

The echocardiographic study of valvar PS should include the following:

1. Morphology of the stenotic pulmonary valve
2. Severity of obstruction

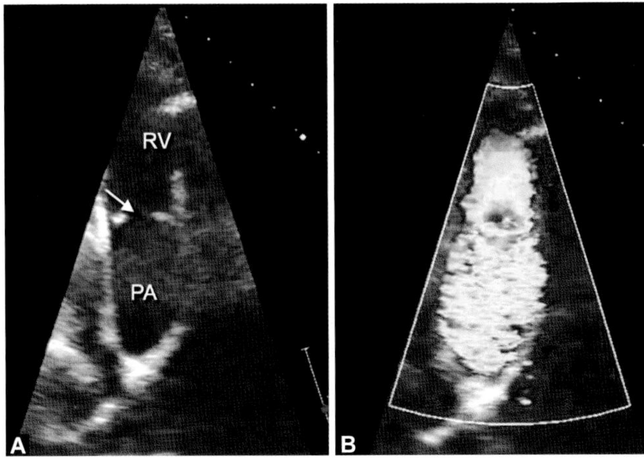

Figs 38.23A and B 2D echo with parasternal short-axis view in a case of pulmonary stenosis. (A) Two-dimensional echocardiograph showing the domed pulmonary valve. (B) Color flow mapping of the same showing the turbulence starting at the level of the pulmonary valve

3. Size and function of the RV, morphology of the tricuspid valve, and tricuspid regurgitation.

Morphology of Stenotic Valve

The stenosed pulmonary valve basically is divided into (a) domed pulmonary valve (90%) and (b) dysplastic pulmonary valve (10%).

Domed pulmonary valve:

- Most commonly identified valve in valvular PS
- Pulmonary valve annulus is usually normal with three well-developed sinuses and commissures.
- Pulmonary valve morphology motion of leaflets during cardiac cycle, and pulmonary annulus all can be well defined from parasternal short-axis view at the level of great vessels, parasternal long-axis view with anterior tilt, subcostal coronal with anterior tilt, subcostal sagittal, and subcostal paracoronal views.
- In PS thickened leaflets are seen.
- During systole, the proximal portion of the leaflets moves through a wide arc, while the distal tips remain relatively close together. This curved configuration of the pulmonary valve leaflets represents systolic doming of the valve and produces an effective narrowing of the pulmonary valve orifice.
- Finally, although during most of the diastole the appearance of the pulmonary valve echoes in patients with valvar PS is indistinguishable from normal, the leaflets frequently move to a fully open or domed position following atrial systole due to elevated right ventricular diastolic pressure in significant PS.
- The pulmonary annulus is measured in the parasternal short-axis and parasternal long-axis views through the right ventricular outflow tract between the hinge points of the valve leaflets in systole.
- Main pulmonary artery and branch pulmonary arteries (commonly left pulmonary artery) are dilated due to jet flow through the stenotic pulmonary valve. The degree of poststenotic dilatation does not correlate with severity of obstruction. Due to dilated pulmonary arteries, the heart shifts rightward displacing the pulmonary valve anteriorly beneath the parasternal window, permitting recording of the pulmonary valve in short-axis view.

Dysplastic pulmonary valve

- In patients with PS due to dysplastic pulmonary valve, two-dimensional echocardiography shows thickened pulmonary valve, redundant leaflets, hypoplastic pulmonary valve annulus.
- Stenosis occurs due to hypoplastic valve annulus, and restricted/immobile valve leaflets.
- Usually, there is absence of poststenotic dilatation of pulmonary arteries due to absence of jet flow.
- Common syndromic association with dysplastic pulmonary valve is Noonan syndrome.

Color Flow Mapping

Although valvar PS is usually diagnosed by two-dimensional echocardiography, Doppler methods are helpful with poor transthoracic windows and will always be required to determine the severity of valvar PS.

- In valvar PS the color Doppler stream accelerates within a centimeter of the valve and its flow velocity increases, reaching its maximum just distal to the orifice at the vena contracta.
- The size, shape, and direction of the flow stream are determined by the severity of stenosis.
- The diameter of the flow stream visibly narrows and the bolus of color flow gives a rough correlation with the severity of stenosis.
- As severity increases the velocity of the narrow turbulent jet increases and the jet is directed more toward the left pulmonary artery.
- The pulmonary artery flow is normally equally divided between the left and right pulmonary arteries; however, its ratio may change in severity (70:30) in stenosed valves.

Severity of PS

- The normal velocity across the pulmonary valve is 0.7–1.1 m/s. The maximal Doppler velocity measured within the jet, downstream the stenotic valve, predicts the gradient across the valve.
- Best alignment for Doppler interrogation of pulmonary valve is obtained from subcostal coronal view with

anterior tilt, subcostal sagittal view, apical four-chamber view with anterior tilt, parasternal long-axis view with anterior tilt.

- Due to poststenotic dilatation of main pulmonary artery, pulmonary valve position is shifted anterior and to right so it may be difficult to get an acceptable Doppler alignment from parasternal short-axis view in some cases.
- Color Doppler display of the PS jet helps in alignment of the Doppler beam parallel with flow in the jet. To obtain an adequate frame rate, a small sector within the 2D image should be defined to calculate the flow information.
- The Doppler sampling volume is then scanned across the pulmonary valve until the maximal frequency shift as determined by a well-defined outline of the envelope and audible signal is obtained.
- The Doppler signal is considered satisfactory when there is a clear envelope.

Right Ventricle

RVH:

- The RV hypertrophies in response to the increased afterload in right ventricular outflow obstructions.
- Quantitative assessment of the RVH is done by measurement of the thickness of the free wall of the RV. The RV free wall is measured in the parasternal long-axis view.

Right ventricular function:

- The systolic function is preserved in the majority of patients of pulmonary valve stenosis.
- *Diastolic dysfunction*:
  - Valvular PS leads to RVH. In the presence of significant pressure overload hypertrophy right ventricular diastolic function becomes abnormal.
  - Abnormal filling pattern of the right ventricular is seen at Doppler echocardiography.
  - The children with PS have a higher peak "a" velocity, and hence the ratio of peak "E" to peak "A" is altered signifying increased ventricular filling in late diastole.

Critical PS in neonates:

- Two-dimensional echocardiography shows thickened pulmonary valve, restricted opening, and usually hypoplastic pulmonary annulus.
- Interatrial septum bulging toward LA with PFO or small ASD.
- Right ventricle is usually severely hypertrophied, tricuspid annulus, and RV may be normal sized or may be hypoplastic.
- With critical PS, usually there is right ventricular dysfunction and bowing of interventricular septum toward LV with suprasystemic RV pressure.
- This group is a continuum of critical PS with normal sized/mildly hypoplastic RV to the pulmonary atresia with intact interventricular septum with normal sized to hypoplastic RV.
- Color flow mapping shows presence of right-to-left atrial shunt, mild-to-moderately severe tricuspid regurgitation, very small antegrade flow, the ductus arteriosus is patent with left-to-right shunt.
- Doppler interrogation in neonate of infants with critical PS reveals severely elevated right ventricular pressure (by interrogation of tricuspid regurgitation jet), increased peak velocity at the level of pulmonary valve. In many cases, peak velocity across the pulmonary valve may not be very high as right ventricular outflow is low due to severe right ventricular dysfunction, and right-to-left atrial shunt leading to decreased right ventricular stroke volume.
- Another important feature, which needs to be assessed in neonates with critical PS, is presence of ductus arteriosus. Widely patent ductus will cause elevation of pulmonary arterial pressure and one can underestimate the PS. So it is very important to define the detailed anatomy by two-dimensional echocardiography, then use of color flow mapping and Doppler interrogation.

Plan of Management and Timing of Intervention for ACHD

With the advent of improved percutaneous techniques more and more lesions are being treated in cardiac catherization lab. Management of the common ACHD is mentioned below:

L→R Shunts

Patent ductus arteriosus in the premature newborn may pose problem and indomethacin can be given in first few weeks in the dose of 0.1–0.2 mg per kg body weight 8 hourly for three doses. Alternatively three doses of ibuprofen may be given. If this is ineffective surgical correction is done.

The PDA in the full-term babies not resulting in CHF can be electively closed percutaneously or by surgery around 1 year of age. If with large PDA, there is CHF surgical correction can be done at any age.

Atrial level shunts generally do not cause CHF in the infancy and elective closure can be done around 2–3 years of age by percutaneous device or surgery. VSD may be closed by surgery or by VSD Device closure percutaneously. Ventricular septal defects if large result in CHF and failure to gain weight after 4–6 weeks of life with the fall of pulmonary vascular resistance. These defects need early surgical correction in infancy after stabilization with medical therapy. In moderate-sized VSD if the weight gain is adequate and the pulmonary arterial pressures are <75% of systemic the VSD closure can be deferred till 6–8 months of age. If the weight gain is adequate and the pulmonary artery pressures are normal but the L →R shunt is more than twice the systemic elective VSD closure can be done around 2 years of age.

Aortic Valvular Stenosis

Patient with isolated aortic valvular stenosis with peak gradients across the aortic valve of >75 mmHg of or mean gradient of 50 mmHg or more, even if asymptomatic need relieve of the obstruction. In presence of symptoms, CHF and left ventricular failure intervention is needed irrespective of gradients. The ideal treatment is percutaneous balloon dilation. The procedure is successful in 88–96% of cases. The re-stenosis rates in 5-year follow-up are 10–12% in pediatric age groups.

Coarctation of Aorta

Balloon dilation is the procedure of choice for isolated discrete coarctation of aorta with gradient of above 20 mm of Hg or associated CHF for less than 9 years or 30 kg weight. The procedural success is 80–90%. However, the recurrence rate is high in neonates and infants but low in later age group. For grown up patients coarctation stenting yields good results.

Pulmonary Valvular Stenosis

Isolated pulmonary valvular stenosis with a peak systolic gradient of 50 mmHg or more is best treated with percutaneous balloon dilation. The procedural success reported is 86–98%, with minimal complication and good long-term results.

BIBLIOGRAPHY

1. Arciniegas F, Farooki ZQ, Hakimi M, et al. Surgical closure of VSD during first 12 months of life. J Thorac Cardiovasc Surg. 1980;80:921-8.
2. Awasthy N, Ambadkar P, Radhakrishnan S, Iyer KS.Lutembacher syndrome with unroofed left superior vena cava: a diagnostic dilemma. Pediatr Cardiol. 2012;24:1e2.
3. Awasthy N, Radhakrishnan S. Stepwise evaluation of left to right shunt by echocardiography. Ind Heart Journal, 2013.
4. Castaneda AR, Freed MO, Williams RG, et al. Repair of tetralogy of Fallot in infancy early and late results. J Thorac Cardiovasc Surg. 1977;74:372-81.
5. Chin AJ, Keane JF, Norwood WD, Castaneda AR. Repair of complete common atrioventricular canal in infancy. J Thorac Cardiovasc Surg. 1982;84:515-22.
6. Cnoussal A, Fontan F, Besse P, et al. Selection criteria for Fontan Procedure. In: Anderson FH, Shinebourne EA (Eds). Pediatric Cardiology. White Plains, New York: Churchill Living Stone; 1978. pp. 559-66.
7. Epstein ML, Moller JN, Amplatz K, et al. Pulmonary artery banding in infants with complete atrioventricular canal. J Thorac Cardiovasc Surg. 1979;78:28-31.
8. Gale AW, Danielson GK, Mc Goon DC, et al. Modified Fontan operation for univentricular heart and complicated congenital lesions. J Thorac Cardiovasc Surg. 1979;78:831-8.
9. Glenn WWL, Ordway NK, Talner NS, et al. Circulatory bypass of the right side of heart VI; shunt between superior vena cava and distal right pulmonary artery; report of clinical application in 38 cases. Circulation. 1965;31:172-89.
10. Hanley FL, Fontan KN, Jones RA, et al. Surgical repair of complete atrioventricular canal defect in infancy. J Thorac Cardio Vasc Surg. 1993;106:387-97.
11. Kirklin JK, Kirklin JW, Pacifico AO. Transannular outflow patching for tetralogy, indications and results. Thorac Cardiovasc Surg. 1990;2:61-9.
12. Kirklin JW, Blackstone EH, Kirklin JK, et al. Surgical results and protocols in the spectrum of tetralogy of Fallot. Ann Surg. 1983;198:251-65.
13. Kriklin JW. Current status of corrective surgery for ventricular septal defect. In: Rowe RD, Kidd BSL (Eds). The Child with Congenital Heart Disease after Surgery. Mount Kisco, New York: Futua; 1976.
14. Le Blane J, Ashmore T, Pine de E, et al. Pulmonary artery banding results and current indications in pediatric surgery. Ann Thorac Sur. 1987;44:628.
15. Leung MP, Beerman LB, Siewers RD, et al. Long term evaluation after aortic valvuloplasty and defect closure in ventricular septal defect and aortic regurgitation. Am J Cardiol. 1987;60:890-94.
16. Masura J, Walsh KP, Thanopoulous B, et al. Catheter closure of moderate to large sized patent ductus arteriosus using the new Amplatzer duct occluder. Immediate and short term results. J Am Coll Cardiol. 1998;31:878-82.
17. Mc Paniel N, Gutgwell HP, Nlolan SP, et al. Repair of large muscular ventricular septal defect in infants employing left ventriculotomy. Ann Thorac Surg. 1989;47:593-4.
18. Mullan MN, Wallace RB, Weidman WH, et al. Surgical treatment of complete atrioventricular canal. Mod Technics Surg. 1980;26: 11-13.
19. Murphy JG, Gersh BJ, Mc Goon MD, et al. Long term outcome after surgical repair of isolated atrial septal defect. N Eng J Med. 1990;323:1645-50.
20. Neutze JM, Ishikawa T, Clarkson PM, et al. Assessment and follow up of patients with ventricular septal defects and elevated pulmonary vascular resistance. ANJ Cardiol. 1989;63:327-33.
21. Pacifico A, Kerklin JW, et al. Complex congenital malformations surgical treatment of double outlet. Right ventricle. In: Kerklin JW (Ed). Advanced cardiovascular Surgery. New York: Crane and Stratlon; 1973. p. 57.
22. Pacifico AD. Atrioventricular septal defects. In: Sterk J, de Leval M (Eds). Surgery for Congenital Heart Defect, 2nd edn. Philadelphia, PA: WB Saunders; 1994. pp. 373-8.
23. Pearl JM, Laks H, Stein DG, et al. Total Cavopulmonary anastomosis versus conventional modified Fontan procedure Ann Thorac Surg. 1991;52:189.
24. Rochini AP, Beekman RH, Schachar GB, et al. Balloon aortic valvoplasty. Results of the valvuloplasty and angioplasty of congenital anomaly registry. Am J Cardiol. 1990:65;784-9.
25. Rodhard S, Wagner D. Bypassing the right ventricle. Proc Soc Exp Bio Med. 1949;71:69.
26. Rothman A, Lucas VW, Sklansky MS, et al. Percutaneous coil occlusion of patient ductus arteriosus. J Pediatr. 1997;130:447-54.

27. Shunt RA, Fyler DC (Ed). Nadas' Pediatric Cardiology. Philadelphia, PA: Hanley and Belfus; 1992.
28. Spangler JG, Feldt RH, Danielson GK. Secundum atrial septal defect encountered in infancy. J Thorac Cardiovascular Surg. 1976;71:398-401.
29. Stanger P, Cassidy SC, Girod DA, et al. Balloon Pulmonary valvuloplasty: results of the valvuloplasty and angioplasty of congenital anomalies registry. Am J Cardiol. 1990;65(11):775-83.
30. Tynan M, Finley JP, Fontes V, et al. Balloon angioplasty for the treatment of native coarctation of aorta. Results of valvuloplasty and angioplasty of congenital anomalies registry. Am J Cardiol. 1990;65:790-2.
31. Wilkinson JL, Goh TH. Early clinical experience with the use of the Amplatzer Septal occluder device for atrial septal defect. Cardiol Young. 1998;8:295-302.

39

Approach to Congenital Cyanotic Heart Disease: Is It Entirely Surgical Approach?

Rajat Gupta, Savitri Srivastava

The magnitude of congenital heart disease (CHD) is great in our country. It becomes clear from the fact that 1% of normal newborn and 2% of premature babies have CHD. With India's population of 1,270,980,000 and birth rate of 22.7/1,000, roughly 3–4 lakhs of CHD patients are added to the existing pool of CHD cases every year. Congenital heart disease constitutes 80–90% of pediatric heart disease cases seen in tertiary care centers of which approximately 25–45% cases have cyanotic congenital heart disease (CCHD). Timely recognization these cases is important because if appropriate treatment is not given, the attrition rate, development of complications and the lesions becoming inoperable is very common. In a child presenting with "cyanosis", it is first important to confirm the presence of cyanosis and rule out peripheral cyanosis by physical examination revealing cold, clammy periphery, and low perfusion. This can be confirmed by pulse oximetry showing normal saturation with peripheral cyanosis and low saturation with central cyanosis. After confirming the presence of central cyanosis one should differentiate whether it is of cardiac or pulmonary origin. Babies having severe pulmonary lesion may present with cyanosis. Response to oxygen is a simple test (hyperoxia test), if the blood gases on giving oxygen for 10 minutes show PO_2 of >200 mm Hg presence of CCHD can be ruled out, if the PO_2 rise to <150 mm Hg the possibility of cyanotic CHD is there, if there is no significant change in PO_2 the cyanotic CHD is confirmed (Table 39.1). If the facilities for blood gas estimation are not available, a marked increase in saturation by pulse oximetry indicates a pulmonary cause of cyanosis. In most cases, the cyanosis is uniform, but some cases may show cyanosis in lower limb and not in upper limb. This will indicates severe pulmonary hypertension with reversal of flow across the patent ductus arteriosus (PDA). Rarely upper limbs are blue without cyanosis in lower limbs and this is diagnostic of reversal of flow across PDA with dextrotransposition of great arteries (dTGA).[1]

Table 39.1 Hyperoxia test—response of 100% oxygen for 10 minutes

PO_2	<70 mm Hg	70–150 mm Hg	150–200 mm Hg	>200 mm Hg
Impression	CCHD very likely	CCHD likely	±	CCHD unlikely

Abbreviation: CCHD, cyanotic congenital heart disease.

In some cases, cyanosis can be aggravated by the pulmonary lesion like chest infection or diaphragmatic hernia. This should be kept in mind.

In a neonate or infant, the most important step is to recognize if the lesion is duct dependent because in these cases the sudden spontaneous closure PDA can result in catastrophic collapse of the baby.

The PDA-dependent lesions can be classified into duct-dependent pulmonary circulation, duct-dependent mixing lesion, and duct-dependent system circulation.

DUCT-DEPENDENT PULMONARY CIRCULATION

Patients with this physiology are sick and cyanosed in neonatal period. They may present with severe cyanosis or with congestive heart failure (CHF).

Pulmonary Atresia with Intact Ventricular Septum

They are very sick patients and present in neonatal life with severe cyanosis and CHF. Their pulmonary blood flow and survival is dependent of the patency of the PDA. As such, as soon as they are detected, they should be started on PGE_1 infusion to keep the ductus arteriosus patent. Subsequently, a detailed echocardiographic evaluation to assess the atrial communication, right ventricular size, inflow, cavity, outflow, and type of atresia—membranous/muscular and dependency of coronary circulation should be done. Patients in whom the right ventricle (RV) is hypoplastic and coronary circulation is dependent on right ventricle will be categorized for single ventricle palliation. Otherwise, if the anatomy is suitable, right ventricular outflow (RVOT) perforation and two ventricle repair are planned.

Two ventricle repair can be done by surgical repair of RVOT with or without Blalock-Taussig (BT) shunt. This can also be done by catheter intervention by laser or radiofrequency (RF) perforation of atretic pulmonary valve followed by balloon dilatation.[2-4] If additional source of pulmonary blood flow is required, it can be done by PDA stenting. First step in single ventricle palliation will be either surgical BT shunt or PDA stenting in cardiac catheterization laboratory.[5]

If this physiology is associated with restrictive patent foramen ovale (PFO), this needs to be enlarged also by balloon atrial septostomy.

Pulmonary Atresia with Ventricular Septal Defect

Degree of cyanosis is inversely proportional to the amount of pulmonary blood flow that is either by PDA or aortopulmonary collaterals or both. Early palliation is required if cyanosis is worsening or for rehabilitation of hypoplastic pulmonary arteries. This can be done either by surgical shunt (BT shunt or central shunt) or stenting of PDA or aortopulmonary collaterals in cardiac catheterization laboratory.[6]

The final correction in this subgroup of patients requires placement of conduit between RV and native or reconstructed pulmonary arteries around 3 years of age. These conduits later need to be replaced, as they calcify and stenose with time. This can be done in cardiac catheterization laboratory by placing bovine jugular vein valve mounted on CP stent (melody valve) in previously placed RVOT conduit and thus avoiding multiple surgeries.

Critical Pulmonary Stenosis with Tricuspid Regurgitation

Some patients of isolated critical valvular pulmonary stenosis (PS) present with cyanosis due to right-to-left atrial shunt generally in new born period or infancy but occasionally later also. They are usually associated with tricuspid regurgitation and CHF. These patients need emergency balloon dilation of the pulmonary valve with very good results (Figs 39.1A to C). In some cases, the dilation is done in staged manner and some of these may need repeat balloon dilation.[7]

Ebstein's Anomaly of the Tricuspid Valve

Ebstein's anomaly of tricuspid valve with right-to-left shunt at atrial level can present in very severe form in neonatal period or it may be diagnosed later. At all the stages, management is surgical except when recurrent tachycardia is present then electrophysiologic study and RF ablation of accessory pathway can be done in cardiac catheterization laboratory.

Tetralogy of Fallot Physiology

Anatomic substrates included in this category are tetralogy of Fallot (TOF), atrioventricular septal defect (AVSD) with PS, dTGA with ventricular septal defect (VSD) and PS, corrected transposition of great arteries (cTGA) with VSD and PS, double outlet right ventricle (DORV) with VSD and PS, single ventricle with PS. These patients may present with severe cyanosis in neonatal period or with cyanotic spells later on. Degree of cyanosis depends on severity of PS/pulmonary atresia (PA), malposition of great arteries, and presence or absence of source of additional pulmonary blood supply, i.e. PDA or aortopulmonary collaterals.

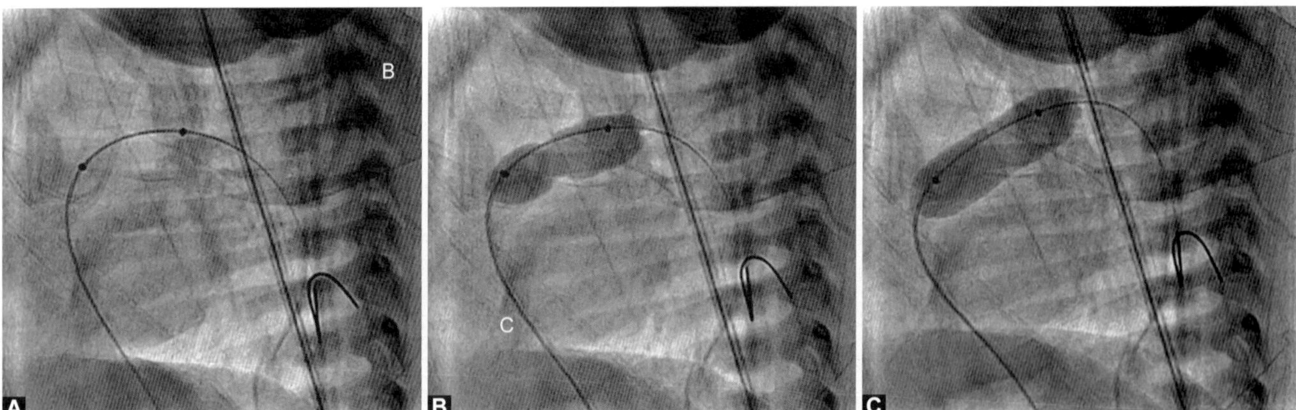

Figs 39.1 A to C Balloon dilatation of pulmonary valve in a newborn done in lateral angiographic projection. (A) Positioning of deflated balloon across the valve; (B) Central waist is formed during inflation; (C) Disappearance of waist on complete inflation

Early palliation if required because of severe cyanosis or uncontrolled spells is generally by BT shunt or central shunt. In patients who are not good candidates for surgery (low weight, sick child), catheter interventions like balloon dilatation (Figs 39.2A to E) or stenting of RVOT, stenting of PDA, or collateral can be done with low procedural risk.[6]

In patients with VSD and PA with same physiology, the final correction involves placement of RVOT conduit after 3 years of age, catheter intervention will be required at a later date for percutaneous pulmonary valve implantation when conduit stenosis become manifest.[8]

Stable patients with TOF, DORV with PS, and AVSD with PS who have adequate anatomy for two ventricle repair are offered corrective surgery at 6–8 months of age.

DUCT-DEPENDENT SYSTEMIC BLOOD FLOW

Critical Coarctation of Aorta

Patients with critical coarctation of aorta have duct-dependent flow to the distal arch and descending aorta and present with circulatory collapse and differential cyanosis as soon as their duct constricts. They should be given supportive care along with PGE infusion. Once stable, they can be taken up for surgical repair of coarctation.

Coarctation of aorta balloon dilatation or stenting can be done even in neonatal period if the patient is a poor surgical candidate, but in such palliated babies surgery will eventually be required. Catheter intervention is also required in patients who develop recoarctation of aorta after surgery.[9,10]

Aortic Arch Interruption

Patients with aortic arch interruption presents in neonatal period with shock when the PDA constricts. Interruption of aortic arch is associated with other cardiac defects, VSD or aortopulmonary (AP) window. Cyanosis can be differential or uniform, it is generally mild because of high pulmonary blood flow.

Initial management includes supportive care along with prostaglandin E1 infusion to keep the PDA open. Response to PGE1 infusion is remarkable and once the patient is stable definitive repair can be done. After surgery catheter intervention may be required if there is restenosis

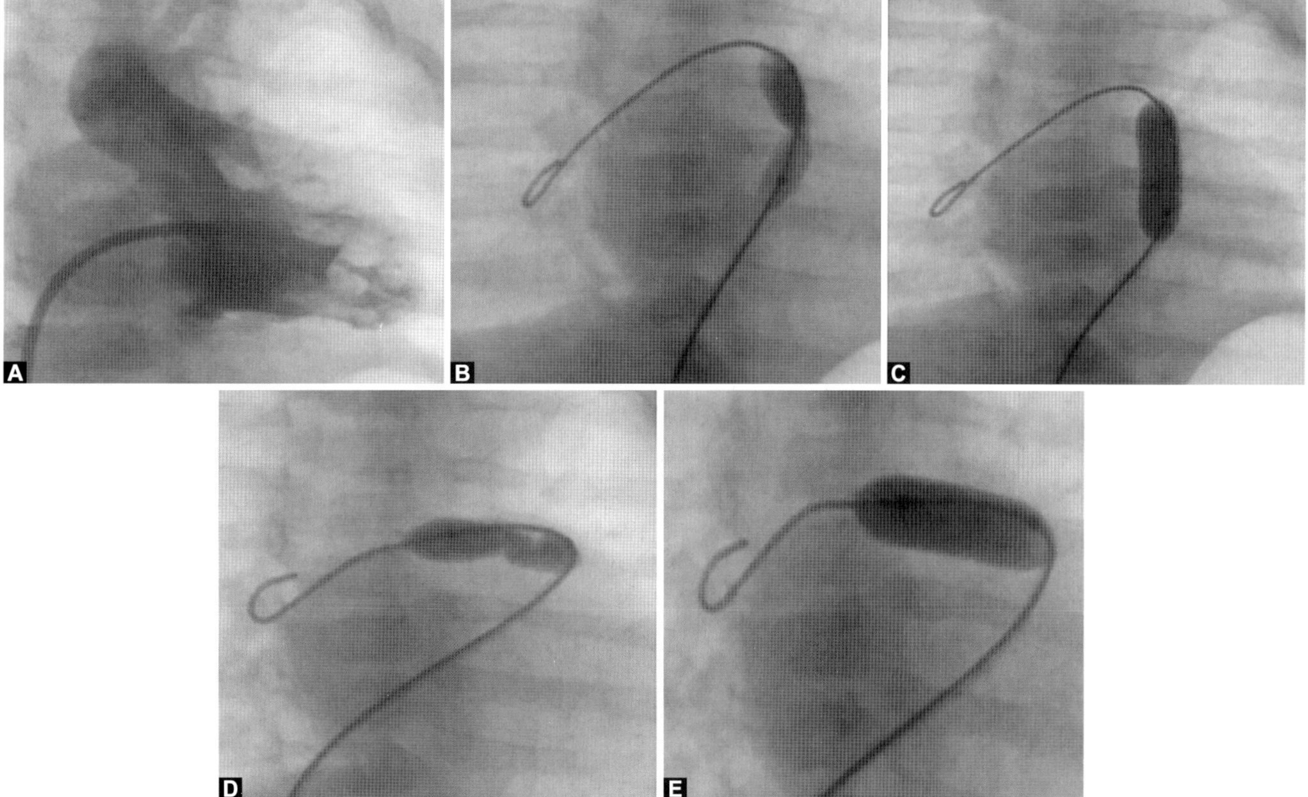

Figs 39.2A to E Balloon dilatation of right ventricular outflow tract in a patient of TOF. (A) Right ventriculogram showing streaky flow across the RV outflow tract (RVOT); (B) Waist formation on the balloon positioned across RVOT; (C) Disappearance of waist after complete inflation of balloon; (D and E) Balloon dilatation of pulmonary valve with complete disappearance of waist

at the anastomotic site, which can be relieved by balloon dilatation.[10]

Hypoplastic Left Heart Syndrome

Patients with hypoplastic left heart syndrome (HLHS) are sick and present in shock when the PDA closes and require PGE1 infusion along with other supportive measures for immediate survival. Norwood stage one palliation is required as a staged palliation toward Fontan surgery. This procedure is now being performed in Hybrid suit where PDA stenting (done for provision of stable source of coronary and systemic perfusion) and stenting of atrial communication (done to ensure adequate mixing and relieve left atrial pressure) is done by catheter intervention and surgeon does the pulmonary artery banding. Balloon atrial septostomy may also be required when atrial communication is restrictive and surgical stage one procedure is planned.[11]

PATENT DUCTUS ARTERIOSUS-DEPENDENT ADMIXTURE LESIONS

Dextrotransposition of Great Vessels

Presentation of patients with dTGA depends upon the presence or absence of associated cardiac defects. Patients with intact interventricular septum (IVS) and small atrial septal defect (ASD) or PFO and a closing duct presents early with marked cyanosis, shock, and metabolic acidosis.

They require supportive therapy and initiation of PGE1 infusion. Balloon atrial septostomy is required if definitive surgery is expected to be delayed. This can be done in cardiac catheterization laboratory or even as bed side procedure under echocardiography guidance (Figs 39.3 and 39.4). Patients with intact IVS should undergo arterial switch operation before 3 weeks of age.[12-15]

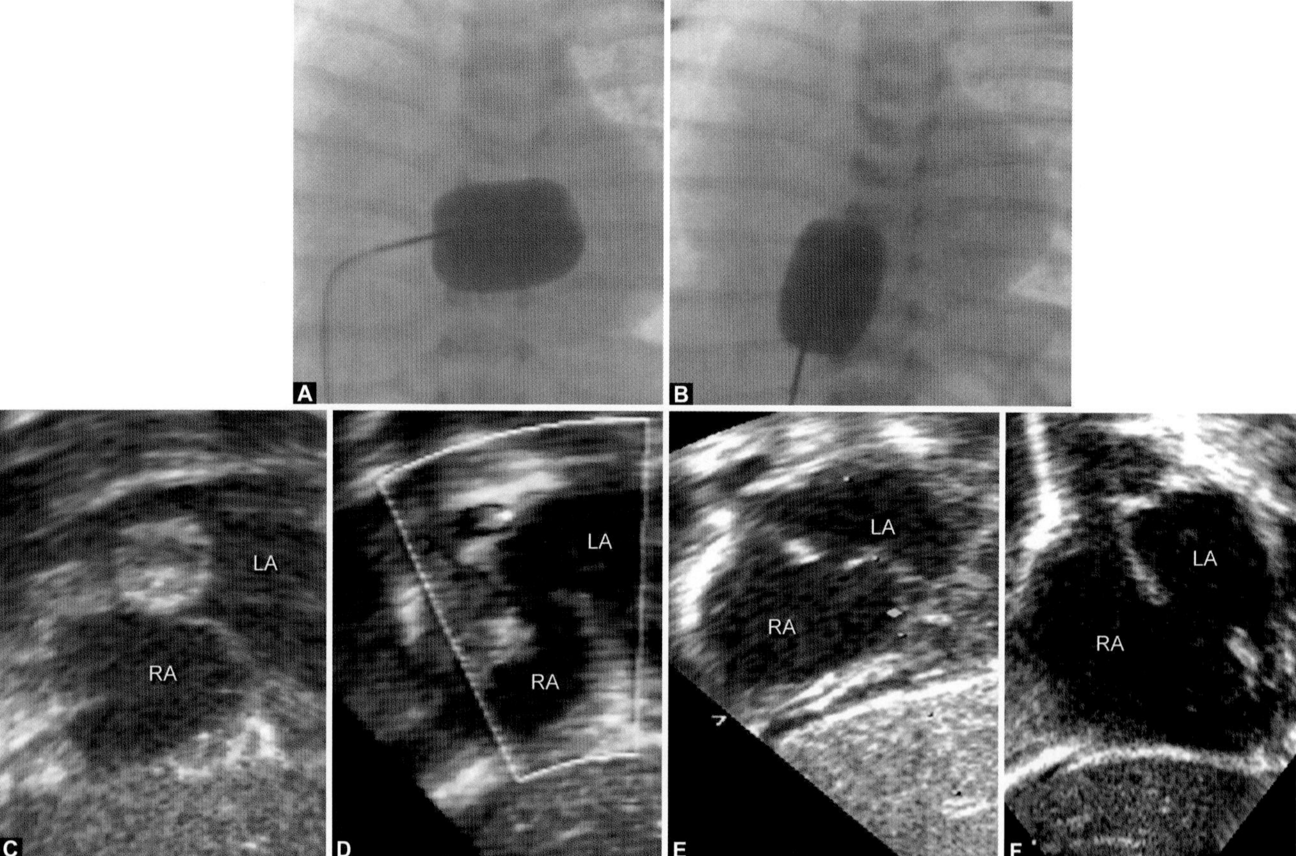

Figs 39.3A to F Balloon atrial septostomy being done under fluoroscopic (A and B) and echocardiographic guidance (C and D) and postprocedure echocardiography showing good result of the procedure (E and F). (A) Balloon is positioned across the atrial septum in left atrium (LA), (B) Balloon in right atrium after it is rapidly pulled; (C and D) Echocardiographic demonstration of position mentioned in parts A, B, E, and F. Echocardiography showing wide atrial communication in coronal and sagittal view, respectively

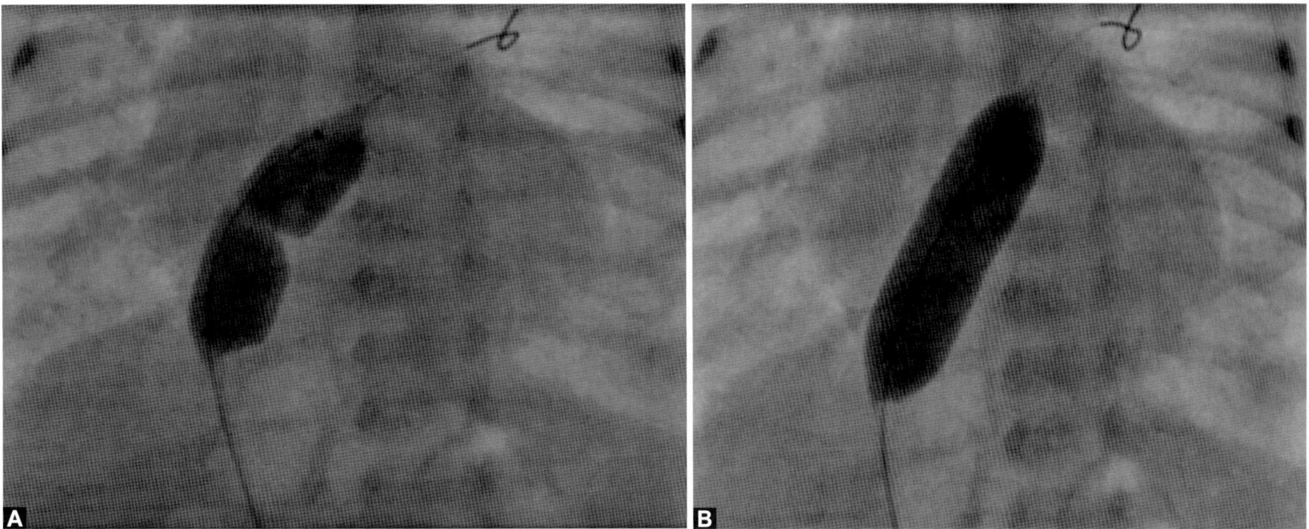

Figs 39.4A and B Static balloon dilatation of the interatrial septum being done under fluoroscopic guidance. (A) Positioning of balloon across the atrial septum; and (B) Full inflation of the balloon

Obstructed Total Anomalous Pulmonary Venous Connection

These neonates are sick at birth with marked cyanosis and respiratory distress. Chest X-ray may not show any cardiomegaly but signs of severe pulmonary venous hypertension are seen. Obstruction is always seen in infradiaphragmatic type but may also be seen in other varieties of total anomalous pulmonary venous connection (TAPVC). Öbstruction can be at the level of vertical vein, individual pulmonary veins, the atrial communication, drainage site of confluence of pulmonary veins. In patients with restrictive atrial communication, balloon atrial septostomy can be done to relieve the obstruction at atrial level on emergency basis and surgery for rerouting of pulmonary veins can be done later. In other cases, emergent surgery is needed. Patients with TAPVC without obstruction should undergo elective surgical repair at 2 months of age.

PULMONARY HYPERTENSION OF THE NEWBORN

In primary pulmonary hypertension of the newborn, there is no identifiable cause of the PAH, and right-to-left shunting at the atrial and ductal level causes cyanosis. Newborn presents with cyanosis with or without tachypnea. Echocardiography shows right-to-left shunting at PFO or PDA. Management is supportive and includes oxygen with or without ventilator support, selective pulmonary vasodilators, e.g. sildenafil and bosentan.

CYANOTIC PATIENTS

Presenting later can be divided into the following groups:

1. Reduced pulmonary blood flow (as discussed earlier)
2. Admixture lesions
3. Severe pulmonary artery hypertension
4. Pulmonary atrioventricular (AV) fistula.

Nonduct-dependent Increase Pulmonary Blood Flow (Admixture Lesions)

These lesions have mixing of blood at atrial, ventricular, or great arterial level. Cyanosis is mild because of increased pulmonary blood flow, and major signs are cardiac enlargement and CHF. On auscultation loud pulmonary component of second heart sound (P2) and flow murmurs are present. Lesions included in this physiology are as follows:

- TAPVC (nonobstructive)
- Truncus arteriosus
- dTGA with VSD
- Single ventricle without PS
- DORV without PS.

Management includes general supportive care and decongestive therapy. Surgical rerouting of TAPVC is done electively around 8 weeks of age or early if severe pulmonary artery hypertension is present. For truncus arteriosus, corrective surgery with VSD closure and RV to PA conduit is done at 6–8 weeks of life as is for TGA and VSD and DORV without PS. Patients with single ventricle and no PS will require PA banding at 4–8 weeks of age and later Fontan pathway.

Eisenmenger's Syndrome

Patients with shunt lesions, such as ASD, VSD, PDA, aorto-pulmonary window, or admixture lesions discussed above, with time will develop severe PAH with reversal of shunt and onset or increase in cyanosis. These Eisenmengerized patients are candidates of nonsurgical medical management only which includes selective pulmonary vasodilators and periodically phlebotomy.[16,17]

Pulmonary AV Fistula

Patients with pulmonary AV fistula are cyanosed but hemodynamically stable. AV fistula can be single and localized, multiple involving one or both lungs, or it may be of diffuse variety. These can be closed successfully in cardiac catheterization laboratory using coils or vascular plugs except the diffuse variety (Figs 39.5A and B).[18,19]

PRE- AND PEROPERATIVE CATHETER INTERVENTIONS

1. Many patients of reduced pulmonary blood flow have significant aortopulmonary collaterals and these have to be closed prior to surgery percutaneously by coil embolization (Figs 39.6A and B).[20]
2. Addressing the stenosis of pulmonary arteries with balloon dilatation or stenting at the time of diagnostic catheterization before Fontan surgery is helpful in preventing postoperative high pulmonary and central venous pressure and thus reducing hospital stay.
3. Presently balloon dilatation of the pulmonary valve in patients of TOF and DORV with normally related great vessels and PS is being done peroperatively so as to avoid transannular patch. This will prevent severe pulmonary regurgitation that is a very common in postoperatively in long-term follow-up of these cases.[21]

HYBRID PROCEDURES

In TOF and allied conditions, when pulmonary artery augmentation is needed pulmonary artery stent can be placed at the time of surgery. In some of these cases, there may be associated apical muscular VSD that is difficult to close surgically, and device closure of such VSDs can be done within the operation theater (OT).[22,23]

Fontan completion is being developed in a way that it can be completed percutaneously. The initial Glenn's operation is done in a modified way so that at the time of Fontan procedure

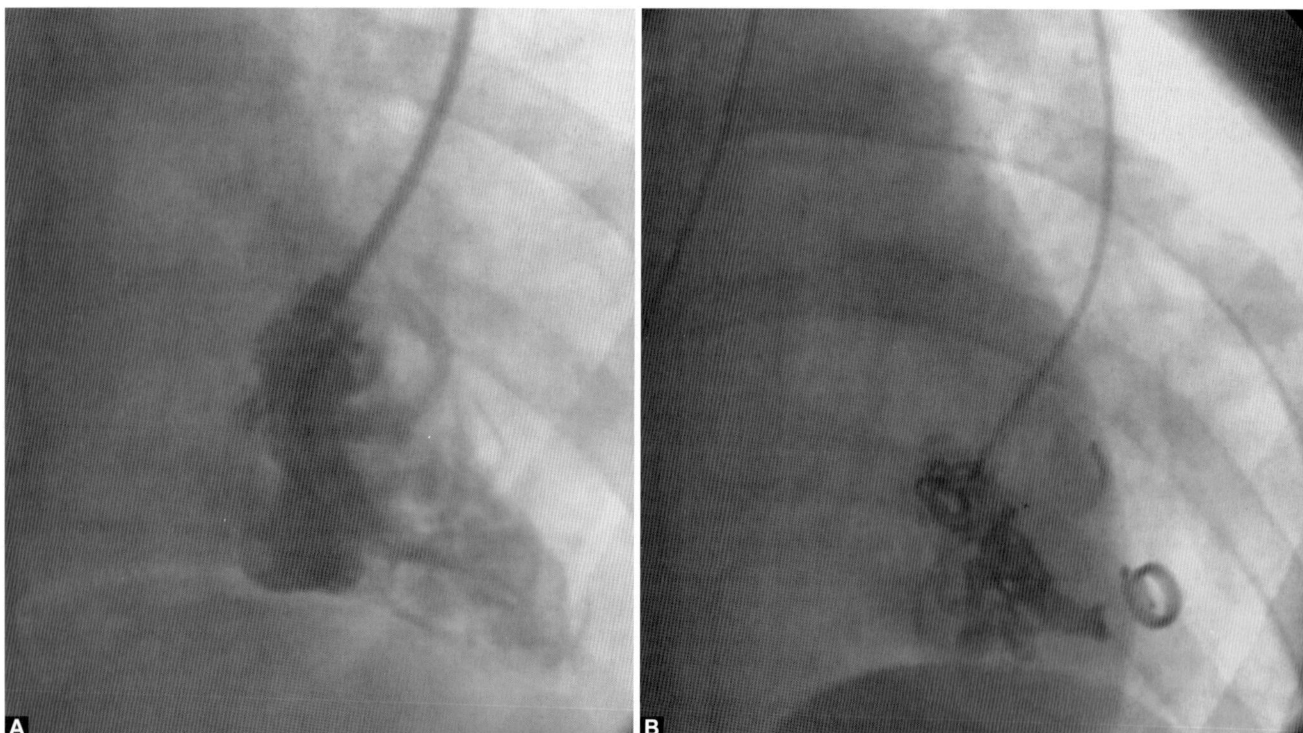

Figs 39.5A and B Coil embolization of pulmonary atrioventricular (AV) fistula. (A) Angiogram of the right lower lobe pulmonary artery showing peripheral pulmonary AV fistula; and (B) Multiple coils used to block the flow through AV fistula

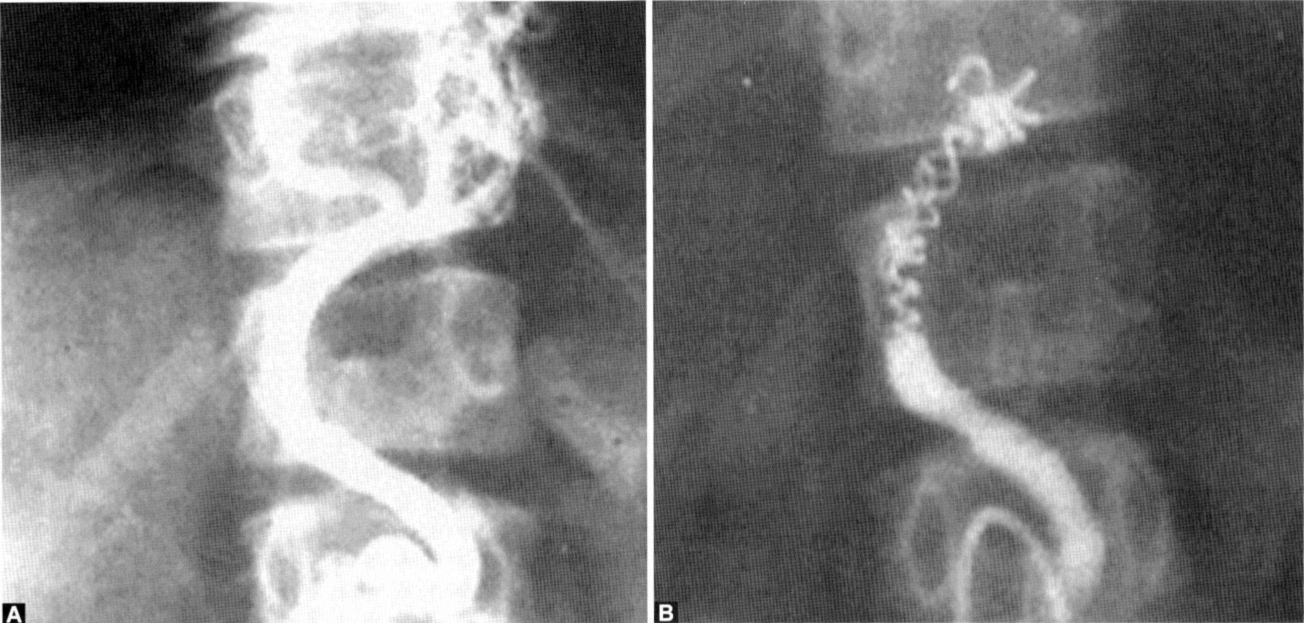

Figs 39.6A and B Coil embolization of aortopulmonary collaterals. (A) Selective angiogram showing large aortopulmonary collateral arising from descending aorta; and (B) Angiogram after coil embolization of the collateral showing no flow across it

the conduit from IVC to PA can be placed percutaneously along with closure of ASD.[24,25]

POSTOPERATIVE CASES

Tetralogy of Fallot physiology cases may need closure of collaterals percutaneously (Figs 39.6A and B) and closure of residual VSD that can be closed percutaneously by device placement.[26] Peripheral PS can be addressed by percutaneous balloon dilatation or stent placement. Senning pathway obstruction can be relived successfully by balloon dilatation. Blocked BT shunt can be opened by thrombosuction and balloon dilatation in cardiac catheterization laboratory (Figs 39.7A and B).[27] Decompressing venous channel after Fontan completion can be coiled or plugged by catheter intervention (Fig. 39.8).[28]

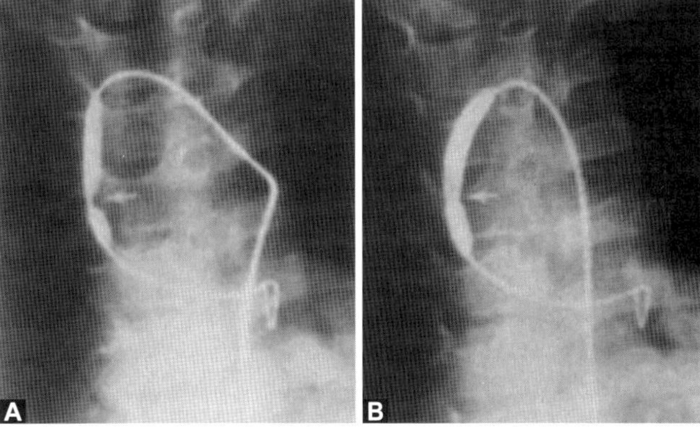

Figs 39.7A and B Balloon dilatation of stenosed or blocked Blalock–Taussig (BT) shunt. (A) Balloon is placed over the wire across the right BT shunt that is stenosed near pulmonary end; and (B) Disappearance of waist after full inflation of the balloon

CONCLUSION

It is very clear that in most of the CHD case, the definitive treatment is surgical at present. Percutaneous catheter interventions are definitive in a few cases only.

However, there is great role of specific management strategies in percutaneous interventional procedures such as residual VSD, peripheral PS, and closure of collaterals. Hybrid procedures are coming up fast, and in many units, there are specialized hybrid cardiac catheterization laboratory.

Pediatric cardiologist and pediatric cardiac surgeons aim at working as a team to obtain the best result for patients with cyanotic CHD.

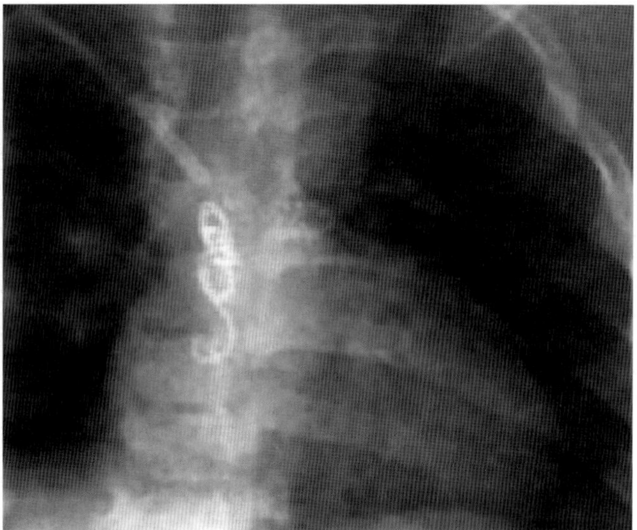

Fig. 39.8 Coil embolization of azygous vein after Glenn operation

REFERENCES

1. Fyler DC, Lock JE, Keane JF. Nadas' Pediatric Cardiology, 2nd edition. Philadelphia, PA: Saunders; 2006.
2. Gibbs JL, Black Bwon ME, Ozum O, et al. Laser valvotomy and balloon valvuloplasty for pulmonary atresia and intact ventricular septum: five year follow up. Heart. 1977;77(3):225-8.
3. Qureshi SA, Rosenthal E, Tynan M, et al. Transcatheter laser assisted balloon pulmonary valve dilation in pulmonary valve atresia. Am J Cardiol. 1991;74:372-81.
4. Humpl T, Söderberg B, McCrindle BW, et al. Percutaneous balloon valvotomy in pulmonary atresia with intact ventricular septum. Circulation. 2003;108:826-32.
5. Santoro G, Gaio G, Palladino MT, et al. Stenting of the arterial duct in newborns with duct-dependent pulmonary circulation. Heart. 2008;94(7):925-9.
6. Learn C, Phillips A, Chisolm J, et al. Pulmonary atresia with ventricular septal defect and multifocal pulmonary blood supply: does an intensive interventional approach improve the outcome? Congenit Heart Dis. 2012;7(2):111-21.
7. Colt AM, Perry SR, Lock JE, et al. Balloon dilation of critical valvar pulmonary stenosis in the first month of life. Cath Cardiovas Diagn. 1995;34:23-8.
8. Kenny D, Hijari ZM. Transcatheter pulmonary valve replacement: current status and future potentials. Intervent Cardiol Clin. 2013;2:181-93.
9. Ebeid MR. Balloon expandable stents for coarctation of the aorta: review of current status and technical considerations. Images Paediatr Cardiol. 2003;5(2):25-41.
10. Elbey MA, Caliskan A, Isık F, et al. Treatment of interrupted aorta in adult patients: a challenge both in surgery and transcatheter intervention. Int J Basic Clin Stud (IJBCS). 2013;1(1):17-23.
11. Honjo O, Caldarone CA. Hybrid palliation for neonates with hypoplastic left heart syndrome: current strategies and outcomes. Korean Circ J. 2010;40(3):103-11.
12. Beitzke A, Suppan CH. Use of prostaglandin E in management of transposition of great arteries before balloon atrial septostomy. Br Heart J. 1983;49(4):341-4.
13. Rashkind WJ, Millier WW. Creation of an atrial septal defect without thoracotomy. A palliative approach to complete transposition of great arteries. JAMA. 1966;196(11):991-2.
14. Baker EJ, Allan LA, Tynan MJ. Balloon atrial septostomy in the neonatal intensive care unit. Br Heart J. 1984;51:337-6.
15. Boehm W, Emmel M, Sreeram N. Balloon atrial septostomy: history and technique. Images Paediatr Cardiol. 2006;8(1):8-14.
16. Brammeli HL. The Eisenmenger syndrome: a clinical and physiologic reappraisal. Am J Cardiol. 1971;28:679-92.
17. Vongpatanasin W, Brickner E, Hills D. Eisenmenger syndrome in adults. Ann of Int Med. 1998;138:745-56.
18. White RI, Mitchell SE, Barth KH, et al. Angioarchitecture of pulmonary atriovenous malformation: an important consideration before embolotherapy. AJR. 1983;140:681-6.
19. Pollak JS, Saluja S, Thabet A. Clinical and anatomic outcomes after embolotherapy of pulmonary AV malformations. J Vasc Intervene Radiol. 2006;17(1):34-5.
20. Perry SB, Radtke W, Fellows KE, et al. Coil embolization to occlude aortopulmonary collateral vessels and shunts in patients with congenital heart disease. J Am Coll Cardiol. 1989;13(1): 100-08.
21. Rao PS, Wilson AD, Thapar MK, et al. Balloon pulmonary valvoplasty in the management of cyanotic congenital heart defects. Cathet Cardiovasc Diagn. 1992;25:16-24.
22. Amin Z, Danford D, Lof J, et al. intraoperative device closure of perimembranous ventricular septal defects without cardiopulmonary bypass: preliminary results with the periventricular technique. J Thorac Cardiovasc Surg. 2004;127:234-41.
23. Metton O, Calvaruso D, Stos B, et al. A new surgical technique for transcatheter Fontan completion. Eur J Cardiothorac Surg. 2011;39(1):81-5.
24. Konstantinov IE, Alexi-Meskishvili VV. Intracardiac covered stent for transcatheter completion of the total cavopulmonary connection: anatomical, physiological and technical considerations. Scand Cardiovasc J. 2006;40(2):71-5.
25. Zhang B, Liang J, Zheng X, et al. Transcatheter closure of postoperative residual ventricular septal defects using Amplatzer-type perimembranous VSD occluders. J Invasive Cardiol. 2013;25(8):402-5.
26. Perry SB, Radtke W, Fellows KE, et al. Acute modified Blalock-Taussing shunt obstruction successfully treated with urokinase and heparin. Images Paediatr Cardiol. 2005;7(3):20-23.
27. Sonomura T, Ikoma A, Kawai N, et al. Usefulness of the Guglielmi detachable coil for embolization of systemic venous collateral after Fontan operation: a case report. World J Radio. 2012;4(9):418-20.
28. McElhinney DB, Reddy VM, Hanley FL, et al. Systemic venous collateral channels causing desaturation after bidirectional cavopulmonary anastomosis: evaluation and management. J Am Coll Cardiol. 1997;30(3):817-24.

40

Pediatric Cardiac Intensive Care: Expectations of the Future

Parvathi U Iyer

INTRODUCTION

Pediatric cardiac intensive care (PCIC) has today emerged as a distinct subspecialty that addresses the highly specialized needs of a unique subset of patients—small infants and children undergoing various complex cardiac surgical procedures. Pediatric cardiac intensive care is a relatively young subspecialty, even in industrialized countries and developed long after pediatric cardiac surgery was born. In the early years, the pediatric cardiac surgeons or adult anesthetists took responsibility for postoperative cardiac intensive care. The growth of pediatric cardiac intensive as a specialty was spurred largely by an increasingly felt need for specialized care of the vulnerable postoperative cardiac infant.

Various key milestones have led to the rapid growth of PCIC as a specialty; these include increasingly complex cardiac surgery on smaller, tinier and sicker infants, surgery for hypoplastic left heart syndrome (HLHS) and various hybrid procedures. With better understanding of small body physiology and perfusion, refinements in diagnostic imaging, and advances in anesthetic techniques, the focus has rapidly shifted to definitive surgery or "more complete correction" rather than palliative surgery, even in the tiny and sick infant. This has meant that highly specialized and skilled pediatric professionals with a thorough understanding of pediatric and small body physiology coupled with an understanding of cardiac anatomy, physiology and the increasingly complex surgical procedures performed, become the "providers of postoperative intensive care". Simultaneously, there has been a plethora of literature on better understanding of cardiopulmonary interactions, various ingenious ways to manipulate the perioperative circulation, and availability of newer drugs for pulmonary hypertension, newer vasodilators and inodilators. An entire new generation of ventilators has become available with different ventilatory modes designed to support the "stiff, noncompliant" post bypass lung. There has also been greatly improved understanding of the open lung concept, lung recruitment, and lung protective ventilatory strategies. All of these developments, which are outside the purview of cardiac surgery, again emphasized the need for a distinct specialty and one which could keep pace with these rapid developments. Thus, the era of adult anesthetists and surgeons as primary providers of postoperative cardiac care was clearly over!

The last decade witnessed a meteoric growth in the field of PCIC with every pediatric cardiac surgical program in the West being supported by a pediatric intensive care team. The last decade also witnessed significant refinements in the use of extracorporeal life support (ECLS), newer forms of mechanical support, and more expedient resuscitation including extracorporeal cardiopulmonary resuscitation, all of which meant that pediatric critical care providers needed to rapidly develop the necessary additional skills.

Refinements in pediatric cardiac surgery along with the routine use of intraoperative echocardiography have led to more and more accurate and speedy surgery with surgeons leaving the operating room with minimal residual defects. This improvement in surgery along with the tremendous support provided by good pediatric intensive care have led to decreasing early and late mortality rates (STS data base overall early mortality rates being under 2%) in this highly vulnerable group of patients.

Thus, in the industrialized world, PCIC is synonymous with multiple technological advances like more efficient management of ECLS, HLHS, complex staged interventions or surgeries in very tiny infants. There is added glamour and excitement in the successful management and heroic salvage of these extremely sick infants with complex problems.

INDIAN SCENARIO AND DIFFERENCE

In India and much of Asia, the story is vastly different: pediatric intensive care is not an exciting specialty associated with the myriad technologic advances that are available to the West, but one associated with innumerable challenges.

Pediatric cardiac intensive care did not exist as a specialty in the most parts of Asia, till recently. In India, the very first unit to have a dedicated pediatric intensivist and a dedicated pediatric cardiac intensive care unit (PCICU) was as late as in 1995. The change in Asia has been slow but over the last few years, many units in Asia have realized the importance of pediatric intensive care and have interacted with Western units to provide a rapid "in-service training" for their pediatricians, so that they could become cardiac critical care providers. Likewise, in India too, change has set in, with many small startup cardiac programs being supported by a PCICU.

Nonetheless, in many parts of India and Asia, cardiac surgeons, adult anesthetists, and cardiologists still continue to provide postoperative care with no dedicated pediatric intensivist or pediatric intensive care unit. Why is this so? This is unfortunately due to the fact that the challenges associated with pediatric cardiac care in emerging economies are perceived to be insurmountable.

CHALLENGES

Pediatric cardiac intensive care is perceived to be an esoteric, glamorous, and expensive specialty irrelevant to daily pediatric practice and unaffordable in India and many parts of Asia. So, many pediatric physicians have no interest in pursuing a career in PCIC. This is despite the huge burden of treatable congenital heart disease: ~2 million children have untreated heart disease and another quarter of a million children with heart disease are born every year in India (Pediatric Cardiac Society of India data). Nearly 90% of these children have the potential for mainstream integration with adequate, appropriate, and timely management.

Late presentation is common with many infants presenting in a sick state with systemic or biventricular dysfunction, severe pulmonary hypertension, or circulatory collapse. Malnutrition, concomitant chest infections or pre-existing gram-negative and fungal sepsis are frequent comorbidities. Other challenges include coexisting hepatitis B, C, and HIV infections. Perennial nursing and medical manpower shortage and relatively inexperienced available workforce make PCIC even more challenging.

Pediatric cardiac intensive care can thus be difficult, wearying and potentially expensive in our country and in most emerging economies. Therefore, there is considerable skepticism in hospital managers about the possibility of "quality pediatric cardiac intensive care" being delivered in a "cost-effective" and meaningful manner.

Despite the overwhelming challenges, a lot is still doable with concerted efforts and unyielding struggle grounded in unwavering hope.

HOME GROWN STRATEGIES

Over the years, we have evolved many strategies to make PCIC more efficient and cost-effective. Our strategies focus on simple, inexpensive, evidence based, or "home grown" innovations.

We have learnt to rely on refinement of simple, inexpensive, evidence-based conventional modalities for management of low cardiac output states and for "near arrest" situations without the use of ECLS. Similarly, we have learnt to "live a life without inhaled nitric oxide" or other expensive vasodilators and manage pulmonary hypertension pre-emptively by "attention to basics" and the use of noninvasive ventilation. Simple, home grown innovations have been used to manage malnourished infants undergoing cardiac surgery.

We have evolved "fast track training modules" for doctors and nurses that we continually modify. Manpower training emphasizes "rapid skill acquisition", soft skills, multitasking and an ability to work with dogged determination in an atmosphere of scarcity and stringent budgeting. We have also implemented a simple, easy to follow, check list of "Early warning signs" as indicators of evolving potential catastrophic events to alert the young and uninitiated medical or nursing staff member. The focus primarily is on "how to survive a shift", a strong safety culture, and on "how to pull together" as a cohesive team.

These strategies have led to manpower performance way beyond expectations:

- *What is feasible?* Our greatest rewards have been our miraculous outcomes. We found that with increasing refinements of intensive care, discharge mortality could be reduced to as low as 1.4–1.8% despite all our challenges. We also found that these outcomes were sustainable despite increasing complexity of surgery. Costs too could be considerably reduced without adversely affecting safety. The long-term outcomes have also been gratifying. Some of the sickest children have been amazingly successful in mainstream integration and have gone on to become successful doctors and engineers and lead meaningful lives.

  In conclusion, PCIC in India has many challenges. However, quality PCIC with a "strong safety culture" is feasible using simple, low cost, home grown strategies, fast track training and better more efficient manpower management. The rewards of PCIC in our country are tremendous—something we can neither easily define nor quantify.
- *So, what does the future hold?* With a population of over a billion the demand for pediatric surgical programs will steadily increase. There will then be an exponential increase in need for strong PCIC support to make these programs viable.
- *Changing PCICU population*: As awareness improves, there will be an emergence of a changing PCICU population with an increasing number of smaller infants undergoing cardiac surgery, interventions, and hybrid procedures. There will also be a steadily growing number of older children and young adults with various arrhythmias or heart failure as a result of various palliative procedures performed in infancy and early childhood.

Thus, there will be an increasing need for pediatric critical care physicians to learn to "change gears rapidly" and be comfortable with both care of the "sick neonate" as well as the "ill adolescent". The nursing and medical staff will have to learn to keep pace with the changing needs of this ever changing PCICU patient population.

- *Cardiac failure, newer drugs and advances*: There would be an ever growing number of adolescents and young adults who would need heart failure management, such as postoperative tetralogy of Fallot, postoperative single ventricle situations, and postoperative Senning procedure. Again, there would be increasing need for pediatric critical care physicians to familiarize themselves with newer drugs, noninvasive home ventilation, and artificial hearts, which may well become the mainstay of the future.

COMPLEX ARRHYTHMIAS

Similarly, complex arrhythmias are expected to evolve over a period of time in single ventricle situations, postoperative tetralogy of Fallot and in situations where the right ventricle is supporting the systemic circulation.

Pediatric critical care teams will have to learn to deal effectively and efficiently with electric storms in the PCICU as well as be comfortable with efficient arrhythmia management strategies as new drugs and interventions evolve.

NEWER MODALITIES IN TREATMENT OF PULMONARY HYPERTENSION

Many operated children may still progress to develop varying degrees of pulmonary hypertension that would necessitate use of newer drugs and other therapeutic modalities. Various innovative therapies, biomolecular strategies, and proangiogenic factors may all eventually become part of a multipronged combination therapy protocol in the intensive care unit.

MANPOWER AND WORKFORCE ISSUES

It is likely that the gap between manpower needs and manpower availability is likely to widen further. Thus, there would be need for further rapid innovation and "rapid or fast track" manpower training and skill acquisition. Telephonic PCICU consultations, videoconferencing, video chats and increasing use of electronic transmission of important patient data would assume a tremendous role in preventing delays in timely intervention in the PCICU.

In summary, challenging times lie ahead with PCICUs being swamped with not only sick preoperative and postoperative neonates and infants, but also with older children and young adults with late sequelae of corrected or partially corrected heart disease. The future will also witness exciting times when advances in medicine, physiology, and critical care will combine with innovations in monitoring technology, information technology, mobile computing, to provide speedy and accurate electronic consultations with steadily improving efficiency in the care of the sick pediatric cardiac infant.

SUGGESTED READING

1. Balachandran R, Nair SG, Gopalraj SS, et al. Dedicated Pediatric cardiac intensive care unit in a developing country: does it improve outcomes? Ann Ped Card. 2011;42:122-6.
2. Chang AC. How to start and sustain a successful pediatric cardiac intensive care program: a combined clinical and administrative strategy. Pediatr Crit Care Med. 2002;3:107-11.
3. Chang AC. Pediatric cardiac intensive care: current state of the art and beyond the millennium. Curr Opin Pediatr. 2000;12: 238-46.
4. Fraisse A, Le Belb S, Masb B, et al. Paediatric cardiac intensive care unit: current setting and organization in 2010. Arch Cardiovasc Dis. 2010;103:546-51.
5. Kulik T, Giglia TM, Kocis KC, et al. ACCF/AHA/AAP recommendation for training in pediatric cardiology. Task force 5: requirements for pediatric cardioc critical care. JACC. 2005;46(7):1396-9.
6. Verma A. Pediatric cardiac intensive care units: the way forward. Ann Pediatr Cardiol. 2011;4(2):127-8.

41

Surgery for Congenital Heart Disease: In Search of Perfection!

Krishna S Iyer

Surgery for congenital heart disease (CHD) is just over six decades old. Soon after the long-standing fear of interfering with the heart was overcome by surgeons in the early twentieth century, attempts to surgically treat CHD began. Extracardiac lesions like patent ductus arteriosus and coarctation of aorta became the first lesions to get a surgical solution. A surgical palliation for the painfully debilitating 'blue baby' syndrome, the Blalock–Taussig shunt was evolved at the Johns Hopkins' Hospital in Baltimore in the early 1940s.[1] This procedure brought symptomatic relief and gave a lease of life to hundreds of children suffering from tetralogy of Fallot (TOF) and other forms of cyanotic CHD. This was one of the first revolutions to occur in the history of surgery for CHD.

It was soon apparent that most CHD would be beyond surgical cure unless surgeons could find a way to open the heart and correct an intracardiac defect while keeping the patient alive with artificial circulation. The use of hypothermia and its potential to enable temporary cessation of circulation was extensively studied in the animal laboratory. Lewis and Taufic performed a series of surgical closures of atrial septal defects using hypothermic circulatory arrest in the early 1950s.[2] However, the time that this technique allowed was too short for repairing anything more complex than the simplest of lesions. Walton Lillehei did some lateral thinking and came up with an out of the box solution using the child's parent as a temporary circulatory support to keep the infant alive and performed a remarkable series of intracardiac corrections, including the first successful repairs of ventricular septal defect (VSD), TOF and atriovenricular canal defect. The technique was called 'controlled cross circulation'.[3] However, the ever-present risk to the life of the parent acting as the oxygenator was clearly detrimental to this method becoming a standard of care. The search for a cardiopulmonary bypass machine for temporary support of the circulation was therefore intense. Several teams across the United States of America and Europe worked towards this goal and the breakthrough came when John Gibbon achieved the first successful closure of an atrial septal defect using a heart–lung machine, which incorporated a screen oxygenator.[4,5] This was the second revolution and thus began the era of open-heart surgery for CHD.

The early heart lung machines were large, cumbersome and prone to breakdowns leading to a high degree of morbidity and mortality. These problems were exaggerated when it came to dealing with the small bodies of infants and young children. The technology available was entirely designed for adult use and was extremely traumatic when used in children. It was also apparent that time related trauma to the blood elements and activation of inflammatory mediators were some of the many reasons for the poor outcomes.[6] Combination of cardiopulmonary bypass and hypothermia soon emerged as a solution and surgical repair of CHD in infancy soon became a reality.[7] Simultaneously, technology improved and the old bubble and screen oxygenators gave way, first, to disposable oxygenators and then to membrane oxygenators. The new technology mimicked the normal lung in that physical contact between blood and gases was avoided, minimizing the level of trauma to blood elements. Today, these oxygenators can support circulation for several days and are actively used in extracorporeal life support systems.

As the morbidity associated with cardiopulmonary bypass was overcome, the focus shifted to refining surgical techniques and evolving strategies for the repair of the more complex surgical lesions. Definitive surgery became the norm for all anatomically correctable lesions. Palliative surgery gradually became limited to surgically uncorrectable lesions like the single ventricle. Neonatal repair was waiting to happen and the advent of the neonatal arterial switch operation in the early 1980s provided just the boost it needed.[8,9] Over the years that followed age and body weight appeared to longer impact surgical outcomes and reports of successful repair in premature babies weighing as little as 1000 grams started appearing in the surgical literature at the onset of the 21st first century.

Surgeons in that pioneering era felt that once the heart defect had been corrected it would affect a 'cure'. The focus was, therefore, on early survival and resolution of symptoms. Little thought was given to long-term outcomes, late complications and quality of life. While avoidance of a major neurological complication was a priority, little thought was given to the effect of CPB on neurodevelopmental outcomes. As surgical techniques were perfected and early mortality and morbidity diminished, intermediate and mid-term follow-up outcomes of surgery began to get published. It became evident that many of the surgical repairs being performed had fundamental flaws and that in many situations surgery did not entirely reverse the secondary changes (e.g. pulmonary vascular disease) that had already occurred. The focus then shifted from early survival to long-term functional results and surgical procedures were modified or even shelved depending on what the follow-up results showed. It became apparent that CHD was not a 'congenital heart defect' but a 'congenital heart disease' that required not just a surgical correction, but a multipronged treatment strategy and life-long follow-up.

With the widespread availability and easy access to surgery for CHD in the developed countries, survival of a child born with CHD was almost assured. Most children born with CHD have their lesions treated before they complete their first birthday, often during the neonatal period. As these children grow into adolescence and adulthood, they face a whole new set of challenges. Residual lesions or onset of new pathology need to be investigated and treated. Arrhythmias are not uncommon, especially following complex or nonanatomical surgery. Issues relating to psychological adjustments to a lifelong disease, employability, insurance, marriage and childbirth in female patients are issues that cry for redress. It became increasingly apparent that neither the pediatric cardiologist, who was predictably unaccustomed to adult needs nor the adult cardiologist, who was often unfamiliar with congenital heart disease, could deal with these issues satisfactorily. This felt need, led to the creation of a whole new specialty—'adult congenital heart disease (ACHD)' or 'grown-up congenital heart disease (GUCH)'.

The timeline of surgery for CHD has been one of constant change and evolution. It is apparent that there have been monumental advances, however, barring the simple lesions, a perfect solution remains elusive for most CHD. The quest for perfection continues with undiminished enthusiasm. The evolution of surgery for two common lesions—tetralogy of Fallot (TOF) and transposition of great arteries (TGA)—illustrate these twists and turns and a brief description follows.

The morphology and physiology of TOF had been well understood in the early nineties following its first description by Etienne Fallot.[10] It remained a debilitating condition with no cure till Alfred Blalock performed, in 1944, the first systemic to pulmonary artery shunt as a palliation for the disorder.[1] The story of the conceptualization of this surgery is now a legend. Helen Taussig, the pioneering pediatric cardiologist, learnt about the technique of subclavian artery to pulmonary artery anastomosis that was being performed in the experimental laboratory in dogs to produce a model of pulmonary artery hypertension.[11] She wondered if the same operation could be performed to increase the pulmonary blood flow in children with TOF and thereby relieve them of their cyanosis. Apparently Robert Gross did not take her seriously when she approached him and she went to Alfred Blalock with her idea. The Blalock–Taussig shunt was born and the rest is history. For the first time a nonanatomical solution had been found to palliate a congenital heart defect. In later years, the classical operation using the turned down subclavian artery would be replaced by the modified one using an interposition graft that preserved distal flow to the limb and overcame many of the late complications. Various other types of shunts were described in this era but failed to match the efficacy of the BT shunt and were discarded. For ten years the BT shunt remained the only treatment for TOF till Walton Lillehei performed the first anatomical correction using the technique of controlled cross circulation. The VSD was closed by direct suture and the right ventricular outflow closed without a patch! It soon became apparent that the malaligned VSD of TOF needed to be closed with a patch and not by direct suture. Complete heart block ensued in a significant number of patients, largely because of the lack of understanding of the course of the conduction bundle in relation to the VSD. This complication needed a solution and led to the development of external pacemakers, followed soon by implantable pacemakers and a whole new field of cardiac electrophysiology took birth.[12]

At that time, it was thought that closure of the VSD and relief of the right ventricular outflow obstruction would completely cure TOF and the operation was euphemistically labeled 'total correction of TOF'. The technique employed a large ventriculotomy and transventricular closure of the VSD. John Kirklin the pioneering surgeon at the Mayo clinic emphasized the need for complete relief of RVOT obstruction notwithstanding the size of the right ventriculotomy required.[13] The ensuing pulmonary regurgitation was assumed to be innocuous and so generous RVOT patches were often placed. Since open heart surgery in infants carried a prohibitive mortality in this era, the concept of staged correction of TOF evolved—initial palliation with the BT shunt in infancy followed by total correction in later years. Surgical outcomes rapidly improved and TOF appeared to be a defect that now had a definitive solution. Interstage mortality remained a worry and the need for doing away with an initial shunt procedure became obvious. He detrimental long-term effects of long-standing cyanosis and the consequences of persistent right ventricular hypertrophy were being more clearly understood. With developments in the use of hypothermia-aided surgery in infants, the age at which TOF was repaired kept coming down. In the early nineties reports of neonatal repair of TOF started appearing, and over the course of the decade, the issue of elective repair of TOF in the neonatal period was hotly debated. Over course of time, TOF evolved from being a condition that was treated surgically in two stages to one that was electively corrected in early infancy![14,15]

The assumption that the pulmonary regurgitation resulting from a long transannular patch was innocuous proved to be vastly erroneous as long-term follow-up of 20 and 30 years became available. It was clear that chronic pulmonary regurgitation led to progressive right ventricular dilatation and dysfunction. Diastolic dysfunction of the right ventricle was increasingly recognized as a major sequel and its pathophysiology was extensively researched. Extensive scarring resulting from a large ventricular incision provided a focus for ventricular arrhythmias resulting in a sharp increase in late mortality and morbidity 20–30 years after surgery. This was a clear demonstration that in CHD good mid-term outcomes alone were not enough to prove the long-term durability of a surgical procedure. The RVOT therefore became an area of intense scrutiny. The classical transventricular approach yielded to the transatrial-transpulmonary approach, which minimized the length of the ventriculotomy and even obviated it in patients who had an adequate annulus. Several techniques were described for the preservation of the native pulmonary valve or to restore its competence. These included creation of pericardial or PTFE monocuspid or bicuspid valves, extension of the native valve cusps, and insertion of bioprosthesis among others. None of the techniques have so far reliably produced durable pulmonary valve competence and so the hunt for perfection in this area continues.

Pulmonary valve replacement was the obvious treatment for chronic pulmonary regurgitation and was recommended for all patients with symptomatic right heart dysfunction.[16,17] Follow-up results soon revealed however that pulmonary valve replacement did not always reverse the effects of chronic pulmonary regurgitation, especially so if the right ventricular dimensions exceeded certain limits. The last decade has therefore witnessed numerous publications devoted to the various electrocardiographic, echocardiographic and MRI findings that predict sudden death and also to the definition of parameters that would indicate the need for pulmonary valve replacement before irreversible right ventricular dysfunction ensued. Interventional cardiologists have made inroads into what was a purely surgical domain by introducing the percutaneous transcatheter placement of a stent mounted pulmonary valve. A less traumatic, albeit more expensive, solution to the problem of chronic pulmonary regurgitation is now at hand.

Clearly, even a common lesion like TOF remains without a perfect surgical 'cure'. Seventy years of pain staking experimental and clinical research have brought about substantial improvements but perfection remains elusive and the quest continues!

The evolution of surgery for TGA has similarly been through many twists and turns. The pre-CPB era witnessed many innovative palliative procedures like the Baffe's procedure,[18] and the Blalock–Hanlon septectomy[19] that enabled some mixing of blood at the atrial level. Ake Senning was the first to achieve a surgical restoration of the circulatory pathway to normal by means of an ingenious atrial switch procedure.[20] The procedure was brilliant in its conceptualization but needed great surgical skill for execution. Little wonder that it did not find too much favor amongst surgeons who took more readily to the simpler atrial partitioning technique devised by Bill Mustard from Toronto.[21] The two surgical procedures served to save the lives of children born with TGA who were lucky enough to survive to late infancy or had had a successful Blalock–Hanlon septectomy. Most newborns with TGA and intact ventricular septum still continued to die in the neonatal period.

The introduction of the Rashkind procedure revolutionized the management of TGA.[22] The procedure helped neonates with TGA survive the critical early months of life and reach an age where they could have a successful atrial switch procedure. Once again, it appeared that a 'cure' had been found for an invariably fatal congenital heart defect. Trouble however was round the corner for the Mustard procedure as a high incidence of baffle related problems became evident. The pericardial patch used for the baffle shrank or calcified and produced systemic or pulmonary venous obstruction. This negative feedback from intermediate-term follow-up of the Mustard procedure prompted a swing back to the Senning procedure, which was based on the use of native atrial tissue and therefore less prone to baffle related problems. Both these techniques, however, still suffered from the drawback that the ventricles still remained connected to the wrong half of the circulation—the right ventricle in the systemic circulation and the left in the pulmonary circulation. As with TOF a major assumption had been made that the morphologic right ventricle would remodel and assume the role of the systemic ventricle for life. As long-term follow-up would show, this was not the case. Right ventricular dilatation and tricuspid valve regurgitation resulted in many after two to three decades of follow-up, and it was evident that the atrial switch procedure was not a curative procedure.

Correction of TGA at the arterial level had always been known to be the appropriate strategy but transfer of the coronary arteries proved to be a stumbling block. It was not until the late 1970s that Jatene from Brazil succeeded in technically performing the arterial switch operation in a child with TGA and VSD.[9] However, while the procedure was successful in patients with TGA and VSD, it failed in patients with TGA and intact septum because the regressed left ventricle failed to support the systemic circulation after the arterial switch procedure. In order for the procedure to work, the left ventricle would have to be reconditioned or 'prepared'. Yacoub devised the means to do this by banding the pulmonary artery, which increased the left ventricular afterload, triggering it to hypertrophy.[23] The arterial switch procedure was then performed after several weeks once cardiac catheterization had confirmed that the left ventricle was capable of supporting the systemic circulation. The left ventricular training process was not always successful and the PA band produced significant distortion of the pulmonary artery and the pulmonary valve making the arterial switch procedure more difficult, and the neoaortic valve more likely to be incompetent. It was clear that this was not the most ideal way to treat TGA with IVS and the atrial switch procedure remained the preferred treatment option.

With confidence in neonatal surgery building up in the early eighties, a breakthrough was achieved with the Boston Children's Hospital group performing the arterial switch operation in the neonatal period.[24] They proved that in TGA with IVS, the neonatal left ventricle was capable of sustaining the systemic circulation immediately after the arterial switch procedure, as long as the surgery was performed within the first two weeks of life. Yet another revolution in cardiac surgery had taken place. Very soon the procedure had been perfected to an extent that survival was close to 100%. The availability of prostaglandin at the same time proved to be a major boon because it allowed neonates with TGA to be stabilized and kept alive till the time they could get an arterial switch operation done. However, patients who missed having an operation in the first two to three weeks were still a problem. The risk of left ventricular failure increased exponentially beyond three weeks of age. Yet again the problem was overcome by an out of the box solution—the rapid two-stage arterial switch procedure. Experimental work had shown that the left ventricular myocardium was capable of very rapid hypertrophy in infancy and could be prepared in a matter of days rather than months as presumed by Yacoub. The preparation of the LV and the arterial switch could then be performed in the same hospital admission without distortion of the pulmonary root that had been the bugbear earlier.[25,26] In later years, even the rapid two-stage procedure was junked in favor of supporting the failing left ventricle on extracorporeal membrane oxygenation, till such time as it prepared itself.

The technique of the arterial switch operation has undergone numerous modifications in response to feedback from follow-up data. A high incidence of neopulmonary artery stenosis, prompted the use of pericardial patch augmentation of the neopulmonary root. The LeCompte maneuver allowed reconstruction of the neopulmonary artery without use of any tube grafts. The trap door technique for coronary artery transfer reduced the incidence of perioperative coronary events. Techniques for dealing with intramural coronary arteries and other coronary anomalies were established such that no coronary abnormality precluded an arterial switch procedure. Despite all these developments, the arterial switch, while providing excellent survival and quality of life in early years, has its fair share of late complications requiring reintervention. These include coronary artery stenosis, pulmonary artery distortion and stenosis, aortic root dilatation and aortic regurgitation and a subclinical limitation of coronary blood flow reserve. Yet again, a lot has been achieved but perfection remains elusive and the quest continues.

The battle to overcome congenital heart disease has taught surgeons one important lesson—even the slightest anatomical deviation from what nature has designed, dooms a procedure to eventual failure. Surgeons are faced with the daunting task of restoring to a sick neonate or infant a normal lifespan. This means that the surgical procedure they perform in infancy has to work without failure for at least 60–70 years. This has probably been achieved for the simpler lesions like ASD, VSD and TAPVC. As the complexity of the lesions increases, the more difficult it becomes to restore anatomical normalcy and less therefore is the chance to restore a normal lifespan. Nevertheless, surgeons will keep striving and keep innovating and refining techniques while learning from past mistakes trying to restore nature's errors. The quest for perfection will ceaselessly continue.

REFERENCES

1. Blalock A, Taussig HB. The surgical treatment of malformations of the heart in which there is pulmonary stenosis or pulmonary atresia. JAMA. 1945;128:189-202.
2. Lewis FJ, Taufic M. Closure of atrial septal defects with the aid of hypothermia. Experimental accomplishments and the report of one successful case. Surgery. 1953;33:52-9.
3. Lillehei CW, Varco RL, Cohen M, Warden HE, Patton RN, Moller JF. The first open heart repairs of ventricular septal defects, atrioventricular communis and Tetralogy of Fallot using extracorporeal circulation by Cross-circulation: A 30-year follow-up. Ann Thorac Surg. 1986;41:4-21.
4. Gibbon JH Jr. Application of a mechanical heart and lung apparatus to cardiac surgery. Minn Med. 1954;37:171-85.
5. Gibbon JH Jr. Artificial maintenance of circulation during experimental occlusion of pulmonary artery. Arch Surg. 1937;34:1105-31.
6. Clarence D, Dwight SS Jr, La Vonne Y, et al. Acute metabolic changes associated with employment of pump oxygenator to supplant the heart and lung. In surgical forum: Clinical congress of American college of surgeons. Philadelphia: WB Saunders; 1952. pp. 165-71.
7. Drew CE, Anderson IM. Profound hypothermia in cardiac surgery: report of three cases. Lancet. 1959;1(7076):748-50.
8. Barratt- Boyes BG, Simpson M, Neutze JM. Intracardiac surgery in neonates and infants using deep hypothermia with surface cooling and limited cardiopulmonary bypass. Circulation. 1971;Suppl 1: 26-30.

9. Jatene AD, Fontes VF, Paulista PP, et al. Anatomic correction of transposition of great vessels. J Thorac Cardiovasc Surg. 1976;72: 364-70.
10. Fallot EA. Contribution à l'anatomie pathologique de la maladie bleue (cyanose cardiaque). Marseilles Med. 1988;25:418-20.
11. Levy SE, Blalock A. Experimental observations on the effects of connecting by suture the left main pulmonary artery to the systemic circulation. J Thorac Surg. 1939;8:525-30.
12. Lillehei CW, Gott VL, Hodges PC, Long DM, Bakken EE. Transitor pacemaker for treatment of complete atrioventricular dissociation. JAMA. 1960;172:76-80.
13. Kirklin JW, Blackstone EH, Pacifico AD, Brown RN, Bargeron LM. Routine primary repair versus two-stage repair of Tetralogy of Fallot. Circulation. 1979;60: 373-86.
14. Barratt-Boyes BG. Primary definitive intracardiac operations in infants: tetralogy of Fallot. In Advances in Cardiovascular Surgery, edited by Kirklin JW. New York, Grune and Stratton; 1973. pp. 155-72.
15. Castaneda AR, Freed MD, Williams RG, Norwood WI. Repair of tetralogy of Fallot in infancy. Early and late results. J Thorac Cardiovasc Surg. 1977;74:372.
16. Cavalcanti PEF, Oliveira Sa MPB, Santos CA, et al. Pulmonary Valve Replacement After Operative Repair of Tetralogy of Fallot Meta-Analysis and Meta-Regression of 3,118 Patients From 48 Studies. J Am Coll Cardiol. 2013;62:2227-43.
17. Geva T. Repaired tetralogy of Fallot: the roles of cardiovascular magnetic resonance in evaluating pathophysiology and for pulmonary valve replacement decision support. J Cardiovasc Magnetic Resonance. 2011;13:1-24.
18. Baffes TG. A new method for surgical correction of transposition of aorta and pulmonary artery. Surg Gynecol Obstet. 1956; 102:227.
19. Blalock A, Hanlon CR. The surgical treatment of complete transposition of aorta and the pulmonary artery. Surg Gynecol Obstet. 1950;90:1.
20. Senning A. Surgical correction of transposition of great vessels. Surgery. 1959;45:966.
21. Mustard WT. Successful two-stage correction of transposition of great vessels. Surgery. 1964;55:469.
22. Rashkind WJ, Miller WW. Creation of atrial septal defect without thoracotomy; a palliative approach to complete transposition of great arteries. JAMA. 1966;196:991.
23. Yacoub MH, Radley-smith R, Maclaurin R. Two-stage correction for anatomical correction of transposition of great arteries with intact ventricular septum. Lancet. 1977;1:1275.
24. Castaneda AR, Norwood WI, Jonas RA, Colon SD, Sanders SP, Lang P. Transposition of great arteries and intact ventricular septum: anatomical repair in the neonates. Ann Thorac Surg. 1984;38:438.
25. Jonas RA, Giglia TM, Sanders SP, et al. Rapid, two-stage arterial switch for transposition of the great arteries and intact ventricular septum beyond the neonatal period. Circulation. 1989;80(3 pt 1): 1203-8.
26. Iyer KS, Sharma R, Kumar K, Bhan A, Kothari SS, Saxena A, Venugopal P. Serial echocardiography for decision making in rapid two stage arterial switch operation. Ann Thor Surg. 1995; 60:658-64.

42

Role of Nurses in Cardiac Sciences

Saramma Thomas

Cardiovascular disease according to literature reviews is an emerging global health issue and a leading cause of morbidity and mortality in developing and developed countries. This disease can lead to serious effects on Quality of Life. This drives for an urgent and high demand for cardiac nurse in the healthcare industry.

Cardiac nurses are the most valued personnel in the cardiac facilities as they play a leading role in cardiovascular disease management and risk reduction. Cardiac nursing practice combines knowledge, human interactions and communication skills in an unique way to solve problems in every possible area of the cardiac facility.

Cardiac nurses are committed to lifelong learning so that they can deliver better evidence-based care in the fast-changing world of healthcare system. They ensure that cardiac patients receive care according to standards, based on best practices. They actively participate in meeting the acute and chronic needs of the patients in the most demanding tertiary care centers. Cardiac nurses are designated as advance nurse practitioners or clinical nurse specialist. Their nursing roles vary according to different settings. All cardiac nurses qualify to perform cardiac care and manage the patient's treatment plan. They are innovators in shaping quality and safety by applying evidence-based practice. Through effective data collection and analytical skills, they improve their own practice as part of broader efforts to improve care. They also actively participate in research activities and help in building the scientific foundation for clinical practice, prevention, and improved patient outcomes.

ROLE OF INFORMATICS NURSING IN CARDIAC SCIENCES

With the advent of technology moving at a fast pace, healthcare trends are transforming nursing roles, responsibilities and their career. The cardiac nurses are the frontiers of the movement in bringing about this change by critically analyzing the benefits of electronic way of monitoring and managing the patient both in care and in documentation. Nurses are embracing technology, as they understand the value of time and the relevancy of optimized care to improve quality.

Cardiac nurse understand patient care delivery work flow system and integration point of automated documentation. They are getting involved in clinical information system cycle. They have more: Buy-in the software, User-acceptance, Positive perception about the system.

Cardiac informatics nurse have evolved in the following areas like order management and communication, staff scheduling phones, pagers, in-house communication devices, online electronic bed management systems, online/integrated patient electronic patient record, integrated hemodynamic monitors (vitals) with electronic medical records, online fully integrated medication administration records, bar code technology, computer organized order entry. Informatics nursing is an evolving and leading part of delivery of health care. They act as navigators in addressing and managing with the complexities of today's healthcare system. This technology provides the team in collaborating effectively in providing care.

NURSING IN CARDIAC SPECIALTY UNITS (HEART COMMAND CENTER/CORONARY CARE UNITS/EMERGENCY ROOM)

Registered nurses working in the adult and pediatric emergency departments, cardiac intensive care units, coronary care units have focused expertise in cardiac advance nursing interventions. Their specific requirement in cardiology are as follows:

- Should be knowledgeable about the disease, pathophysiology presentation.
- Knowledge of vital parameters, pain management, cardiac arrhythmias and its management on individualized need.
- Knowledge and skills in providing advanced cardiac life support and basic life support also attend certification programs approved by recognized associations so as to competently manage cardiac arrest situations.
- Initial nursing assessments and reassessments need to be intermittently conducted, monitored and documented within the time frame of unit protocols.

- Constant monitoring and timely notification of critical alerts of clinical laboratory, radiological investigations, intake output to the concerned cardiologist.
- Knowledgeable about nursing process, which relates to nursing assessment, nursing diagnosis, nursing goals, nursing implementation and nursing interventions of patient with: acute coronary syndrome, heart failure, cardiogenic shock, arrhythmia, structural disorders.
- Awareness on indication and contraindication for use of IV thrombolytic therapy.
- Communicate with inbound emergency medical technicians for cardiac emergencies managed through ground ambulatory services and aircraft services.
- Knowledge and skills in handling of post cardiac care procedures, mechanical supports like intra-aortic balloon pump, cardiac extracorporeal membrane oxygenation which may be needed for heart muscle failure (myopathy) where the heart cannot pump blood around the body effectively.
- Methods of hemodynamic monitoring, management of invasive and noninvasive ventilator monitoring.
- Knowledge on post-care instructions on temporary and permanent pacemakers, automatic implantable cardioverter defibrillator and electrophysiology management.
- Where appropriate or necessary, they must collaborate with other healthcare professionals such as the patient's cardiologist, physiotherapist, or nutritionist, to devise and implement care and recovery plan specific for the patient.
- Cardiac nurse specialist have become more valued members of the team, at times they will lead, sometimes they will follow, they provide ..... to people at really vulnerable times in their life, through reassurances and psychological support for factors such as nutrition, physical therapy, personal hygiene and stress.

ROLE OF CARDIAC NURSE IN PREOPERATIVE UNITS

- Cardiac preoperative care includes assessment of patient knowledge of diseases and evaluating a patient's willingness for surgery. This is done by taking a detailed history and performing a complete head to toe examination.
- This is followed by ordering appropriate laboratory and radiological tests for assessment and prescribing necessary medications for surgery.
- Cardiac nurses are trained to implement the policies on informed and high-risk consents. Patient informed consent or a high-risk consent is obtained through a process defined by the organization and carried out by trained staff in a language the patient can understand.
- The planned care includes surgical or invasive procedures, anesthesia (including moderate and deep sedation), use of blood and blood products or other high-risk treatments or procedures.

ROLE OF NURSE IN CARDIOTHORACIC OPERATION THEATER

The cardiothoracic operation theater is a nursing specialty were nurses work with surgeons, anesthesiologist, surgical technologists. They perform preoperative, intraoperative, and postoperative care primarily in operating theaters for the following surgeries like coronary artery bypass grafting (CABG), suture less valve surgeries, congenital heart surgeries aneurysm repairs, heart transplantation, Left ventricular assist device implantation. The team members are as follows:

Scrub Nurse

The scrub nurse is a perioperative nurse that works directly with the surgeon within the sterile field. The scrub nurse takes care of instruments, sponges, and other items needed during the procedure, maintains sterility, assists with positioning, prepping and draping of the patient, cardiac monitoring maintain hemostasis, help in fixing devices and drains and complete the procedure by cleaning and applying dressings and coordinates with the needs of the surgical team. The operative nurse develops an approach to ensure correct site, correct procedure and correct patient surgery by having essential time out process for all adult and pediatric cardiac and vascular surgeries.

Circulating Nurse

- The circulating nurse assists during surgery. The duties include, a review of patients case. They are involved in supervision of sterilization services. Maintaining adequate levels of supplies of stock and equipment in quantity and quality. This role requires unique knowledge, wisdom and skilled training above the traditional education for becoming a Registered Nurse.
- Three components are being taken care during these three phases, i.e. preoperative, intraoperative and post-surgery. These are the safety goals laid down as per the international guidelines:
  - *Sign in*: Pre-procedural verification process of the correct site, procedure, and patient along with availability of special equipment and/or implants. The process also involves ensuring availability of all relevant documents, images, and studies.
  - *Time out*: A pause, just prior to performing a surgical or other procedure, during which any unanswered questions or confusion about patient, procedure, or site are resolved by the entire surgical team.
  - *Sign out*: It is an assessment done by the cardiac operation theater nurse to ensure equipments, instruments, sponge, needles are in accurate counts, specimens taken for biopsy are counterchecked for correct labels.

ROLE OF NURSE IN CARDIOPTHORACIC-RECOVERY UNITS

Cardiac care nurses in the postsurgical units or recovery units takes an efficient hand off transfer of the patient from operation room personnel's accompanying the patient. These nurses requires a strong understanding of all functions of the cardiac, pulmonary and renal infections.

- The bedside nurse must use proper assessment tools in caring for the adult and pediatric patient following heart transplantation.
- Reporting and recording of the vital parameters to the attending cardiac surgeons and anesthesiologist.
- Need to follow the initial goals of asepsis, hemodynamic management in the postoperative surgical patient, adequate oxygenation and ventilation, control of bleeding, restoration of intravascular volume, optimization of blood pressure.
- Cardiac output to maintain organ perfusion and metabolic stabilization, providing sufficient analgesia for pain control along with atrioventricular pacing.
- Management of cardiac extracorporeal membrane oxygenation, which may be needed after open heart surgery, or managing heart muscle failure (myopathy) where the heart cannot pump blood around the body effectively.

HIGH DEPENDENCY UNITS/STEP DOWN UNITS CARDIAC NURSING

- Cardiac surgery patient after their recovery from immediate postoperative care are planned for transfer out to departments labeled as step down units. The nurse posted in the cardiac step down unit constantly monitors and manages the patients, to ensure patient has stable hemodynamic and achieve a successful recovery.
- The routine activities of monitoring vitals, prevention of wound infection, early ambulation, physiotherapy, health education are accomplished on daily basis.
- Discharge process is initiated by filling all related documents pertaining to discharge, completing the discharge summary and imparting appropriate discharge advices by the patient's surgeon or postoperative physician.

ROLE OF CARDIAC NURSE IN CARDIAC CATHETERIZATION LABORATORY

- Nurses play an important role in cardiac catheterization laboratory, a diagnostic and therapeutic unit for identifying and treating coronary artery diseases.
- They assist for procedures like coronary angiograms/angioplasties/specialized structural procedures such as transthoracic aortic valve implantation (TAVI), patent foramen ovale (PFO), atrial septal defect (ASD) repair, percutaneous ballon mitral valvuloplasty (PBMV) and cardiac device implants/electrophysiology testing or ablation.
- Preparation of patients include assessing patient's vital signs, oxygen levels and heart rhythm before the physician examines the patient. They are under the constant guidance of cardiologist.
- Patients may be awake during the procedure, on conscious sedation which requires the cardiac catheterization laboratory nurse to monitor, help keep them calm and reassured.
- They assist and scrub for the procedures following the guidelines of asepsis.
- Cardiac nurses facilitate information flow through documentation which serves in many ways in the continuity, quality and safety of care.
- Postprocedure care.

Nurses monitor patients during their recovery in the recovery area patient's vital signs, following postprocedure care, administering medications and preventing post care complications like hematoma, excessive bleeding and fever. Timely provide education to patients and their families before discharge about medications, nutrition and care of a surgical site.

PATIENT AND FAMILY EDUCATION

Registered nurses provide instructions and education to patient and their families before discharge from the cardiac recovery units, education to include information on medication, nutrition and care of surgical site.

NURSES ROLE IN CARDIAC REHABILITATION UNIT

Patients admitted to the hospitals with a cardiovascular diasease are followed up in the cardiac rehabilitation unit: The cardiac rehabilitation process of helping people with a heart condition aims to make remarkable changes to their life and get them back on their feet again—physically, emotionally, socially and vocationally. The nursing team in the cardiac rehabilitation unit focuses primarily on individualized patient goals, imparts advices on how to quit smoking, delivers group education sessions for heart disease prevention, symptom management, risk factor management and lifestyle programs.

CARDIAC NURSES AS MENTORS

The cardiac sciences program has continuing education instructors. They hold a responsible position within the program and work together as a team. They participate in hospital-wide education, orientation, basic life support (BLS), advanced cardiovascular life support (ACLS) and a plethora of other initiatives and meetings.

- They update patients' knowledge and their self-care performance. An interactive patient, family and community education approach is successful in influencing compliance of the cardiac patients to follow healthcare advices.
- These nurses are upgrading their care, practice and developing in capacity through continuous nursing education and through participating in certification programs. Throughout their tenure of experience, they work out as mentors or preceptors in providing guidance to their subordinates and non-nursing personnels.
- The education role of the cardiac nurse provides the opportunity to positively affect one-on-one patient care and influence improvement in healthcare systems.

ROLE OF CARDIAC NURSE IN KNOWLEDGE AND SKILL DEVELOPMENT

- Nurses holding baccalaureate, associate, specialy degrees can continue to become a Cardiac nurse. This requires continuing education, skills and hours of clinical practice to become certified and experts to perform the duties effectively and efficiently. Competency assessment for these nurses is based on rigorous training schedules through competency based learning models. Mandatory minimum requirement of credit hours of training related to cardiac diseases or acute cardiac care.
- Cardiac nurses qualify to train as preceptors as they gain one to two years of experience and shows proficiency in care. They organize training programs for novice nurses through The preceptorship programs where a novice nurse is under the guidance of an experienced nurse being of a competent level. They work together on same shifts and the sole objective is that novice nurse achieves competency and develop a positive approach towards learning and caring.

Cardiac Nurse Involvement in Community Outreach Programs

- The aim of the cardiac nurse in the community care is to improve patient outcomes and decrease hospital admissions.
- They involve the patient and their family members in their own plan of care, assessment of their condition, identifying symptoms and understanding their treatment regimen. They actively evaluate their dietary and exercise compliance and its value to treatment.
- Cardiac nurses ensure patient mental and physical well being upon return home through constant follow-up visits.
- The outreach services are initiated in the form of health talks, seminars and training sessions in villages, schools, professional institutions, vocational camps, community or care homes.

ROLE OF CARDIAC NURSE IN MANAGING END OF LIFE ISSUES

- Cardiac nurses identify the prognosis of patients and provide invaluable emotional support to critically and chronically ill patients and their family members.
- They interact with the patient and family through counseling sessions, skilled in handling the patients and family's reaction to health and the potential for pathological grief reactions. They provide comfort and stability at the required moments of coping.
- The nurses also facilitate in providing information to patients and relatives about how to choose to donate organs and other tissues during meeting the requirements of end of life issues.

The cardiac nurses act as pioneering leaders helping in improving outcomes in individuals and communities as a whole. Challenges are evidenced, key strategy is to continue providing quality nursing care for better outcomes. The cardiac services of these nurses need to be incorporated into part of nursing researches, which will help in promoting an importance of the role being played by them in patient care. To ensure this, cardiac nurses need to take leadership roles in shaping health care, increasing efforts to train cardiovascular nurse to become efficient forerunners and strive in controlling the global burden of cardiovascular diseases. Our global aim is to help people who have suffered a heart-related illness work towards healthier lifestyles.

At the end of her life, Florence Nightingale said, "May we hope that when we are all dead and gone, leaders will arise who have been personally experienced in the hard, practical work, the difficulties and the joys of organizing nursing reforms, and who will lead far beyond anything we have done."

BIBLIOGRAPHY

1. *http://www.ehow.com/about_5663810_role-nurses-cardiac-surgery-patients.html*
2. *http://www.ehow.com/about_5553254_duties-cardiac-care-nurse.html*
3. *http://www.ehow.com/about_5231997_role-clinical-nurse-specialist.html*
4. *http://www.oxfordradcliffe.nhs.uk/cardiac/cardiacmedicine/specialistnurses/icd.aspx*
5. *http://www.wales.nhs.uk/sitesplus/documents/986/BHF%20Nurse%20Impact%20Re*
6. *http://www.americannursetoday.com/article.aspx?id=7086&fid=6850*
7. *http://www.oxfordradcliffe.nhs.uk/cardiac/cardiacmedicine/specialistnurses/chestpain.aspx*
8. Journal of Cardiovascular Nursing. 2011;26(4):S56-S63.

43

Ethical and Legal Issues in Cardiology

Vibhu Ranjan Gupta

INTRODUCTION

With the increasing complexity in medical care and in the doctor–patient relationship, it is important to keep in mind ethical issues in medical practice and their medicolegal implications. Yet each one carries the reader forward toward a better appreciation of the subject. Problems can arise because of poor communication, lack of knowledge of cultural and other aspects, inability to convince patients about a modality of therapy, etc. The elaboration of the cardiac cases will be of particular interest to practicing cardiologists, but some scenarios are of general clinical interest too. While cultural and other issues may somewhat color the cases one has to deal with, there can be no doubt that the essential matrix is lucid. With rapid advancement in medical science, technology, and skills comes a myriad of legal, ethical, and moral problems. Almost daily, items of ethical and medicolegal significance are appearing in the media. A basic understanding of the medicolegal and ethical issues in health care is essential for safe, responsible, and ethical practice in daily clinical work. Today, patients tend to be well- or ill-informed about the disease and health. Before a healthcare provider delivers care, ethical and legal standards require that the patient provide informed consent.

CONSENT

All patients/individuals desirous of undergoing treatment in a hospital have the right to autonomy and self-determination. An informed consent is a mechanism to provide them with relevant information about the procedure/test/intervention they are advised to undergo. This information lead to awareness of the planned procedure, its risks, expected benefits, known complications, and alternatives; and helps them make an informed choice and participate in decision making. A consent form serves as a tool to document that the necessary information has been conveyed to and understood by the patient/representative and that she/he is willing to undergo the said procedure/test/intervention. Informed consent is the legal embodiment of the concept that each individual has the right to make decisions affecting his/her well-being.

Implied versus Expressed Consent

On admission to the hospital for treatment, the patient and his/her family would agree to abide by the rules and regulations of the hospital. This includes allowing the hospital to conduct the physical examination (inspection, palpation, percussion, auscultation), basic tests to plan treatment, to allow administering drugs prescribed as per the treatment plan.

***Voluntary informed consent*:** A patient's consent is informed when the patient has been given sufficient information so that he/she understands the nature of his/her condition, the nature and purpose of the proposed treatment, the risks and consequences of the procedure or treatment, the feasible alternative procedure or treatment, and the prognosis if the procedure is not performed nor any treatment given.

***General consent*:** When the nature and probable risks of the procedure or treatment are of such a common and ordinary nature so as to be within the patient's understanding and knowledge.

***Implied consent in an emergency*:** Consent in emergencies may be implied if the condition of the patient precludes his/her ability to make a decision regarding treatment or procedures.

An emergency is a situation where delay for the purposes of obtaining consent may reasonably be anticipated as endangering the life of the patient or significantly increasing the harm to the patient's health.

Informed Consent

Informed consent can be defined under "right to know" as an agreement to proceed with a particular treatment/procedure/test based on understanding of the following:

- Nature and character of the proposed treatment/procedure/test

- Material facts involved
- Anticipated results and expected benefits
- Possible risks and complications (anything with a risk of >1% in scientific literature should be mentioned)
- Available alternatives including the option of declining treatment/procedure/test.

Material facts are facts to which a reasonably prudent person would attach significance in deciding whether or not to participate in the proposed treatment/procedure/test.

A patient's consent is considered informed when the patient has been given sufficient information so that he/she understands the nature of his/her condition, the nature and purpose of the proposed treatment, the risks and consequences of the procedure or treatment, the feasible alternative procedure or treatment and the prognosis if the procedure is not performed nor any treatment given.

It is the policy that separate informed consent is taken for various activities. Person/team member who will be performing the procedure/test for which consent in being obtained:

- *For surgical/invasive procedures*: Doctor carrying out the named procedure/test or a team member who shall be physically present during the said procedure/test
- *For anesthesia*: Anesthetist in-charge of the case or his/her assistant
- *For procedures in ward/ICU*: Treating consultant or registrar or ward RMO
  - Counselors appointed for specific purposes (e.g. HIV testing, blood donation, etc.).
  - Nursing staff are NOT responsible for obtaining consent but share the responsibility (with treating clinical staff) of ensuring that consent is completed as per protocol.

This is ensured that all patients undergoing operative and invasive procedures are allowed to participate in care decision. All patients with planned or emergency operative, invasive procedures, diagnostic or therapeutic procedures, blood transfusion and internal examination will be provided with adequate information related to the planned procedure, risks, benefits, alternatives, and potential complications (all these clauses are included in the consent form). After adequate information has been provided, an informed consent will be obtained from the patient/patient's relative:

- Informed consent is obtained for all procedures as required by the law. Any procedure under any form of anesthesia/sedation
- Any form of anesthesia including conscious sedation and monitored care
- All invasive diagnostic tests and procedures
- Other diagnostic procedures like stress test, contrast imaging
- Angiographic procedures
- Angioplasty and intravascular catheter procedure
- All interventional procedures (including pacemaker insertion, tumor embolization, etc.)
- Aspirations [including fine needle aspiration cytology (FNAC)]
- Biopsy and bone marrow aspiration
- Catheterization of major vessels [arterial cannulation, central line, peripherally inserted central catheter (PICC)]
- Endoscopy procedures (gastrointestinal, respiratory, or others)
- High-risk consent where appropriate
- HIV testing
- Restraint
- Dialysis
- Chemotherapy
- Blood transfusion
- Nuclear medicine tests
- Radiology investigations (CT, MRI, fluoroscopy, etc.)
- Radiation therapy including brachytherapy
- Discharge against medical advice (DAMA)
- Admission/general consent
- Blood donor consent
- Termination of pregnancy
- Dental procedures like tooth extraction
- Invasive cosmetic procedures including piercing of ear lobes
- Disposal of anatomical remains
- Release of confidential information except as permitted or required by law
- Any treatment/procedure/test where the treating doctor feels the need to obtain consent
- Consents pertaining to clinical research and drug trials.

Consent is not required in the following conditions as per law:

- Medical examination of persons brought for this purpose by police. Consent is needed for treatment
- When arrested person(s) are brought for collection of evidence (e.g. blood sample)
- Medical examination directed by the court (examination of genitalia in case of rape victim needs consent in writing)
- Medical examination needed for statutory purposes (e.g. armed forces).

All patients with planned or emergency operative, invasive procedures, diagnostic or therapeutic procedures, blood transfusion, and internal examination will be provided with adequate information related to the planned procedure, risks, benefits, alternatives, and potential complications (all these clauses are included in the consent form). After adequate information has been provided, an informed consent will be obtained from the patient/patient's relative.

As per the existing laws and norms defined by the hospital, should be replaced by hospital policies the informed consent will be taken prior to the procedure/treatment.

Staff members will clearly explain the proposed treatment or procedure to the patient or his legal guardian (in case of minors, i.e. under 18 years of age).

In case if a medical emergency, the consent is also taken telephonically from the patient's family and recorded.

The explanation should include and not limited to the following:

- Potential drawbacks, outcomes, and benefits
- Potential problems related to recuperation
- The likelihood of success
- Possible results of nontreatment
- Alternatives if any
- Adult patient (conscious, sound of mind) will give the consent him/herself
- In case the patient is unconscious/delirious, a minor or mentally incapable of making the decision by himself or if the patient indicates that she/he would prefer to have someone else give consent the signature of designated person will be taken
- In case of mentally challenged patients signature will be taken from legal guardian.

The senior consultant or his designee shall discuss in lay terms about the procedure, its risks, benefits, and alternatives with the patient or the patient's surrogate decision maker. The senior consultant or his designee shall document the discussion by obtaining the patient's or his surrogate decision maker, written informed consent on the appropriate form.

In a life-threatening emergency, consent shall be implied; therefore, the patient's signature is not required. In such situations, the senior consultant/consultant shall document in the patient's medical record both the nature of the emergency and the inability of the patient or surrogate decision maker to consent.

It is the responsibility of the person obtaining the consent to ensure that the consent form shall be properly filled prior to signing. All entries shall be in ink.

Any available adult who shall be identified on the form by title or relationship to the patient shall be witness to the patient's signature or the signature of the surrogate decision maker. The date and time of signing shall be clearly indicated.

The consent form must be signed by the senior consultant/consultants or his designee, anesthesiologist, patient or his decision maker, and the witness prior to entry into the surgical suite and before any premedication and at least 3 hours after the administration of sedatives.

If the senior consultant/consultant or the anesthetist's signature is not on the consent form, the procedure shall be postponed or canceled.

The decision regarding the patient's ability to make an informed consent shall be the ultimate responsibility of the senior consultant/consultants.

A patient or the surrogate decision maker may revoke the consent for the procedure at any time before it is carried out. In such an event, the senior consultant/consultants or his designee shall discuss the procedure again and if the patient or the decision maker still wishes to revoke the consent, then the procedure shall not be carried out. The patient or decision maker shall sign a note to the effect on the signed consent form. The senior consultant/consultant or his designee shall document this in the progress notes.

A separate high-risk consent is obtained for procedures defined as high-risk by the hospital. This consent is in addition to the procedure consent obtained for all patients.

CONSENT PREREQUISITES

- Name and signature of person explaining the procedure and obtaining consent
- Name of the person who will perform the procedure for which consent is being obtained
- Name and signature/thumb impression of person providing the consent (patient/surrogate)
- Name and signature/thumb impression of person witnessing the consent (not applicable for HIV testing and some other consents)
- Name and signature/thumb impression of interpreter (if applicable)
- Date and time of consent
- Name of procedure/treatment/test for which consent is being obtained
- Documentation of risks, expected benefits, potential major complications (anything with a risk of >1% in scientific literature), and alternatives
- No abbreviations used.

TIMING OF CONSENT

- Informed consent is obtained prior to performing any procedure listed above or as per discretion of the treating doctor/team
- For planned surgical or invasive procedures, consent is obtained within 24 hours in advance of the procedure (also see point 3)
- For planned surgical/invasive procedures, consent is obtained before the patient is wheeled out from the ward to the OT
- In case the planned procedure is delayed or rescheduled, a fresh consent is obtained.

SPECIAL CONSENTS

- *Organ retrieval*: The transplant coordinator shall take informed consent of the next of kin for the removal of organs/tissues from the deceased donor. A separate consent signed for adult and minor along with donor and recipient details and photographs.
- *Organ transplantation*: Legal consents taken on organ donation and transplantation as per Transplantation of Human Organs and Tissues Act (THOA).
- *Discharge against medical advice (DAMA)*: If a patient refuses to comply with the treatment plan proposed by his/her physician, OR decides to leave the hospital

without completing his/her treatment, the patient would be given a DAMA discharge, wherein consent is signed by the patient or relatives, taking responsibility of their actions to refuse treatment.
- *Consent for HIV testing*: Consent must be obtained only from the individual undergoing the test. Witness must be avoided to respect patient confidentiality. Surrogate consent is not allowed except in case of "provider initiated testing" where the following conditions are fulfilled:
  - The treating doctor strongly suspects AIDS based on clinical signs and symptoms
  - Patient is not in a condition to give voluntary consent (see section "Surrogate consent").

VALIDITY PERIOD OF CONSENT

A consent is valid until:
- Revoked by the patient, or
- Circumstances have changed such that the nature/risks of procedure and/or the alternatives to the procedure for which consent was obtained are no longer valid, or
- 30 days for procedures that require to be repeated regularly (see above "specificity of consent").

ETHICAL CONCERNS

One of the main ways that patients are involved in their care decisions is by granting informed consent. To consent, a patient must be informed of those factors related to the planned care required for an informed decision. Informed consent may be obtained at several points in the care process. For example, informed consent can be obtained when the patient is admitted for inpatient care in the hospital and before certain procedures or treatments for which the risk is high. The consent process is clearly defined by the hospital in policies and procedures. Relevant laws and regulations are incorporated into the policies and procedures.

Patients and families are informed as to which tests, procedures, and treatments require consent and how they can give consent (e.g. given verbally, by signing a consent form, or through some other means). Education by hospital staff is provided to patients and families as part of the process of obtaining informed consent for treatment (e.g. for surgery and anesthesia). Patients and families understand who may, in addition to the patient, give consent. Designated staff members are trained to inform patients and to obtain and to document patient consent.

LEGAL CONCERNS

There is also a legal angle to this concept. No one has the right to even touch, let alone treat another person. Any such act, done without permission, is classified as "battery" physical assault and is punishable. Hence, obtaining consent is a must for anything other than a routine physical examination. Various laws and court judgments have addressed consent and its documentation. Some of the important laws/guidelines related to consent are as follows:
- Medical Termination of Pregnancy Act
- Pre Natal Diagnostic Techniques Act
- National Aids Control Organization
- Transplantation of Human Organs Act
- Medical Council of India Act.

DISCLOSURE OF INFORMATION

In doctor-patient relationship, the onus of disclosure of information lies with the doctor and the right to decide the manner in which his/her body will be treated lies with the patient:
- Consent is obtained by the person/member of the team responsible for performing the procedure for which consent is being obtained.
- The patient/surrogate is explained the following in detail in a language understood by him/her. An interpreter is used in case of language barrier:
  - The diagnosis, if known
  - The nature and purpose of the proposed treatment or procedure
  - The risks and benefits of the proposed treatment or procedures
  - Alternatives (regardless of costs or extent covered by insurance)
  - The risks and benefits of alternatives
  - The risks and benefits of not receiving treatments or undergoing procedures.
- The person taking consent verbally explains about the procedure. Informed consent may be supplemented through printed educational material that gives further information relevant to the patient's condition.
- The person taking consent ensures that the patient/surrogate has had the opportunity to ask questions.
- The consent form is signed by the following and date and time are documented:
  - The person who has made the explanation for obtaining the informed consent
  - *Patient/surrogate*: If surrogate gives consent reason for obtaining consent from the surrogate and contact details/relationship with patient are documented
  - Interpreter (if applicable)
  - Witness (not applicable to HIV testing and certain other consents)
- The original signed informed consent is placed in the patient's medical record.

Patient should be given opportunity to ask questions and clarify all doubts. There must not be any kind of coercion. Consent must be voluntary and patient should have the freedom to revoke the consent. Consent given under fear of injury/intimidation, misconception, or misrepresentation of facts can be held invalid.

ETHICAL AND LEGAL ISSUES IN EMERGENCY CARDIOVASCULAR CARE

Ethical and cultural norms must be considered when beginning and ending a resuscitation attempt. Although physicians must play a role in resuscitation decision making, they should be guided by scientifically proven data and patient preferences.

Principle of Patient Autonomy

Patient autonomy is generally respected both ethically and legally. It assumes that a patient can understand what an intervention involves and consent to or refuse it. Adult patients are presumed to have decision-making capability unless they are incapacitated or declared incompetent by a court of law. Truly informed decisions require that patients receive and understand accurate information about their condition and prognosis, the nature of the proposed intervention, alternatives, and risks and benefits. The patient must be able to deliberate and choose among alternatives and be able to relate the decision to a stable framework of values. When decision-making capacity is temporarily impaired by factors such as concurrent illness, medications, or depression, treatment of these conditions may restore capacity. When patient preferences are uncertain, emergency conditions should be treated until those preferences can be clarified.

Advance Directives, Living Wills, and Patient Self-determination

An advance directive is any expression of a person's thoughts, wishes, or preferences for his or her end-of-life care. Advance directives can be based on conversations, written directives, living wills, or durable powers of attorney for health care. The legal validity of various forms of advance directives varies from jurisdiction to jurisdiction. Courts consider written advance directives to be more trustworthy than recollections of conversations.

A "living will" is a patient's written direction to physicians about medical care the patient would approve if he or she becomes terminally ill and is unable to make decisions.

Surrogate Decision Makers

When a patient/individual cannot give Informed Consent, the consent is obtained from one of the following classes of persons in the following order of priority (i.e. "the consent hierarchy"):

- The patient's/individual's guardian or parent if the patient is <18 years of age
- An individual whom the patient has nominated at the time of admission to give consent
- The patient's spouse
- Children of the patient who are eighteen (18) years of age or older; son and daughter in order of preference
- Adult brother or sister of the patient in order of preference
- The patient's parent
- Adult grandchildren
- Significant other (e.g. close friend) may give consent only in case of emergency
- No person may provide informed consent to health care:
  - If a person of higher priority has refused to give such authorization; or
  - If there are two or more individuals in the same class and the decision is not unanimous among all available members of that class.

The name, relationship with the patient of the signatory will be recorded on the consent form. When guardians, family members, or others listed in the informed consent hierarchy are unavailable, the head of the hospital in his or her custodial capacity may authorize the proposed treatment or procedure for a patient if necessary to safeguard the health, safety, or well-being of the patient. The treating doctor indicates in the medical record that it is his clinical determination that the patient's condition represents a life-threatening emergency and it is in the best interest of the patient to proceed without obtaining informed consent. If there is no time for the surgeon to note this in the medical record, the treating team must obtain verbal information from the surgeon related to his/her determination. The verbal information should be objectively documented in the medical record as soon as practical postoperatively. The head of the hospital and a peer physician/surgeon of the same specialty will countersign this.

If the patient is mentally sound but physically incapable of giving a written consent, his consent is obtained and recorded in the consent form as verbal consent and signed by two witnesses (one from the hospital side and one from the patient's side). Such consent form is marked "verbal consent" and complete contact details of the witnesses are documented on the form.

Verbal consent is also sufficient for procedures which the patient has to undergo for a long time (e.g. dialysis), provided an informed consent has been obtained initially. A fresh written informed consent is obtained whenever fresh information is provided or once in 30 days, whichever is earlier.

SOCIETY FOR CARDIOVASCULAR ANGIOGRAPHY CODE OF ETHICS

Society for Cardiovascular Angiography (SCAI) recognizes that ethical issues surrounding medical practice are more complex and critical than ever. The society also recognizes its responsibility to promote the highest possible ethical behavior by its members. The SCAI members must recognize their responsibility to patients, to society, to other physicians, and to other health professionals.

To that end, the SCAI code of ethics defines the principles and standards of conduct the society believes essential to the practice of invasive/interventional cardiology at the highest level, and defines standards for ethical, honorable behavior by SCAI members.

It is the policy of SCAI that members will comply with the following code of ethics. It is also SCAI's policy to counsel members as appropriate, assist them to comply with these principles, and, when necessary, apply the society's enforcement and disciplinary process in a fair and impartial manner. In the case of alleged and proven violations of this policy, such violations will be adjudicated through application of SCAI's separately published enforcement and disciplinary process policy.

Patient Care

The patient's welfare and best interest will always be first and foremost in the member's clinical decision making and dedicated to providing competent, appropriate, evidence-based medical care with compassion and respect for human dignity and welfare.

A member's interactions with patients will occur without inappropriate external influence with the expectation that the patient's quality of life will be improved and/or the risk of postprocedure adverse outcomes will be reduced. Prior to the member performing a procedure, the patient will be given an explanation regarding details of the procedure, potential risks and benefits, and all reasonable alternatives to the procedure, so the patient can make as fully an informed decision as possible.

Maximizing a patient's safety and comfort will be a priority before, during, and after the procedure, a member's decision to perform an invasive/interventional procedure will be based upon what is in the best interest of the individual patient will accept the importance of independent, impartial and periodic peer review, and cooperate fully with this as a critical component of continuous quality improvement and appropriateness review. Performing inappropriate procedures on patients is profoundly unethical and any member doing so will suffer permanent loss of membership in the society.

Professionalism

Member will interact honestly, professionally, and respectfully at all times with patients, patients' families, the member's colleagues, and other healthcare professionals, respect the rights of patients, families, colleagues and other healthcare professionals, and will safeguard patient confidentiality within the letter and spirit of the law.

Member will recognize and fulfill a responsibility to participate in professional activities contributing to the best possible patient care and fulfill a responsibility to maintain awareness of appropriate peer-reviewed published guidelines and standards, with integrity and report results honestly and fully. No claim will be made to research or intellectual property that is not his/hers. Plagiarism, falsification of results, or the use of others' research without proper citation is unethical.

Continuing Education and Disclosure

Member will maintain her/his invasive and interventional skills and keep up to date with medical knowledge by participating in educational meetings, conferences, or other educational programs, and by keeping abreast of appropriate peer-reviewed publications, continually apply and advance scientific knowledge, make relevant information available to patients, colleagues and the public, obtain consultation, and use the talents of other health professionals when indicated. In advance of serving on SCAI committees, educational programs or writing groups, a member will fully disclose industry relationships and other potential conflicts of interest in accordance with the Society's current disclosure/conflict of interest policy.

LEGAL IMPLICATIONS OF MEDICAL RECORDS

Medical records serve as communication between healthcare providers regarding the patient's health history, injuries, illness, care plans, response to treatment, tests results, and much more. In addition to providing records that manage and document the patient's care, medical records are used in reimbursement, research, and legal issues. Because the medical record is a legal document, many rules and regulations apply, including regulations on documentation, record retention, privacy acts, and disclosure.

Medical Records Contents

- Registration no.
- Date and time
- General consent form
- Initial assessment (shall also include screening for nutritional needs)/triage sheet
- Reason for admission, diagnosis, plan of care
- Reassessment (patient progress notes)
- Tests/investigations prescribed and done with their findings
- Medications prescribed
- Medications administered (with time also mentioned)
- Adverse drug reaction wherever applicable
- Written consent (as applicable) (refer to consent policy)
- Preanesthesia assessment record (applicable for patients to be anesthetized)
- Record for immediate re-evaluation (done immediately before OT) for anesthesia

- Adverse event if any related to anesthesia
- Postanesthesia status
- Preoperative assessment/provisional diagnosis for surgical patients
- Operation/procedure performed
- Operative notes (made before transferring the patient out of recovery area)
- Postoperative order sheet
- Batch no. and serial no. of implantable prosthesis wherever applicable
- Consent to operation/anesthesia/others
- Consent to HIV testing
- Consent for blood transfusion
- Preoperative orders sheet
- Preoperative check list
- Preanesthetic checkup (PAC) record
- Patient restrain notes if applicable
- Glucose monitoring chart
- Investigation ordered sheet
- Laboratory reports (bio/micro/bb/clinical/histo)
- Catheterization laboratory report [angio/percutaneous transluminal coronary angioplasty (PTCA)/percutaneous coronary intervention (PCI)]
- Report (X-ray/USG/CT scan)
- Reports of cardiac diagnostic
- ECG report
- Critical care flow sheet
- Routine monitoring (TPR chart and other applicable)
- Perfusion record
- Record of implants
- Investigation flow chart
- Nutritional assessment
- ICU progress notes
- In-house transfer form
- Clinical chart
- Nursing admission assessment
- Patient education record
- Daily nurses flow sheet
- Postevent analysis in case of blood transfusion reaction (if applicable)
- Postevent analysis in case of cardiopulmonary resuscitation (CPR) (if applicable)
- Transfusion administration record sheet
- Sentinel event if any
- *In case of transfer*: A case summary, date of transfer, reason of transfer, and name of receiving hospital
- *Discharged patients*: Discharge summary: DAMA summary/transfer summary
- *In case of death*: A death certificate having cause of death, date and time of death
- Autopsy/biopsy reports if applicable
- Lama consent form if applicable.

Each and every entry made in the medical record of any patient shall be named, dated, timed, and signed by the person making that entry.

CONCLUSION

The honest and fair communication to patients by healthcare providers is an ethical imperative. Excellent communication eliminates or reduces the likelihood of misunderstandings and conflict in the healthcare setting, and also may affect the likelihood that a patient will sue. We conclude that focusing on the whole decision-making process, effective communication, proper documentation of medical record, and a proportionate and individualized approach to consent could go some way to improve the experience of many patients in cardiology and reduces the medicolegal cases.

BIBLIOGRAPHY

1. Beauchamp TL, Childress JF. Principles of Biomedical Ethics, 5th edition. Oxford: Oxford University Press; 2001.
2. Etchells E, Sharpe G, Walsh P, et al. Bioethics for clinicians: consent. CMAJ. 1996;155:177-80.
3. Francis CM. Autonomy and Informed Consent, Medical Ethics, 2nd edition. New Delhi: Jaypee Brothers Medical Publishers (P) Ltd. 2004. pp. 54-65.
4. Joga Rao SV. Medical Ethics: A Ready Referencer, 1st edition. Bangalore: Legalaxy Publications; 2004. p. 84.
5. Madhava MNR. Medical ethics and health care—issues and perspectives. Karnataka Med J. 2000;71:2-9.
6. Medical Ethics Manual. World Medical Association, Inc; 2005. p. 105.
7. Medical Ethics Manual. World Medical Association, Inc; 2005. pp. 42-50.
8. Policies and SOPs based on JCI 4th Edition and NABH 2nd edition.
9. Snyder L, Leffler C. Ethics and Human Rights Committee, American College of Physicians. Ethics Manual, 5th edition. Ann Intern Med. 2005;142:563.
10. Srinivas P. Consumer Protection Act and Dermatological Practice, a Dermatologists' Perspective of Medical Ethics and Consumer Protection Act. In: An IADVL Book, 1st edition. 2007. pp. 7-21.
11. Trehan SP, Sankhari D. Medical Professional, Patient and the law: The Institute of Law and Ethics in Medicine, 2nd edition. Bangalore: National Law School of India University; 2002. pp. 57-68.

Index

Page numbers followed by *b* refer to box, *f* refer to figure, *fc* refer to flow chart and *t* refer to table

A

B

C

D

E

J

K

L

M

N

O

P

R

S

T

U

V

W